MR

Mother and Baby Health

Mother and Baby Health

THE A-Z OF PREGNANCY, BIRTH AND BEYOND

Dr Yehudi Gordon and Harriet Sharkey,
Andy Raffles and Felicity Fine

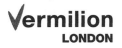
Vermilion
LONDON

1 3 5 7 9 10 8 6 4 2

Published in 2007 by Vermilion, an imprint of Ebury Publishing

A Random House Group company

The Random House Group Limited Reg. No. 954009

Addresses for companies within the Random House Group can be found at
www.randomhouse.co.uk

A CIP catalogue record for this book is available from the British Library

The Random House Group Limited makes every effort to ensure that the
papers used in our books are made from trees that have been legally sourced
from well-managed and credibly certified forests. Our paper procurement
policy can be found on www.rbooks.co.uk/environment

Printed and bound in Great Britain by
Mackays of Chatham plc, Chatham, Kent

ISBN 9780091912857

Copies are available at special rates for bulk orders. Contact the sales
development team on 020 7840 8487 for more information.

To buy books by your favourite authors and register for offers, visit
www.rbooks.co.uk

Preface

Mother and Baby Health holds a deep respect for babies and families. This continues the philosophy and the feel of *Birth and Beyond,* which we wrote in 2002. We hope this book will empower you to trust your instincts, find the information and the support you need, and enjoy your baby and family, and your own journey as a parent.

We know there is always more than one way to approach a problem, so we have aimed to offer enough detail to allow you to make choices that feel right for you on any given day. This book covers the primal period from conception until a year after birth but much of it relates to everyday life and we hope it will be your companion for years to come.

USING THIS BOOK

Mother and Baby Health offers advice on basic life issues – ranging from caring for yourself and your baby, and supporting your emotional wellbeing and your relationships, to feeding, sleeping, exercising and preventing aches and pains. It covers health concerns that may arise for mothers or babies in pregnancy, birth and beyond. We also offer advice for fathers. Throughout, we give mainstream medical and complementary options for care, as appropriate. The combination is 'integrated healthcare', where physical, emotional and lifestyle elements are all considered and complementary therapies may be used with the safety net of modern medicine.

We've used an A–Z format for easy access, and there's an extensive index at the back of the book to help you find what you're looking for. While our aim is to give comprehensive advice, this book does not have all the answers: it has been written for you to use in conjunction with support and guidance from your medical and complementary specialists and your community of friends and family.

OUR TEAM

It has been a pleasure for us to come together again as a team and share the insights we have gained as parents and in the course of our work. Yehudi writes from his experience as a father and grandfather and as an obstetrician and gynaecologist. His strong vision has inspired us all. His acknowledgement and acceptance of each baby and mother as sensitive and aware underlies everything we write. Yehudi recognises that physical and emotional wellbeing are always intertwined and this holistic approach informs every area of his work, and is at the core of our book.

Harriet and Yehudi have been writing in partnership for 10 years. They have had a great time exploring pregnancy, birth and parenting and the way babies experience life. For this book they have been delighted to go deeper into a subject they are so passionate about. Harriet's love of babies, her appreciation of human nature and her interest in health filter into the book throughout. She has been pivotal in ensuring the book is personal, comprehensive, practical and easy to read. Andy brings insights from 30 years in the field of medicine and especially paediatrics, where he is called upon daily to support and guide babies, children and parents. Andy has a wonderful knack of being to the point, practical and reassuring, and helps us keep the tone light but safe. Felicity, who has been practising as a homeopath for over 15 years, has an astounding ability to make homeopathy applicable and accessible. Her compassionate approach in her work and family life has been a constant influence throughout the writing of this book. Over the years, many other people have contributed to this book; we give them personal thanks on page 574.

We have loved working on *Mother and Baby Health* – it has been a pleasure and privilege for us to work as a team, and to create a book that celebrates our amazing babies and gently guides and supports us as parents. Above all, *Mother and Baby Health* is what it is thanks to the many mothers and babies who have been part of our lives. They have inspired us and taught us so much. Thank you!

Yehudi, Harriet, Felicity and Andy
November 2007

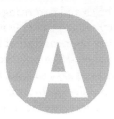

Abdominal pain

See also Pain, mother.

During pregnancy, your uterus grows and reaches your rib cage. The muscles, ligaments or joints in your abdomen stretch, and ligaments supporting your spine and pelvis and the surrounding muscles soften and expand. Your bladder is pushed forwards and up, and your bowel is pushed up. Therefore, it is hardly surprising that many women experience aches and pains. Discomfort may also arise from internal organs (uterus, bladder, kidneys, stomach, colon), or from the muscles and ligaments, or the joints in your back, abdomen or pelvis.

Pain in the uterus and ovaries: urgent attention

* Severe pelvic pain in early pregnancy at the front of your abdomen, often low down on one side and perhaps intense and knife-sharp, may indicate an ECTOPIC PREGNANCY. This is a rare occurrence but may be life-threatening because there is internal bleeding.
* Strong contractions in early pregnancy may indicate a threatened MISCARRIAGE if the pain is accompanied by bleeding. In premature labour, the symptoms may be similar.
* Spreading, severe pain in later pregnancy is very rarely a sign of placental abruption (page 444) where there is bleeding between the placenta and the wall of the uterus. The pain is over the front wall of the uterus and is usually constant, unlike contractions that

come and go. Medical advice is essential, particularly if you feel shocked and are bleeding.

Pain in the uterus and ovaries: common pain

* Mild to moderate pain in early pregnancy, usually on one side of the pelvis and abdomen, often arises from the ovary after normal ovulation. Your ovary can be observed during an ultrasound scan. Pain may be quite intense but diminishes by Week 10.
* Contractions in pregnancy are normal, as the muscle wall of your uterus contracts in Braxton-Hicks or 'practice' contractions (page 357). The pain perception associated with them varies enormously. They are usually not felt but there may be runs of discomfort lasting for hours, more commonly in late pregnancy. Each contraction is over in 30 to 60 seconds.
* Labour contractions are more likely to feel painful. In labour the intensity of pain increases (page 380).
* The round ligaments that run from the top of the uterus to the inguinal area in the groin lengthen in pregnancy. Sometimes tension gives discomfort on the upper part of the uterus, often on one side. The pain may radiate into your groin.
* FIBROIDS may exist without symptoms, but there may be pain over the area of the fibroid that lasts for days or weeks and then gradually fades.
* After the birth, your uterus reverts to non-pregnancy size by contracting, a process that gives rise to 'afterpains' for a week or two. Afterpains are stimulated when you

breastfeed, and are often more intense with subsequent births. You may be able to ride through them by focusing on your breathing, as you did in labour, or you may require painkillers or HOMEOPATHY.

Bladder and kidney pain

The ureters are tubes that transfer urine from your kidneys to your bladder. During pregnancy they swell due to hormonal changes and pressure from your uterus, and may cause discomfort, often on the right. Pain may radiate from your groin up towards the kidney area at the back of your abdomen under the lower ribs.

- Around 5 per cent of women are susceptible to urinary tract or kidney infections in pregnancy. If there is a bladder infection, the main symptoms are a need to pass urine frequently and burning as the urine emerges. Pain in the ligaments and joints of the pubic symphysis (page 43) in front of the bladder may mimic cystitis but the pubic joint is tender to the touch and this distinguishes the two.
- If infection extends up to the kidneys, which is rare, you may feel tenderness extending into the back of your abdomen. A severe kidney infection (page 171) may cause pain and a fever.

Stomach, bowel and anal pain

Severe pre-eclampsia (page 69) may cause upper abdominal pain in late pregnancy and needs urgent attention.

Stomach and bowel pain may be caused by digestive problems, such as nausea, HEARTBURN or INDIGESTION. Pains in the lower abdomen may arise from spasm in the wall of the colon or the rectum. For a small number of women, this may occur as part of an underlying bowel disorder, such as IRRITABLE BOWEL SYNDROME (IBS). It may also be associated with CONSTIPATION or DIARRHOEA. Contractions of the lower colon wall can feel like uterine pain and give rise to fear of premature labour.

Sometimes pain in the anal area is associated with PILES.

Back pain

Sometimes pain arising from the ligaments or the muscles on the front of the spine is referred forward into the abdomen as tummy pain. It may mimic pain arising from the uterus. For more on back pain, see page 43.

Action plan

✚ Red flag

Contact your midwife or doctor urgently if you have:

- acute/sharp pain that has started recently, particularly if it is severe.
- abdominal pain associated with bleeding.
- upper abdominal pain in late pregnancy.

Talk to your midwife or doctor at your next visit if you have ongoing or low-level pain. For tips on what you may do, see page 431.

Because dysfunction or strain in one area of the body can cause pain in another area, provided you have ruled out any physiological problem in your uterus or pelvis, it may be worth considering other issues such as back pain (page 43), and whether posture could contribute.

Abscess

See Breastfeeding, difficulties.

Abuse

See Child protection and abuse; Violence and abuse, mother.

Accidents and first aid, baby

Children do and will have accidents. Their curiosity and spirit of adventure is healthy, but does sometimes lead to minor cuts or bruises, or the insertion of small objects into orifices (such as a button up the nose). Some babies take minor injuries in their stride, while others get extremely upset from the shock of even a little bump. Whatever your baby's reaction, your care will make him happier as he recovers. If he has a serious accident it will be distressing for everyone, but again, as a parent it is your role to make him comfortable, remove any danger, and seek appropriate medical care. He may be very frightened and will rely on you for reassurance and support. If an accident is serious, don't hesitate to call 999.

This guide gives basic tips. It is also worthwhile familiarising yourself with baby first aid in theory and in practice by attending a class at a local clinic. Information and advice does change and it is optimal to go to a class or course every nine to 12

The ABC of resuscitation

The following is for guidance only and is directed to the care of a baby under one year old. In order to effectively follow the ABC it is always best to attend a first aid class.

If your baby stops breathing or is unconscious and cannot be roused
Call for help. Make a quick call to a neighbour, friend or relative – even a passer-by. Stimulate your baby by gently shaking him.

If there is no response, act quickly and as calmly as you can:

A – Airway
Ensure the airway is clear. If you see something, lie your baby along your forearm with his head supported on your hand and lower than his chest. Give five firm slaps on the back to dislodge any foreign object.

B – Breathing
Check for breathing movement of the chest. If there is none:

Position your baby's head 'nose to ceiling' – chin lifted and head tilted back slightly.

Give five rescue breaths: put your mouth over your baby's mouth and nose and blow just hard enough to make his chest move, as though he is taking a deep breath for himself. Take a breath for yourself between breaths.

C – Circulation
Check your baby's circulation by raising his foot or hand above the level of his heart. Pinch the big toe or thumb for a count of 10, and watch as the colour floods back. If the colour seeps back, check again. If there is no flush of colour, or a staggered return of colour, give chest compressions (below) to boost the heart and to maintain blood supply to the brain.

- Use two fingers and place them in the centre of your baby's chest, roughly two finger-widths below his nipples, and press hard enough to depress the breastbone 1–2cm (½–¾in)
- Give 30 chest compressions at a rate of 100 per minute to two mouth-to-nose rescue breaths.
- Continue resuscitation (30 compressions to two rescue breaths) without stopping until help arrives or your child starts breathing.

If your child starts breathing again
Turn him on his side so that secretions can run out of his mouth.

Keep watching his breathing rate to make sure it continues.

Keep checking these until help arrives, and be prepared to restart the ABC if his breathing rate falls or stops.

months so you can keep up to date, and learn skills that are relevant to your child's age. The suggestions for homeopathic first aid (page 11) apply equally to adults and babies.

Is it an emergency?

Many minor injuries can be handled at home. If you are ever unsure about whether an injury needs emergency care, treat it as an emergency. Call 999 or your GP right away. The following situations require emergency attention:

- Difficulty breathing – shortness of breath, unable to feed or speak.
- Blue or purple colour to lips, skin or nail beds.
- Chest or stomach pain or pressure.
- Sudden dizziness, weakness or change in vision.
- Change in consciousness level – such as loss of consciousness, confusion, or difficulty waking.
- First seizures – a FIT or convulsion of any type.
- Any bite by an animal or human.
- Pain or loss of use of a limb, which might indicate broken bones.
- Broken bones.
- BLEEDING that does not stop with direct pressure.
- Burns or scalds larger than your baby's palm or any burn or scald to the face.
- Puncture wounds to the skin at any site, due to sticks or sharp points.
- Head, neck, back or eye injuries.
- Signs of allergic reaction such as nettle rash (urticaria), swelling of the face, lips, eyes, or tongue, fainting, or difficulty breathing or swallowing, or wheezing (see page 16).
- Swallowed drugs or household cleaners.

If you do provide first aid treatment for your baby, call your GP to see if any follow-up care is needed.

Accidents and first aid, baby
Broken bones and fractures

It is very unusual for small babies to break a bone because their bones are strong and flexible, and the forces required to break a bone are great. Common causes are being dropped from a baby buggy, car seat, table or changing mat on a high surface, or being carried by an adult who falls. Because a break usually results from the involvement of older people, it is common for parents to be visited by a member of social services to exclude the possibility of child abuse (page 131).

If a break happens, it may be immediately obvious, or only brought to light when your baby is less settled than usual. Note: there may not be bruising or swelling. Once set in a cast, recovery will be speedy. If your baby stops using a limb or seems in pain when a limb is moved then take him to your nearest hospital accident and emergency (A and E) department. An X-ray is the only sure way to diagnose a fracture.

- A broken bone will usually be set in a cast for roughly three weeks for an arm bone and six weeks for a leg bone. If the bone needs to be straightened, your baby will be given an anaesthetic.
- Once the cast is in place, the fracture is unlikely to give much pain, but if your baby seems uncomfortable, you may use infant paracetamol suspension (page 429). If he has a large fracture, your doctor may suggest other pain relief medications.
- Modern casts are lightweight. To bath your baby, wrap the cast in a plastic bag, and seal the bag with tape. Alternatively, give your baby a 'top and tail' wash with a flannel or cotton wool and water. Keep the limb out of the water if at all possible. If the exposed part of the limb begins to swell and/or the digits start to change colour, seek medical attention.

Homeopathy

- You may give Aconite (30c) as soon as you can, to treat shock.
- Arnica (30c) may be given for shock and pain relief and to begin the healing of muscles and tissues – one dose every 15 minutes for an hour, then three times a day for up to four days.
- When the fracture has been set, you may give Ledum (30c) three times a day for four days in conjunction with Arnica.
- After the initial pain and swelling have reduced, Symphytum (6c) speeds the bone healing process – from one week after the accident you may use three times a day for one week, then twice a day for up to three weeks.
- If the fracture has not healed after using Symphytum, you may use Calc Phos (6c) twice a day for two to three weeks.
- If the ribs are broken, you may use Bryonia (30c) twice a day for up to two weeks.

Accidents and first aid, baby
Bumps and bruises

Your older baby will almost certainly get one or two bumps and bruises as he learns to sit, and later to crawl, as tumbles are an inevitable part of the learning process. Try to minimise injury by removing obstacles and offering a carpeted area in which to play. Never leave your baby unattended on a raised surface – such as a sofa, bed, table or chair. Never put his car seat on a raised surface (such as a table or worktop) with him in it.

If your baby tumbles and has a light bruise or bump, give loving care. He may let you rub the area slightly – this eases the pain, increases circulation and begins the healing process.

Witch hazel is good to use in the first instance to reduce bruising, if the skin is not broken.

Homeopathy
- *Arnica* is the No.1 remedy for mild shock following an injury or accident, and for trauma and bruising, and can be very effective. You may use 30c every 15 minutes for four doses then three times a day for up to three days. If the skin is not broken, you may apply *Arnica* cream twice a day for a few days.
- When an area thinly covered by skin is bruised (such as an elbow or shin), or bruising follows a fracture, dislocation or sprain and *Arnica* does not help, you may use *Ruta* (30c) three times a day for up to three days.
- *Ledum* is the other remedy to consider if *Arnica* does not help and the bruise may feel cold to the touch. Again, you may use in the 30c potency three times a day for up to three days.

Accidents and first aid, baby
Burns and scalds

Burns and scalds are the most common cause of serious injury in babies, due to hot liquids, flames or hot ashes, electricity, friction, chemicals or even radiation. Adventurous mobile babies pull tablecloths and kettle wires, and may knock cookers or tables, unwittingly spilling hot liquid. Even a small baby may be scalded if mum or dad spills a hot drink.
- In a superficial burn the skin may appear red or form a blister filled with fluid. It usually recovers well without scarring.
- A deeper burn or scald will cause the skin to come away. Recovery may be prolonged and there will be scarring. Occasionally, skin grafting is necessary.
- Even deeper burns result in blackening of the skin.
- Inhalation of hot liquids or gases can cause damage to the airway – seek emergency help immediately.

If your baby is scalded, the immediate treatment is:
- Remove him from the source of the heat.
- Remove clothing if necessary (clothes hold hot water onto the skin).
- Pour cold water over the injured area.
- Keep the skin area exposed, allowing it to cool.
- A loose covering can be applied, cling film is ideal, especially if you are moving your baby to hospital – do not apply greasy dressings.
- If the burn is smaller than the palm of your baby's hand, use a proprietary burn cream. If it is bigger, seek help and do not apply cream.
- Infant paracetamol suspension is ideal as a pain reliever. Use the dose recommended on the bottle (page 429).
- Seek help.

Homeopathy
Homeopathic treatment is useful for minor burns. For severe burns that are larger than the palm of your baby's hand with blistering and whiteness or black tissue visible, seek immediate medical help.
- *Aconite* (30c) may be given for the shock, every 15 minutes for three doses or until the situation is under control.
- For minor burns, scalds without blistering or with minimal blistering where there is stinging, soreness and redness, bathe the affected area in a diluted tincture – 10 drops of *Urtica Urens* to 250ml (½ pint) boiled, cooled water. This is especially effective for scalds from boiling water.
- To minor burns or scalds you may apply *Combudoron* burn ointment (available from most chemists).
- If the burn is more severe and very painful you

5

may use *Cantharis* (6c) alongside medical treatment twice a day for up to a week.

- Burns to the tongue or burns that look healed but still hurt respond well to *Causticum* (6c) three times a day for up to one week.
- After initial healing, you may use *Calendula* cream twice a day for up to two weeks – it soothes and can help to minimise scarring.
- If an infection appears, consult your homeopath for an appropriate remedy.

Sunburn

Even very short exposure to strong sun can cause redness and blistering of a baby's sensitive skin. Prevention is best, but if there is burning:

- Paracetamol or infant ibuprofen suspension can help relieve pain.
- After-sun lotion or simple emollients such as E45 stop burned skin from drying out.
- A weak hydrocortisone cream (0.5–1 per cent) available over the counter will reduce the pain and discomfort of mild sunburn, where the skin is red but not blistered.
- *Calendula* cream may be soothing.
- *Combudoron* cream, also used for scalds, may be effective.
- The homeopathic remedy *Belladonna* (30c) three times a day for two days may help to take the heat out of the sunburn.

Accidents and first aid, baby
Cat scratches

Cats usually avoid babies but babies are very curious and can annoy them. Apart from the discomfort from a scratch – worst if on the face or eyes – there is the risk of cat scratch infection, which is usually only contracted from kittens. After being scratched, redness spreads up the arm or leg, and then settles down. Later the lymph nodes ('glands') in the groin or armpit on the affected side flare up.

- Simple antibiotic treatment settles the condition over a two- to three-week period.
- Homeopathy: you may use *Calendula* tincture – 10 drops in 250ml (½ pint) water – to bathe and clean the scratch, and apply *Calendula* cream to soothe and promote healing.

Accidents and first aid, baby
Choking

If your baby chokes on something he will struggle for breath, may become red in the face, cough, grasp his neck and seem terrified. You will need to act quickly. The cause is likely to be food or a toy stuck in the airway.

- Call for help.
- Check your baby's airway and give him five back slaps (page 3).
- Check if the airway is clear and he is breathing.
- If not, turn him over to face you.
- Place the heel of your hand on the lower part of his chest and give five firm thrusts.
- Check his airway is clear and he is breathing.
- If not, give five rescue breaths (page 3).
- Check for circulation and start chest compressions if necessary (page 3).
- Keep repeating this cycle until your baby improves. Call 999 if you were not able to do this immediately.

Accidents and first aid, baby
Cold injury

Babies are very vulnerable to extremes of temperature, both hot and cold. Cold injury occurs when the usual colour of the skin does not settle after warming up. Hands and feet remain blue and the skin appears mottled, even when the body temperature is normal. This is a sign of HYPOTHERMIA and needs medical attention.

Accidents and first aid, baby
Cuts and abrasions

Cuts among babies are unusual, although broken glass on the ground or a sharp knife left in reach might cut fingers. Stumbling, falling or being knocked, particularly onto an open cupboard or a table corner, can cause a nasty cut to the head. In babies cuts bleed easily.

Minor cuts

- Apply firm pressure and the bleeding will usually come under control within five minutes.
- Wash the affected part.
- When bleeding has stopped do not disturb the injury, as this will often start the wound bleeding again. Apply a firm dressing or plaster if possible.
- If the cut continues to bleed ask for help in a pharmacy, or visit your doctor.
- Homeopathy: *Calendula* cream is good – you may also bathe the graze or cut with 10 drops of *Calendula* or *Hypercal* tincture dissolved in 250ml (½ pint) boiled, cooled water to guard against infection and promote healing. For a deeper cut, you may give *Hypericum* (30c) three times a day for up to three days.

Deep cuts

- Act quickly.
- If your baby has lost consciousness or appears to be in shock, ask someone to call the emergency services while you begin first aid.
- Lie your child down with his feet elevated about 15cm (6in). This increases blood flow to the brain and reduces the risk of shock. If possible, elevate the site of bleeding, as well, as that helps reduce blood flow to the injured part.
- Use a sterile bandage or cloth to apply firm pressure directly to the wound. If nothing else is available, use the palm of your hand (after washing your hands, if possible). Maintain steady pressure until the bleeding stops. If an artery has been cut, it will take at least 10 minutes of constant pressure. If blood soaks through the bandage you're using, don't remove it. Instead, just add another layer on top. Try to keep calm and to calm your baby (anxiety will pump more blood to the site).
- Once the bleeding stops, leave the bandage or cloth in place. If more blood seeps through, apply another bandage or cloth on top. Don't remove the first bandage; that could cause more bleeding. To maintain pressure, wrap cling film or tape tightly around the bandages and the injured area.
- If your child is awake and alert, take him to the nearest hospital accident and emergency department as soon as possible. If he is woozy or unconscious, call for an ambulance.

Accidents and first aid, baby
Dog bites

Dog bites are common, and are usually no more than a playful nip. Severe dog bites can cause serious injury, including fractures and deep cuts, and the wound can become infected.

- Clean the bite with water, and apply a dressing to stop the bleeding.
- Seek expert help from your GP or hospital accident and emergency department. Professional care is essential because the risk of infection is high.
- Homeopathy: you may give *Ledum* (30c) hourly for the first two hours followed by *Hypericum* (30c) hourly for the next two hours. *Hypercal* tincture – 10 drops in 250ml (½ pint) water – may also be used to bathe and clean the bite.

Accidents and first aid, baby
Drowning and near drowning

A young baby can drown in very little water, in a bath or a shallow pond or paddling pool. Prevention is certainly better than cure – do not leave your baby unattended in or near water. Many children do, however, survive drowning intact (without brain damage), especially if they are very cold because this slows down the body's system and it can operate without oxygen for longer.

If you find your baby face down in water, not breathing, lifeless and perhaps blue and cold:

- Call for help.
- Shake him gently and see if he responds.
- If there is no response give five rescue breaths (page 3).
- Check for breathing or response.
- If there is no response, continue to give rescue breaths and give chest compressions (page 3).
- Continue until help arrives.

Accidents and first aid, baby
Falling down stairs

Every year many babies are injured by falling down stairs, usually in the home. Prevention is the best approach. Always carry your baby down stairs in your arms, never on your shoulders. Keep a stair gate in place at all times – at the top and bottom of the stairs. This keeps your baby out of danger of falling and also helps to stop pets and toys ending up on the stairway and tripping you up.

If you fall down the stairs holding your baby or your baby falls down without you:
* Check Airway, Breathing and Circulation (page 3).
* If your baby is unconscious – call for help.
* If your baby is awake, make sure he is using all limbs fully and equally. Check for bumps and bruises. Notify your doctor or go to a hospital accident and emergency department if you are concerned.

Accidents and first aid, baby
Inhaled and swallowed objects or liquids

If you think your child has swallowed a medicine tablet or dangerous fluid:
* Clear chewed tablets/liquid from the mouth.
* If your child is drowsy do not make him sick. Never give salt water.
* If he has drunk a toxic liquid (household cleaner) do not make him sick, he will probably vomit anyway.
* Call an ambulance.
* If he is choking, take the appropriate action immediately (page 6), and then call an ambulance.
* Look around on the floor for tablets that have been dropped rather than swallowed, or spilt liquid.
* What quantity was originally in the pack/bottle? Take any remaining medicines and containers with you, especially of household cleaners, when you go for medical help.
* If your child has vomited, collect a sample of vomit for the medical team to check.

Foreign body in your child's nose – using the 'parent's kiss'
It is common for children to get a foreign body lodged in the nose. If you cannot touch or grasp the object, the first line of first aid is to try the 'parent's kiss'. Gently cover your child's mouth with your mouth and at the same time press against the nostril opposite the side where the foreign body is stuck. Then gently but firmly blow into your child's mouth. This may either blow the foreign body out or move it so you can see and grasp it. If this does not work, it is important to seek medical care.

Accidents and first aid, baby
Injury to ears

If your baby is bleeding from the ear, treat it as directed on page 62. It is important never to poke anything into the ear. If something is pushed into the ear do not try to remove it as it is likely to be pushed in further. Take your baby to the local hospital accident and emergency department or to your GP. It may be necessary for a specialist to remove the foreign body.

Homeopathy
Seek medical help and en route you may administer one dose of *Silica* (30c), which will facilitate the removal of the object. After it has been removed you may give one dose of *Hypericum* (30c). *Arnica* (30c) three times a day for the next two days will help reduce any swelling.

Accidents and first aid, baby
Injury to eyes

The eyes are very well protected behind the bony ridges of the eye socket and serious eye injuries are very uncommon. If your baby does injure his eye, take him to your GP or local accident and emergency clinic – it is important to be very careful.
* If you can see something in your baby's eye, such as an insect, an eye lash or a piece of grit,

use a clean cloth or tightly rolled piece of cotton wool and gently encourage it to come out. You can also try using plain water to flush it out. If he is crying it may come out of its own accord.
- If you cannot get to the foreign object, resist poking and prodding.
- If his eye appears swollen and you are unaware of any accident, he may have an EYE INFECTION or be displaying an ALLERGY OR INTOLERANCE.

Homeopathy

Any eye injury needs medical attention.
- If a small foreign body is stuck in the eye, you may give *Aconite* (30c) for shock and fear and then *Hypericum* (30c) hourly for three hours, which reduces pain and sensitivity. Once the foreign body is out of the eye, you may bathe the closed eye with a mixture of eight drops *Euphrasia* tincture to 250ml (½ pint) boiled, cooled water every three hours until there is relief. Never use undiluted tincture. Hold your baby in front of you so he is facing you, soak cotton wool in the diluted solution and gently squeeze it over the eye area. You may also give *Euphrasia* (30c) three times a day until the eye settles.
- If your baby has a knock to the nose or face and gets a black eye, you may give *Arnica* (30c) immediately and then hourly for three hours. You may also use *Arnica* cream provided the skin is not broken. If the bruising is painful and is soothed by cool compresses, you may give *Ledum* (30c) two hourly for six hours then three times a day for two to three days.
- For a minor cut to the eye area you may use *Calendula* (30c) three times a day for a few days and *Calendula* cream rubbed lightly around (but not on) the cut. You may combine this with *Hypercal* tincture (10 drops to 250ml/½ pint boiled, cooled water) and bathe the area three times a day.

Accidents and first aid, baby
Injury to hands, fingers, feet and toes

Small babies love to explore and often get minor cuts and grazes (above), particularly on the hands. Sometimes a finger or toe may be caught in a door, and as a result a nail or tip will be crushed or torn.

- Wash the affected part and look at the damage. Even small cuts may bleed heavily.
- Apply firm pressure and stop the bleeding (page 7).
- If the nail has been torn it will probably need removal by the local accident and emergency department or hospital minor injuries unit. Once removed, future growth depends on how much damage there has been to the base of the nail.
- If a finger or toe tip has been crushed, the bony tip may be exposed. A few stitches are needed to close the cut, and the digit will heal well.
- If the tip has been amputated, find it, place it back on the finger or toe and go to the local accident and emergency department or minor injuries unit. It may be sewn back on. These kinds of injuries have good rates of recovery.
- Babies can get thread wrapped around a toe or finger, and if this is not noticed for a few days then the digit can turn black. If possible unwind the thread, but it may be buried in the swollen skin. Go to the local accident or minor injuries unit for help.
- Homeopathy: *Arnica* (30c) every 15 minutes for the first hour may be used to treat shock and *Hypericum* (30c) given hourly for three hours may be useful to alleviate pain and repair nerve endings.

Accidents and first aid, baby
Injury to head

Most children who injure their head suffer no ill effects. Even in the case of a skull fracture a child will usually make a full recovery. Common injuries in children include being hit by a swing seat, falling from a low height onto a hard (or even soft) surface, or receiving a kick to the head from an animal (especially horses).

A common cause of serious brain injury is shaking. Because the head of a baby is heavy and the neck muscles are weak, even two or three shakes of a baby under 12 months of age can lead to brain damage caused by bleeding into the brain. If you believe your baby may have been shaken and is behaving abnormally, you must seek expert help immediately.

If after a head injury, however trivial, your baby behaves in any way differently from normal, consult your doctor. While most children survive injury with no harm, symptoms may be delayed for a few hours, so watch your baby closely.

* Seek medical attention if your baby is conscious but drowsy, pale and listless; vomiting, crying incessantly, abnormally quiet and unresponsive.
* While you are travelling to hospital or waiting for your doctor to arrive, one dose of *Arnica* (30c) may be an effective initial treatment.

Accidents and first aid, baby
Injury to mouth and nose

The soft tissues of the face are so well supplied with blood that any injury to the mouth, nose or ears tends to bleed a lot. The bleeding will probably stop in a few minutes.

* If the nose is bleeding, don't squeeze it – it will be bruised.
* Lips and tongue bleed easily, and the volume appears greater because it's mixed with saliva.
* Recovery from a mouth injury can take time, particularly if there is bruising or if mouth ulcers develop. Avoid acid drinks and foods for the first few days.
* Homeopathy: *Arnica* (30c) every 15 minutes for the first hour may be used to treat shock and to curb the bleeding, then *Hypericum* (30c) hourly for the next three hours. You may also bathe the area in a solution of *Hypercal* tincture – 10 drops to 250ml (½ pint) boiled, cooled water.

Accidents and first aid, baby
Insect bites and stings

Insect bites and stings are a common problem for babies, particularly in the summer and in temperate regions. The best treatment is prevention (page 522).

The commonest biting insects are mosquitoes and midges whose bites usually cause intense itchiness and a raised spot, often with a dark centre. The swelling is due to a release of histamine. After a few hours the skin may become hot and swollen, and redness may spread

around the site of the bite. Very often there is a crop of bites within a small area. The spots and swelling can become fluid-filled blisters. Symptoms usually disappear within 48 hours but you can treat the bite with proprietary creams and/or with oral antihistamines (such as Piriton) available over the counter, particularly if the swelling is significant: 2.5ml (½ tsp) of Piriton syrup or 0.5–1 per cent of hydrocortisone cream can be used to reduce swelling and itching. If the bite(s) become infected ANTIBIOTICS are usually effective within five to 10 days.

If your baby is bitten by a wasp or bee, keep a close eye on him. Rarely these stings can cause serious allergic reactions (page 16). If your baby develops swelling of the face or mouth, noisy or difficult breathing or difficulty swallowing, he needs urgent medical care.

Bee stings are often left in the skin. The chemicals in the sting can be neutralised with an ammonia pen, available from all chemists, and you can pull the sting out with tweezers.

For a bee sting you can dab a diluted mixture of bicarbonate of soda and water on the site. Vinegar soothes wasp stings.

Homeopathy
If your baby is in shock, you may give *Aconite* (30c) immediately. Then you may give the most appropriate remedy (30c) every 15 minutes for the first hour, reducing to one dose every two hours for the next six hours.

* *Ledum* if the skin is punctured and the skin becomes puffy and swollen yet feels cold, and is soothed by cold compresses.
* *Hypericum* if pain is shooting upwards from the site, and it feels tender, numb, tingly and hot.
* *Apis* for ant, bee or wasp stings leaving hot, puffy, red skin and burning, prickling or stinging pain.
* *Urtica Urens* for itchy, blotchy skin, like a nettle rash that feels better for rubbing. This is a specific remedy for jellyfish stings.
* *Rhus Tox* if the sting comes from a plant and scratching the skin makes it worse, or it is worse at night or from warm bathing.
* You can also bathe the irritated skin in a tincture of *Hypercal* or *Urtica* (10 drops to 250ml/½ pint water).
* If you have *Pyrethrum* spray in your first aid kit (opposite), you may use it two hourly for the first six hours.

First aid kit for your baby and family

Keep a first aid kit easily accessible and replace anything you use as soon as possible. Specifically for your baby a kit requires:

- List of useful telephone numbers.
- Thermometer (see page 239 for different types and for details of recognising a fever).
- Tweezers.
- Paracetamol suspension and suppositories (page 429).
- Children's ibuprofen for night use and more severe pains not helped by paracetamol (page 429).
- Teething gel or homeopathic teething granules.
- Oral rehydration sachets (such as Rapolyte), to use if your baby has DIARRHOEA or VOMITING.
- Barrier cream for severe nappy rash.
- Antiseptic cream (suitable for your baby's age).
- Small sticking plasters.
- Small roll of adhesive tape to stick down dressings for scalds and burns.
- Antihistamine syrup (such as Piriton).
- Cotton wool balls – for cleaning skin, but not for a dressing as they stick to the damaged skin surface.

Homeopathic remedies

- You may buy family first aid kits and your homeopath may prescribe anything that is not included but suits your particular needs. *Aconite* (30c) is best given straight away for shock and is also handy for parents as it reduces panic and fear. Useful applications include *Calendula* cream and *Combudoron* cream for burns, Bach flower rescue cream, *Hypercal* tincture for cuts and grazes and *Pyrethrum* spray for bites and stings.

Accidents and first aid, baby
Prevention and safety for your baby

Even before you bring your baby home it is a good idea to prepare for his needs and anticipate the dangers that everyday objects can present. Being accident aware – and taking effective preventive steps – involves judging everything from your baby's point of view, and remembering that his abilities and vulnerability alter with age. He may do something you don't expect (like roll for the first time or touch something you thought was out of reach), so try to stay one step ahead. Saying 'No' is not enough – it is a parent's responsibility to ensure that danger in the environment is kept to a minimum.

Most childhood accidents happen in the home. It is the easiest place to guard against accidents, yet also the easiest place to overlook dangers.

What your baby breathes

Do not smoke around your baby or expose him to smoky environments (page 37). Ensure that all your gas and heating appliances – most importantly gas boilers – are checked annually by a Corgi-registered gas fitter. You may decide to fit a carbon monoxide detector close to your gas appliances.

Choking hazards

Small objects such as peanuts, batteries, pens, 5p coins, pins and nails can be swallowed or may lodge in an airway and may become life threatening. Keep them away from your baby. Don't give your baby toys with small parts.

Surfaces and falling

- Never leave your baby on a raised surface when you leave the room or even turn your head. Babies can fall from beds and sofas very quickly. If you need to lay him down out of your arms, or if you have to leave him unattended, even for a minute, place him on the floor or in the safety of his cot or pram.
- Always strap your baby into his car seat before lifting it off the floor.
- Never leave the car seat on a raised surface with your baby in it.

- Always strap your baby into his rocking chair, pram or pushchair.
- Once your baby is sitting, a lightweight rocking seat is no longer appropriate – he has the strength to tip it over.
- Guard the top and bottom of stairs with a stair-gate as soon as your baby is mobile. A baby who can crawl may not have an awareness of the danger of stairs and may fall from the top. Babies can climb stairs before they learn to come down safely, and even younger babies can roll.
- Don't leave your baby unattended in a baby bouncer or walker.
- When your baby is cruising keep obstacles out of the way so they can't trip him up.

Inside

- Use a fire guard around a fire or any radiator or hot water pipe that may scald.
- Cover all electric sockets – plug covers are widely available. If possible use safety plugs, which are fused, and a trip switch to prevent electrocution.
- Keep all electric wires out of your baby's reach.
- Avoid free-standing shelves. Use brackets to fix shelves to the wall securely.
- Remove unsteady stools or tables until your baby is much older.
- Put all glass-topped coffee tables in storage or give them away.
- Use locks for cupboards containing anything dangerous.
- Avoid standing lamps, including table lamps.
- Fit window locks to all windows that may be accessible to a child.
- Use non-slip socks or soft shoes for your baby so he doesn't slip when pulling himself to standing.
- At other people's houses watch for hazards – even tablecloths when pulled could bring down a hot cup of tea. When visiting friends who don't have small children be baby aware.

Bathroom

- Never place your baby in a baby bath resting on a raised surface.
- Never leave your baby unattended in the bath or in the bathroom.
- Always run the hot tap last, and watch your child while the water is running.
- Support your baby in the bath.
- If bathing with your baby, place a towel on the floor and lift your baby out before you step out of the water, to avoid slipping. Ideally, have another adult with you who can help.
- Wash the bath thoroughly after using essential oils.
- Keep all toiletries and medicines out of reach.
- Do not use talcum powder – it can cause harm if your baby inhales it.

Kitchen

- Your baby may pull a jug, cup of tea or a plate of hot food off the table. More babies get burned by cups of tea and coffee than by anything else.
- Turn all pot handles away from the edge of the cooker, and use the rings furthest from you as often as possible.
- When your baby is mobile, use a guard on your cooker.
- Keep all dangerous substances out of your baby's reach and fit cupboard locks.
- Keep sharp knives out of reach.

Food

- Avoid the risk of choking – never prop up your baby's bottle.
- At meal times always stay with your baby, especially with soft lumpy foods.
- Watch any toddlers around your baby and help them understand that tiny babies only eat milk so that they don't offer food, however friendly they are trying to be.
- Don't give your weaned baby small morsels that carry a risk of choking. Avoid peanuts, and cut pieces of fruit, especially grapes, into small pieces. Be aware of risks such as fish bones and unevenly distributed heat.

Bedroom

- Avoid overheating and the risk of suffocation. Don't put pillows around a bed that your baby is sleeping or playing on; avoid placing cot bumpers and collections of soft toys in your baby's cot (page 487).
- Keep your baby's cot away from shelves because he may reach up and pull things onto himself.

In the car

- Always use a car seat for your baby and fix it where it is safe with the correct seat belt and away from fitted airbags. Upgrade the car seat to suit your baby as he grows.
- Use sun shades to prevent overheating.

- Use child locks.
- Never start the engine before your baby is fully strapped in.
- Never leave your baby alone in a parked car.

Outside
- Keep your child dressed appropriately for the weather and time of year.
- Watch what your child picks up, or where he puts his hands – they will almost certainly go into his mouth frequently.
- Always strap your baby into his pushchair or pram. Don't ignore the middle strap in a pushchair that passes through the legs.
- It's safest not to use a pushchair on an escalator. Take a lift if possible, or alternatively take your baby out and hold him. Another adult may help by carrying or supporting the pushchair for you.
- Always use the brake on a pushchair or pram when you are stationary, no matter how flat the surface appears to be.
- Be careful of open water, including ponds, buckets and water butts. Even very shallow water poses a risk – babies can drown in just a few centimetres of water.
- In playgrounds, your baby likes to copy others and his curiosity may drive him to do something he is not capable of. Stay with him at all times.
- If you cycle, do not fit a child seat until your baby is big enough to sit in it safely and wear a protective helmet. Buggies that attach to the back of a bike and have a full body harness are safer.
- In public sand pits check for animal faeces and broken glass.

Sun safety
- Keep your baby out of direct sunlight if possible.
- Keep his legs and arms covered in loose clothes and encourage him to wear a sun hat.
- Use an umbrella for shade in the buggy or pram.
- Always apply a high sun protective sun cream (factor 25 or higher), especially if at the seaside or beside a swimming pool.

Pets
- Family pets may get jealous – watch them carefully and don't leave them alone with your baby. Even familiar dogs may bite.
- Don't let your dog lick your baby's bottles.
- If you arrange your space so your baby is never physically lower than your dog, he will remain the boss. When he is on the floor, keep your dog in another room.
- Prepare your pets, especially cats. If they sleep in your bedroom move them to another room a few weeks before the birth.
- When your baby has arrived, use a cat net over doors and you may fix a stair gate on some doorways so you can close it if you want to keep your dog out of a room. Put a cat net over the pram when your baby is sleeping in it.
- Try to keep your pets' routine as normal as possible, as this can reduce jealous reactions.
- Be wary of other people's pets.

Poisonous substances
Most cases of poisoning in children are with household cleaners, unused tablets (commonly iron tablets and painkillers among new mums), and tablets taken from grandparents.
- Keep all detergents, shampoos, medicines, fertilisers and any other poisonous substances out of your baby's sight and out of reach.
- Medicines should be kept locked up in a medicine cupboard. Take any tablets and medicines that are not being used or are past their best-before date to your local pharmacist, who will dispose of them safely.
- In the garden or park don't let your baby eat any berries or leaves he finds. Most are harmless, but some are toxic. Watch your baby closely.
- Alcohol can be dangerous even in small amounts. Don't leave alcoholic drinks within your baby's reach.
- When grandparents or other visitors call, ask them to keep their handbags tightly closed – they are a good source of colourful tablets and other dangerous items.

Acne

See Rashes and spots, baby.

Active birth

See Labour and birth, mother, active birth.

Acupuncture

Acupuncture is a branch of traditional Chinese medicine based on the concept of *qi* (or *chi*), which is sometimes translated as 'vital energy'. Acupuncture treatment involves stimulating minute points on the body surface where *qi* is concentrated, or the meridian pathways along which *qi* flows. Every part of your body is associated with a certain type of *qi* that has a specific quality and function. In illness, some types of *qi* may be deficient or excessive, and the resultant imbalance leads to symptoms, which might be physical, psychological or spiritual.

Through altering the flow of *qi* and releasing blockages, acupuncture treatment affects body and mind. It can be used to treat acute problems and deep-seated issues. The same principles can be applied using finger pressure, known as acupressure. Acupressure is used for babies. The acupuncturist may combine acupuncture or acupressure with moxibustion (which involves the burning of herbs) and massage.

There is as yet no single scientific explanation for acupuncture, although it is known to work via the central nervous system and to stimulate the production of pain-relieving chemicals called endorphins, which act in the brain. This may help explain why it can be effective for pain relief in labour (page 381). It also increases the rate of wound healing and it probably releases body chemicals that promote healing.

▍APPLYING ACUPUNCTURE

- *Using needles.* The acupuncturist inserts one or more very fine needles at the relevant acupuncture points. Many people find this painless, or only slightly and briefly uncomfortable, and often feel harmonised and relaxed. The needles may be taken out immediately, or left in for 20 minutes. Pre-sterilised disposable needles are used to prevent the transfer of infection.
- *Moxibustion.* A herb, known as 'moxa' (traditionally *Artemesia vulgaris*), is burned and used to warm a specific acupuncture point or an area of the body. Moxa is traditionally used to

turn a breech baby. It is also used in women who feel the cold unduly.
- *Acupressure* can be very effective for self-treatment and for people who fear needles or do not need strong stimulation. It also underpins massage therapy, which takes many forms. In Chinese medicine it is called *tuina*. *Shiatsu* is a Japanese form of massage based on Chinese medicine.

Alcohol

See Drugs, alcohol.

Allergy and intolerance

See also Asthma and wheezing, baby; Asthma, mother.

An allergy is an abnormal reaction of the body's immune system to certain substances or 'allergens'. Allergic individuals suffer symptoms when exposed to substances that are harmless to non-allergic people. The word allergy is derived from the Greek words *allos*, meaning different, and *ergos*, meaning action. Another word for allergy is atopy, and an allergic reaction may be referred to as atopic.

This term is generally used by health professionals to describe reactions involving a specific part of the immune system – IgE antibodies (also known as type E immunoglobulin – see below). The immune system remembers the allergen(s) it is exposed to and becomes 'sensitised' so that on subsequent exposures there is a rapid antibody response, giving a reaction. The term 'sensitivity' is used to refer to body reactions that do not involve IgE antibodies. Sensitivities can be caused by other parts of the immune system such as immunoglobulins A and G.

The term 'intolerance' refers to a severe reaction to a particular food, usually because of the lack of the enzyme needed to digest it. Deficiency of the enzyme lactase, for example, which digests lactose (found in milk), will cause bacterial fermentation in the intestine, leading to problems such as frothy motions and wind. Intolerance to foods is a common problem in babies. Deficiency of lactase is also relatively common in adults.

Intolerance is far more common than allergy but with similar symptoms it can be difficult to distinguish between the two. Both are usually treated by avoiding the substance that triggers the condition. Some forms of intolerance may improve if the food or chemical is removed for a few months, and only encountered infrequently from then on. A true allergy can remain a problem for many years or for life.

Allergy, sensitivity and intolerance may cause similar symptoms, including itching, rash, abdominal pain, prolonged diarrhoea and breathing problems. In babies, symptoms commonly involve some aspect of bowel function. While true allergy is less common than intolerance, many more people today are affected by both than was the case 20 years ago.

Sometimes parents incorrectly suspect allergies in their children because many common illnesses in young babies have symptoms similar to those connected with allergy, sensitivity or intolerances. It may require careful observation and considerable time to obtain a clear picture.

Living with allergy and intolerance
If you are affected, or your baby is, the key to reducing or eliminating symptoms is to discover the particular substance or substances that are triggering the symptoms. Avoiding a trigger is usually the most effective prevention.

Most allergies cause only mildly uncomfortable reactions yet these may become tiresome. Any one person's symptoms can impact upon an entire family, particularly if a baby's allergy is distressing and he cries a lot, and/or the allergy presents practical challenges (such as avoiding certain materials or foods). Some reactions cause acute symptoms requiring urgent attention (see anaphylactic shock, overleaf). If an allergy is severe, or there are several allergies, your lifestyle may change considerably.

Intolerances often pass with time, particularly if the trigger is discovered, avoided and is re-introduced on an occasional basis. And although some allergies persist for life, many children do 'grow out of' allergic symptoms in five to 15 years.

▨ CAUSES AND SYMPTOMS
The range of triggers for allergies is almost limitless, as each person's system is different. An allergy can run in the family, but it is also possible to develop an allergy when there is no family history. If you know your baby may be at risk through genetic inheritance you may choose to take preventive measures (page 21).

An adult may carry the genes responsible for an allergic reaction without having any apparent signs of allergy. Similarly, a baby may inherit the genes but it may be years before the allergy appears, if it appears at all. Allergies do not always cause the same symptoms. If your mother has hay fever, you may have asthma, and your child may develop a severe rash – all from having an allergic reaction to the same food.

Contact
The skin will absorb certain allergens. Allergic contact dermatitis is an inflammation of the skin caused by a local allergic reaction to the absorption of substances such as latex (rubber), the dyes and chemicals in washing powder, plants, metals (especially nickel) in jewellery, and cosmetics.

Food
Foods and food components are common causes of allergic-type reactions. These are covered in more detail on page 19.

Inhalation
Pollens, mould spores, dust mites, animal dander (flakes of dead skin and hair) and industrial and traffic pollution are some of the many potential allergens in the air. Usual symptoms are hay fever (allergic rhinitis), asthma and conjunctivitis. Babies under one year old are seldom sensitive to inhaled allergens.

Injection
The most severe reactions can occur when allergens are injected and gain direct access to the bloodstream. Commonly this is through an insect bite or sting but some people react to medications (such as penicillin). Allergic reactions to vaccines are extremely rare.

Illness
An intolerance may follow an illness that increases sensitivity. For instance, following viral

infection of the respiratory tract resulting in a bad cough, the airway may remain sensitive for some time. After a bout of diarrhoea or gastroenteritis, the intestine may become temporarily intolerant to sucrose or lactose. Such an intolerance almost always passes in time.

Emotions

When a person is anxious or stressed the associated hormones can make intolerances more likely. This is particularly true of irritable bowel syndrome (IBS) symptoms and food intolerance, nervous system reactions (such as headaches) and general fatigue.

Symptoms

The body's immune system is highly efficient at protecting against foreign materials, such as bacteria and viruses, by producing antibodies. Protective antibodies, called immunoglobulins, help destroy a foreign particle by attaching to its surface, and this makes it easier for other immune cells to destroy it.

An allergic baby develops a specific type of antibody called immunoglobulin E, also called IgE, in response to a foreign substance. When an allergic reaction occurs, various chemicals, including cytokines and histamine, are released and cause inflammation in various parts of the body. The response causes allergic symptoms involving one or more areas, such as the:

- digestive system (bowel), with abdominal pain, bloating, colic or irritable bowel syndrome, diarrhoea or constipation, nausea and vomiting, or gastro-oesophageal reflux.
- skin, leading to rashes and eczema.
- lungs, nose, ears and eyes, leading to coughing, asthma or hay fever with a runny nose and excessive mucus, sometimes running down the throat to cause a cough, as well as sore eyes and wheezing (page 36).
- nervous system, leading to a range of symptoms, including tiredness, hyperactivity, irritability, migraine, depression or insomnia.

When allergens are eaten, inhaled or absorbed they may enter the bloodstream and travel around the body. In this way a single allergen can affect multiple organs. For example, a food allergen may cause digestive problems, asthma and tiredness. The effects on distant organs may make the trigger difficult to spot.

Symptoms in a baby

Allergies and intolerances usually become evident by about six months of age, often in response to a food that has been introduced in the weaning diet. However, this is not always the case: extremely sensitive babies may have a reaction in the first days or weeks to even small amounts of foreign proteins – cow's milk proteins consumed by the mother and present in breast milk, for example. It is also possible for an allergic baby to display a sensitivity in the womb (evident by raised levels of IgE in umbilical cord blood).

Some symptoms appear a few minutes after contact or ingestion of an allergen. Others appear within a few hours and sometimes, especially where diarrhoea or constipation is involved, symptoms may not appear for two or three days.

▓ DIAGNOSIS AND TREATMENT

If you suspect an allergy, book an appointment with your doctor. You may be referred to a specialist to discuss diagnosis.

If you have or your child has a severe allergic reaction – breathing difficulties, fainting, listlessness, pale or blue skin, swollen throat, unconsciousness – call an ambulance. If the reaction is less severe, but you are very worried, for instance your child is crying uncontrollably and seems to be in great pain or has excessive vomiting, diarrhoea or even constipation, call your doctor immediately.

✚ Red flag

Anaphylaxis and anaphylactic shock: an emergency

Anaphylaxis is a rare but acute allergic reaction that affects the whole body and requires immediate medical attention. It may involve relatively mild symptoms, or more serious symptoms involving facial swelling, particularly around the eyes and mouth, and collapse. If swelling occurs in the throat, there may be difficulty breathing and swallowing. Very rarely, anaphylactic shock may be fatal. There are three recognised levels of allergic reaction, and three levels of response:

Level 1

Skin and mucous membrane reactions – usually mild. A skin rash appears, lips tingle, and eyelids may swell. Other symptoms may include coughing, itchy skin, joint swelling, nausea, abdominal pain or bloating, headache and collapse.

- Treatment for all age groups: antihistamine by mouth (such as Piriton).

Level 2

A wheeze and cough with shortness of breath in addition to level 1 symptoms. No colour changes nor reduction in consciousness.

- Treatment: as above, with the addition of 10 puffs of salbutamol (Ventolin) or similar, can be repeated every 10 minutes.
- Call your doctor or the NHS Direct service.
- In the case of a young baby, go straight to hospital.
- Begin taking oral steroids and continue for three days.

Level 3

As above but with life-threatening wheeze, and blue colour change due to lack of oxygen. This is true anaphylaxis.

- Treatment: as above, with addition of epinephrine injection.
- The emergency medical team will give oxygen and intravenous steroids and immediate transfer to hospital.

If you or your baby has had a level 3 response you should carry an adrenaline syringe, of which the best known brand is called Epi-pen, and wear a medical information bracelet or tag (such as Medic-alert). A quick, decisive adrenaline injection can be a life-saver.

Diagnosis options

An allergy is diagnosed by asking detailed questions about wellbeing and symptoms (called 'taking a history'), conducting skin and blood tests, and finally exposing the person to the suspected allergen (a 'challenge') to see if recorded symptoms are repeated. In many cases so-called 'allergic symptoms' are never confirmed in this way, and people may be unnecessarily excluding foods from their diet when no true allergy exists.

For you or your baby, observation – linking symptoms with what has been eaten, drunk or inhaled – is the first step. Remember, it may take two or three days, or longer, for a reaction to become apparent. You may wish to have further tests with a specialist.

Self-testing – exclusion and challenge

You can carry out your own test by avoiding a single possible allergen for a period of time ('exclusion'), and observing your reaction to see if your symptoms improve. If your symptoms return when you reintroduce the allergen (performing the 'challenge'), this helps confirm the diagnosis. However, your doctor may ask you to note the pattern several times before making a firm diagnosis, since symptoms such as diarrhoea or rash often come and go, particularly in babies.

You may not see the results immediately. In the case of intolerance, symptoms may get worse before they get better and it may be a week before they diminish. If symptoms do not change you could then look for another possible cause.

If your baby's allergic reaction is severe it is best to seek the advice of a specialist. You may be advised to refrain from introducing the food until your child is three to five years old. If the allergy persists you will need to exclude the food for life.

Further diagnosis to determine whether the reaction is based on an allergy or intolerance may be carried out with clinical tests. These tests are not always definitive and clear diagnosis may take a long time.

Specialist tests

Allergy tests are constantly developing and being modified. To date they give an indication that you may be allergic to a specific substance but they are not absolutely reliable. Many tests are available, offered by allergy specialists (also called allergists) and clinical ecologists. The scientific validity of many of the easily accessible tests in health food shops and clinical ecology centres has not been subject to extensive clinical trials. Nevertheless, they may be useful for you. Your choice depends on your own situation. Conventional allergy testing, with skin prick and RAST (a blood test which measures IgE levels in response to specific allergens), is available through the NHS. Other tests are not. A baby needs to be three to six months old before any tests can be conclusive.

Treatment options

● There are few long-term medical cures for allergies. Some individuals respond well to other treatment methods, such as homeopathy (see complementary care, below).
● The best, easiest and least-expensive treatment is to avoid the allergen(s).

Treatment for you
If it is difficult for you to avoid the trigger for your allergy, you may require medication, so check with your doctor or pharmacist that it is safe.
● Inhaled corticosteroids and bronchodilators (for ASTHMA) taken by the mother are considered safe for babies in pregnancy and during breastfeeding. It is best to use minimum doses for all corticosteroid drugs.
● Corticosteroids used on the skin for eczema are safe – there is very little absorption into the bloodstream. The same is true for corticosteroid enemas used to treat colitis. Nevertheless, use the minimum you need to control symptoms.
● Antihistamines have been used for decades to treat nausea in pregnancy and to date they have not been shown to harm the developing baby. After the birth your breastfed baby may be sleepy as small amounts of antihistamine filter through.

Treatment for your baby
● If it is not possible to avoid an allergen, for instance where hay fever persists through spring and summer, it is important to do what you can to make your child comfortable. This may include use of antihistamines and local skin sprays for itchy bites, and the use of a salbutamol (Ventolin) inhaler and occasionally steroids.
● Make sure that everyone who cares for your baby is aware of his allergy, knows how to avoid it and what to do if symptoms arise. This also applies to drugs that he may be given on prescription. It is important for older children to understand as much as possible about their allergy.

Desensitisation
Allergy desensitisation or 'allergy immunotherapy' stimulates the immune system with gradually increasing doses of the allergen. The doses are given by injection. The aim is to modify or stop the allergic response by reducing the strength of the antibody IgE. This form of treatment is very effective for allergies to pollen, mites, cats and, especially, stinging insects. It usually takes six months to a year to work and further desensitisation injections are usually required for three to five years. The injections are commonly reserved for use when there is a severe life-threatening allergic response to wasp and bee stings, although they may occasionally be used in treatment of allergy to house dust or some grass pollens. They are not easily available in the UK, except from specialists in allergy treatment.

There are a number of other treatments that may desensitise an allergic person so that they can tolerate allergens. They are still experimental and consist of placing a dilute solution of the allergenic food under the tongue.

Complementary care
More and more people are turning to complementary therapies such as homeopathy, acupuncture or herbal medicine. Their efficacy for you or your baby depends on your individual constitution, the nature of your sensitivity, and the skill of the person caring for you. It is essential to visit a specialist, as self-treatment is not appropriate, and you may need to commit to several visits over a period of months. Complementary therapies can often be used in conjunction with conventional medication, and when effective may help to reduce medicine dosage.

■ ENVIRONMENT AND LIFESTYLE

If you discover that your child is allergic to an airborne allergen such as pollen or animal dander, you will need to do all you can to avoid exposure. Smoking is a significant factor. Never smoke around your baby or expose him to other people's cigarette smoke.

Reducing house dust or mites requires simple measures, such as using a special vacuum cleaner that removes fine dust particles, cleaning curtains and furniture coverings regularly, keeping soft toys and clothes in drawers, avoiding feather pillows and quilts, replacing carpets with linoleum or wood-type flooring, and improving ventilation in the house. Avoid blown-air heating.

If your child is sensitive to pollen you may need to install air conditioning to keep the house cool instead of opening windows.

Where there is a pet allergy it might be possible to reduce or stop contact with the pet and to keep the pet clean and well brushed. Sometimes the only option is to find another home for the pet – this is often the case with allergy to cat saliva, which forms a fine dust when dry and can get everywhere.

When there is sensitivity to a metal, fabric, or a chemical used in everyday washing, for instance, you may need to replace them with hypo-allergenic products. These are produced without the use of substances that cause allergic or sensitivity reactions in a significant number of people. Even so, hypo-allergenic products, such as baby-wipes or shampoo, still contain chemicals that can irritate a baby's sensitive skin.

■ FOODS

Food is a common cause of allergic reactions and intolerances in babies and children, and it is perhaps not surprising that reported cases are on the rise. We eat a huge range of food sourced from around the world. Much of the processed food we eat has been grown with the use of chemicals, enhanced with modifiers, flavouring and colouring, and preserved with yet more chemicals. Many people are sensitive or intolerant to specific components in the food, such as monosodium glutamate (MSG), and sulphites used to enhance crispness and prevent the growth of mould.

There are many different chemicals responsible for food sensitivities, for example naturally occurring histamine in raw fish, which may cause diarrhoea or wheezing, or additives and preservatives, which often give rise to rashes. Because symptoms may result from a chemical added to a certain food, you may wish to use organic produce as often as possible.

The following entries consider the more common food allergens. After milk, wheat is the most common, but there are many possibilities, and food combinations may cause a reaction even though a single food on its own does not. If your baby displays an allergy to any food it is best to avoid the food, and then try the food challenge test (page 17) three or four months later, as some allergies and intolerances may have passed in the meantime. However, if you already know your baby has an allergy or intolerance, you need to avoid the problem food completely. If there is a chance your baby may be allergic to peanuts, for example, avoid all contact with them as even minute traces on your hands may cause a reaction in your baby.

The food challenge

Excluding a food and observing whether symptoms reduce is the easiest way to diagnose a food allergy. And only by re-introducing the food in a 'food challenge' (page 17) can you discover if an allergy or intolerance has passed.

Cow's milk protein

The most common abnormal reaction to food among young babies is to cow's milk. A true cow's milk allergy, where the immune system produces IgE antibodies that attack proteins in the milk, affects around 5 per cent of babies and adults. Reactions not involving the immune system are better described as an intolerance to cow's milk. For example, a baby with lactose intolerance does not produce lactase, the enzyme needed to digest the sugar, lactose, found in milk (overleaf). This intolerance is more common than true allergy.

The two main protein components in milk that trigger allergies are whey and casein, and an individual may be allergic to either or both. Casein is the curd that forms when milk is left to curdle, and whey is the watery liquid that remains. Casein is the most significant allergen in cheese. When milk is heated it may alter the whey proteins, so a whey-sensitive adult may be able to tolerate evaporated, boiled or sterilised ('long life') milk and milk powder. These milk-substitutes are not suitable for babies.

Most babies do not encounter cow's milk proteins until they are given formula milk or dairy products. For a tiny number of very sensitive breastfed babies, small amounts of cow's milk protein from the mother's diet may pass into breast milk and cause allergic symptoms.

Your doctor may recommend a milk substitute, perhaps a soya or hypo-allergenic formula (page 79). You may be able to get this on prescription. It is not recommended to use goat or sheep milk for babies under one year. If an alternative is required this should be in the form of a pre-digested cow's milk, called a hydrolysate – such as Pepti or Pregestamil – or a soya-based milk, which is suitable after six months of age. Another alternative is a totally synthetic milk – made up of amino acids and supplemented with fats and vitamins – such as Neocate.

Although some babies seem to get relief by switching to other types of formula, it is likely that they will either develop a sensitivity to the alternative milk, or that they are intolerant rather than truly allergic to the original milk. If your baby reacts to the alternative formula your doctor will prescribe a specialised milk.

Once your baby begins to eat solid food you will need to take care to avoid foods that contain milk ingredients. Advice from a nutritionist or dietitian will help you ensure your baby gets a nutritionally adequate diet. Because your child is susceptible you may notice other food allergies or intolerances, most commonly to wheat.

Gluten intolerance (coeliac disease)

Coeliac disease is an inherited disorder in which eating gluten in foods leads to the formation of antibodies that damage the lining of the small intestine. This results in malabsorption of nutrients and vitamins. Gluten is one of the proteins found in many cereal grains – mainly

wheat, rye and barley. A similar protein is found in oats. Rice, maize, sorghum and millet do not contain gluten.

More than 5 per cent of the population of Europe have an intolerance to gluten (it is more common in families of Mediterranean origin) and there are 10 times as many 'carriers', who are at risk of becoming intolerant.

Babies with gluten intolerance are unlikely to show symptoms before they eat gluten for the first time. Therefore gluten-containing products should be kept out of a baby's diet as a matter of routine until at least six months of age, irrespective of whether there is a family history of coeliac disease.

A baby with coeliac disease is likely to have frequent bowel movements producing bulky, putty-coloured stools with a highly unpleasant smell. Left untreated, coeliac disease can lead to protein and fat deficiency, and inadequate absorption of vitamins and trace minerals. In severe cases, malnutrition may lead to weight loss, muscle wasting, distended abdomen, anaemia, listlessness, irritability and immature bone development.

Gluten intolerance is initially diagnosed by excluding gluten from the diet and observing an improvement in symptoms. Confirmation may be made by blood test and possibly a biopsy (removal of a sample of tissue) from the wall of the small intestine. You will need specialist nutritional advice for a gluten-free diet that still provides adequate nutrition, including roughage. Coeliacs need to stay on a gluten-free diet for life.

Lactose intolerance

Lactose is a sugar found in all milks. An enzyme, lactase, usually breaks down lactose in the bowel, allowing it to be absorbed. If this enzyme is absent or reduced then large amounts of lactose remain in the bowel. Bacteria in the bowel then get to work on it resulting in diarrhoea and frothy stools, the characteristic signs of lactose intolerance. Breastfeeding your baby encourages the activity of lactase. Rarely, a baby does not have sufficient lactase despite being breastfed, and reacts to the lactose in breast milk. Lactose intolerant babies need a specialised milk formula.

Adults may have relatively little lactase in

their gut. Although they may tolerate some lactose, if they drink too much milk they may react in the same or a similar way, revealing an intolerance. This is more common among people of Asian or African heritage.

Lactose intolerance is diagnosed through detection of an excessive amount of sugar in a baby's stool (there is more sugar because it has passed through the bowel without being digested).

Colief (lactase) drops are available from a chemist. These add a small amount of the missing lactase enzyme to the milk, and can relieve many of the symptoms. Always consult your doctor before self-treating your baby.

Nuts

In the UK around 1 per cent of people have a nut allergy and this may cause very serious or fatal reactions (page 16). It's advisable to keep nuts out of your child's diet for the first few years. If you are prone to allergy, it is best to avoid eating nuts in pregnancy and when you are breastfeeding. If you are not prone to nut allergy it is okay to eat them.

It is very rare indeed for babies of under one year to have any reaction to peanuts or other nuts, as they rarely come across them in their diet. In the rare case where a baby does react, the most likely symptom is a skin reaction due to contact with a peanut oil (often listed as 'arachis' on the label). A small dose of antihistamine is usually effective.

Around 10 per cent of children sensitive to peanuts are also sensitive to tree nuts. (Peanuts are not strictly speaking nuts – they are legumes from the same family as peas and beans.)

▓ PREVENTIVE MEASURES

With sensitivities on the increase, many parents are keen to do what they can to reduce their children's chances of developing allergies or intolerances. The most pro-active approach you can take in pregnancy is to look after yourself, eat a balanced healthy diet and avoid family allergens and smoking. If there is no history of allergy in your family or your partner's family, there is no need to avoid certain foods in pregnancy simply because they are potential allergens.

Breastfeeding

The best food for your baby is your breast milk. Breastfeeding reduces your baby's exposure to potential allergens, such as the protein in cow's milk, and has a protective effect. This is particularly significant if your baby is born prematurely or there is a family history of allergy.

* Breastfeeding for longer than one month without other milk supplements offers significant protection against food and respiratory allergy at three years of age.
* Six months of breastfeeding may delay the onset of genetically inherited eczema until the end of the first year.

You might want to keep a record of the foods you eat with notes on your baby's symptoms. It may be possible to determine which foods cause your baby distress, and then you have a choice to limit or avoid them. If your baby reacts to something you have eaten you will need to exclude it and continue to breastfeed.

Solid food

It is best to delay weaning your baby until six months (page 557). If you have a family history of allergy to certain foods, avoid these until your baby is one year old. If your baby was born prematurely, apply these timescales after his expected date (not actual date) of delivery. This can reduce the chances of an allergy developing, and if the allergy does occur may reduce the severity of symptoms.

Ambiguous genitalia

See Genitalia, ambiguous.

Amniocentesis and CVS

If your baby has a high risk of having a genetic or chromosomal abnormality, or another condition that can be detected before birth, you might consider antenatal screening using amniocentesis or chorionic villous sampling (CVS). These tests involve obtaining cells originating from your baby and analysing them in a laboratory. The results will either put your mind at rest, because they will confirm that everything is fine, or, if an abnormality is diagnosed, will help you to make plans for the future. For some conditions, treatment can begin in the womb. Amniocentesis is also used to treat anaemic babies with a blood transfusion in the womb.

The tests are 'invasive' (requiring entry into the womb environment) and carry a small risk of miscarriage. In amniocentesis this is around 0.5 per cent (or around one in 200) when carried out at Week 16 (the risk is higher before Week 15) and for CVS the risk is around 1 per cent (around one in 100).

Less commonly, other invasive screening techniques may be carried out including cordocentesis, to remove blood cells from the umbilical cord, and foetoscopy, allowing detailed viewing of a foetus in the womb.

Why carry out the tests?

Invasive testing is usually only carried out when a significant risk has been identified. The most common conditions looked for are:

- *Chromosomal abnormalities.* A missing or an extra chromosome in a baby's genetic make-up can have significant effects on development, leading to a CONGENITAL ABNORMALITY. The most common chromosomal abnormality is DOWN'S SYNDROME, which is caused by having an extra chromosome 21 (hence the condition is also called 'trisomy 21', meaning three copies of chromosome 21). With improved ultrasound scans and blood tests for Down's syndrome, the use of amniocentesis has decreased.
- *Inherited genetic diseases.* If the parents are known to have, or are at a high risk of having, a genetic disease, their baby may be tested in the womb. Examples include TAY-SACHS DISEASE, CYSTIC FIBROSIS, and sickle cell anaemia and thalassaemia (page 476).

There are a number of congenital abnormalities that cannot be detected through amniocentesis or CVS because they are not related to the chromosomes or genes. These include heart defects and cleft lip. The second trimester scan, around 18–20 weeks, takes a close look at organ development to attempt to find these abnormalities. Despite this, a small number of babies are born with abnormalities that are not detected in pregnancy.

What happens

Both amniocentesis and CVS are performed in the ultrasound scan room by a foetal medicine specialist obstetrician. During the whole procedure your baby can be seen clearly on a monitor and this ensures your baby is unlikely to be harmed. You will be able to see the image on the screen.

An amniocentesis is carried out around Week 16 and allows a sample of amniotic fluid to be collected. The fluid contains cells that have been shed from your developing baby's skin. A fine needle is inserted through your abdominal wall and the obstetrician will withdraw 10–20ml (2–4tsp) of fluid. The amniotic fluid removed represents 5–10 per cent of the total volume and will be replaced by your baby within six hours.

The procedure takes only a few minutes and you can go home within an hour. You may be more anxious before the needle is inserted than during the procedure. The feeling of the needle is similar to having a blood test in your arm, but fear of injury to your baby may increase your sensitivity. Some women feel no pain; others feel a needle prick.

CVS is carried out between Weeks 11 and 14. A small amount of chorionic villi from the placenta are removed using a needle inserted into the placenta and gentle suction, under ultrasound guidance. The cells from the chorionic villi are cultured in a laboratory so the chromosomes or the function of the genes can be analysed. Depending on the location of your placenta, your doctor may insert the needle through your abdominal wall or through your cervix. In the transcervical approach, a speculum, which is usually used when taking a cervical smear, is used to widen the vagina in order to view your cervix and the needle is inserted via the cervix, still under ultrasound guidance. It may be more uncomfortable than amniocentesis.

Analysis and results

The sample is sent to a laboratory where it is divided in two. One half is examined using a DNA probe test. Cells are treated with specific probes, which make the chromosomes visible under a light microscope. Normal cells have two chromosomes in each group. If the DNA test reveals a trisomy (three chromosomes in a group), the results are reliable. False positives do not occur. There is, however, a tiny chance (one in 1,500) that the initial test result will show a normal chromosome complement even though a problem remains undetected (false negative). Because of this, the second half of the sample is incubated and the cells grown over two weeks for amniocentesis or four days for CVS, then the chromosomes are counted. The result on the incubated cells is totally reliable.

If the test is being done for a specific gene disorder, for example cystic fibrosis, the cells will be examined in the laboratory to check whether that gene is functioning correctly or not.

Cordocentesis and foetoscopy

Later in pregnancy, a sample of your baby's blood may be taken from the umbilical cord, any time after Week 16. This is called a cordocentesis. The advantage is that the cells can be grown more quickly than with amniocentesis but there is a higher miscarriage risk. As more centres offer amniocentesis results in three days, this test is used very infrequently. This technique is also used for intrauterine transfusions for anaemia or low platelet levels.

If an ultrasound scan detects a developmental problem that may benefit from surgery in the uterus, a foetoscopy may subsequently be carried out. This is only done in specialist centres and involves inserting a small camera with a light source into the uterus.

Action plan: after the test

After the procedure the needle puncture site seals in a few minutes. A single dose of homeopathic *Hypericum* (200c) may be useful to assist healing of the puncture site. You will be asked to stay for 30 minutes and take it easy for the next 24 hours and avoid intense physical activity and sexual intercourse.

- The most significant risk is miscarriage and you will be asked to be aware of any bleeding, cramping or leaking fluid from the vagina. Around 1 per cent of women experience these symptoms and they do not usually result in miscarriage. Bleeding is slightly more common in CVS.
- In an amniotic fluid leak it may track between the amniotic membrane and the wall of the

uterus, down to the cervix and emerge from the vagina as a clear urine-coloured discharge. Leakage usually stops within 48 hours as the membrane seals. Continuous prolonged leakage, however, may lead to a miscarriage.
- If you have these symptoms, call your doctor immediately for advice.

Infection following the procedure is very rare. Harm to the foetus is very unlikely because with the aid of ultrasound the obstetrician can see and can control the needle. CVS before Week 10 may be associated with a higher incidence of foetal limb abnormalities. There is a small risk of Rhesus sensitisation (page 67) if you are Rhesus negative and your baby is Rhesus positive. An anti-D injection (page 68) after the procedure will usually eliminate this risk.

A repeat test is rarely needed, but more common after a CVS (around 1 per cent). If you need a second test this is not usually because there is something wrong with the pregnancy. It may simply be that the cells have failed to grow, or results were unclear and a fresh sample is needed.

If the test reveals an abnormality

If the test reveals a chromosome or genetic abnormality, your foetal medicine specialist will discuss the implications. You are likely to feel shocked and may be faced with a very difficult decision. Termination of pregnancy may be an option. Most parents appreciate genetic counselling (page 267). It often helps to talk to other parents who have had children with similar conditions before making a firm decision about the future.

Amniotic fluid

See also Labour and birth, mother, spontaneous and premature rupture of membranes.

Amniotic fluid is the name for the watery liquid that surrounds and cushions your baby in the womb. It is this fluid that is released when your 'waters break'. The amniotic fluid is in dynamic balance and is replaced and topped up every four to six hours by the placenta and by your baby swallowing and urinating. The fluid remains sterile and all your baby's waste by-products are removed by the placenta.

The amniotic fluid is held securely within the amniotic sac. This sac is made up of two separate membranes. The outer one is the chorion, which extends to the edge of the placenta and lines the entire womb. Inside this is the amnion. The chorion originates from placental cells and the amnion develops from your baby's cells. Together, these two membranes form a strong boundary around the waters of protection in which your baby bathes.

During antenatal examinations your midwife routinely estimates the volume of amniotic fluid surrounding your baby. It can also be visualised by means of an ultrasound scan.

In most pregnancies, the protective membranes 'rupture' shortly before labour begins, or during labour. Early rupture of the membranes is one of the most common triggers for premature birth (page 393). The amniotic fluid is clear (not urine coloured) and has a slightly sweet smell. Rarely, the membranes remain intact and a baby is born within the sac. This is known as being born 'in a caul'. In some traditions, this is considered to be a sign of blessing and good luck.

▓ EXCESS FLUID

An excess of amniotic fluid is called polyhydramnios. In most instances of suspected polyhydramnios, the baby is normal and healthy; the excess fluid is mild and not a cause for concern.

If the excess is severe, the additional pressure could cause BREATHLESSNESS, HEARTBURN AND INDIGESTION as well as abdominal discomfort (see ABDOMINAL PAIN). More seriously, the increased pressure may lead to PREMATURE BIRTH. Another possible effect is that with extra space your baby may lie in an awkward transverse lie position (page 345). During labour, if your baby's head remains high and the membranes rupture there is an increased risk that the umbilical cord may prolapse (displace downwards) in front of the head. This potentially serious complication is discussed on page 339.

What happens

Your baby may be large (page 396). If you have DIABETES and your blood sugar is not well controlled, your baby may swallow and urinate excessively leading to the increase in fluid. Fluid volume will be high if you are carrying TWINS – and even more so if the twins are identical. In very rare instances fluid may accumulate when a baby has difficulty swallowing, either because there is an obstruction in the oesophagus or because of a neurological difficulty, and the amniotic fluid cannot be recycled.

Action plan

A detailed ultrasound scan will identify twins and check your baby's anatomy. Your baby's weight can be estimated on a scan and from your midwife's examination. A glucose tolerance test may be performed to exclude maternal diabetes, particularly if your baby is large. If a cause cannot be found on the scan this is a good sign and your baby is likely to be normal. Draining the amniotic fluid by inserting a needle into the uterus is not a worthwhile option and may precipitate premature birth.

Lifestyle and nutrition

- When the excess fluid is significant you may be encouraged to give up work and rest frequently during the day to reduce the risk of premature birth.
- If you have diabetes, meticulous control of your blood sugar levels through good dietary control and/or medication will reduce the amniotic fluid volume.
- If there is no diabetes it is useful to reduce your intake of sugar, sweets and fizzy drinks and fruit juices as a protection against excessive foetal growth (page 262).

Medical care

When labour begins, or if the membranes rupture, contact the hospital immediately. Your medical team will watch carefully for umbilical cord prolapse, a very large baby or transverse lie. If any of these is present you will need a CAESAREAN SECTION.

After birth, your baby will be thoroughly checked and a soft tube may be inserted via her mouth into the stomach to check for a blockage of the oesophagus. The long-term outlook is usually good, largely depending on the underlying cause of the polyhydramnios, and whether birth was premature.

▓ REDUCTION IN FLUID

A reduction in amniotic fluid is known as oligohydramnios. The amniotic fluid volume usually peaks at 36 to 40 weeks, and if your baby is late the volume may naturally reduce, particularly after 42 weeks. Fluid volume is one of the main factors your midwife or doctor will check after 40 weeks. Amniotic fluid protects the umbilical cord from being compressed, so low fluid volume in labour increases the risk of umbilical cord compression, which can lead to FOETAL DISTRESS.

Usually when there is suspected oligohydramnios the baby is healthy. In some instances a baby may be healthy but a little small. In other instances placental function is reduced and the baby may have INTRAUTERINE GROWTH RESTRICTION (IUGR).

What happens

Often, there is a reduction in volume when a baby is normal. If the reduced fluid is due to insufficient placental function and there is slow growth, you and your baby will need to be monitored closely. In rare instances, oligohydramnios occurs if a baby is unable to pass urine because the kidneys have not developed or there is an obstruction to the flow from the bladder. When this is the case, reduced fluid is usually obvious on an ultrasound scan from Week 20.

Action plan

If there is a slight reduction in amniotic fluid and your baby is otherwise healthy, no treatment is needed.

Medical care

- The natural reduction in the volume of amniotic fluid in late pregnancy may occur earlier than usual and your team will check your baby's health closely.
- If there is IUGR and reduced placental function

you will need frequent checkups using clinical examination, ultrasound scans and possibly foetal heart monitoring.
- If your baby has a kidney or bladder problem, treatment will be based around the individual problem.
- If the reduction is large your doctor may advise INDUCTION of labour (see LABOUR AND BIRTH, MOTHER) or a caesarean section before term, particularly if there is severe IUGR.
- If the reduction is moderate you may be advised to have your baby by Week 40. The timing of the induction will depend on the fluid volume and the wellbeing of your baby.
- In labour, particularly after the membranes rupture, your baby's heartbeat will be monitored frequently to check for umbilical cord compression and foetal distress.
- After the birth, a paediatrician will examine your baby, taking into account all the information gathered in pregnancy. Your baby's outlook will depend on the cause of the oligohydramnios. If it was due to insufficient placental function this can be corrected with early and frequent feeding after birth.

Anaemia, baby

See also Bleeding, baby; Blood screening, baby.

In the womb, your baby produces her own blood with a special type of foetal haemoglobin, the protein that carries oxygen and gives blood its red colour. It is needed because oxygen levels received via the placenta are lower than those obtained when the baby breathes air after birth. After birth, haemoglobin changes as the adult type gradually replaces the foetal type. Anaemia occurs when there is an abnormally low level of haemoglobin in the blood.

▓ PRENATAL FOETAL ANAEMIA

Anaemia before birth is rare. The most frequent cause is Rhesus disease (page 314). A tiny number of babies have anaemia in the womb due to an infection, especially parvovirus, although TOXOPLASMOSIS and cytomegalovirus may also be a cause, or because of the complication of foeto-maternal transfusion (page 26), or a severe strain of inherited thalassaemia (page 477).

Anaemia after birth

Full-term babies are born with a haemoglobin level of 16–20 gm/dl (gram per decilitre – roughly 33 per cent greater than adults) and often look very red at birth. After birth, the extra red blood cells break down, giving rise to the yellow pigment, bilirubin. This may cause jaundice. The released iron is stored in the body for later use. By two to three months the haemoglobin level is 9–12 gm/dl, which is roughly 30 per cent below adult levels, and this is normal. Haemoglobin builds up to adult levels over the next six months.

If the umbilical cord is clamped more than three minutes after birth (page 334) extra blood cells will be able to enter the baby's circulation and she is less likely to be anaemic. This is especially important for low-birth-weight babies.

Babies born early are particularly prone to iron-deficiency anaemia because iron stores are laid down in the last four weeks of pregnancy. Premature babies may require transfusion for anaemia when there is difficulty breathing or feeding. Iron deficiency in babyhood infrequently leads to severe anaemia.

In the first year, the two most common causes of minor anaemia are inadequate iron intake due to the use of inappropriate milks (page 79) and excess iron loss. This is usually due to the continuous but small loss of blood from the bowel because of inflammation resulting from cow's milk intolerance (page 19). When the haemoglobin level is 10 gm/dl or less, compared to 12 gm/dl, a baby may look pale. Rarely, anaemia may be due to an inherited condition (page 476).

Action plan

If iron-deficiency anaemia is suspected, treatment is generally simple and improvement can be expected over a one- to two-month period, after which your baby will look less pale and feel better.

- Replace inappropriate milk with a baby-milk fortified with iron. Follow-on milks, which contain extra iron, can be used after six months when iron is better absorbed.
- Remove any food causing an intolerance.
- Iron supplements designed for babies may also be given.

▦ FOETO-MATERNAL TRANSFUSION

When your baby's blood circulates through the placenta, it does not usually mix directly with your blood, although a small amount can cross into your bloodstream during birth and in pregnancy. In very rare circumstances, with no known cause in pregnancy, a baby may lose a significant amount of blood in this way. Moderate loss usually results in anaemia, and if this is ongoing it may lead to INTRAUTERINE GROWTH RESTRICTION (IUGR) and even heart failure. If the loss involves 30 per cent or more of a baby's blood volume, this is called a foeto-maternal transfusion and there may be foetal distress before or during labour showing a specific alteration in the heart rate that necessitates urgent delivery. If haemoglobin is below 10 gm/dl, a blood transfusion may be needed at birth. In very rare cases, foeto-maternal transfusion occurs without warning signs and it is a rare cause of stillbirth (page 501).

Anaemia, mother

See also Sickle cell disease and thalassaemia.

Haemoglobin in your red blood cells carries oxygen around your body and to your placenta and baby. Adequate haemoglobin levels are normally maintained when you consume a balanced diet containing sufficient iron, in combination with other minerals and vitamins. Anaemia occurs when the concentration of red blood cells and/or their haemoglobin component fall.

If you are anaemic you may look pale and feel tired, be short of breath or feel faint. Mild anaemia in pregnancy is not harmful for your baby.

Before pregnancy the normal haemoglobin level is over 11 gm/dl.

Anaemia in pregnancy

During pregnancy, the number of red cells in your blood increases. However, the amount of fluid in your circulation also increases, so it is perfectly normal to have a slight drop in haemoglobin concentration. The level usually stays above 10.5 gm/dl. In pregnancy, it is normal practice for anaemia to be diagnosed if the haemoglobin count falls below 10.5 gm/dl, although many women have a count of between 9 and 10.5 gm/dl and do not experience any symptoms of anaemia. Women carrying large, healthy babies often show haemoglobin levels slightly below 10.5 because there is more fluid in the mother's circulation and the baby absorbs more iron and mineral elements from the mother's blood.

It is routine to check the haemoglobin level in the first 12 weeks and again after Week 30. If the level is low, laboratory tests will be carried out to investigate the cause and treatment will be geared towards raising the levels.

A normal haemoglobin level indicates that the oxygen supply to the placenta is normal, and you have adequate reserves of red blood cells should bleeding complicate birth.

Anaemia after birth

Your haemoglobin level may be tested on the second or third day after birth. The amount of fluid in your circulation diminishes after birth but you will still have the extra red blood cells that formed during pregnancy so the concentration of haemoglobin will actually increase, usually at a rate of 1 gm per week for three or four weeks. If you lose a lot of blood in labour, however, you may become anaemic.

What happens

Vitamin and mineral deficiency is by far the commonest cause of anaemia. In pregnancy you need more iron and minerals and your baby uses an increasing quantity as pregnancy progresses. During the last months of gestation, your baby's store of iron increases. This will get him through the first few months of life when iron intake will be low.

Some people are more susceptible to mineral deficiency, perhaps because of poor nutrition before conception, heavy menstrual periods, difficulty absorbing nutrients because of a bowel disease or because of a previous eating disorder (page 200). The commonest deficiency is iron but many women with low iron stores are also low in other minerals, mainly zinc, cobalt, selenium and vitamins B12, B6 and folic acid. Sometimes deficiencies in these nutrients can cause anaemia even where iron levels are normal.

You are more likely to become anaemic if you are carrying TWINS or a LARGE BABY or if you have had babies in close succession. Some women inherit an anaemic tendency (page 476). After birth, levels of haemoglobin depend on the amount of blood lost during birth, your nutrition and any underlying anaemic tendency.

Action plan

It is important to raise low haemoglobin levels because tiredness and low energy may reduce your enjoyment of parenthood and could contribute to DEPRESSION and to low milk flow. Laboratory tests investigate the cause, and treatment will be geared towards raising the levels.

If you are at risk of anaemia from sickle cell disease or thalassaemia (page 476) you may need specialist care, and dietary measures alone will not correct your anaemia.

Diet and supplements

Stick to a nutritious diet (page 253). Iron- and mineral-rich foods include meat, seaweeds (including laver bread), green leafy vegetables, raw vegetables and salad, beans and peas, pulses, tofu and soya beans, millet and lentils. Other foods that you might not think of eating that are particularly rich in iron include apricots, cane molasses (take a dessertspoon daily), coriander and parsley.

Although you can get lots of iron and minerals in your diet (page 263), you may also need an iron supplement. Your doctor will advise. The main drawback of iron supplements is constipation and this is reduced by taking the iron before a meal. As anaemia can result from a lack of iron as well as other minerals, it is best to take iron together with vitamin and mineral supplements formulated for use in pregnancy (page 264). Iron is best absorbed if taken on an empty stomach with diluted fruit juice or vitamin C, followed by food one hour later. Take the other vitamin and mineral supplements at a different time of day. Black (Indian) tea blocks the uptake of iron, so avoid drinking tea for one hour before and after taking supplements. Nettle tea can improve mineral absorption and also contains iron.

Continue all the supplements for three to six months after birth.

Homeopathy
To aid the absorption and assimilation of iron take *Calc Phos* (6x potency) and *Ferrum Phos* (6x) daily, morning and night, in addition to having a nutritious diet. It's a good idea to consider constitutional treatment under the help of a qualified homeopath.

Medical
If your haemoglobin levels do not rise after taking supplements, the doctor will carry out further blood tests to look for rarer causes of anaemia, particularly sickle cell disease and thalassaemia. If your iron and ferritin (stored form of iron) levels remain low this indicates either that you are not taking iron, or that you are not absorbing it. If you are not absorbing it, a different type of supplement may help, such as iron EAP (page 264). Rarely, injections of iron may be needed to boost stores.

If haemoglobin levels drop below 8 gm/dl after birth you may be offered a BLOOD TRANSFUSION, which will bring levels up immediately. The alternative is to take iron and mineral supplements combined with a good diet, and let your levels rise gradually over a period of days or weeks. You may feel a lack of energy until the levels rise.

Anal fissure

See Piles (haemorrhoids) and anal fissure.

Anorexia

See Eating difficulties, mother.

Antenatal tests

See also Caring for you.

Antenatal tests have been designed and modified over the years to detect, treat and prevent problems and improve safety for mother and baby. It is up to you which tests you have. It is a legal requirement that every woman gives her consent, albeit verbal, to have a test done.

Expectant parents vary greatly in their desire to know details. At one end of the spectrum there are people who prefer no monitoring. At the other end are people who ask for every test available. In between, the choice varies widely. Many parents find tests reassuring and helpful for bonding with their baby. For others, the anxiety of the test and the wait for results can be difficult, and pregnancy may seem like a problem rather than a natural process. If testing raises emotional or ethical issues for you, it may diminish your joy of pregnancy.

If you are concerned about the safety of tests, such as ultrasound (page 33) and amniocentesis (page 21), you may wish to talk to your midwife or doctor and research the latest information before making your choice. In most cases, tests bring reassuring results. Less commonly, they highlight an issue that indicates a need for more attentive care to improve safety.

Some blood tests give an actual result such as your blood group. Some scans are also increasingly accurate as technology develops. There are also tests that do not give definitive results but are designed to 'screen' for a condition and calculate a risk factor. If the risk is significantly raised, further testing or treatment may be suggested. An example is screening for Down's syndrome (page 30), where early ultrasound scans and blood tests may indicate a higher than average risk and an amniocentesis is required to give a definitive result. A 'false positive' result is when a test indicates there may be a problem but your baby turns out to be healthy. A 'false negative' result is when the test misses a problem. As screening tests improve, the number of incorrect results diminishes and invasive tests are needed less frequently.

What happens

Throughout your pregnancy (or 'period of gestation') your antenatal visits keep you in touch with your midwives and with your hospital or healthcare centre. These visits provide important opportunities for you to ask questions and discuss your feelings, and may involve a range of tests, listed on the following pages. It is your choice how many times you visit your healthcare professional. Many women have up to 10 visits – more if closer monitoring is advised. If you have any concerns in-between routine appointments, the usual approach is to book additional checks with your GP or midwife or visit the maternity department of your local hospital.

As soon as you have confirmed your pregnancy, you can arrange to see your midwife at your hospital or local surgery. This is your 'booking visit' when you'll discuss your due date, the tests on offer and your choice of hospital or home birth, among other things. If you have chosen to have consultant-led care, or you have a high-risk pregnancy, some or all of your antenatal visits may be with an obstetrician.

Routine antenatal visits are typically spaced at monthly intervals until Week 28, then every two weeks until Week 36 and finally every week until your baby is born. At routine visits, your midwife will ask to examine you and your baby as well as checking your blood pressure and usually your weight and testing a sample of your urine. In addition, you may book in for ultrasound scans (page 33) and blood tests.

At each routine visit your midwife will talk to you about how you are feeling and about how things are going for you. You may discuss your family and partnership, working, diet and supplements, and your network of support. She will examine you and your baby by placing her hands on your abdomen to check your baby's growth and the amount of amniotic fluid. She will note any test results.

From about Week 14, your midwife will be able to hear your baby's heartbeat with an ultrasound monitor that allows you to hear it too. From Week 28 on she can feel whether your baby is head down and facing your back or your side and whether his head is engaged in your pelvis. She will check your baby's size and amniotic fluid at each visit. An apparently low or excessive growth rate may mean you have closer surveillance and more frequent visits.

Record keeping

Your notes record your background medical and family information and the results of all antenatal tests and examinations. Eventually they will contain a record of your birth and your postnatal care. In most hospitals, you will be given a copy to bring to every visit. You may also carry it with you if you are travelling. A lot of information is recorded in shorthand. If you're confused, don't be afraid to ask.

Common abbreviations and medical terms used in maternity notes are listed below:

EDD	Estimated date of delivery
LMP	Last menstrual period
Primagravida or Para 0	Your first pregnancy
Multigravida or Para 1 or more	You have had more than one pregnancy lasting over 24 weeks
7/52	Seven weeks
FMF/ FMNF	Foetal movements felt/Foetal movements not felt
FHH/ FHNH	Foetal heart heard/Foetal heart not heard
Alb	Albumin – a protein that may be detected in your urine
BP	Blood pressure
Hb	Level of haemoglobin in your blood, an indicator of ANAEMIA
Fe	Iron tablets (prescribed if you are at risk of anaemia)
MSU	Midstream urine sample
NAD or nil	Nothing abnormal detected (often related to urine sample)
Oed	Oedema – swelling of the hands, feet or face (page 504)
PET	Pre-eclamptic toxaemia (high blood pressure) (page 68)
TCA	To come again
VE	Vaginal examination
Ceph or Vx	Cephalic or Vertex – your baby has his head down
Br	Breech – your baby has his bottom down
ROA or LOA	Right occiput anterior or left occiput anterior. Your baby is lying with the back of his head facing the front and pointing right or left
ROP or LOP	Right or left occiput posterior – your baby is lying with the right or left side of the back of his head facing your back
E/Eng	Engaged – your baby's head has moved down into your pelvis
NE	Not engaged
Height of fundus or SFP (symphysis fundal height)	The height of the top of your uterus (the fundus), measured from the top of your pubic bone

▥ BLOOD PRESSURE

Your midwife will ask to measure your BLOOD PRESSURE at each antenatal visit. The test is simple and it measures the pressure in your arteries as your heart pumps blood around your body. The systolic pressure shows pressure during a heartbeat. In your notes this figure is the upper of the two numbers in your blood pressure reading. The lower figure is your diastolic pressure, which is the blood pressure between heartbeats.

The average blood pressure for adult women is 110/70 mmHg (millimetres of mercury). A reading between 130/90 and 90/60 mmHg is considered normal. If your pressure is low or raised your midwife will discuss the implications and whether you need more intensive checking. If the pressure is raised with signs of pre-eclampsia (page 68), it needs prompt treatment.

▥ BLOOD TESTS, MOTHER

The analysis carried out on your blood depends on your medical history, the stage in your pregnancy, your choices and normal practice in your region. Your midwife will ask to take your first sample at your first booking visit. She may refer to it as the FTMSS (first trimester maternal serum screen), before 14 weeks, or STMSS (second trimester maternal serum screen), between 14 to 27 weeks. Further tests may be arranged depending on your hospital policy and your individual situation.

* *Your blood group.* It's important to know your blood group. In the rare event that you need a blood transfusion (page 72), it will help to ensure blood that matches your type is available.
* *Rhesus factor.* The rhesus factor is a protein attached to red blood cells. If you lack the factor (as do 15 per cent of the population in Europe) you are 'Rhesus negative'. If you are Rhesus negative and your partner and your baby are Rhesus positive, there is a small risk you may develop antibodies that could cause an unborn baby in subsequent pregnancies to become anaemic. Treatment during pregnancy and after birth prevents the antibodies developing (page 68).

* *Haemoglobin.* This is the protein pigment in red blood cells that transports oxygen. If your levels are low, this indicates you may be anaemic (page 26). If you have anaemia, your haemoglobin level and the number of red cells in your blood can be increased by treating the cause. Haemoglobin is routinely checked in the first and third trimesters.

Congenital conditions

You may decide to have one or more of the following tests, depending on your personal and family circumstances.
* *Sickle cell anaemia* and *thalassaemia* (page 476).
* TAY-SACHS DISEASE.
* *Cystic fibrosis and Down's syndrome* (page 31). These conditions may also be screened for using blood tests as part of a wider screening process, known as integrated screening (opposite). Screening for other rarer genetic disorders (page 266) may also involve blood testing.

▥ DOWN'S SYNDROME AND SPECIALIST TESTS

See also Congenital abnormalities; Genes and genetics.

Two common congenital (present from birth) conditions screened for in pregnancy are DOWN'S SYNDROME and CYSTIC FIBROSIS. Down's syndrome is a chromosomal abnormality, thought to be caused by a fault occurring during cell division in the fertilised egg. It is rarely a genetic fault and so cannot usually be inherited. Cystic fibrosis is a genetic condition and so can be inherited. Other less common congenital conditions can be screened for when a family history suggests there may be an increased risk, and the parents would like to know.

Tests for Down's syndrome
Though Down's syndrome is rare it is the most commonly detected chromosomal abnormality. The risk of a baby having Down's increases as a mother's age rises. Nevertheless, many more younger women have babies so most Down's

children are born to mothers under 35 years old. If you choose to be screened for Down's syndrome, the most reliable test is 'integrated screening', using a combination of ultrasound scan and a blood test. If the screen shows your baby is at high risk then, for confirmation, an amniocentesis or CVS is needed (page 21). Some women choose to have an amniocentesis or CVS without blood tests.

Integrated screening

Here an ultrasound scan is performed at Weeks 12–13 to check the thickness of the skin behind your baby's neck called NT ('nuchal translucency'). The information is available immediately. You also have a blood test between Weeks 10 and 16. The blood and scan results are fed into a computer and combined with accurate dating of the pregnancy and facts about your age, weight and height and previous history. Then a single risk factor is calculated. This factor is much more accurate than predicting Down's syndrome using your age as the sole guide.

Availability of this 'integrated testing' is promised on the NHS from 2007. It detects over 90 per cent of Down's syndrome babies, and has a relatively low 'false positive' rate of 3 per cent (where the test reveals a problem but your baby is healthy). Even with this test, some couples still choose amniocentesis or CVS if they are older than 38 years or have a deep anxiety or a previous history of problems in the family.

In the rare cases that the test indicates a calculated risk higher than 1 in 250, it is usual to offer an amniocentesis or CVS. This allows a sample of your baby's cells to be obtained and studied to accurately determine the chromosome count. You will be offered advice and counselling about the test and the choices you may face. If the risk is increased, it is common for expectant parents to feel anxious

but for the majority the chromosomes are normal.

Cystic fibrosis

Around 1 in 24 UK Caucasians is a carrier of the defective CFTR gene, which causes cystic fibrosis. The proportion of carriers is lower among Asians and people of Afro-Caribbean origin. If you choose to, you will have a blood test. If you are found to be a carrier, your partner will be similarly tested. If both of you are carriers you will be offered genetic counselling and amniocentesis or CVS (page 21) to check your baby's genes. If both parents are carriers, there is a:

* 1 in 4 chance the baby will have cystic fibrosis,
* 1 in 2 chance the child will be a carrier, but not have the disease, and a
* 1 in 4 chance that the child will not have cystic fibrosis nor be a carrier.

Tests for other chromosomal or genetic abnormalities

There are many other genetic or chromosomal tests available but these are offered only if your personal or family history indicates your baby is at increased risk of a problem. Your doctor or midwife will ask you for information about your history and give you advice about the need for additional blood or amniocentesis or CVS tests. The tests available include those looking for sickle cell disease and thalassaemia (page 476) and Tay-Sachs disease (page 507). If there is a possibility of a rarer condition, you will be referred to a foetal medicine specialist for advice and counselling.

▓ INFECTION AND IMMUNITY TESTS

* *HEPATITIS.* This is a viral infection of the liver. Hepatitis B and C can infect a baby at or after birth. If your test shows you are infected with

Risk factor for Down's syndrome

AGE	RISK	AGE	RISK	AGE	RISK	AGE	RISK
26	1 in 1,286	31	1 in 796	36	1 in 307	41	1 in 85
27	1 in 1,208	32	1 in 683	37	1 in 242	42	1 in 65
28	1 in 1,119	33	1 in 574	38	1 in 189	43	1 in 49
29	1 in 1,018	34	1 in 474	39	1 in 146	44	1 in 37
30	1 in 909	35	1 in 384	40	1 in 112	45	1 in 28

hepatitis B your baby may be given a vaccine within 24 hours of delivery and again at one and six months to prevent infection. Your blood may also be tested for hepatitis C.

- *HIV*. All health authorities offer screening for HIV. Even if you do not suspect that you have been at risk of infection, you may wish to take the test. Treatments can greatly reduce the risk of passing HIV to an unborn baby.
- RUBELLA (German measles). This is a viral infection that can seriously affect the health of an unborn child if the mother becomes infected in the first 16 weeks of pregnancy. If your blood reveals you are not immune, you cannot be vaccinated until after your baby is born, but you can be aware and avoid coming into contact with infected people.
- SYPHILIS. This sexually transmitted infection is rare. It can pass unnoticed for years, yet it does threaten foetal and maternal health. Infection can be treated with antibiotics and any risk to the growing baby greatly reduced or eliminated.
- TOXOPLASMOSIS. This infection is commonly passed on through soil, uncooked meat and cat faeces. Infection in pregnancy poses a risk to a developing baby. Testing is available but it is not routine in UK. It is commonplace in France.
- *Vaginal infection*. Common vaginal infections include GROUP B STREP (GBS), VAGINOSIS and CHLAMYDIA. Screening for these bacterial infections is not routine but if you have previously had a vaginal or sexually transmitted infection, then it is a good precaution to have a swab sample taken. This is tested in a laboratory and if bacteria are found, treatment may be recommended during pregnancy (vaginosis or chlamydia) or in labour (GBS) to reduce the risk to your baby.

▓ INTERNAL EXAMINATIONS

For many women there is no need for any internal examination in pregnancy. An internal examination is no longer routine in the UK. In France and Japan it is standard at most antenatal visits. Urine tests now accurately confirm pregnancy, and dates can be estimated from a woman's knowledge about conception and from ultrasound scans.

Internal examinations are used to assess

your cervix and the position of your baby's head. They may be recommended if there is concern that your cervix may not be competent (page 127), the membranes rupture (page 393) or if you have a vaginal discharge (page 541). If you decide to induce labour (page 375), induction is likely to work well if your cervix is ripe – an internal exam assesses ripeness. In some hospitals, a cervical smear test is carried out in pregnancy. If labour is suspected, your midwife will check internally to establish if labour has begun.

▓ URINE TESTS

At each antenatal visit you'll be asked to provide a sample of urine. A sample collected midway through emptying your bladder will give the clearest results. The urine is tested with a strip of treated paper and if something shows up in your urine test, your midwife will discuss the implications with you.

- *Blood*. Blood in urine is not a common finding. It may indicate a bladder infection (page 533) or more commonly bleeding from the vagina (page 63). It may very rarely be due to a kidney or bladder problem.
- *Glucose*. The presence of glucose may be caused by a normal increase in blood flow through your kidneys, which is related to pregnancy. The reason for testing is to detect underlying DIABETES or the onset of gestational (pregnancy-related) diabetes (page 179). If your urine glucose levels are raised on two consecutive occasions, you may be offered a blood glucose tolerance test to confirm diabetes.
- *Ketones* (page 179). These are produced by your body when body fat is used for energy. Ketones appear if you have been vomiting or had a poor appetite. If the levels are high, this may indicate you are not getting adequate nourishment or have developed gestational diabetes.
- *Protein*. If your test reveals protein in your urine it may indicate a urinary tract infection (page 533). In late pregnancy, it is one of several signs that may indicate pre-eclampsia (page 68). Rarely, protein may indicate an underlying kidney disease.

■ ULTRASOUND SCANS

Ultrasound scanning is an imaging technique that uses sound waves to build up a picture of internal organs and other structures in the body. It is particularly effective in viewing a baby in the womb. The sound waves are reflected back from the baby and analysed to create an image on a screen. These images can be printed off so that medical staff – and parents – can have a record.

Ultrasound scanning has radically changed antenatal care. Scans are now used as the primary source of information about a baby's age, size and gender, and are becoming increasingly reliable as tools for detecting problems relating to baby or mother. In most hospitals, it is routine to offer two or three scans. In the vast majority of cases, scans indicate that pregnancy is progressing well.

Many people enjoy the opportunity to see their baby before birth, kicking, turning or sucking his thumb. Pictures are kept as treasured keepsakes and sent to friends and family. It is now possible to detect a baby's gender on a scan – it's your decision whether to find out or not. The intimate revelations of a scan often make dads feel the pregnancy is more real. Some parents are nervous that scanning may harm their baby or intrude into the baby's space, or that a scan may create anxiety about development where there is not a problem, or they would prefer not to know. Some people feel it is not natural and don't want to spoil the surprise of discovering their baby's sex at birth. You are entitled to decline scans that are offered to you, if this is your preference.

What happens

Your bare abdomen will be smeared with a warm jelly and the ultrasonographer (ultrasound operator) slowly passes a transducer or probe over your skin, pressing down slightly and moving in all directions. If the scan is carried out through your vagina (called a trans-vaginal scan) you will be asked to draw up your knees with your feet flat on the bed, while the probe (like a tampon) is inserted into your vaginal opening. Trans-vaginal scans can provide more detailed images, especially in early pregnancy.

The computer creates an image from the ultrasound echoes. While your baby is small you may see his complete body, including his face and tiny fingers. When your baby is larger – or if the ultrasonographer zooms in – you may not see everything in perspective. The ultrasonographers often try to keep up a running commentary, but their chief task is to study the changing image carefully and bring into view each limb and organ to confirm that all is in order.

Your ultrasonographer may also be able to view blood flow in your baby's body and the placental blood vessels using Doppler ultrasound. This detects the movement and flow of blood, which is displayed on the computer screen as colour superimposed on the normal ultrasound image. It provides a dynamic picture of your baby's health and the function of the placenta.

You will be offered still or DVD images to take home. In some hospitals, 3-D images give a clearer look at the baby's face and body. These also improve the accuracy of diagnosis.

Ultrasound and safety

To date, there has been no proof that ultrasound scanning can cause harm to an unborn baby. The waves are of low intensity and have no impact on development. Some studies investigated a possible association between 'serial' ultrasound scans (six or more in one pregnancy) and low birth weight (page 322), but ultrasound scanning is to date not believed to be a significant cause of intrauterine growth restriction. Because scans are mainly used for diagnosis there is a strong argument that it is safer to have them because if a problem is discovered it may be treated or alleviated. The final choice rests with you. You do not have to have all or any of the scans on offer.

How many scans might you have?

The number of scans you are offered will depend on your hospital and how your pregnancy proceeds. If you want early confirmation, have been undergoing fertility treatment, are concerned about an ectopic pregnancy, or have a history of miscarriage, you may have a trans-vaginal scan at some time between Weeks 5 and 8.

More commonly, the first trimester scan is

given at Weeks 12–13. This confirms viability, number of babies and pregnancy dates. It is called the nuchal scan and is the most important screening test for DOWN'S SYNDROME and some other disorders.

A second trimester scan between Weeks 18 and 22 is the main check for growth and possible abnormalities. At this stage, ultrasound enables very close examination of all parts of your baby, including internal organs and gender, and of the placenta and amniotic fluid. In experienced hands, ultrasound scanning is an increasingly reliable way to detect high-risk pregnancies (page 33). During the scan most couples are reassured that everything is going well. Examining the flow in your uterine arteries at this stage (using Doppler ultrasound) can also predict your risk of high blood pressure and pre-eclampsia (page 68).

You may be offered a third trimester scan (Weeks 32–8), which will confirm how your baby is lying and growing and estimate his weight. The site and appearances of the placenta and the volume of amniotic fluid around your baby can be clearly analysed. Doppler ultrasound scans allow measurement of blood flow through the umbilical cord to reflect how well the placenta is working, can help assess your baby's welfare, and may be used with the second trimester scan to calculate the risk of growth restriction (IUGR). If labour is delayed you may be offered a scan after the due date to evaluate your baby's wellbeing and the function of the placenta so you and your birth team can make informed decisions about induction (page 375).

If there is a suspicion that your baby is at risk, for instance if growth appears to be slow (IUGR), your obstetrician or midwife may advise 'serial' ultrasound scans to monitor your baby regularly and frequently. These assess your baby's rate of growth and the volume of the amniotic fluid, and include Doppler ultrasound to assess placental function and blood flow to your baby's brain, liver and abdominal organs.

▓ WEIGHT MONITORING

Weighing may be part of antenatal monitoring. Your midwife will check your starting weight and the weight gain. She may calculate your BMI (body mass index), as an indication of the weight that suits your body build. The measurements provide an objective record of your rate of gain. If you gain too much or too little weight, you will be able to implement a plan for the duration of pregnancy (pages 253–65).

Antibiotics, treatment

If you are diagnosed with an infection and prescribed antibiotics in pregnancy, or while BREASTFEEDING, or they are prescribed for your baby, the type of medication will be chosen to suit your needs. Antibiotics target and destroy harmful bacteria. Symptoms from the infection may begin to improve remarkably quickly. At the same time, the antibiotics may also reduce populations of beneficial bacteria that are important for health, and you may experience side effects such as TIREDNESS and loose motions or DIARRHOEA. Sometimes if levels of beneficial bacteria fall too low, this can allow fungal (CANDIDA) organisms to thrive, and you may develop thrush. Taking simple measures to nurture the helpful bacteria can reduce the impact of any side effects, and assist your recovery. Some antibiotics, particularly tetracycline and streptomycin, may harm a developing baby and are not taken in pregnancy.

Action plan

- Ensure you eat a balanced diet and drink sufficient water. The information on pages 253–65 offers guidelines.
- It's particularly important to keep refined sugars and sugary foods to a minimum, as they feed a number of harmful organisms (such as *Candida albicans*) and may cause them to multiply at a time when your gut's natural defences are low.
- It may help to increase your daily intake of vitamins and minerals (page 263) to improve your energy and boost your immunity.
- Rest – your body needs to recover from the illness. Begin exercising at a gentle pace and within your own comfort zone.
- If you are breastfeeding and are prescribed antibiotics it is still advisable to continue feeding. There is no conclusive evidence that small amounts of antibiotics passed in breast

milk do any significant harm, although they may lead to diarrhoea and/or oral thrush in a baby. You may reduce these risks by taking probiotic supplements yourself, beginning as soon as you wish.

Probiotics

* *Lactobacillus acidophilus* and *Bifidobacterium bifidum* are 'friendly' bacteria that are good to have in your system. These are among a family of 'probiotics' that exist naturally and promote health but whose numbers may fall in the presence of antibiotics. Taking probiotic supplements, or consuming them in live yoghurt, is believed to help repopulate your intestines with friendly organisms. Probiotics may help restore the normal bacteria in the bowel and perhaps reduce the diarrhoea and oral thrush (oral candidiasis) that antibiotics can lead to. There are two schools of thought – one that it is worthwhile to begin taking probiotics during a course of antibiotics, one that it is effective to begin taking them once the course of antibiotics is completed. There are numerous preparations on the market – for example, in tablet or capsule form and in live 'bio' yoghurts – that help to boost friendly bacteria into the gut. If you take yoghurt, it is preferable to avoid sweetened types. Certain medications may interact with probiotics and it is always important to discuss your individual situation with your doctor.
* If you have adequate levels of friendly bacteria while you are pregnant or while you breastfeed, they will also benefit your baby.
* When your baby is born, within hours her body is covered in bacteria, and within days her bowel is full of bacteria. This early colonisation with bacteria occurs naturally, and the balance that occurs for your baby can be influenced easily. For example, BREASTFEEDING will help to colonise her bowel with beneficial levels of friendly bacteria, whereas antibiotic use may swing the balance in favour of harmful bacteria. Breastfed babies have high concentrations of protective Bifidobacteria and Lactobacillus, while in formula-fed babies high levels of the harmful *Streptococcus fecalis* and *Escherichia coli* are more likely.
* Giving your baby probiotics routinely is not advisable.

Homeopathy

In addition to taking a probiotic supplement, your homeopath may advise a detox programme, usually *Sulphur* (30c), one dose in the morning for three days, and *Nux Vomica* (30c), one dose in the evenings for three days. This may be followed by constitutional treatment to re-balance your system with remedies prescribed personally for you.

Anxiety

See Depression and anxiety, pre- and postnatal.

Apnoea

See Breathing difficulties, baby.

Aromatherapy

Aromatherapy is based on the use of essential oils extracted from plants. Each oil is thought to contain the plant's active constituents – its 'life force'. When applied to the skin, or inhaled, the constituents of the oil are absorbed. The effect can be deeply relaxing or revitalising, depending on the oil used. Oils can also be chosen to trigger healing, strengthen organs, reduce stress and enhance emotional balance.

Provided the oils chosen are suitable for use in pregnancy or while breastfeeding and the correct guidelines are followed (see box, overleaf), aromatherapy oils are simple, safe and effective to use. Many women find them helpful during pregnancy, labour and birth, especially for aiding relaxation. When used appropriately, oils can also relax your baby. You may wish to visit an aromatherapist for a relaxing massage and find out which oils best suit you. Alternatively, you can use them in your own home. Always ensure that you follow instructions, because excessive doses may be harmful. Oils to help alleviate particular problems can be found in relevant sections throughout this book.

▨ HOW TO USE ESSENTIAL OILS

* To bring the scent of an oil into the room, put several drops in water in an oil burner or vaporizer, or onto a tissue or into a bowl of water placed near a radiator.

- Put a couple of drops on cotton wool, and place this in your pillowcase or your shirt pocket.
- For a relaxing massage, mix with a nourishing carrier oil (almond, grapeseed or wheatgerm for instance) and massage into the skin. During pregnancy, use in the ratio of 20 drops of essential oil to 100ml (3fl oz) of carrier oil. You can prepare some oils in advance for use in labour (page 364).
- After the birth you can increase the ratio to 40 drops of essential oil to 100ml (3fl oz) of carrier oil.

Using oils safely

- Do not use aromatherapy until after the first 13 weeks of pregnancy, unless advised to do so by a qualified aromatherapist or midwife.
- Avoid bay, basil, clary sage, comfrey, fennel, hyssop, juniper, marjoram, melissa, myrrh, rosemary, thyme and sage during pregnancy.
- Always follow the instructions provided with oils and, wherever possible, seek advice from a qualified aromatherapist.
- Never add more oil than the stated dose.
- Never take oils internally.
- If you have a history of miscarriage, avoid using chamomile until after the first 16 weeks of pregnancy.
- Lavender oil is best avoided until after Week 24.
- Don't apply oils to your breast while you are breastfeeding as they are easily absorbed by the skin and can be passed to your baby in your breast milk. An exception is if you are treating a problem (such as engorgement), in which case it's important to apply the compress at the end of the feed so the oils are fully absorbed and integrated into your body before you feed your baby again.
- For babies, use five to 10 drops of essential oil per 100ml (3fl oz) of carrier oil.
- In your bath, use four to six drops of essential oil, preferably mixed with a tablespoon of carrier oil. In a baby's bath, use just one or two drops. Add the oils to the warm full bath only once you have turned off the taps, as agitation of the water destroys the oils. Stay in the bath for five to 15 minutes to relax and to nourish your skin. You can use a single oil or blend two or three oils in order to enhance each other's properties. But don't use more than four oils at a time.
- For long-standing pain (or early labour pains) you can use a hot compress. Fill a basin with water as hot as your hand can bear and add four or five drops of oil. Fold a clean absorbent cloth and dip it into the water to absorb the essential oil from the surface. Wring out the surplus water, cover the cloth with plastic and place it on the painful area. Replace it with a fresh one when it has cooled to blood heat. Hot compresses are especially good for backache and other muscular pains.
- Cold compresses are good for headaches, acute breast engorgement, mastitis and sprains. They are made in the same way as hot compresses, but with the water as cold as possible. Add ice before use.

Asphyxia

See Foetal distress and asphyxia.

Asthma and wheezing, baby

See also Allergy and intolerance; Breathing difficulties, baby; Coughs and colds, baby.

Wheezing is a whistling noise in the chest made when breathing out. It happens when the airways become constricted (narrowed) and there may also be a build-up of mucus, restricting airflow. The restriction in airflow may also cause breathlessness. Wheezing is extremely common, particularly under the age of two years, and generally needs no treatment. It may be triggered by infection or allergy or the cause may be unknown. A diagnosis of asthma may be suggested when there are repeated episodes of wheezing, and/or the wheezing is linked with allergy.

Viral-triggered wheeze
Viral-triggered wheeze is by far the commonest reason for wheezing. It occurs in about 25 per cent of babies and children under five years of age, and is three times more common in boys. Children who develop a cold or cough in response to a common virus, usually RSV (page 155), go on to develop a wheeze at least once in their lives. This happens because the infection may trigger sensitivity in the membranes of the entire respiratory system. This is sometimes referred to as hyperactive or irritable airways. Fortunately, the sensitivity decreases with age. The younger the baby is when the first wheezy episode occurs, the more likely he is to grow out of the tendency to wheeze.

Each episode of a viral-triggered wheeze may last for six to eight weeks, during which time your baby's sleep may be disturbed and his cough may worsen when excited or upset. If your baby gets another cold before recovering fully, the cycle may repeat. This gives the impression of a respiratory infection lasting all winter, when in fact it is actually a prolonged period of lung sensitivity.

Post viral respiratory sensitivity
Following a cold, up to 25 per cent of infants and children under five wheeze or cough, often for eight weeks or more. This is called post viral respiratory sensitivity and can be highly aggravating, particularly at night, as it disturbs sleep.

Wheeze resulting from passive smoking
Some wheezy babies are born to mothers who smoked in pregnancy, or are exposed to smoke as babies. The tobacco smoke has the effect of reducing lung capacity and making them more sensitive to viruses. Babies affected by smoking commonly develop a viral-triggered wheeze. The symptoms improve with age but the affected lungs never achieve optimal function, and viruses may trigger wheezing attacks in later

life. As the lungs age, they have less reserve capacity than those of adults who were not exposed to cigarette smoke before birth.

Asthma and allergy associated wheezing
Asthma is the term commonly used when a baby has repeated wheezy episodes; and when wheezing is connected with an allergy. It is now recognised that at least three different forms of asthma can be found in babies. A wheeze associated with allergy is much less common than a viral-triggered wheeze, at any age. When an allergy is present there may be other symptoms, in particular eczema, and possibly sensitivity to foods (which may become apparent after six, 12 or more months (page 19).

* It can be difficult to distinguish an allergy associated wheeze from a viral-triggered wheeze when there are no other allergic symptoms. The important difference is that children who have an allergy-related condition take longer to grow out of it, if they ever do. The symptoms do, however, get milder with age.
* Environmental allergens don't usually affect a child until the toddler years. So a susceptible baby who lives with a cat, for example, won't start to develop allergy or asthma symptoms until he's at least six months old, and probably older than that.
* BREASTFEEDING reduces the risk of asthma, especially if you breastfeed for the first six or 12 months. This protective effect may delay the onset of allergy-related asthma and possibly reduce the risk of asthma developing at any time. There is more on the protective effect of breast milk on page 81.

Action plan
Usually, no treatment is needed, although you may take preventive measures, and help ease any discomfort if your child is wheezing. Sometimes doctors prescribe asthma medications to control symptoms, but these, if effective, should be stopped when the symptoms have improved (the same medications are often prescribed for wheezing, whatever the underlying cause, as for diagnosed asthma when allergies are one of the key triggers). Antibiotics may be helpful if the wheezing is accompanied by illness and a raised temperature. Do consult your GP if you are concerned about wheezing.

HOMEOPATHY can be very effective and in this case needs personal advice. While you wait to see your homeopath, you may find a remedy on page 158 to ease the problem.

Asthma is more common in babies whose mothers smoke or who have a family history of the condition. You cannot change your family's genes but you can protect your baby from tobacco smoke before and after pregnancy.

Asthma, mother

If you are an asthma sufferer you may be concerned that BREATHLESSNESS, a natural side effect of pregnancy, indicates an attack. If you become anxious, breathlessness may worsen and you may begin to wheeze. Yet severe asthma is rare in pregnancy and in labour, and for two out of three women it improves. One reason may be a physiological increase in production of cortisone during pregnancy.

Asthma is often caused by an ALLERGY. It may also be a reaction to a viral chest infection. Very occasionally, asthma occurs for the first time in pregnancy. When this happens it usually clears completely after birth, although it can signify an allergy or intolerance.

What happens

Asthma involves spasm and inflammation of the smooth muscles lining the bronchioles, the small air passages in the lungs. This is called a bronchospasm. The bronchial passages become narrowed, making breathing difficult, and this may induce wheezing.

An asthma attack may last for anything from a few minutes to many days. In pregnancy it will have little effect on your baby, although in very rare circumstances uncontrolled prolonged asthma can produce complications such as PREMATURE BIRTH and INTRAUTERINE GROWTH RESTRICTION (IUGR) if there has been a reduction in the oxygen content of the mother's blood.

Action plan

If you are an asthma sufferer, the most important step is to prevent attacks where possible. If you are aware of the triggers, avoid

them. If you are not, pregnancy may be an opportunity to re-assess your environment and consider potential triggers such as pollens, and irritants in your home, food and drink. Your asthma is under good control if you are free of symptoms, sleeping well and obtaining your personal best peak air flow.

Mild asthma

* In pregnancy, your doctor may want to monitor your lung function by measuring 'peak expiratory air flow rate'. Ideally, you will maintain normal or near normal lung function.
* Your obstetrician may assess your baby for early warning of IUGR.
* Some doctors advise physiotherapy to reduce excessive coughing and the strain this puts on the abdominal muscles.
* If your asthma is mild you will not need medication but there are agents that can be used safely during pregnancy and while breastfeeding. Ask your doctor for advice.

✚ Red flag

Severe asthma

If you have a severe attack you will need prompt attention, such as a broncho-dilator (a drug that widens the airways) and perhaps oxygen, because the oxygen level in your blood may fall, and your baby may become hypoxic (low in oxygen). This is dangerous for you both. Take your usual medication for relief when the first signs appear and continue taking regularly scheduled medications for the time it takes to see a doctor. If you have an acute attack, call an ambulance.

Medications

* Occasionally it may be necessary to use corticosteroid ('steroid') drugs if asthma is severe. If the steroids are inhaled, very little is absorbed into the bloodstream or passed to your baby.
* Inhaled bronchodilators and inhaled anti-inflammatory steroids do not appear to affect breast milk. Antihistamines, however, can cause sleeplessness and irritability in babies and

reduce production of breast milk and so are best avoided.

- If asthma symptoms develop while you are in labour, someone from the medical team will measure your peak flow rates. You may be given intravenous fluid as a precaution against dehydration. Adequate pain relief and continuing regular medication will limit the risk of bronchospasm. After birth you may need more medication than usual, either in higher doses or more frequently.

Lifestyle, diet and exercise

- Aerobic exercise helps by expanding your lungs and draining secretions from the chest and sinuses. It is good to exercise with guidance from a trainer or from your doctor.
- Bronchospasm can be avoided or reduced by taking medication before exercise, warming up and cooling down, and not exercising in cold air.
- Avoid trigger foods. Focus on foods containing B vitamins (such as green leafy vegetables and pulses), magnesium (sunflower seeds, fish and figs), antioxidants (citrus fruits, soya beans, olive oil and apricots) and omega oils (fish and seeds).
- Avoid smoking and being in smoky atmospheres.
- Do what you can to avoid chest infections, which may spark an attack of asthma.
- After birth you may find that the normal demands of caring for a new baby increase your asthma, and attacks may make you more tired than usual.

Homeopathy

Although homeopathy has a great deal to offer in the treatment and management of asthma, it is best to consult a qualified homeopath, who will give you individual advice.

Autistic Spectrum Disorders (ASD) and developmental concerns

All babies exhibit challenging behaviours at some time. In the vast majority of cases, this is part of normal development. The persistence of some types of challenging behaviours may be a marker for one of a range of developmental difficulties, loosely called the disorders of communication, and including the term autistic,

or autistic spectrum disorder (ASD). Autism is not a medical diagnosis, or even a medical illness. It is a collection of difficulties in development that forms a pattern which, if recognised, defines the diagnosis.

ASD is not usually diagnosed until a child is three or four years of age. However, many experts agree that there are features within the first year of life that may make earlier diagnosis possible. Many children who are later diagnosed as having one of the autistic spectrum disorders do exhibit challenging behaviours in the first year, including difficulties with sleep, excessive crying, difficulties in being consoled and even feeding difficulties. It is important to remember that these same symptoms are expressed in many children who do not have any developmental problems.

What happens

ASD and Asperger's syndrome

ASD is present in six to nine per 1,000 children (roughly ½ to 1 per cent). Autism is four times more common in boys than girls. Asperger's disorder, also called Asperger's syndrome (AS), is recognised as one of the autistic spectrum disorders, sometimes also referred to as pervasive developmental disorder. The main features of Asperger's disorder are social interaction impairment and repetitive patterns of behaviour and activities. It is different from the disorders at the more severe end of the autistic spectrum, in that children with Asperger's do not have the same difficulties in acquiring language that children with autism have. The distinguishing features of AS are problems with social interaction, particularly reciprocating and empathising with the feelings of others.

Attention deficit disorder (ADD)

Attention Deficit Disorder (ADD), or Attention Deficit Hyperactivity Disorder (ADHD), is another developmental disorder of childhood, which probably continues into adulthood but is as yet unrecognised in adults. ADD or ADHD affects up to 5 per cent of some populations, and typically shows itself in early childhood. It is characterised by a persistent pattern of inattentiveness, irritability and sometimes hyperactivity. Often there is forgetfulness, poor self-control and temper outburst, poor organisation and associated impulsivity and distractibility.

CAUSES

Many theories are in circulation about the possible cause or causes of ASD, but none yet explains the widely different degrees of expression, even between siblings who are both affected. The only theory with firm credibility is the genetic explanation: strong scientific evidence supports that, in part at least, genetic make-up is a strong determinant. However, the environment, including the way a child is parented, is also significant – every child's behaviour reflects, to some extent, his experiences (page 46). Dietary and chemical factors may be implicated, but these are relatively weak components in what is essentially a genetically determined, environmentally influenced condition.

DIAGNOSIS

Currently there is no generally applicable test for ASD – particularly as there are no specific indicators in the first year after birth and some possible symptoms may be linked with other types of developmental or learning difficulties. Often it is not possible to make a reliable diagnosis until the age of two or later. Some children with ASD are not diagnosed until late primary school, or their teenage years.

Even so, 60 per cent of parents whose children are later diagnosed with a degree of ASD notice that something 'doesn't feel right' and tell one or more healthcare advisors about their concerns. If you are worried, it is better to talk to someone for your own peace of mind, and to receive extra support if you or your baby needs it. Current recommendations are for any parental concerns to be investigated (see below).

There are some factors that may be linked with ASD and if these are present they need to be considered together with a thorough and specialised assessment if any early diagnosis is to be reliable. There are some early warning signs for a pre-school child (up to the age of five years) that should prompt referral to a specialist. They are listed below.

It is important to recognise that children

who subsequently do not demonstrate any long-term autistic features will at some time show some, or even all, the features listed. This is because at certain developmental stages it is normal for these features to appear and then disappear again. It is when these features persist beyond the age when they would normally be expected to disappear that a more serious problem may be suggested. For example, the throwing of objects, or casting, which is entirely normal from six to 12 months, should have stopped by the age of 18 months and been replaced by releasing objects back to an adult. If it persists beyond 21 months it would be considered abnormal.

Communication: possible indicators

Deficient non-verbal communication, such as:
* lack of pointing,
* difficulty following a point,
* failure to smile socially,
* failure to share enjoyment, and
* failure to respond to the smiling of others.

Impairment in language development, such as:
* impaired comprehension,
* poor response to name, and
* unusual use of language.

Communication: absolute indicators for referral
* No babbling, pointing or other gesture by 12 months.
* No single words by 18 months.
* No two-word spontaneous (non-echoed) phrases by 24 months.
* Any loss of any language or social skills at any age.

Social impairments
* Limitation in, or lack of imitation of, actions (for example, clapping). Babies mirror from birth (such as mouth movements) and by smiling at an early age, and it is considered normal for a baby to imitate clapping by four to six months. If such patterns of motor skill and social skill developments are limited, or do not develop within three months of their expected appearance, then these may be early warning signs of developmental difficulties.
* Lack of sharing toys or other objects.
* Lack of interest in other children.
* Odd approaches to other children.

- Minimal recognition or responsiveness to other people's happiness or distress – for instance, lack of smiling in response to another's smile is a sign of poor social responsiveness.
- Limited variety of imaginative play or pretence, especially social imagination (that is, not joining with others in shared imaginary games).
- Being in his own 'world'.
- Failure to initiate simple play with others.
- Failure to participate in early social games.
- Preference for solitary play activities.
- Attachment that seems either excessive or reduced. At the age of seven to nine months, many babies become wary of strangers (page 221). Your baby may resist staying with anyone other than you, but if this seems an excessive response it may be an early sign of some developmental difficulty. However, babies who seem inseparable from their mothers at this age often have no long-term difficulties.

Impairment of interests, activities and other behaviours

- Over-sensitivity to sound or touch.
- Aggressive physical mannerisms such as biting and hitting.
- Aggressive behaviour towards peers.
- Responding badly to a change in routine or location.
- Repetitive play with toys (for example, lining up objects) persisting beyond the usual expected age.
- Turning light switches on and off, regardless of scolding.
- Persistently disregarding adult requests, such as repeatedly saying 'No'. This may be normal, and there will be an influence from the style of parenting, but should improve between the ages of one and two years. Persistence after the age of two, and certainly beyond three years, would raise concern among healthcare specialists.

In an older child the diagnosis is made according to factors in three main areas of development – social, communication, and thought and behaviour. In particular:

- *Social*. Delayed or atypical social development, especially interpersonal development.
- *Communication*. Impaired language and communication (verbal and non-verbal skills, including understanding as well as expression).
- *Thought and behaviour*. Rigid thought and behaviour, poor social imagination, obsessive behaviour, reliance on routines, delay in pretend play.

Professional concerns about more able children (such as those with Asperger's syndrome/so called 'high functioning' autism) may not develop until children are exposed to the greater social demands of the school environment.

■ LOVE, CARE AND PROFESSIONAL SUPPORT

If you raise concerns, this begins a process of expert assessment, along with a period of review and re-assessment. A whole team of specialist workers are needed to make a diagnosis, if one is possible. These may include specialist language therapists, educational advisors, educational psychologists, clinical psychologists, child psychiatrists and other therapists.

If a diagnosis is considered your child will be followed up until either it becomes apparent that he has progressed developmentally out of the possible diagnosis, or that a firm diagnosis can be made. Often this takes several years, and even after a diagnosis is made there may be progress resulting in changes to the expected outcome.

Knowing the underlying reasons for your child's behaviour is important in helping you and other professionals to devise strategies for educational and emotional and family support. It is important to remember that ASD is just one of many factors that influence your child's moods and behaviour, and any supportive measures that suit him will work best when the whole picture is taken into account. Other factors include his personality and interests, the environment he is in, the family characteristics, and the behaviour of the adults and other children in his life.

It is also common for children with ASD to have the disorder in combination with other conditions. Your child is likely to feel most content when he is lovingly accepted and can pursue his interests in an environment of safety and encouragement. You will often benefit from extra support and as your child grows it may be possible to form a more comprehensive profile of his individual needs and strengths, so that you and others can be there for him in an appropriate way.

Without a formal diagnosis it may be more difficult to access specialist nursery provision, and later on to get help in the school or other educational setting.

Your reaction

Receiving a diagnosis may be distressing for you (page 45) although in the long term a clear diagnosis has many benefits, enabling your child to be well supported, loved and encouraged. With appropriate support the potentially stressful impact on your family may be reduced.

Often the main difficulty is identifying and arranging support and appropriate resources, and this often leaves parents angry and tired.

If your child's behaviour is difficult for you, and/or you are struggling to arrange the support he and you need, you may become anxious, short-tempered and tired. It is important for you to care for yourself and ask others to care for you (page 121). You may also want to spend time with a family therapist or a local group as you deal with your own feelings and develop effective ways to nurture your child, minimise your anxiety and cope with difficulties.

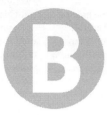

Back and pelvic pain

See also Pain, mother.

Many pregnant women get low-back pain and pelvic pain. It can usually be addressed and relieved with attention to POSTURE, EXERCISE and relaxation (page 451). Some women have severe pain that may continue after the birth and this may have an underlying cause. If you have had back pain before, you are more likely to have discomfort in pregnancy.

Lumbar pain
Lumbar pain involves the lumbar vertebrae behind the lower part of the abdomen and can occur with or without spreading to the legs. It may stem from the joints between the vertebrae, the intervertebral discs, the surrounding muscles or ligaments, or the nerves that run from your lumbar spine into your lower abdomen and legs. Rarely, low-back pain may be caused by a herniated vertebral disc. This is a serious problem that requires specialist care.

Sometimes tension arises from deep muscles on the front of the vertebrae and may cause symptoms that mimic uterine or bowel pain. This is because the nerves adjacent to the muscles may be irritated and the pain is then interpreted by your brain as arising from an abdominal organ rather than from the muscle in your back.

Pelvic pain
The pelvic girdle is made up of three large bones, the sacrum (base of the spine) and two pelvic bones. They form three joints: one at the front, the symphysis pubis, and two sacroiliac joints at

the back. The coccyx or tailbone is attached to the sacrum. In pregnancy the pelvic and lumbar spine joints soften and widen. The symphysis pubis widens from 5mm to 12mm. As it widens, the pubic and sacroiliac joints can be painful when pain-sensitive ligaments are stretched.

Sacroiliac joint pain
This is felt in the buttock, usually on one side, and may radiate down the back and outer side of one thigh, usually to the level of the knee and, rarely, to the calf. It is four times more common than lumbar pain. Without treatment symptoms of sacroiliac joint pain can continue several months after delivery.

Dysfunction of symphysis pubis (DSP)
This may cause pain over the pubic joint, in the vagina, groin and lower abdomen, or over your bladder. If the sacroiliac joint is involved it can radiate down to the thighs. It is usually worse when walking, rolling over in bed, parting the legs (for example, when getting into a car) or putting weight on one leg (such as when using stairs).

Sometimes, on movement, a clicking can be heard or felt. DSP occurs if softening of ligaments allows excessive movement and an abnormally wide gap in the pubic joints. Following delivery, the space decreases within days but the supporting ligaments take three to five months to return fully to their normal state and pain may continue. DSP pain is increased if one or both sacroiliac joints are unstable and this leads to extra stress on the symphysis joint.

Sciatica

This involves the sciatic nerve. It is rare and accounts for a tiny percentage of low-back pain or discomfort in the sacroiliac joint in the buttock region or deep in the vagina. You may feel it more on one side and the pain might radiate down the back of one thigh. In late pregnancy, sciatica may bring on sharp pains. Babies tend to lie more heavily to one side of the uterus, so the discomfort can be stronger in one side. If pain is associated with loss of sensation or tingling in your thighs or feet, or muscle weakness, a prolapsed intervertebral disc may be considered and specialist advice is essential to reduce long term weakness and pressure on the nerve.

Nocturnal pain

This occurs in the low back only at night in bed and may follow daytime DSP and sacroiliac pain. There are many theories about night pain that include muscle fatigue after exercise in the day, stress from imbalanced posture and changes in circulation.

Postnatal backache

This is very common as joints and ligaments take months to return to normal after birth. Sacroiliac strain can increase if you have a forceps- or ventouse-assisted delivery (page 373). Your abdominal muscles may take up to a year to regain pre-pregnancy tone, and before this they do not provide maximum support for your back. The way you carry, hold and feed your baby may compound the problem. If you have intense symptoms it is best to treat them before attempting to become pregnant again.

Action plan

+ Red flag

Beware of pain radiating into your leg or foot, tingling, numbness or weakness of the muscles. This may indicate pressure on your sciatic nerve and you need specialist advice.

Medical care

* It is best to discuss your pain with your midwife or doctor, particularly if it is severe or there are other symptoms that concern you.
* You may be advised to use a TENS machine (page 386) or take paracetamol in safe doses (page 408).
* Osteopathic treatment (page 424) can be a very powerful aid.
* You might be referred to a physiotherapist who can give you specific exercises and postural advice. Some recommend the use of support straps, corsets or belts.

What you can do

Be aware of your posture (page 451) and care for yourself. You can also try:

* A warm bath or a hot-water bottle for lower back pain.
* A massage.
* Lying on your back on the floor with your calves and feet supported on a low chair approximately 60cm (2ft) above the floor for about 20 minutes, once or twice a day. Do not do this if you feel faint.
* Exercise and yoga, but with DSP don't open your legs wide.
* PILATES helps strengthen your back muscles and often reduces the pain.

Try not to get downhearted. If you have back pain in pregnancy this won't necessarily make labour harder, and if your pelvic joints have opened wide this could mean that labour is in fact easier. If you are feeling low, your emotions may affect the way your body feels and increase the pain, and could also make you slouch, exacerbating imbalance. You may benefit from emotional advice and support.

Homeopathy

In addition to attention to your posture and lifestyle, homeopathy may help to relieve general back pain. Recommended dosage of a suitable remedy is 30c potency, three times per day, for one week, and then re-assess.

* *Kali Carb* if your back feels weak, stiff or bruised with dragging pains in the lumbar region and the coccyx, you wake regularly at 3am and sweat at night, feel worse sitting for any length of time or walking, and feel better for lying on a hard surface or with pressure on your back.
* *Rhus Tox* if you have stiffness in your lower back, feel as if the muscles seize up when you rest, and get better for movement and warmth.

- *Arnica* is generally used to alleviate bruising and may help pain in the back if you have no clear symptoms.
- If back problems persist you may take *Calc Phos* and *Calc Fluor* 6x potency in a combination remedy morning and night for two weeks, only after the twelfth week of pregnancy, and re-assess.

One of the following remedies may help DSP, in 6c potency three times per day for five to seven days, before re-assessing:
- *Calc Phos* when your sacroiliac joint and hips feel stiff, cold and a bit numb, and the condition is worse when climbing stairs or lifting and in cold weather and better for resting and warm weather.
- *Aesculus Hip* for general aching, stiffness and weakness, when your sacrum and hips feel bruised, and it's difficult to get up from sitting, and the condition is worse when walking, standing or bending.
- *Bryonia* when there is tearing pain, and movement of any kind aggravates. You may feel better for applying pressure to the painful area.

Bad news

See also Emotions; Loss of a baby.

If you are told that something may be wrong with your baby, or something happens to you or your baby, you are likely to be sensitive to every comment. It is helpful to know how vulnerable everyone feels at this time. You may feel out of control, or angry at the situation, at yourself or at the medical team.

You may have guessed that there could be a problem. If this happens it is best that an explanation follows soon. You will need an opportunity to talk with someone who allows you to feel safe to express your thoughts and feelings, whatever they may be. Most hospitals have a supportive team. You will then need time to assimilate the information and have a follow-up appointment to discuss it. You may also seek help from another source (such as another doctor for a second opinion). Everyone prefers to receive bad news in a comfortable setting. It is not surprising that people often remember how bad news was told to them.

If you are told bad news when you are alone, a follow-up appointment is essential with your GP or consultant when your partner or another adult can be with you. Your immediate response – 'No!' – may block your ability to hear what is said. It may be really helpful to have someone else with you who can ensure you can be present for the conversation, and discuss it with you afterwards. You may find it useful to write things down.

How you may respond

There are many different reactions but most people have a series of responses that take time to evolve:
- You may be in shock, unable to believe what has happened.
- You may react in many ways that include feeling confused, angry, accepting or enraged and even violent.
- You may then adapt – recognising the information and the significance of what happened.
- You may then start incorporating the information, getting back to daily life and making plans for the future.

Being informed

Most people find it easier to take in information in small chunks. It is important to understand something before you move on, so do not be afraid to ask until you understand it. If you feel lectured to, or you cannot understand the medical words, say so and ask others to phrase things in a different way.

Understanding the information may take a long time, and in some instances there may be no clear explanation. The best way to communicate is when the medical team shares the information openly. Midwives and doctors are encouraged to be honest with you even when things have happened that in hindsight may have been avoidable. If you feel that you have been given different answers to the same questions, having another adult with you allows you to discuss the differences.

If you feel you are not being understood or that information is being withheld, contact the director of the midwifery, obstetric or paediatric service and arrange to meet them. This will enable the director to make inquiries on your behalf. All hospitals have a formal complaints procedure.

Although you may want to avoid upsetting the medical and midwifery team it is important to express your feelings and worries. The doctors and midwives are supported to process their own feelings and they are there to look after you.

Planning for the future

Once you have gathered information it is easier to move to the next level of discussion: what's to be done. You and the care team will need to consider the causes, the treatment options and the outlook, as well as support options.

It is helpful to be clear about timing appointments and what to expect next from your medical team. It is best to establish this at the end of each consultation. Making a step-by-step plan will help you feel in control. The support you need may come from the hospital medical team, your GP or health visitor, or your family and friends.

The rest of your family

You may find it difficult to share bad news with your family. Grandparents and other relatives can be deeply affected by the news, but being informed is preferable to not knowing and it is usually best for factual information to come from you to reduce the risk of misinformation. Your relatives will also need support to come to terms with their own feelings, and it may be important for you to establish some boundaries so that you do not take full responsibility for them while you are also in need of love and care. Other children in the family may have very strong emotional reactions, and can have surprising clarity. The honesty of a three year old can be very healing.

Love and support

Bad news, a traumatic event or illness will undoubtedly affect you. Many people find it incredibly hard to focus, and some parents lose confidence in themselves and in the future. You may find some of the advice on caring for yourself (pages 121–4) helpful as you approach a particular problem or after a period of disarray and confusion. You and your partner are there for one another, although you may feel pressure on your relationship and it is usually helpful to have other sources of loving support from your family and wider community.

Homeopathy

The following remedies may be useful immediately after a shock. You may use the most appropriate in 30c potency and repeat the dose 15 minutes later.

- *Aconite* if shock is accompanied by panic, fear and restlessness, with fear paramount. The event is often unexpected.
- *Arnica* after a physical trauma or shock to the system – it is the No.1 remedy after an accident or operation.
- *Ignatia* after hearing bad news, such as a difficult medical diagnosis or a death, and you feel numb, perhaps have a lump in your throat and want to be alone.

Behaviour, baby

See also Autistic Spectrum Disorders and developmental concerns; Emotions; Growth and development, baby.

Your baby's behaviour is spontaneous; an honest and unfiltered expression of who he is and what he feels from moment to moment. It is influenced by his genes, his experiences in the womb and by how he is mothered and cared for after the birth. Babies who experience a warm, accepting and loving environment tend to learn quickly to delight in and trust themselves and the people around them, and express themselves with joyful spontaneity.

In terms of developmental stepping stones, progressive physical and vocal control and cognitive development, your baby follows a predictable route (for example, sitting before walking, arm control before finger control, sounds before words). This is covered in detail on pages 270–8. At any time, your baby's behaviour reflects his stage of development as well as how he feels emotionally (page 206). He is driven by a powerful need to be in a relationship and feel held, to be fed and talked to, to sleep, rest and play, and to be warm. His behaviour communicates this. Some aspects of behaviour may be predictable (such as making eye contact from birth, or being able to laugh and clap later on) but these are only snapshots of the whole person who is your unique baby. No two babies behave in the same way, not even TWINS.

For the vast majority of babies, behaviour is not a cause for concern about development or health. On the contrary, it tends to be a cause of celebration and pride among parents and the wider family. Sometimes, you may be challenged by your baby's behaviour. Challenges are a normal part of every parent–baby dance and when there is love, acceptance and patience, they seldom persist. On rare occasions, difficulties are an indication of a physical illness or a problem causing pain. Even more rarely it may be a sign of brain or body dysfunction, perhaps 'congenital' (page 148) or acquired through injury after birth. For this reason, it's important to get professional advice if you are concerned.

Difficult behaviour is explored in the following entry. Here, we look at the huge range of 'normal' behaviour and what it might mean for your baby and for you.

I need ...
Your baby is a powerful communicator. Lots of eye contact and smiling, for instance, is a request for you to tune in and reflect his smiles. Lots of CRYING means your baby needs something. Every baby has basic survival needs and intense emotions, and your baby needs to feel 'held' emotionally and physically while he expresses these.

Your baby's family
Your baby's behaviour also reflects what is happening in the family around him. Contentment, stress, arguments, illness, loving support or relationship tensions have an impact on everyone who is present. Although he may not be actively engaged in adult conversations, he is sensitive and responds to the family emotions. If your baby is cared for by grandparents, childminders or in a crèche, what he experiences there will be significant.

Parents' perceptions
There is no right or wrong way for your baby to behave: what is considered normal in one culture, country or family might be considered strange or abnormal in another. What happened to you as a child in your family of origin will affect what you expect from your baby. The views of your friends and peer group will affect you, too. Some parents believe in strict routines and times during the day and night when their baby is expected to do certain things such as sleep or eat. In other families, infant-led parenting (page 432) is the norm and strict routines are not. Each individual approach is based on a point of view, rather than any absolute measurement of right or wrong, good or bad.

Adults tend to be very judgemental about babies. Parents are also competitive. The main behaviours scrutinised are eating, sleeping, crying, pooing and smiling. One of the first things many people ask about a baby is, 'Is he good?' Roughly translated, this usually means: does he sleep for long periods, does he cry, is he 'easy' to care for? Any such judgements belong always and only to adults. Babies are neither 'good' nor 'bad', nor can a baby under one year old be naughty, 'lazy' or 'spoilt'. It may be interesting for you and your partner to ask – what does 'good' mean for me and for us? What are our expectations? Is our love and acceptance dependent on how our baby behaves?

Your baby's relationships
A baby who feels accepted and safe, and discovers that his needs will be met when he expresses them, learns that relationships can feel good, loving and trusting. The mother–baby dyad is the prime model from which your baby learns. His early relationships, particularly with you, set a standard for his feelings and behaviour in other relationships as he grows up.

Experiences in early relationships can be difficult, such as being isolated or in persistent pain without comfort, being repeatedly left to cry, being frequently called naughty, wrong or difficult. When this happens, some babies become quiet and suppress the expression of their needs – behaviour that will endear them to their carers. They may be labelled 'good'. Yet a baby who becomes compliant to gain favour may lose the ability to trust and act out his own feelings, and in adulthood may be a 'pleaser' who rarely enters into conflict, and may be self-doubting. Some babies may react to a similar situation by being demanding, unsettled and upset and may be labelled 'difficult'. In adulthood, argumentativeness and rebellion may continue to protect a lack of self-confidence.

Babies who experience neglect, verbal abuse or physical violence are likely to mirror their carers' behaviour by showing extreme behaviour – ranging from excessive quietness to vigorous anger. Later in life, they are prone to repeat a pattern of abuse.

These examples are part of a broad spectrum in which behaviour is a reflection of personality and life experience. It is human nature to survive, and so protective behaviour patterns form unconsciously. Patterns can be like armour around a vulnerable inner child who may have 'gone into hiding', frightened of coming out for fear of being hurt.

Love and acceptance

Your own baby is a unique individual and you can help him feel good about himself, and form trusting, loving relationships by providing an environment in which he feels loved, held and accepted. The importance of this in the sensitive early months of life cannot be overstated.

Behaviour, baby, difficult

Each baby brings his own style and has unique feelings to express. Wide variations in normal behaviours – sleeping, eating, pooing, and so on – are natural. What seems difficult or challenging for one parent may not be a problem for another. When your baby's behaviour seems difficult, it might be helpful to ask yourself 'is the glass half full or half empty?' In other words, are you looking at your baby in a positive light or are expectations or illusions of perfection making things seem negative?

Your baby invites you to be lovingly accepting and supportive, to look at the practical issues that are part of everyday family life, and to consider your own expectations and feelings (including anger, disappointment and guilt). If your perception alters, you may be more accepting and relaxed and your baby's behaviour may change. If you are worried, seek professional advice. Occasionally, diagnosing an underlying cause reveals an issue that can be relieved with appropriate treatment.

Challenging behaviour

It is inevitable that your baby will challenge you as he expresses himself, explores his world and pushes boundaries. It is essential that he does this and it is an important sign of normal development. He will automatically behave in a way that gets you to focus on him and meet his needs.

You may think your baby should behave differently because of what you have learnt from your family or your peer group, but these models may not be appropriate for him. You may expect him to behave in a way an older child or an adult would, or to behave just like you. This is to 'adultify' your baby. It is not appropriate to assess your baby's behaviour according to criteria that are suitable for adults. Asking friends or a trusted health professional about what is normal for your baby's age and stage of development may help you to let go of your fears and any urge to control your baby's behaviour. A simple shift in attitude can be profound and transform your relationship.

Developmental concerns

If your baby is in pain from an underlying issue, such as reflux (page 554), or is having difficulty feeding (page 91) or sleeping (page 485), this may be the root cause of upset, and medical advice is important for you all. Some behaviours reflect a developmental issue affecting the nervous system. The issue may be minor or severe, such as CEREBRAL PALSY. Some behaviours come about when a baby has an autistic spectrum disorder (page 39) that can only be confirmed later in the early toddler years. It is important, therefore, to ask for professional advice if you are concerned.

If your baby is angry

* It is perfectly normal for your baby to be angry and to express this through his body. Anger is one of his fundamental feelings (page 208). As he grows, you can help him learn about behavioural boundaries. For example, it is okay to be angry but it is not okay to bite his brother. Be loving, clear and consistent.

* If your baby has an outburst of angry kicking or shouting you can offer safety and loving support and stay with him as he calms down. He may not want you to touch him but being with him still offers a feeling of safety and gives the message that you still accept him, and are there for him. Without your help, his body and mind may not be able to 'unwind', and a future outburst may become more powerful, which is very frightening for him. The practice of shutting a baby or child in another room or a 'naughty corner' away from the rest of the

family (the equivalent to solitary confinement) can never be calming or reassuring, and is never appropriate in the first year.

- You may find it helpful to bring yourself back to your centre by focusing on your breathing (page 105) and give yourself a few moments to feel grounded. If you find it hard to stay with your child when he is angry, it is important to get support; perhaps an adult to be with you both, or an adult who can spend time with your baby while you have time out. Above all, try to be loving and accepting of yourself and your child. You will both have days when your behaviour is difficult.

Your older baby

- When your baby is older he has greater conscious control over his behaviour. Nevertheless, he is far from being an adult and needs to try out his feelings, actions and boundaries, and will still be wonderfully spontaneous. He needs you or another adult to help him feel safe as he explores himself and his world.

Caring for yourself

It is important to acknowledge your responsibility for your baby and part of this is to ensure you are well cared for. You may need extra support, particularly when you feel stressed and tired – this is all part of CARING FOR YOU. It is equally important to remind yourself that you cannot take sole responsibility. Your baby has a unique take on life and you cannot control his experiences, feelings or behaviour. What you can do is offer a supportive environment. For instance, with regular feeding you can help him avoid discomfort from hunger. With lots of contact time, he is less likely to have separation anxiety (page 220). If you are feeling emotionally stressed this may make things worse – confiding in someone may help you relax. Many parents feel guilty when their babies are difficult. Knowing that your baby has his own feelings (which are not the same as yours) and that you cannot take all responsibility may help you avoid guilt and explore practical options that will help your family. The suggestions on page 208 may help you be there for yourself, and your baby, during the good and the bad times. Guilt is explored on page 213.

▮ GENITAL TOUCHING

Experiencing bodily pleasure is a delight for babies. In the womb, pleasurable sensations come from the feeling of fluid on skin and the rhythmic contractions of the soft surrounding walls. After the birth, loving skin-to-skin touch, BREASTFEEDING and MASSAGE are all pleasurable.

As your baby builds bodily control he will enjoy feeling and seeing his hands, face, toes and legs as he gets to know himself. Every baby is different, and some seem to like the feeling of touching their genital areas or the sensation they get by rocking or rubbing against something. This is similarly common among girls and boys.

There is nothing naughty about this and a small baby does not associate genitals with sexual practices. Behaviour that stimulates the genitals is explorative and is not masturbation in the same sense as it is understood for adults. There is no need to worry, nor to ask your baby to stop, nor to label the habit as dirty or wrong. It will pass of its own accord and is a natural part of exploration. Just ensure that you keep your baby's nappy area and hands clean.

Older children may rub themselves against objects – and this is usually just a passing habit. It is best not to draw attention to it.

▮ HAIR PULLING

Hair pulling is usually a self-comforting habit. It often goes along with thumb sucking (page 512). Your baby may recline with his thumb or fingers in his mouth and twist his own hair or yours with the other hand. This can be very relaxing and your child may often do it before falling asleep or when he feels upset or nervous.

Some babies may break off bits of hair, and this may leave a bald area or a patch of short stubs. When the pulling or plucking stops, your child's hair will grow back normally. Some babies eat the hair they pull off. This rarely occurs before the age of six months. If your baby does this it is unlikely to cause any health problems, although swallowed hair may become a tight hair ball (bezoar) and could cause digestive problems. Cutting your baby's hair may stop the habit but this depends on the cause. The habit may reflect his anxiety or feelings of insecurity and reduce as your baby feels more settled – some of the advice on page 208 may give useful guidance if you think your baby may be anxious. Sometimes hair pulling and eating is associated with iron deficiency, so it would be a good idea to get this checked at your local baby clinic.

HEAD BANGING

Head banging is surprisingly common. Up to 20 per cent of babies and toddlers bang their head on purpose, although boys are three times more likely to do it than girls. Head banging often starts between six and 12 months of age and peaks between 18 and 24 months. A head banging habit may last for several months, or even years, though most children outgrow it by the age of three.

What happens

It is not always immediately obvious why a baby or toddler bangs his head. The action may be purely physical, it may be emotionally driven, or a combination. There are some recognised reasons:

- He may find it relaxing and do it rhythmically as he's falling asleep, when he wakes in the night, or perhaps when he's asleep. Some rock on all fours as well.
- He may be in pain, for example, from teething or an ear infection. The banging distracts from the pain and the rhythmic motion may be soothing.
- If he bangs his head during temper tantrums, he's venting intense anger and frustration. He's using physical actions to express his feelings and he may be comforting himself. The banging is a sign that he wants your attention and he may need your help to calm down (page 48) or to meet a basic need (such as a wet uncomfortable nappy, hunger or a sore tummy).
- He may need you to notice him, and have learnt that head banging gets the attention he wants.

Head banging is usually a normal part of child development but rarely it may be associated with autism and other developmental disorders (page 39). Specialists generally only consider this when there are other factors, and it would not be a diagnosis on its own.

Action plan

Assessing the situation

- Follow your instincts and ask for professional advice to ascertain whether your baby is in pain. A check by your doctor is useful to also exclude any underlying developmental issues.
- Ask yourself how your baby may be feeling emotionally, and what he needs to feel safe. There are many ways to support him when he is having intense feelings (page 208).
- Ask yourself what practical help your baby might need – including time spent with you and other adults, playtime, rest time and a feeling of loving safety. He might enjoy being carried a lot as you go about your day. Kangaroo care works well for young babies (page 518) and a sling is very versatile, even for toddlers. Make sure he gets lots of physical exercise during the day, too, to help him burn off the nervous energy.
- If you and your partner are arguing, your baby's behaviour may be due to this. You may need to talk things through (page 462) and/or seek professional emotional support.

Being there for your baby

- Give your baby lots of positive and loving attention. Babies love attention and tend to repeat behaviour that gets them noticed. Showing delight and giving encouragement for his behaviour throughout the day may fulfil this basic need and strengthen the bond between you.
- Don't scold or punish your baby. He's too young to rationalise and your disapproval will make him feel bad. It is likely to reinforce his behaviour, or encourage other difficult behaviours.
- If your baby enjoys rhythmic repetition he may get this with you – rocking in your arms, being strapped to you while you go walking, joining in playful games, for example.
- Help him find other outlets for his love of rhythm. Try dancing, marching, and drumming or clapping to music together. A metronome in his room might give him the comfort of a steady rhythm – and you might try some gentle music, too.

Making bedtime safe

* Protect your child from injury. For example, if he is in a cot, check the screws, hang fabric or a quilt between the cot and the wall to reduce the noise of the banging. Don't put pillows or blankets in his cot because these are a suffocation hazard, and make sure any cot bumpers are securely tied to the cot railings. If your baby shares your bed (page 487), ensure he cannot slip between the bed and the wall, and that he cannot injure himself by falling off the bed. You may want to extend your bed safely with an extra mattress at the same height, or move your mattresses onto the floor where there is no danger of falling (but if you use more than one mattress ensure they are well secured so your baby cannot slip between them).
* If the banging happens at night, as a way of 'coming down', start or re-assess a soothing bedtime routine. A warm bath, a MASSAGE, calmly rocking your baby in your arms, and a quiet song may all help. The structure of a fixed bedtime routine can be very comforting for babies (page 490).

Complementary therapies

Cranial OSTEOPATHY may make a huge difference to your baby. Repetitive physical behaviours can reveal underlying structural imbalance or discomfort, and some people believe they may reflect a baby's experience during birth and a need to release tension or pain. Osteopaths are skilled at locating and releasing tension. Cranial osteopathy is very gentle and does not involve manipulation. MASSAGE is another soothing technique. If you would like to use HOMEOPATHY it is important to get an individually prescribed remedy that takes account of your baby's personality, birth experience and current behaviour.

▨ HITTING, BITING OR PINCHING

As your baby grows older and gets more mobile, more social and mixes with other children, hitting, biting or punching may begin. These behaviours are his way of communicating and defending his territory. Before your baby is one year old he does not plan ahead – apparently aggressive behaviour is a natural and spontaneous expression of his feelings, and a way of exploring what is and is not acceptable.

Your baby needs you to help him when he has feelings that are uncomfortable and when he feels threatened (for example, when playing with other children, or simply because you are not with him). He may need your intervention to protect him, and your guidance as he learns about relationships. Guiding your baby lovingly and being consistent may help him learn that when he hurts other people this does not feel good for them.

What happens

Your child might be angry about something. This is a normal and frequently occurring emotion (page 218) and each child expresses it uniquely. Exercising control over other children might be your child's way of expressing his power as well as his anger.

Babies and children learn from what others do (rather than what is said), and you may need to consider whether another adult's or child's behaviour could be a model for aggression or bossiness in your child. It may take a lot of courage to look into and accept your own actions and feelings.

For some babies biting and hitting occur if there are communication skill difficulties, such as delayed language. This is often part of an individual child's normal development. Unusually delayed skill in communication may be one of a collection of problems that may prompt consideration of autistic spectrum disorder (page 39).

Action plan

* When your baby bites, hits or pinches, focus on him and tell him lovingly and without anger that what he is doing is painful. Tell him how important it is to stop. Let him know the behaviour is not acceptable and you love him – you are setting boundaries that help him learn (page 433).
* Consider what he may be feeling and if something is frightening him or making him angry. This may prompt you to make some simple changes that have widespread benefits (for example, spending more time with him, slowing to his pace, taking more time handing

over to a childcarer, or adjusting the way you approach bedtime).

- Be consistent, and allow your baby space and time to express his feelings safely in your presence. If he is angry he will need your help to calm down (page 51).
- Reacting with your own tap or slap is likely to reinforce the undesirable behaviour.
- Ensure that everyone who cares for your baby behaves in a consistent way.

SECURITY OBJECTS

Your baby experiences his mother as an extension of himself and being with mum is to be with his favourite thing. A security object (or transitional object) serves a mother-like role, providing familiarity and comfort when there is no contact with mum. Not all babies use such an object, but many do find them extremely comforting. It might be a soft toy, a blanket, an item of clothing or something similar.

A security object relieves tension and anxiety and is a positive, rather than a negative, attachment. A common time to form a strong attachment to something soft and cuddly is between six and nine months, at the time your baby begins to realise that he is separate from his mum. This realisation may be a problem for your baby and he may become clingy. As well as wanting you or another loving adult, he may want to have his object with him all the time, or want it most when he is upset, is going to sleep or when he is away from you.

Any security object is hugely important to your baby while he makes the transition towards independence. A security object provides a safe place that your baby can rely on as his explorations take him further from you. It is best to keep it close and give it to him when he asks for it. Unless it gets really dirty, refrain from washing it (the smell is reassuringly familiar). Some families have two similar objects, or divide a security blanket in two – so there is always a spare if the original goes missing or is left behind.

Birth

See Labour and birth, baby; Labour and birth, mother.

Birthmarks

A birthmark, or naevus, is a mark on the skin that is apparent at birth or appears within the first few weeks. The commonest birthmark is a vascular naevus, a salmon patch or 'birth stork mark' over the nape of the neck or over the eyelids. This forms because of dilated blood vessels and tends to disappear within the first year. The mark is not related to the birth process.

A port wine stain is a flat, red mark. It is rare, affecting one in 500 newborns. The mark tends to persist, unchanged, during childhood and may be associated with dilated and malformed blood vessels under the skin. If your baby has a large port wine stain she will be referred to a dermatologist (skin specialist) and perhaps a plastic surgeon.

Haemangiomas (strawberry marks) consist of dilated blood vessels that are rarely present at birth but appear within four weeks in around one in 10 babies (commoner in pre-term babies). A haemangioma begins as a barely visible small red mark that grows over weeks to form a bright red compressible area of dilated small capillary blood vessels. Growth usually stops by 12 months of age, but may continue longer. The marks usually shrink and disappear without treatment during the first few years.

Laser treatment is available for both types of birthmark and may be effective in reducing the blood flow and altering the colour of the skin. It is usually reserved for either cosmetic purposes – when the naevus is very obvious, on the face for instance – or is interfering with the closing of eyelids, for example.

Birth partner

See Labour and birth, mother, birth partner.

Birth plan

See Labour and birth, mother, birth plan.

Birth trauma, baby

See also Labour and birth, baby, being born; Pain, baby.

It is very unlikely that your baby will be injured at birth. With modern obstetric care severe injury, or birth trauma, is extremely rare, affecting 2–7 in 1,000 babies. Minor bruising is more common. If your baby is injured, he is likely to recover completely with your loving care, good paediatric care and his own natural healing capacity.

What happens

Some babies are more likely to be injured during birth. They include:
- PREMATURE babies, born before Week 37, who have more fragile bodies. Bruising is the most frequent form of birth injury among babies born early.
- LARGE BABIES, whose birth weight is over 4.4kg (9lb 8oz). They are more likely to need assistance with FORCEPS OR VENTOUSE (see LABOUR AND BIRTH, MOTHER) or experience a delay in the birth of their body or SHOULDER DYSTOCIA, all of which may cause injury.
- Babies who are not positioned optimally, such as those in the BREECH (bottom downwards) position.

If your baby is considered to be at risk of injury, your birth team will pay close attention to your progress in labour. Using an upright position (page 350) for birth can reduce the possibility of injury occurring. If you need intervention, your obstetrician will take care to avoid injury to you and your baby and may decide that a CAESAREAN SECTION is preferable.

Action plan

Baby
- If your baby requires medical attention treatment is likely to be straightforward and physical recovery is normally complete within days or weeks. When one injury is discovered, it is usual practice for a paediatrician to examine your baby in detail for other injuries.
- In the early days your baby will feel discomfort from his injury – the extent depends on the

injury. He may be in pain, shocked and/or angry about what happened. His emotional and physical discomfort may be heightened if he has been separated from you.
- Above all else, your baby needs to be with you as soon as possible. If this is not possible, it is best for your baby to be with his father or another caring adult.
- Your baby's level of pain may be reduced with skin-to-skin contact and frequent feeding – the sucking action is very soothing for head pain, in particular, and breast milk has painkilling properties comparable to morphine. Being lovingly held is important, including when he may be crying, as it helps him feel safe.
- Simple pain relievers such as paracetamol (page 429) often help, but sometimes stronger morphine-based drugs may be required, for the first few hours after birth. Usually all pain relief can be stopped within 48 hours.
- You may want to use other healing tools such as cranial OSTEOPATHY, MASSAGE or HOMEOPATHY.

Mum and dad
If your baby's injuries are mild he may show little sign of discomfort and you may feel okay with the birth. If you feel upset or shocked or if your baby is not well and requires ongoing treatment, you will benefit from practical support at home to ensure you eat well and can rest, plus the loving support of friends, family or professionals to help you accept and process your emotions and cope with the situation in hand. The range of reactions after birth is explored on page 394.

▓ BONE INJURIES

The collarbone (clavicle) is the most common bone to fracture, most often when a baby is large and there is difficulty delivering the shoulders during the birth (shoulder dystocia). Around 2 per cent of large babies (weighing over 4.4kg/9lb 8oz) do fracture the clavicle. With this bone broken, your baby is unlikely to move the arm on the injured side and there may be bruising over the broken bone. The paediatrician will also check for damage to your baby's spine and the nerves associated with the muscles of the arm and hand (Erb's Palsy, page 56).

The bone usually heals after 7–10 days and requires no specific treatment. If movement of the arm causes your baby distress you can make him more comfortable by pinning the sleeve of the babygro to his chest on the side of the injury: this acts as a splint. You may be able to feel a bump at the site of the fracture. This will usually remodel over the following few years.

More rarely the humerus (upper arm) and femur (upper leg) bones may be damaged. On extremely rare occasions the obstetrician feels or hears a snap during birth. If your baby does not appear to be moving his arm or leg this may be an early sign, followed by swelling and pain when you move it for him. An X-ray will confirm the diagnosis.

A fractured humerus needs to be treated by an orthopaedic specialist and a plaster cast may be needed for 14–21 days. Fractures of the femur can be treated with traction using a weight hung from a bandage round the leg for 14–21 days – the weight encourages healing.

If there appeared to be little trauma during labour and birth, yet a baby still has a bone injury, the diagnosis of brittle bone disease (osteogenesis imperfecta) may be considered, although this is extremely rare.

▓ HEAD AND FACE INJURIES

A baby's skull bones are capable of overlapping and 'moulding' to ease the passage through the mother's pelvis and birth canal. The extent to which this happens, and how long the moulding remains prominent after birth, varies according to each baby's position and the duration and intensity of labour. Bruising is the most common facial injury, and skull bone fractures are very rare.

Soft tissue damage and bruising

In some newborns, the facial skin appears blue from tiny pinpoint bruises caused by bleeding into the skin as a result of the pressure of birth. The blueness is often present if the cord has been tightly wrapped around the baby's neck. These bruises are harmless and will fade after a few days. If the bruising affects the eyelids they may swell. The bruising may also affect the conjunctiva, the clear membrane that covers the eyes. If a small amount of bleeding occurs, the conjunctiva will

appear red. After a few days this will fade to brown and eventually disappear. There is no long-term harm to the eye or to vision.

A few weeks after delivery, a pea-sized lump may appear in the cheek or elsewhere under your baby's facial skin. This is usually due to a small lump of fat that has changed from its natural liquid state to a more solid state because of pressure during birth. It will disappear within a few weeks.

Sometimes a foetal scalp electrode, used in foetal monitoring, may leave a small cut or spot on a baby's scalp. This will heal in a few days, but does occasionally become infected. The faint scar will disappear beneath the hair. Scalp electrodes are used infrequently (page 336).

Swelling and bruising of the scalp

Swelling of the scalp does not require any specific treatment.

Caput succedaneum

Usually just called caput, this is a swelling of the soft tissues of the scalp. The natural condition develops as your baby travels through the birth canal and helps to protect the skull bones and the brain. It usually disappears after 36 hours but some babies also have associated bruising under the skin. Babies delivered with the help of forceps, or more commonly the ventouse (page 373), may have more pronounced caput and bruising.

Cephalohaematoma

This is an area of bleeding and bruising underneath the lining membrane of one of the cranial bones in the skull. It often appears several hours after birth as a raised lump on the head. It is more common with ventouse deliveries. The bruise tends to get bigger over the first weeks and then, as the blood is reabsorbed, it shrinks. A large bruise may take up to three months to disappear but smaller swellings will reduce in a week or two. Draining the blood that causes the swelling is unnecessary and may introduce infection. If the area of bleeding is very large an excess of bilirubin, a yellow pigment, may be produced when the red blood cells have broken down and JAUNDICE (yellowing of the skin) may develop. If the jaundice is severe your baby may require treatment.

Sub-aponeurotic haematoma

This condition is extremely rare but more serious, with bleeding that crosses over various skull bones and can spread down to the face, leading to bruising that lasts for weeks. It may be caused by a ventouse delivery. The bruised area is larger than a cephalohaematoma and may cause a fall in BLOOD PRESSURE that leads to more intense jaundice and requires treatment. It usually disappears completely with time.

Damage with bleeding (haemorrhage) into the brain

See also Foetal distress and asphyxia.

The most common reason for a bleed into the brain (intracranial haemorrhage) is bleeding from fragile blood vessels in the brain of a premature baby if there is a period of low oxygen levels, or even with minor trauma at birth. Some babies have abnormal blood vessels in the brain that bleed. In a full-term baby bleeding may be linked with the forces applied during forceps or ventouse assistance, usually if there has been a prolonged labour with difficulty navigating the pelvis, or foetal distress (page 249) with reduced oxygen levels.

The risk of an injury to the brain ranges from one in 1,000 for an operative (FORCEPS OR VENTOUSE) delivery or CAESAREAN when in labour to one in 3,000 for non-operative delivery or caesarean section when not in labour. The risk associated with forceps and ventouse is slightly greater than a caesarean in labour.

A baby who has had a brain injury resulting in bleeding may have anything from the most minimal of symptoms, such as poor feeding and irritability, to major complications such as neonatal FITS and even unexpected death. If symptoms are mild or absent and the bleed is mild, there may be no consequences. If there has been significant bleeding into the brain and the blood accumulates, symptoms may be obvious and the baby will be extremely ill. Alternatively, the effect may become more obvious over a few weeks and the head may visibly enlarge from hydrocephalus (water on the brain).

If bleeding is suspected, your baby may be given electroencephalography (EEG) and ultrasound or MRI scans. If the injury leads to a fit, anti-convulsant medication may be given. Your baby may also be tested for infectious and genetic or blood clotting abnormalities. He will be closely monitored to ensure that hydrocephalus does not develop.

Often the blood is naturally absorbed over a period of weeks or months. Only rarely does it need to be removed surgically, if the blood clot is causing pressure on the brain. The outlook for babies with haemorrhage of any cause is very variable. It is determined by the size of the bleed, which part of the brain is involved and the underlying cause. While there may be no lasting effect, rarely the injury may lead to learning difficulties or physical disability.

Subdural haemorrhage

The dura consists of the outermost lining membranes of the brain. Subdural haemorrhage usually occurs in babies born at full-term from birth trauma. With improved obstetric practice, these have become much less common. The tentorium is a part of the dura membrane and tentorial tears may cause blood to collect in the brain stem, an area that controls breathing and consciousness. Very rarely this may lead to severe damage.

Subarachnoid haemorrhage

Blood may pass into subarachnoid space under the innermost of the lining membranes of the brain. It occurs after damage resulting from low oxygen flow to the brain (page 301) and after birth trauma but the cause may be unclear. The effects and symptoms may be severe.

Intraventricular haemorrhage

This is bleeding into the fluid-filled ventricles of the brain. It mainly occurs in premature babies because the ventricles have a very fragile network of tiny blood vessels that bleed easily. The haemorrhage may be suspected if a baby is unwell, and confirmed on an ultrasound scan of the baby's head. If the bleeding is severe it can have long-term effects.

Intraparenchymal haemorrhage

Bleeding into the brain substance can be due to birth injury, malformed blood vessels, abnormal blood clotting or low oxygen levels. The effects vary according to the extent of the bleed and it may lead to long-term nerve damage.

Damage to the ears

Ear injury is not common. With a forceps delivery the ear lobes can be caught behind the blades of the forceps and bruised. The bruising disappears in a few days. If the ears are crinkled from pressure in the uterus before labour they are not injured during birth and usually open out soon. Occasionally, the folding stays and a simple foam-covered spring can correct the ear shape.

Eye injuries

One or both of the eyes may have a bright red area or red spots on the white area surrounding the iris. This is called a subconjunctival haemorrhage and is the result of breaks in the small blood vessels on the surface of the eyeball and small amounts of bleeding into the white lining. This is very common. The blood is absorbed over several weeks and there is no harm to the eyes or to vision.

■ NERVE DAMAGE

Nerve damage cannot always be attributed to injury during labour or birth and may be present before birth as a CONGENITAL ABNORMALITY. A congenital condition is one the baby is born with. This is especially so for nerve injuries such as facial nerve palsy, the majority of which are found after an uneventful, unassisted delivery.

Facial nerve palsy

Facial nerve palsy is thought to be due to the congenital absence of some of the fibres of the nerve associated with the facial muscle. It usually results in a lopsided cry and one eyelid not closing completely. More rarely it is caused by the facial nerve becoming compressed during a forceps birth. The facial nerve controls the muscles of expression and the eyelids. If the affected eye cannot blink or close, it is sometimes necessary to use eye drops to stop the eye from becoming dry until the nerve recovers naturally. The nerve recovers within a few days for most babies, but occasionally takes months. Some babies need to be referred to a plastic surgeon and recovery may not always be complete.

Erb's or Klumpke's Palsy

The nerves from the spinal cord in the neck (the brachial plexus) supply the muscles of the arm and shoulder. When these are bruised or damaged there may be limited or no movement in the shoulder, arm, wrist or fingers after birth. Depending on which nerves are injured, this is called Erb's or Klumpke's Palsy.

The most frequent cause is delay in delivery of the shoulders (shoulder dystocia) when traction, used to assist with the birth, stretches and damages the nerves in the neck. There may also be a broken clavicle. Usually recovery is complete and takes just hours or a few days. Less than 15 per cent of affected babies need physiotherapy and the attention of a paediatrician and may need months to recover. If recovery is incomplete within one year, an operation to rejoin the nerves is often successful.

Cerebral palsy

Cerebral palsy has a serious and long-term impact on a baby and his family, and is covered in more detail on page 124. Cerebral palsy is not nerve damage. It is damage to the nervous system, in particular to 'mature' areas of the brain in a near term or term baby. In most cases, cerebral palsy is a congenital abnormality present from some stage in pregnancy and cannot be prevented. A small minority of babies with cerebral palsy may have had a birth injury related to FOETAL DISTRESS AND ASPHYXIA with oxygen deprivation. Modern obstetric and midwifery care is designed to minimise oxygen deprivation and poor blood flow.

Biting

See Behaviour, baby, difficult.

Bleeding and blood-clotting disorders, baby

■ HAEMOPHILIA

Haemophilia is the general term for a range of blood-clotting disorders. It is due to a deficiency of one of the components of the blood called 'factors' which are responsible for causing the blood to clot following an injury. Babies with haemophilia do not bleed any faster than non-sufferers but because the blood does not clot, bleeding is markedly prolonged. There are many different blood-clotting disorders. The most common is haemophilia A, also known as 'classical haemophilia' (due to a deficiency of clotting factor VIII).

Other forms include haemophilia B (also called Christmas disease or factor IX deficiency) and haemophilia C (factor XI deficiency).

Haemophilia is an inherited disorder in 40 per cent of childhood cases, with an identifiable family history. In the remaining 60 per cent of newly diagnosed children, it is a new genetic change, resulting in haemophilia with no preceding family history. In the majority of genetic cases a boy baby has a faulty gene on the X chromosome he inherits from his carrier mother. Boys have only one X chromosome, and so, unlike girls, do not have a normal gene to compensate for the faulty one. Very rarely, females inherit haemophilia because the faulty gene is on both sides of the family. Female carriers of the haemophilia gene can be 'symptomatic carriers' and have mild or very mild haemophilia, perhaps only detected by sensitive blood-clotting tests.

What happens

If a baby has haemophilia it is unlikely that the problem will be diagnosed or even suspected within the first six months, because very few babies sustain an injury that causes bleeding in this time. If male haemophiliac babies have a circumcision (less than 1 per cent of all circumcised babies) only 30 per cent bleed excessively.

- Occasionally a baby may have repeated and prolonged bleeding from the nose as a symptom, and occasionally blood in the stool arising from bleeding into the bowel.
- More rarely, for 1–2 per cent of haemophiliac babies, there may be intracranial haemorrhage, or bleeding in the brain (page 53).
- At any time, if a baby undergoes surgery the decrease in blood clotting will be apparent.
- Bleeding into the joints (haemarthroses) is one of the more common signs in a previously undiagnosed haemophiliac. Blood in the joint will cause swelling, pain and reduced movement

(and is sometimes difficult to diagnose in a young baby who is not yet fully mobile).
- Some children with a less severe clotting disorder (such as haemophilia B or C) may only show symptoms with heavy menstrual periods or bruising as teenagers.

Once a baby becomes mobile, falls and bumps are inevitable and bruises may be more profuse, larger or more noticeable than usual, and in unusual places. Any cuts to the mouth may bleed excessively. Unfortunately, bleeding may prompt suspicion of child abuse before a diagnosis is made. It is a matter of routine to check a baby's clotting before saying an injury was non-accidental. An initial test that does a general screen for blood-clotting deficiencies gives results within an hour. If it reveals an abnormality, further screening looks for the missing or reduced factors.

The degree of clotting factor deficiency determines the frequency and severity of the bleeding episodes. Mild deficiencies result in prolonged bleeding only after surgery or trauma. Severe deficiencies cause bleeding to occur spontaneously, without trauma.

Children with a suspected clotting problem are referred to a haemophilia centre for diagnosis and treatment with blood-clotting factor replacement. Most children can be treated at home with the assistance of homecare nurses or with a short hospital stay.

▨ THROMBOCYTOPAENIA

Thrombocytopaenia is a rare condition, affecting fewer than one in 5,000 babies. It is a reduction in the number of platelets (a type of small blood cell) below the normal level (which is 50,000 to 3,000,000 platelets per cubic ml of blood). It can also mean a total absence of platelets from the blood. Platelets are responsible for clotting, so a shortage or absence results in bleeding into the skin, the mouth, nose and ears, and can be quite severe.

What happens

- The commonest cause of a low platelet count is infection, where bone marrow is put under stress and platelets are used up more quickly than they can be produced.

- If you have a low platelet count your baby is unlikely to be affected. Only rarely does a mother with thrombocytopaenia pass an antibody against the platelets to her baby in the womb. If this happens, the baby's platelets are destroyed.
- Occasionally, often following a viral infection, a baby's body may destroy its own platelets (idiapothic thrombocytopaenic purpura).
- Very rarely, it is associated with von Willebrand's disease (see below).
- Most rarely a low platelet count is a marker for bone marrow failure due to leukaemia and other rare diseases that involve the bone marrow.

Action plan

Specialist treatment depends on the cause and involves the use of blood products. For example, immunoglobulin may be used to mop up the antibody that is causing the platelets to be broken down. If the mother's platelet count is low during pregnancy, the baby will need careful monitoring after birth. If bleeding or bruising is a problem, platelet transfusion may be needed and corticosteroids may be given.

With treatment, the condition usually improves over a 10–21-day period. The outlook is excellent, providing a baby does not suffer a major bleed – the risk of this happening is very small, at around one in 10,000 cases of thrombocytopaenia.

▓ VON WILLEBRAND'S DISEASE

Von Willebrand's disease (vWD) is not common, but is the most frequently occurring bleeding disorder among babies in the UK, affecting 1–3 per cent of the UK population. It is passed from parent to child in the genes.

Von Willebrand's disease rarely causes problems in newborn infants, male or female. Later in life bruising (bleeding into the skin) is the most common problem, rather than bleeding into the joints and muscles, which is more commonly associated with classical factor VIII deficient haemophilia A (page 57). With the more severe forms there may be bleeding from the bowel, urinary tract or mouth. Bleeding can happen after surgery.

What happens

Von Willebrand's disease occurs when the body does not produce enough of a protein called von Willebrand factor (vWF), or produces abnormal vWF. This factor is involved in the process of blood clotting. People with vWD have difficulty in forming blood clots and as a result may bleed for longer. In most cases the bleeding is due to an obvious injury, although it sometimes occurs spontaneously. There are three types of vWD:

- Type 1 is the most common and mildest form and results when the body produces slightly decreased amounts of normal vWF.
- Type 2 is when the body produces an abnormal type of vWF and may be associated with a low platelet count.
- Type 3 is the rarest and most severe form when the body does not produce any detectable vWF.

Action plan

Von Willebrand's disease is most commonly treated by replacement of vWF with blood products or with desmopressin, which increases the amount of factor VIII and vWF in the blood. Treatment is given if there is bleeding or before surgery or dental work. The treatment chosen depends on the type of vWD. All families or patients with the condition should be under the care of specialist centres, and will carry cards identifying their health condition and treatments.

Bleeding and blood-clotting disorders, mother

See also Bleeding and blood-clotting disorders, baby.

A complex system ensures that your blood clots when necessary, following an injury, for example, and stays fluid the rest of the time. Blood clotting requires special cells that make up the blood clot, called platelets, a sticky protein called fibrin, which mixes with the platelets to make the clot, and other components known as 'factors'. When a person has a blood-clotting disorder, this process does not function efficiently.

▣ EXCESS CLOTTING (THROMBOPHILIA)

Throughout pregnancy, a mother's normal ability to produce blood clots is slightly suppressed, and this changes as soon as the placenta is delivered. Some women have an increased tendency for the blood to clot. This is called thrombophilia. Thrombophilia is rare and requires specialist care, either from an obstetrician or a blood-clotting specialist haematologist. If it is severe, it requires more intensive treatment in pregnancy than if the effect is mild. It may be genetic and inherited, as in factor V (Leiden), protein C and S, or homocysteineaemia and will be more severe if one abnormal gene is inherited from each parent than if one normal and one abnormal gene is inherited. Alternatively, a reduced clotting ability may be acquired, as in antiphospholipid syndrome, associated with lupus erythematosus, an autoimmune disorder in which the body's immune system attacks its own tissues.

What happens

Soon after the embryo attaches to the uterus, placental cells come into contact with the mother's blood vessels, which are the only source of nourishment. Thrombophilia can cause the blood to begin to clot and thus reduce blood flow and nutrients to the embryo. This may happen early or late in pregnancy. In a mild form, it may have no effect. Untreated, though, it may cause complications such as MISCARRIAGE and recurrent foetal loss, pre-eclampsia, INTRAUTERINE GROWTH RESTRICTION (IUGR), placental abruption, deep vein thrombosis or in very severe instances STILLBIRTH. If you or other members of your family have experienced any of these conditions, you may consider being tested for thrombophilia because treatment greatly reduces the risks.

Action plan

Medical care

Treatment depends on the specific condition. In severe cases it is best to begin treatment soon after conception. Any agents that reduce blood clotting can cause internal bleeding and need to be used with caution and with specialist advice.

- Low-dose aspirin (75–150 mg) can be continued throughout pregnancy. Rarely, it may cause side effects, such as gastric irritation, heartburn and internal bleeding, so it is best to take aspirin with food. You will need to be monitored. The aspirin needs to be stopped by 36 weeks so that any effect on your baby's blood platelets and clotting system is no longer present at birth. If you take aspirin it is important not to use supplements of omega essential fatty acids as these may increase the blood-thinning effect of the aspirin.
- Heparin is more powerful than aspirin for severe thrombophilia. Heparin is administered by injection and you can inject yourself. The doses will be monitored by your obstetrician. Heparin has the advantage that it does not cross the placenta and so cannot harm the baby, but the disadvantage is that long-term use can lead to bleeding or reduced bone mineral density and OSTEOPOROSIS. It is a powerful drug and the main side effect is internal bleeding, if you are sensitive to the medication. It is used less commonly than aspirin but it is very effective when used appropriately.
- If you have thrombophilia it is best to choose a non-hormonal method of contraception and consider taking low-dose aspirin daily. You may need to take heparin after surgery, including caesarean section.

▣ REDUCED CLOTTING

In some cases, the blood is slow to clot after an injury. This can lead to bruising and excessive blood loss, in severe cases.

What happens

There are different types of disorders that lead to reduced blood clotting.

- Inherited (genetic) types, of which the best known is haemophilia (page 56), mainly occur in males. In some families, women are born with a deficiency that may lead to bruising, heavy periods or bleeding after a cut, surgery or tooth extraction. Sometimes a clotting problem appears for the first time in pregnancy. If you have a family or personal history of clotting problems, your blood-clotting factors may be screened before pregnancy. It is difficult to screen for individual coagulation factors during pregnancy because the levels alter. Blood tests are also available to check clotting in an emergency. Replacing the appropriate clotting factors corrects a blood-clotting disorder.

- Very rarely during pregnancy the clotting system may be stimulated and the factors depleted and the blood is then unable to clot normally. This may occur in severe pre-eclampsia, with bleeding caused by placental abruption, or severe infections, immune disorders or kidney or liver disorders. The abnormal clotting is treated as part of the underlying condition.
- Thrombocytopaenia (reduced blood platelet cells) may be related to pregnancy.

Action plan

If you are already known to have a blood-clotting disorder, your care in pregnancy, birth and the postnatal period will reflect this. However, sometimes excessive bleeding after birth may be the first sign that you have a clotting disorder.

If your clotting factors or platelets are low they may be replaced before labour for your safety. If you have excessive bleeding during or after birth they will be replaced by an intravenous infusion of blood or the clotting factors. If you do not have an underlying disorder, since your liver makes the clotting factors, they will be replaced within hours. Being well nourished maximises your blood's clotting ability.

▨ THROMBOCYTOPAENIA

Thrombocytopaenia is a low blood platelet cell count. Platelets are important for normal blood clotting and a low count increases the risk of bleeding, particularly at birth. Sometimes thrombocytopaenia is caused by antibodies in the mother's circulation and these may cross the placenta and reduce the platelet count in the baby. Thrombocytopaenia in babies is discussed on page 57.

What happens

Pregnancy thrombocytopaenia

In 5–8 per cent of pregnant women, platelet counts drop and the cause is not known. It does not cause symptoms, occurs in late pregnancy

and the problem clears spontaneously within two weeks of birth. It does not affect the baby's platelets.

Idiopathic thrombocytopaenic purpura (ITP)

This may cause lower platelet counts and begins before or early in pregnancy. It is a very rare immune disorder with antibodies directed against platelet cells. The baby can be affected. The platelet count is monitored and the condition only needs treatment with steroids if the platelet count drops excessively.

Pre-eclampsia

Thrombocytopaenia may develop in very severe pre-eclampsia (page 57). It resolves when the pre-eclampsia is resolved, usually after the birth.

Systemic lupus erythematosus (SLE) and thrombotic thrombocytopaenic purpura

These are very rare causes of thrombocytopaenia requiring specialist diagnosis and treatment.

Action plan

If your platelet count is below 150,000 but above 50,000 on a routine blood count in pregnancy, there are no signs of bleeding or bruising and you are well, the cause is likely to be pregnancy thrombocytopaenia and no treatment is needed. Your blood will be checked frequently until the birth. If the count is below 50,000 or there is bleeding or bruising, you will need specialist care to investigate whether you have antibodies in your blood that are reducing platelet numbers.

Caesarean section is not usually needed for low platelet counts. In many centres an epidural anaesthetic is not used if the platelets are under 100,000 because of the small risk of bleeding into the epidural space, around the spinal cord.

The main concern is that a baby could be affected, and if birth is traumatic there is an increased risk of birth injury with brain haemorrhage. This is very rare.

If you have idiopathic thrombocytopaenic purpura then steroids may be needed. They require three to seven days to take effect and not everyone responds. If the platelet count remains low, a platelet transfusion may be needed in labour to prevent or control bleeding.

Your baby's platelet count will be analysed from a blood sample taken from the cord at birth and, providing treatment begins early to avoid major bleeding, the outlook is excellent. The count may be checked a few weeks later if you have platelet antibodies in your blood that could have crossed to your baby and reduced the count.

Bleeding, baby

See also Accidents and first aid, baby; Birth trauma, baby.

Nothing can be as worrying as seeing your baby bleed, from any part of the body, and any amount. Fortunately, mature term babies have an efficient blood-clotting (coagulation) mechanism and this usually prevents any bleeding from becoming severe or dangerous.

+ Red flag

If your baby has any bleeding it is important to seek medical help immediately. Often the blood does not indicate a serious problem but it is always best to be reassured or to get early treatment if your baby needs assistance.

For many babies who do have a significant bleed, there is an underlying health-related problem, such as the mother being on anticonvulsant or anti-tuberculosis treatment, or the baby having a malfunction of the liver or a major infection. PREMATURE babies are more prone to infection (sepsis) which may lead on to bleeding, and their clotting systems are less mature. Only very rarely does excessive bleeding indicate a deficiency in blood-clotting ability (page 58).

The following entries cover the most common incidences of bleeding.

▓ BLOOD IN STOOLS

Blood in the stools, when it occurs with no other symptoms, is usually much less significant than the same symptom in an adult. It is important, though, to seek help early if the bleeding suddenly occurs or your baby appears to be ill and has other symptoms.

Common causes and remedies

- If your baby is breastfed the most likely cause of blood in her stools is that you have cracked nipples. Even without obvious cracking, your baby's suck may be strong enough to cause bleeding and you may not be aware of it. The blood does no harm and you can continue to feed. With closer attention to the way your baby is positioned at your nipple, and by treating any cracks in your nipples promptly (page 97), your baby is less likely to consume blood.
- If blood is bright red and coats the outside of your baby's motion this could be due to a small tear in the skin of her anus (anal fissure). This has probably occurred through passing a large or hard stool. You may not be able to see the tear but there may be a small tag of skin. Fissures heal of their own accord if steps are taken to avoid CONSTIPATION.
- By far the most common reason for blood in the motion of an otherwise well baby is some form of allergic colitis (inflammation of the large bowel due to food intolerance). Common foods that cause this allergic symptom are milk, rice and wheat. The diagnosis is simple to make if the blood clears when a food is excluded. Treatment is to avoid the food while taking advice from a nutritionist to ensure your baby receives adequate nutrients. This can occur even in solely breastfed infants, due to wheat or rice or protein causing the sensitivity crossing from the breast milk. If your baby is sensitive she may show other symptoms such as diarrhoea or a rash, and this may be intermittent depending on the food you eat (or she eats if weaned).
- Blood mixed with a motion and diarrhoea may indicate infection in the bowel. A viral infection is typically associated with vomiting. Less commonly, the infection is bacterial and likely to cause pain. Treatment suggestions for infection are discussed on pages 182 and 553.

Intussusception

Rarely, bloody stools indicate intussusception, a condition that is dangerous but can usually be effectively treated if diagnosed early. With intussusception, a portion of the bowel folds in on itself. The tissues in the bowel wall contain blood vessels that support the bowel and these get trapped and strangulated, and the tissue swells. Bloody mucus may appear in the stool, and vomiting may develop. If the diagnosis isn't made quickly and treated, the section of bowel may die, causing the child to go into shock.

Together with bloody mucus in the stools, your baby is likely to have a sudden pain, initially coming in waves, and may have diarrhoea and begin to vomit. If the diagnosis is delayed and the condition worsens she may have abdominal swelling and increasing or continual pain.

Intussusception generally occurs between the ages of three months and six years, more often in the first two years. The discomfort usually causes a baby to strain and cry loudly, preferring to lie very still during an episode of intense pain.

The treatment is often surprisingly easy. If intussusception is suspected early, a barium enema is usually carried out to confirm it, and will often cure it, too. The pressure of the barium-containing fluid used for the test is often able to cause the intussusception to pop back out and cure itself. If that doesn't work, it can be surgically repaired.

▓ FROM THE NOSE, SKIN AND EARS

Bleeding from the nose or ears is unusual, except when a baby has a cold. If your baby has a bloody discharge from the nose and it lasts longer than a normal cold, then there may be something lodged in the nose, such as a button or piece of paper, and you may be able to see it. Don't try to remove it unless it is close to the nostril opening. If removing it is likely to be difficult, take your baby to the local accident and emergency department. Your baby may need an anaesthetic while the object is extracted. Another common cause of nose bleeds is a blow to the nose (page 10).

Bleeding from the skin usually results from a cut or graze requiring first aid. A less common cause is a condition called purpura that leads to bleeding into the skin that results in a rash. If your baby has a rash that does not disappear when a glass is pressed against her skin, and she appears unwell, this may indicate a severe infection with a bacterium called meningococcus (page 409). Call your doctor if you suspect this. In most cases, a severe infection scare is a false alarm, but it is best to be sure.

Very rarely haemophilia, or von Willebrand's disease, can appear as skin bleeding, but these conditions more usually cause bruising.

▓ FROM THE VAGINA

It is quite common for baby girls to have a little bleeding from the vagina after they are born. Your own hormones, including oestrogen, will circulate in your baby while she is in the womb and will act on her body. As oestrogen levels in your baby's body fall after birth, her womb may bleed as the lining is shed. The bleeding may appear pink or red and is usually mixed with mucus. It commonly stops after one week.

Any further or persistent bleeding from the vagina may need to be investigated as it may suggest your baby has a birthmark called a vascular haemangioma, and this has begun to bleed having been damaged by contact with a nappy.

Another very common symptom that is alarming yet misleading is the presence of pink discolouration on the nappy. This is not blood, but a deposit of urate crystals from the urine. The crystals can glow pink, particularly under fluorescent light. It is harmless and goes away by itself.

▓ VITAMIN K DEPENDENT BLEEDING (HAEMORRHAGIC DISEASE OF THE NEWBORN)

Vitamin K is required by the liver to make factors essential for clotting the blood. Vitamin K dependent bleeding (haemorrhagic disease of the newborn) arises from a deficiency in vitamin K. The deficiency can be prevented if additional vitamin K is given in the newborn period when levels are naturally low. The vitamin is manufactured in the bowel by bacteria acquired after birth. Although breast milk is the ideal nutrition for babies, it is low in vitamin K.

Vitamin K dependent bleeding is rare. It can cause bleeding from the mouth, nose and gut in the first weeks after birth, and affects around one in 10,000 babies in the UK each year. The condition is serious, with a high risk of death or disability if bleeding occurs into the brain. Unfortunately, in roughly one of every three babies affected the vitamin K deficiency bleeding occurs without prior warning or known risk factors. For this reason, additional vitamin K is given routinely. Studies in the UK, the USA, Germany, Switzerland and Sweden have concluded that intramuscular vitamin K prevents haemorrhage completely, and that oral vitamin K offers a very significant degree of protection.

Administering vitamin K after birth

It is routine to offer all babies vitamin K at birth. A single injection is the most frequent treatment offered in the UK. Fewer than one third of babies are given oral vitamin K at birth. Oral treatment requires a repeat oral dose at 1 week, and again at 1 month. The injection offers the most reliable protection for babies born prematurely, babies whose risk is increased because of maternal medication taken in pregnancy (e.g. drugs to treat epilepsy or TB; blood-thinning drugs such as aspirin, or warfarin); babies whose mothers have liver disease; and babies whose birth was traumatic and/or incurred bruising.

Weighing the risks

In the late 20th century there were some concerns about a link between childhood cancer with intramuscular vitamin K injection. This link has not been proven and there are no established risks. If you are concerned about as yet unproven risks, you will need to consider these against the known risk of bleeding with potentially fatal or damaging outcomes if either no vitamin K is administered or even if the oral route is chosen. The oral administration has not been in place for many years and there is a chance of some as yet unknown risk that may become apparent with time.

It has been estimated that if vitamin K were given only to high-risk babies, among 646,000 annual births in the UK, there might be:

- 60 babies who suffer a bleed,
- 15–20 babies suffering a bleed into the brain,
- 4–6 babies who die from the bleed into the brain, and
- 10–20 babies who may be brain damaged because of the bleeding.

▨ VOMITING BLOOD

Even a small amount of blood in the stomach is likely to make your baby sick. The most likely source of the blood, if your baby appears well apart from the vomit, is that you have cracked nipples. The blood is altered by stomach acid and may appear dark brown. Although this is alarming, it is harmless, and the best thing to do is to continue feeding and treat your cracked nipples (page 97).

Some babies with severe reflux (page 554) may occasionally vomit flecks of red blood. Again this is alarming but usually harmless, and you need to treat the reflux. If vomiting of red blood is associated with dark or black motions, this may indicate that there is blood passing through the bowel, and it is important to seek your doctor's advice.

The only other cause for concern of blood in the vomit is that your baby may have a rare clotting disorder. The commonest is vitamin K dependent bleeding (page 62). If your baby vomits some blood, and even if she is well, if you have chosen not to give vitamin K to your baby at birth please bring this to the attention of your doctor or health visitor.

Bleeding, mother, during pregnancy

See also Ectopic pregnancy.

Vaginal bleeding may occur at any time during pregnancy and should always be reported to a doctor or midwife.

✚ Red flag

If bleeding is heavy and there is pain and/or evidence of clots, this is an emergency. Visit your doctor or the nearest hospital accident and emergency department.

Worrying though it is, light bleeding that is not accompanied by other symptoms may not affect your baby. The medical team can conduct tests to put your mind at rest. If there is a problem, early diagnosis and treatment will reduce risk to your baby.

Bleeding in early pregnancy

Many normal pregnancies are associated with light bleeding, also referred to as 'spotting', during the first 12 weeks. Some people believe that hormonal changes can cause bleeding at times when a period would have occurred but this has not been substantiated. A common cause arises from small blood vessels in the uterus that open as the placenta implants, usually in the first six weeks. Implantation bleeding is usually light and does not indicate problems with the baby.

As a sign of a threatened MISCARRIAGE, bleeding often stops and pregnancy continues normally. If the pregnancy is definitely miscarrying, bleeding is profuse and is accompanied by pain and the passing of clots and embryonic material. Although rare, an ECTOPIC PREGNANCY may be associated with bleeding and severe pain. Bleeding may also be due to a vaginal infection, which has no effect on a baby's wellbeing, and may also occur later in pregnancy.

Bleeding in mid- and late pregnancy (antepartum haemorrhage)

Light spotting in the second half of pregnancy is usually not a cause for concern and pregnancy continues normally. Bleeding is not a symptom of a developmental abnormality in the baby. In the last weeks of pregnancy it may be a 'show' (page 360), consisting of blood mixed with mucus, and is a sign of imminent labour.

Occasionally, bleeding may be connected with a condition that requires medical care.
- It may be linked with cervical erosion or vaginal infection (bright red blood). Neither poses a risk to your baby. An erosion needs no treatment and an infection can be effectively treated.
- More seriously, a possible cause is a placenta praevia, or low-lying placenta (painless bleeding, bright red) (page 442). If you have this condition your baby may need to be delivered by CAESAREAN SECTION, especially if the bleeding is heavy or your pregnancy is full term.
- More seriously, but also very rarely, bleeding can be linked to placental abruption where the placenta separates from the wall of the uterus and emergency care is essential (usually dark red blood and abdominal pain). A severe abruption is very dangerous for you and your baby and an immediate caesarean section may be needed.
- Very rarely, bleeding in mid-pregnancy is a sign of late miscarriage (heavy loss, often containing clots) or early premature labour.

Action plan

Heavy bleeding requires emergency medical attention. You will be asked when the bleeding started and whether it is persistent or intermittent, its colour and quantity and if you have any pain.

You will be given a clinical examination and an ultrasound scan that allows a doctor to observe the position and function of the placenta and check the wellbeing of your baby. In late pregnancy, your baby's heartbeat will also be monitored. Then a plan of treatment can be recommended. This usually begins with resting and taking it easy. Further treatment depends on the underlying cause of the bleeding and the urgency of the situation.

Bleeding, mother, following birth

See Labour and birth, mother, bleeding following birth.

Bloating and flatulence

Feeling bloated and passing excessive wind is very common in pregnancy because of slower movement of food through the intestine combined with a change in diet, particularly if you eat something that your body is sensitive or allergic to (see ALLERGY AND INTOLERANCE). An excess of wind usually occurs after eating and is worse in the afternoon and evening. Sometimes, more often in late pregnancy, flatulence is accompanied by a feeling of swelling and bloating and uncomfortable INDIGESTION.

What happens

- Swallowed air is one cause of flatulence. You may swallow air quite unconsciously: as you talk, especially when you are upset or nervous, eating or drinking in a hurry, chewing gum or if you smoke.
- Some foods are not digested in the stomach but pass into the colon where they are processed by intestinal bacteria that produce gas. Common examples include:
  —foods rich in soluble fibre – such as fruit, beans, corn, peas, oats and wheat bran.
  —foods containing the simple sugar fructose, including figs, dates, prunes, melons, pears and grapes and, in lesser quantity, onions, asparagus, broccoli, cauliflower, Brussels sprouts, artichokes.
  —spicy foods.
  —wheat-containing foods (when there is an intolerance).
  —artificially sweetened 'diet' drinks or fizzy drinks.
  —lactose, a sugar found in milk, if you are lactose intolerant (page 20), and any dairy products may bring on flatulence.
- Flatulence can also accompany nausea or morning sickness, often because of swallowed air or a change in diet to alleviate the nausea.
- Intolerances and allergies, and irritable bowel syndrome (IBS) often cause flatulence in addition to the usual symptom of diarrhoea and/or constipation and may occur for the first time in pregnancy.
- CANDIDA infection in the gut can cause wind.
- After labour, wind may be caused by tearing of the anal sphincter, a valve that normally acts to prevent the involuntary release of gas (page 318).

Action plan

If you are worried that excess wind is hiding an underlying problem with your baby then a clinical examination or an ultrasound scan will put your mind at rest.

It is worth looking into your eating pattern. You may alter some habits with positive effects lasting a lifetime.

Diet

- Eat and drink slowly in a calm environment. Chew your food thoroughly before you swallow.
- For a few days, avoid foods most likely to cause flatulence (above). Then gradually add them to your diet again, one by one, while keeping track of your symptoms and noting which foods are a problem for you. You may find that a combination of foods triggers symptoms, rather than a single food in isolation.
- If you have dramatically increased the fibre in your diet, try cutting back and then increase the level more gradually until you find the optimum level (page 152).
- Try peppermint, chamomile or fennel tea after eating.
- Cut down on fizzy drinks and alcohol.
- Aduki beans are thought to reduce wind, particularly if they are well cooked. You may find adding more garlic, onion and ginger to your cooking helps.
- Try bio-yoghurt.
- A variety of herbs can aid digestion – try cooking with lemon balm, rosemary, sage, thyme, caraway or fennel.

Homeopathy

You may take one tablet (30c potency) four times a day for three to four days, then re-assess.

- *Carbo Veg* for gas in the upper abdomen, acid reflux, if your tummy rumbles, loud belching relieves the problem, you feel heavy and full, sluggish, chilly, and worse 30 minutes after food, and from wearing tight clothes.
- *China* if you are belching excessively with no relief, there is bloating, rumbling and gurgling in your tummy, colicky pains, particularly in the afternoon, a good appetite but food tastes bitter, you crave sour fruits and feel better from pressure on your abdomen.
- *Lycopodium* if you feel bloated all the time, hungry but quickly feel full and worse after eating cold food or beans, cabbage, onions or sweets, and much worse between 4 and 8pm.
- *Nux Moschata* when flatulence begins immediately after eating and there is a feeling of bloating with cramping pressure in the abdomen, your mouth and throat remain dry yet you are not thirsty, you crave spicy foods and may feel a bit spaced out and chilly.
- *Nux Vomica* if you want to pass wind but can't, feel pressure in an upward motion, colicky

spasms, lower back pain and nausea, worse about two hours after eating, crave spicy foods, feel uptight, irritable and stressed.

Blocked milk ducts

See Breastfeeding, difficulties.

Blocked nose, baby

See also Coughs and colds, baby.

A young baby's natural instinct is to breathe through the nose, even when it is blocked. So if your baby's nose is blocked, this may disrupt his sleep as well as breast- and bottle-feeding. His nose may be blocked because the lining membranes have swollen and not necessarily from excess mucus production alone. A stuffy nose may linger for a few weeks even when a cold has passed.

A blocked nose in a baby aged 4–6 months in the absence of a cold may be a sign of a food or pollen ALLERGY, although this is rare, and would need expert assessment.

Some babies seem to have a very sensitive lining to the nose and upper airways that is always swollen and producing excess mucus. This occurs when the function of blood vessels that feed the tissues is somehow impaired. See your doctor if your baby's blocked nose is causing you concern.

Snoring
Your baby may snore at night. This is usually perfectly normal, and nothing to worry about. Young babies tend to be noisy breathers in general because their airways are narrow and filled with lots of secretions. The air passing through these secretions causes vibratory sounds. Most of the time, these sounds gradually subside as a baby's airways grow and as he learns to swallow excess saliva. If your baby has a cold or a stuffy nose, his snoring may be louder.

Sleep apnoea
In the first year it is relatively unusual for the tonsils or adenoids to cause problems, and even more unusual for a doctor to recommend removal. Sometimes the enlarged tonsils or adenoids can affect feeding, as well as causing sleep difficulties. Often this is associated with a pre-existing problem affecting the skeleton or function of the head, neck and mouth, such as cleft lip or palate (page 142). It is not usual for tonsils and adenoids to be removed until later in childhood, as normal growth and development often significantly improve matters. Sleep-related apnoea (page 102) due to enlarged tonsils and adenoids is very rare in children aged under two years, and such a diagnosis requires assessment at a specialist centre.

Action plan
To help your baby breathe properly, clear his nasal passages by one of the following methods:
- Stand in a warm shower with your baby to allow the moist air to loosen excess secretions in his airways. Do this just before bedtime, since noisy breathing from clogged airways is mostly a problem during sleep.
- It may help to humidify the air where your baby is sleeping, using a warm-mist humidifier. This can be especially helpful if central heating has dried the air, or the air is cold.
- You might try saline nose drops, available from your local pharmacist.
- You may be advised to try a simple suction system (called an aspirator, and stocked by chemists), which removes mucus, but its usefulness is questionable as it may actually aggravate your baby's mucus-producing cells.
- Corticosteroid nose drops may sometimes be presented.

Massage
Gently massaging your baby's face, or giving him a light chest massage, may help. Appropriate techniques, together with other suggestions for making your baby comfortable, are discussed on page 158.

Homeopathy
The remedies below are specifically for use if your baby's nose is blocked. If you're using remedies for a cold, there may be some crossover. You may give the most appropriate remedy in 30c potency three times per day for three days and then re-assess.
- *Sambucus* for snuffly newborns who need to breathe through the mouth as the nose is dry and congested with thick mucus, when feeding is difficult and your baby may wake from sleep

suddenly as if desperate for breath. Congestion is worse from lying down, at midnight and from 2 to 3am and better from being held upright.

- *Nux vomica* for blocked nose, especially at night, with mouth breathing, the nose is running during the day; your baby may be irritable and difficult to settle and is worse in a warm room and at night.
- *Lycopodium* for a completely blocked nose when mucus is visible, your baby is mouth breathing and snoring, may have colicky symptoms, and the blockage is worse between 4 and 8pm.
- *Pulsatilla* when your baby's mucus is abundant and yellow, he is clingy, weepy and distressed, better for gentle motion and in the fresh air and worse for lying down and in a stuffy environment.
- *Kali Bich* for snuffles with thick, stringy mucus, your baby is worse on first waking and better for warmth and rest.

Blocked tear ducts

See Eye infection and swelling, baby.

Blood group and rhesus factor, mother

As part of your antenatal serum screening (page 30) your blood group and rhesus factor are checked. This picks up any discrepancy between your blood type and your baby's, and allows your team to take measures to prevent any potential effects for your baby.

ABO INCOMPATIBILITY

ABO incompatibility disease refers to the disease in the newborn that occurs because of a difference between the baby's and the mother's blood groups. The incompatibility may occur in babies with blood types A, B or AB whose mothers are of a different blood type. The most common is when the mother is blood group O and a baby is group A or B. This is similar in nature to Rhesus incompatibility (see below), but it cannot be prevented. Ordinarily this is a less severe problem than the Rhesus type of disease although it may be a cause of JAUNDICE after birth.

Usually women with group O blood have antibodies against A and B blood types that circulate in their bloodstream but are too large to pass across the placenta into the foetal circulation. However, some foetal red cells often cross into the mother's circulation. These foetal red cells stimulate the formation of a smaller type of anti-A or anti-B antibody, which can pass into the baby's circulation and cause the destruction of foetal red cells.

The degree of seriousness cannot be predicted from antibody levels alone. Very often the antibody levels are high but have no effect on the baby. In other cases, there is increased destruction of red cells that leads to jaundice after birth. Jaundice may need to be treated with phototherapy. The jaundice or destruction of the baby's red cells is usually complete by four to six weeks of age, and sometimes a BLOOD TRANSFUSION is required. Once jaundice has been treated, as well as any anaemia arising in the first six weeks, there is no other long-term effect.

If you have had one affected baby, the condition should be tested for at the birth of any subsequent babies, by analysing a sample of the cord blood.

RHESUS FACTOR

Most people (around 85 per cent) have a protein in their red blood cells called Rhesus factor. If you have it, you are Rhesus positive (Rh+). If you do not, you are Rhesus negative (Rh–). Rhesus factor has three components: C, D and E. The D is the most important.

Rhesus factor must be taken into account to ensure the correct blood is given in blood transfusions and for tissue typing. But otherwise Rhesus carries no implications regarding a woman's general health. It may be significant in pregnancy, however. Roughly 15 per cent of women are Rhesus negative. If the baby's father is also Rhesus negative, the baby will definitely be Rhesus negative and there will be no problem. But if the mother is Rhesus negative and the father is Rhesus positive there is a 50 per cent chance that the baby will be Rhesus positive, too.

If some of the baby's blood enters the mother's bloodstream, the mother's body will react to the baby's apparently foreign blood cells and produce anti-Rhesus antibodies. The antibodies usually have no effect on the first baby. But in a future pregnancy, if that baby is also Rhesus positive, the antibodies can cross the placenta and destroy some of the baby's red blood cells. Depending on the severity, this can lead to foetal ANAEMIA and JAUNDICE after birth. Fortunately, this is preventable.

Foetal cells may enter the mother's circulation:
* in small amounts during pregnancy,
* during amniocentesis or CVS,
* after antenatal bleeding or miscarriage,
* most likely during the birth as the placenta separates,
* if a Rhesus negative mother receives a blood transfusion of Rhesus positive blood.

Action plan

Any effect on a future baby can easily be prevented if you have an injection of anti-Rhesus D. The anti-Rhesus D mops up any red blood cells that may have travelled from your baby into your blood and prevents the development of destructive maternal antibodies.
* During pregnancy, the injection is given at Weeks 28 and 34 and also after amniocentesis or CVS antenatal bleeding. It is also given after MISCARRIAGE.
* After the birth, the cord blood from your baby will be tested to find the blood group and your blood will be checked for the presence of foetal red blood cells. If your baby is Rhesus positive you will be injected with anti-Rhesus D within 72 hours of birth, which ensures that you do not make antibodies that may affect a future Rhesus positive baby.

In the extremely unlikely event that you are Rhesus negative and have developed antibodies before pregnancy, this will be detected in an antenatal blood test. There is a chance that your baby may be affected. She will be regularly monitored by foetal medicine specialists using ultrasound scans, and the concentration of the antibodies in your blood will be checked every four weeks.

If your baby is severely affected and develops anaemia and resulting HYDROPS FOETALIS, a blood transfusion may be needed in the uterus before birth, or, if pregnancy is sufficiently advanced, labour may be induced and your baby will receive treatment for jaundice (phototherapy or even exchange transfusion) or anaemia.

Blood pressure, high and pre-eclampsia

Normal blood pressure is less than 140/90 mm of mercury (mm/Hg). Raised blood pressure is called hypertension. There is a specific type of hypertension that is linked to pregnancy known as pre-eclampsia or toxaemia of pregnancy.

High blood pressure in pregnancy has a number of causes:
* Pre-eclampsia, where it is pregnancy-related and disappears after birth (most common in first baby).
* Underlying hypertension present before conception, although it may not have been diagnosed. Usually the hypertension is familial in origin but rarely it is due to kidney disease.
* Sometimes a family tendency is brought to light by the pregnancy.

Mildly raised blood pressure may have little or no effect on you or your baby. A severe rise in blood pressure in pregnancy can have serious effects, including eclamptic convulsions (seizures or fits) and reduced blood flow to the placenta with reduced placental function and INTRAUTERINE GROWTH RESTRICTION (IUGR).

Pre-eclampsia occurs in around 5 per cent of first pregnancies and is usually mild. It can occur in later pregnancies. Commonly it does not begin until Week 34 and blood pressure usually goes back to normal after birth. If it is severe, however, it may begin earlier, and sometimes it does not arise until labour, or even a few days after birth.

'Eclampsia' is derived from the word 'eklampo', used by the ancient Greeks to mean 'lightning strike', and may have referred to the bright flashes that women see during seizures or to the fact that seizures sometimes strike without warning in apparently healthy pregnant women.

If you have essential hypertension (that is, of unknown cause) before you conceive the underlying hypertension may not change in pregnancy, but you are at higher risk of a further elevation. If existing high blood pressure is complicated by pre-eclampsia this is called essential hypertension with superimposed pre-eclampsia and needs careful monitoring, as it is more dangerous.

What happens

Symptoms of pre-eclampsia may not appear in the early stages. This is the reason for testing your blood pressure and urine throughout pregnancy so that treatment can begin early. Rarely, eclampsia can strike without pre-eclampsia signs.

Mild pre-eclampsia

- Blood pressure rises to 140/100 mm/Hg and there is slight swelling of the feet or hands and the urine contains no protein.
- Women often feel well and are surprised when a midwife takes the rise seriously.
- Early treatment can help to prevent a further rise.

Severe pre-eclampsia

- Blood pressure may rise above 160/110 mm/Hg and protein appears in the urine. This shows that the condition is having an effect on the kidneys and on blood vessels throughout your body, including the placenta.
- Other symptoms may include headache, dizziness, blurred vision, restlessness and irritability or drowsiness. There may be pain high in the abdomen and nausea (related to a swollen liver), bruising or bleeding (effects on blood clotting), and excess fluid retention with intense puffiness of the limbs or the face and excess weight gain.
- Severe pre-eclampsia becomes eclampsia when fits or convulsions occur (indicating effects on the brain). This may be preceded by severe headache, blurred vision, confusion and pain in the abdomen. It may lead to coma. This life-threatening condition for mother and baby is unlikely to happen with modern obstetric care, which ensures that treatment begins before eclampsia occurs.
- If pre-eclampsia becomes severe there is an increased risk of bleeding related to placental abruption (page 444), and immediate delivery may be necessary.

What may cause pre-eclampsia?

The exact cause of pre-eclampsia is unknown. There may be a genetic predisposition. It is likely that the condition is related to the immune system reacting to the placenta or the baby. Researchers believe that pre-eclampsia may be part of a spectrum of disorders that begin in the first few weeks of pregnancy as the placenta implants and invades the arteries in the wall of the uterus. Incomplete invasion may lead to a number of conditions, including pre-eclampsia where the baby is growing normally, or reduced foetal growth (page 322) with or without pre-eclampsia. A recent theory is that the placenta may release an excess of 'FLT' protein that affects the cells lining the mother's arteries and leads to high blood pressure. Pre-eclampsia is more likely if you are carrying TWINS.

If you have a strong family history of high blood pressure or had high blood pressure before pregnancy you may experience a further rise during pregnancy. A diet deficient in nutrition and vitamins and minerals before and during early pregnancy may increase the likelihood of a rise in blood pressure. High blood pressure may also accompany an existing kidney disorder.

Action plan

The key preventive measure is to ensure you are well nourished (page 253) and you are getting an adequate balance of exercise and rest. If you are genetically predisposed it is still important to stick to a nutritious diet.

- Most pre-eclampsia is mild and babies of affected mothers are usually big and healthy. Often the only difference in care is closer monitoring.
- If you have mildly raised pressure, relax, look after yourself and continue to be monitored.
- Be aware that excessive weight gain or swelling may be signs of a further rise.

+ Red flag

If you have protein in your urine or are diagnosed with severe pre-eclampsia or you have headaches, blurred vision or abdominal pain you will need intense treatment and monitoring.

Medical care

- If pre-eclampsia is mild your blood pressure and urine will need to be checked twice a week, or on a daily basis, depending on the level of pressure. You may test your urine protein levels at home and use a portable electronic machine to check your blood pressure. If you are nervous of hospitals the level may be falsely high when you are checked by the midwife; this is called the white coat syndrome.

- You will also be given blood tests to assess kidney and liver function and blood-clotting ability. This is particularly important if your hypertension is familial or you have a kidney problem.
- Your baby's wellbeing will be assessed: you will be examined and asked to note the movements and may be given additional ultrasound scans.
- If pre-eclampsia is severe, you will be admitted to hospital and checks will be made more frequently.
- If blood pressure remains above 150/100 mm/Hg, particularly if there is protein in your urine or hypertension has been present before pregnancy, anti-hypertensive medication may be needed. The drugs are usually taken as tablets but if the situation is urgent the anti-hypertensives are given by intravenous infusion in hospital. If the pre-eclampsia is severe this may be given in combination with anti-convulsant medication, such as magnesium sulphate, to prevent eclamptic fits. It is preferable not to use benzodiazepine (valium) as an anti-convulsant to avoid affecting your baby's breathing and alertness after birth. The medicines are powerful agents and you will require frequent blood pressure and urine checks and blood tests. If anti-convulsant medication is needed for more than a few hours it is usually necessary to deliver the baby urgently.

Lifestyle, diet and complementary therapies
These therapies are very useful in conjunction with medical monitoring and may help to keep blood pressure manageable until your baby is mature and to reduce pressure if severe pre-eclampsia is developing.

- It is sensible to rest: reduce strenuous activities and stop or cut down on work.
- If the pressure is very high, bed rest may be advised.
- If you have mildly elevated blood pressure, exercise within your comfort zone will improve circulation and can stabilise levels. Gentle yoga stretches may help.
- Meditation and visualisation are useful.
- Continue to take vitamin and mineral supplements and omega essential fatty acids. In cooking, use plenty of garlic. It may improve circulation and help reduce high blood pressure.
- Reducing salt in the diet is useful as a preventive measure.

- Acupuncture can help to reduce high pressure.
- Homeopathy can have powerful effects but qualified advice must be taken. Remedies for swelling may be an effective way to reduce fluid retention and swelling, but do not tackle the underlying cause of raised blood pressure.
- Aromatherapy oils that may help include orange, petitgrain, tangerine, sandalwood, ylang ylang and bergamot, and low doses of rose and melissa. All use needs to be guided by an aromatherapist and after consultation with your doctor. Use the oils in the bath or mixed with a base oil for massage (as described on page 36). From Week 24 lavender can be used.

When early birth is necessary
- You can safely wait for labour to begin spontaneously if hypertension is mild, provided your baby is healthy.
- Where hypertension is significant and your baby is mature, induction of labour may be advised (page 374), and you and your baby will both be monitored closely.
- If pre-eclampsia is severe and there is INTRAUTERINE GROWTH RESTRICTION or a risk of eclampsia, a PREMATURE BIRTH either by induction or CAESAREAN SECTION may be safer for you and your baby.
- If you have very severe pre-eclampsia or are having eclamptic convulsions, immediate caesarean section is the best option.

Treatment during labour
You and your baby will be closely monitored during labour, with frequent checks of your blood pressure and urinary protein levels and your baby's heart patterns.

- Epidural anaesthesia (page 383) may reduce high blood pressure and anti-hypertensive drugs will be used if they are needed.
- If contractions are weak or ineffectual the usual drug used to enhance them, oxytocin, needs to be administered with caution because in high doses it may elevate blood pressure.
- Ergometrine, which is often used after the birth to reduce bleeding, must be avoided because it may significantly raise blood pressure.

After the birth
Blood pressure usually begins to drop within a few hours of birth.

- Your baby will be carefully examined to check for any effects of reduced placental function and intrauterine growth restriction. If he has been born prematurely, care will reflect the stage of pregnancy and his condition at birth.
- When pre-eclampsia has been severe the risk of eclamptic convulsions continues for up to seven days after the birth, so observation and treatment need to continue.
- The midwives will monitor your blood pressure postnatally because occasionally pre-eclampsia can begin in the first few days after birth.

Blood pressure, low and fainting

Low blood pressure (hypotension) is usually a sign of good health in pregnancy. If you have naturally low blood pressure it may drop lower and return to normal as soon as your baby is born. The level naturally falls in the middle trimester by 10 mm/Hg. If pressure drops significantly, however, it may cause dizziness or faintness. A level below 90/55 mm/Hg is significant, although many fit athletes have levels below this. Your midwife will assess the significance of your blood pressure in the context of your personal lifestyle and changes to the levels as pregnancy progresses.

Action plan

Excessively low blood pressure is usually completely avoidable with a balanced diet, regular gentle exercise and yoga, and by avoiding sitting or standing for too long. Drinking appropriate amounts of fluid also helps to improve circulation. If you have low blood pressure and feel faint or dizzy you will need to address the cause.
- Sit down straight away: this will help blood flow back to your heart, and if you do faint you will avoid being injured by falling.
- As you stand up from sitting or lying or when you have to stand or sit for a long time, you can prevent fainting by contracting and releasing the muscles in both calves, thighs and buttocks for two to three seconds each time. As the muscles contract they pump blood back to your heart, the circulation to your brain is restored and you no longer feel faint.

- Standing for prolonged periods or getting up suddenly may cause blood to pool in your legs, and the lack of blood flowing to the brain makes you feel faint. Sitting for a long time may have a similar effect. The effect is stronger if you are unfit, if you have varicose veins (wear support tights), if you have consumed alcohol or taken drugs to lower blood pressure or when in hot temperatures. It reduces if you move around regularly.
- In mid- to late pregnancy, if you lie flat on your back, the weight of your uterus and baby presses on the arteries and veins that run along the back of the abdominal cavity and this may reduce the amount of blood flowing back to your heart. This occurs only in a small percentage of women. You may find it more comfortable to lie on your side in bed, particularly in late pregnancy.
- If you have a low level of sugar in your blood, called hypoglycaemia (page 261), you may feel faint and also have low blood pressure. This is completely avoidable with a balanced diet – eat regularly and consume a balance of slow-burning (starchy) carbohydrates with vitamins, minerals, roughage and plenty of fluid.

On rare occasions, loss of blood from BLEEDING in pregnancy can lead to a severe fall in blood pressure, known as clinical shock. This is an emergency that requires urgent intravenous fluid replacement.

Homeopathy for fainting
You may take the most appropriate remedy in 30c potency immediately and repeat half an hour later. Rescue Remedy may be hugely beneficial as well.
- *Aconite* for fainting accompanied by anxiety or fear, usually at night. It is often the first remedy to choose if you get up 'too quickly' and feel faint, and if you feel better from fresh air and moderate temperatures.
- *Carbo Veg* for fainting with weakness, when you are pale and feel clammy and cold, and feel better from being fanned and from fresh air. This remedy is extremely helpful just as you are coming round from a faint.
- *Sepia* if you faint from weakness and exhaustion, if your blood pressure falls because of the way you've been standing or sitting, and if you feel great heat followed by chilliness.

71

• *Belladonna* if you faint after becoming over-heated, you feel dazed, agitated and flushed, with no tolerance for bright lights, noise or jarring motion, and you are very thirsty.

• *Bryonia* if fainting comes on with dehydration or sudden movement, your mouth is dry, you're thirsty and irritable, feel better for sweating and having a cool drink or moving to a cooler environment.

Blood screening, baby

See also Anaemia, baby; Bleeding, baby.

■ HAEMOGLOBINOPATHY SCREENING

The haemoglobinopathies are a group of diseases ('-opathies') of haemoglobin, the red pigment in blood. In these blood conditions, the way oxygen is carried around the body is altered and as a result there can be serious health problems. The two main diseases, although rare, are sickle cell disease and thalassaemia. There are two screening tests for these:

• antenatal maternal blood sampling (and paternal sampling if the mother is a carrier), and
• postnatal newborn blood spot screening.

In some parts of the country, the routine blood spot test performed using a simple heel prick six to eight days after birth (page 338) is screened for the haemoglobinopathies. Bigger cities are considered to have enough families at risk to warrant all infants having blood spot analysis, while other areas are more selective. Your local antenatal clinic will be able to tell you if you will be offered the tests at booking and at birth. You should receive a leaflet detailing the different blood spot tests when you book for your pregnancy.

Blood transfusion, mother

Blood transfusion is only used where there is an emergency or where your haemoglobin level is very low, usually below 8 gm/dl (page 26). The donor blood will be obtained from your local blood transfusion service and emergency supplies are kept in the hospital. Your blood group is known from antenatal blood tests. A repeat blood sample is taken and the laboratory will cross-match it with the donor's blood to ensure the two are compatible. Rhesus (Rh) and other blood groups will be checked to ensure the new blood will not cross-react with antibodies in your circulation.

The donor blood is also checked for infections, particularly HEPATITIS and HIV. The possibility of being infected is very remote with modern cross-checking and has been estimated at less than one in a million.

The procedure takes about four hours but can be speeded up to a matter of minutes in an emergency where there is shock. It is given intravenously with a drip and you can sit up in bed during the transfusion. After a transfusion it is best to take iron supplements to replace your iron stores for the next six months.

Blues

See Emotions, sadness and happiness.

Body image and self-esteem

Your body image is how you feel in your body, and how you think you appear to others. Whether it is positive or negative depends on what's happening in your life at the moment (including whether you feel tired, sore, clean, physically toned or well dressed). It also rests on the way you value yourself, or your self-esteem.

Your self-esteem involves your opinion of whether you are good enough, whether you feel loved, precious and important. It is based on experiences over your lifetime, beginning in infancy. As a baby you may have felt loved, valued and affirmed, and enjoyed close bonds in your family. If so, it is likely you developed a sense of self-worth. Alternatively, you may not have felt loved, or welcomed, or you may have been criticised or hurt. If so, your self-esteem may have been lower. Your early foundations are part of your emotional make-up (page 206). For many people, the level of self-esteem established in infancy remains in childhood, adolescence and adulthood, although along the way relationships, situations or personal choices can alter it.

Wherever you start from, your self-esteem may soar and plummet during the primal period (the period between conception and your baby's first birthday). Many things affect the way you feel about yourself – love, smiles, laughter, tiredness, pain, a crying baby, fluctuations in weight, irregular meals, social life, and so on. Self-esteem may dip without familiar props such as work; equally it may rise in the presence of your loving baby and as your parenting skills improve.

If your self-esteem is low, it may be useful to consider how well you are caring for yourself. This includes being with people who love you, eating and exercising well, receiving support, being guided by your feelings and regularly assessing what works well for you and your family (page 124). The key to boosting your self-esteem will be unique to you – maybe friends and family might help you feel better, you may join a group or opt for counselling or psychotherapy (page 162). You may also turn your attention to your outer appearance.

Feeling good, looking good

Both before and after birth, many mums feel positive when they dress up and pamper themselves. Just doing your makeup or hair, or getting out of your house clothes into a different outfit, can help you feel good. You may have a friend who can give tips on enhancing your good points or you could treat yourself to a day with a stylist.

In pregnancy
* Resist the temptation to swamp yourself in tent-like dresses or squeeze into things that are too small.
* Low-waist trousers and stylish tracksuit bottoms are comfy and flattering.
* Avoid tops with horizontal stripes if you are feeling big. Low-slung tops or V-necks are flattering.
* Until the last few months of pregnancy you may be able to wear non-maternity drawstring trousers and tunics in your normal size. As soon as these get too tight, it's time to move into maternity clothes. Non-maternity clothes

two sizes larger than you used to wear will not flatter.
* Wear a good bra, changing size as you grow. If you are unsure of your size, ask to be measured. Most good clothes shops have trained staff who can do this.
* If your feet are swollen, invest in a comfortable pair of shoes or boots. Keep high heels for special occasions.
* There are specialist lingerie shops and websites for beautiful underwear in pregnancy. Feeling sexy is fun.
* A light foundation or subtle bronzer can improve your skin tone if hormones make your face blotchy or spotty, or if nausea leaves you pale. A subtle gloss or lipstick may be very flattering.
* A dash of mascara is often all that is needed to highlight your eyes and transform your face.
* If you feel heavy, a hair cut may lift your face and your spirits.

After the birth
* Gather some comfy clothes to wear at home that wash and dry easily.
* Choose tops made for breastfeeding, and/or a selection of button-fronted shirts/dresses and cardigans.
* A good bra is really important.
* Rest a muslin cloth over your shoulder to catch your baby's dribbles.
* Absorbent washable breast pads help to keep your tops clean and dry.
* Allow yourself time to get into pre-pregnancy trousers and tops. It is okay to downsize gradually – what's important is to feel comfortable.

'Bodymind'

Whatever happens in your body is always linked to the way you feel emotionally, and the same applies in reverse – all your emotional feelings have a physical presence in your body. Something in your body can affect your emotions, just as an emotional feeling can impact your body. As hormones change, for instance, or when you get hungry or when you exercise, your mood alters. Equally, if being with another person is making you happy or agitated, your body reflects this (you may become relaxed or tense, have tummy or back pain, develop a headache, and so on). There is also a spiritual element (page 73), which may be very important for you. The term 'bodymind' reflects this integration. It is an essential concept that reflects the philosophy of this book.

The concept of body and mind being inter-related is as relevant today as it was in the time of the ancient Greeks. It has been accepted in many systems of medicine across the world for many thousands of years. 'Bodymind' implies the 'whole' person and applies to everyone – including you and your baby.

Sometimes, physical problems have their root cause in an emotional issue (for example, depression often manifests with altered sleep patterns, chronic pain, bowel disturbances, etc.) The body never lies. Sometimes, emotions reveal a physical issue (for instance, irritability when hormones or blood sugar are out of balance). The mutual 'bodymind' influence is ongoing from second to second.

In pregnancy, women and babies are further influenced by one another. Your baby and the placenta affect your body and your emotions, and what is happening in your 'bodymind' influences your baby's environment. There are many ways you and your baby communicate in pregnancy, including through hormones (page 307), movement and sound.

Many people believe that the integration of body and mind means our bodies hold memories and emotions on an unconscious level. There are numerous fields of study relating to this. Some focus on the brain; some focus on the wider nervous system; others look at hormones; others at chakras; others at genes; others at a wider holistic picture. All concur that what happens in each person's life, from conception onwards, becomes part of that person's uniqueness – his or her physical make-up, self-esteem, emotional sensitivities, memories, health tendencies, and so on.

Caring for yourself means attending to your physical, emotional and spiritual wellbeing. If something feels out of balance it's worth considering several aspects of you (page 123). Caring for your baby follows the same principles – nurturing him well involves caring for his emotional *and* his physical needs, and respecting his spirit or his

individuality with love and acceptance. The suggestions on page 208 are simple tips for being emotionally nurturing and there is advice throughout this book on the many elements of wellbeing.

Bonding

See Emotions, bonding and attachment.

Bottle-feeding

Breast milk is the best food for your baby. It is protocol in most hospitals for mothers to be given information detailing the benefits of breast milk and supported to have undisturbed time, preferably with skin-to-skin contact, to try BREASTFEEDING from birth. A bottle of formula should not be given to your baby from birth except for medical reasons, or after a full discussion with you.

Current recommendations for optimal nutrition and mother–baby bonding are to breastfeed exclusively for six months. For a small number of women and babies, bottle-feeding needs to begin from birth because breastfeeding is not an option (for example, because of HIV infection) and there are some women who elect not to breastfeed. For mothers who do breastfeed from birth, bottle-feeding may be introduced weeks or months later and the reasons for this are wide ranging. For example, sometimes a baby indicates a preference, or sometimes it's the mum's choice. A minority of women never bottle-feed at all.

Formula milk cannot give your baby all the goodness of breast milk – yet it does contain a balanced quota of nutrients, including vitamins and minerals, and most babies thrive on it. When you bottle-feed, you and your baby can enjoy lots of close contact, and feeding time may be intimate for you both. Creating a relaxed environment, helping your baby to suck at her own pace by angling the bottle in her favour, and being aware of your own comfort will help both of you to relax. Skin-to-skin contact makes most babies feel good, and is simple when you bottle-feed. You can hold your baby naked (except for a nappy) against your body, covered with a soft blanket or towel.

Formula milk and weight gain

A number of research studies have linked bottle-feeding with the rise in childhood obesity. It is easier for babies to consume more calories than they need from formula milk because the formula does not respond to a baby's requirements for calories, protein and fluid as well as human breast milk does. There is a belief that babies who are formula-fed too much or too frequently may develop the propensity for gaining weight later in life. If you tune into your baby and follow her signals – just as you would if you were breastfeeding – and take advice if you are unsure how much milk to give as your baby's weight increases, you will be offering your baby a good start. Your health visitor will monitor your baby's growth and development and let you know if the gain is too high or too low (page 559).

■ BONDING AND EMOTIONS

See also Emotions.

Baby

Your baby's emotional response to feeding from a bottle will be unique to her. Many babies make a very smooth transition to the bottle and don't complain, and each feeding time may offer precious contact and a chance for bonding more deeply. Eye contact and touch enhance bonding and your baby will feel good if you are relaxed and focused on her. Providing she is comfortable, and has lots of love from you, she is likely to enjoy feeding times and will continue to get the nutrients she needs for growth. Bottle-feeding may be a great chance for your baby to bond more deeply with a range of adults – she may get a lot of pleasure from spending more time with her dad, aunts and uncles, and perhaps with siblings. She may feel most safe and relaxed if held skin to skin.

If the person feeding your baby is distracted, or being bottle-fed means your baby misses out on regular contact with you, she may be upset or angry. She may not show this vocally. Creating quality time and responding to your baby's cues allows her to communicate her needs and to receive the touch, love and food that she requires.

Mother

Bottle-feeding your baby may bring up a range of emotions for you. You may be happy that you and your baby are well and enjoy feeding this way. If you were previously having difficulties breastfeeding, or if your baby seems more settled now you have introduced a bottle, you may feel relieved. Other members of your family – particularly your baby's dad – may be delighted that they can enjoy feeding times.

Some mothers feel quite low when breastfeeding ends, both as a result of hormonal changes and because they miss the intimacy. Fortunately, there are many ways to stay close and bottle-feeding does not mean you cannot be together, skin to skin, or sleep together, if this is what you both enjoy. You may feel guilty if bottle-feeding is not what you had hoped to do or if you have gone against your baby's preferences. If you have lots of quality time with your baby, your baby is putting on weight and thriving, and you are also feeling well, your guilt may soon disappear. If you continue to feel guilty (page 213) weighing up the pros and cons for you, your baby and your family may help you accept the way things are and enjoy the positive aspects of bottle-feeding.

If you are in a social situation where you are frequently defending yourself or justifying your choice this can be tiring. Peer pressure sometimes makes women who choose to bottle-feed feel like failures – but there is a distinction between the view of other people and your own gut feelings. It may be helpful to talk to someone who supports your choice.

■ COMBINING BREAST AND BOTTLE

Combining breast and bottle may be a practical option for you and your baby. You may use formula feed or expressed milk (after Weeks 6–8). This may allow you time to rest, go to a regular class, to work, or to have an unbroken night's sleep; and your baby may respond well if the formula milk satisfies her for longer (it does take longer to digest than breast milk). Occasionally, supplemental bottle-feeding is advised to increase a baby's intake if her weight gain is slow and this has been confirmed by a health professional (page 559).

Success depends on a few factors: your own milk supply, your baby's preference for breast over bottle (or vice versa) and consistency. It is not advisable to introduce a bottle before your milk supply is well established. It is optimal to exclusively breastfeed for six months before you begin to offer bottles. At the earliest, it is best to wait until after Week 6. This is because for the first six weeks the milk-making hormone prolactin regulates your milk supply, in response to your baby. After this its flow maintains the supply. Prolactin is also at its highest during night feeds, so if you wish to continue breastfeeding it is best not to skip these and potentially reduce your supply. Some mothers do find that once they begin supplemental bottle-feeding their breast milk supply reduces. Generally, your breasts and your baby will accommodate the change most easily if you offer a bottle at the same time(s) each day and keep feeding your baby at night and for the first morning feed.

If your breasts become uncomfortable when you reduce breastfeeding, you may need to take precautions against engorgement (page 93).

Working women sometimes express in their lunch hour to maintain their milk supply, and this makes it simpler to breastfeed exclusively on days when they don't work. Employers in the UK are required by European Union Law to provide women time off and appropriate facilities to express breast milk.

If your baby rejects the bottle

If your baby rejects the bottle you may decide that she has made a good choice, and follow her lead and breastfeed exclusively for longer. If your initial choice was made because you were feeling tired or overwhelmed there may be several things you can do to rest and to have time to yourself. The advice on page 81 may help you maintain your energy.

Alternatively, you may feel that on balance you have no choice (for example if you have to return to work), or you have been advised by your doctor that it is important for your baby to consume extra calories from formula milk. The first thing to try as you encourage your baby is gentle persistence, helping her get used to it. She probably misses breastfeeding. You may need to try a range of teats. Some parents find it easiest for a dad or grandparent to offer the bottle at first, giving their baby a chance to get used to the bottle without the distracting smell of mum's breasts. If this works, once your baby

is happy drinking from a bottle, she is likely to enjoy taking the bottle from you and you can still have precious contact during feeding time.

▨ HOW MUCH AND HOW OFTEN TO FEED?

It's important to ensure your baby receives sufficient nourishment – neither too little nor too much. The suggestions below are guidelines. There is huge variation between babies, and your own baby's appetite will fluctuate.

Feeding on demand

It is important to be aware of your baby's needs and follow her cues instead of placing all the emphasis on finishing a bottle. This is infant-led care (page 432) in practice. If you give her what she asks for, rather than what you think she should eat, you will avoid having a hungry baby, or a baby who is gaining weight too quickly. The early days are for learning how your baby signals her needs, and in time you will learn her language. Beyond seven or eight months, some parents and babies develop simple sign language (such as thumb in mouth) to indicate thirst or hunger.

If your baby is still hungry after a feed, she will be restless or cry, although she may also cry because of wind or COLIC. If she has had enough, she'll show her lack of interest by CRYING or turning her head, or may hit the bottle with her hands. She may continue sucking if you press her, even if she isn't hungry. If your baby seems to ask for more milk, it may be time to try a small increase (below). On hot days she may just be thirsty and pre-boiled, cooled water may satisfy her.

The first days

Your baby needs to eat little and often at first. She may be hungry every one or two hours, and drink only 50ml (between 1 and 2fl oz) at a time. The exact amount depends on her size and these guidelines apply if your baby is born at full term. In the early days, feeding on demand ensures your baby will feed when she is hungry.

By two or three weeks

The gaps between feeds may now get longer, and she may take 100ml (3fl oz) per feed. Again, the precise amounts vary according to your baby's size. You will soon recognise her hunger cries.

After a number of weeks

Over time a pattern may fall into place. Generally, bottle-fed babies take a drink of milk roughly every three hours for a total of six to eight feeds a day. As your baby grows, the number of feeds each day may not change but the amount will increase. By four weeks she may drink 140ml (4fl oz) and by 12 weeks your baby may drink 210ml (6fl oz), although there's no need to worry if she still only takes 140ml (4fl oz) and is gaining weight adequately. If you make 35ml (1fl oz) more than your baby usually drinks she will leave a little, and when she begins to drain the whole bottle, increase the amount by a further 35ml (1fl oz). Continue to do this in stages. The maximum amount for a single feed is 280ml (8fl oz).

Your baby's feeding rhythm

Formula milk takes longer to digest than breast milk, and many bottle-fed babies soon establish a reasonably regular feeding schedule, although this isn't universal and some do not. The ideal is to follow your baby's lead and to work together in partnership, rather than to force her into a structure. The benefits of flexibility and of rhythm over routine are discussed on page 436.

Even the most predictable baby has unexpected hunger in the middle of the night or a voracious appetite one day and wants less the next. Like all babies, yours will have growth spurts and may have unsettled or hungry patches on a regular basis, so keep your routine flexible.

Wind and colic

- If your baby is very windy after feeding or appears to have tummy pain or colic (page 144), you may be able to ease her discomfort by altering her position during a feed. There are also teats designed to reduce air-swallowing.
- If your baby seems to be guzzling and milk escapes her mouth and runs down her chin, it's quite likely the flow is too fast and this may give her wind. A different shape of teat with a slower rate of flow may suit your baby better. There are many types available, including teats

for newborns. Tilting the bottle differently may also help – less of an angle puts less pressure on the milk and helps decrease the flow. Try it out on your hand: is the milk dripping slowly or squirting out?

- An important element of feeding is the environment. When you are relaxed and not rushed, and your baby feels closely connected with you, having eye contact and perhaps being skin to skin, she may eat less hurriedly and enjoy time to relax and digest in your arms. She may need to break often during a feed, and when you are in tune with her, and not in a hurry to finish a feed, it is easier for her to take the time she needs.

▨ NIGHT FEEDS

For many months, your baby needs milk in the early hours of the morning (between midnight and 7am) as well as last thing at night (around 10 or 11pm). Do what you can to keep night feeds as *un*interesting as possible. Some time after the eighth week she might drop the early morning feed, but this is not a rule and many babies continue to enjoy this feed for longer. Her preferences depend in part on her digestive system and how peacefully she sleeps, and in part on how you guide her. Whether she wakes for a feed may reflect how she eats and sleeps during the day.

After 12 weeks, if your baby is waking frequently and drinks only 35ml (1fl oz) before falling asleep, she may be waking for comfort rather than hunger. She may have a powerful need to be with you, to suck, and to feel your touch and hear your heartbeat and your voice. It may be worth looking at your daytime routine – if you are out during the day, and not with your baby as frequently or for as long as she needs, spending more time together may reduce her craving for you at night. You may decide to alter your daytime commitments, and/or to co-sleep if you cannot have quality time together during the day.

Never resort to adding extra formula to a bottle or mixing it with baby cereal in an attempt to get your baby to sleep for longer. When a baby eats solid food before her digestive system is sufficiently mature there is an increased risk of some childhood illnesses and the extra calories may contribute to excessive weight gain (for more see weaning, page 557).

▓ PREPARING BOTTLES

Cleaning and sterilising

Your baby has a very sensitive digestive system and for the first year is particularly susceptible to bacterial infection, so it is important that everything that she sucks and drinks is sterile.

Always clean bottles thoroughly in hot soapy water using a bottle brush that is not used for ordinary washing up. Make sure all milk deposits are cleaned off. Turn the teats inside out and squeeze them lightly to test for blockages. Thoroughly rinse everything, then sterilise using one of the methods below. If your bottles or teats become damaged or torn, throw them away, as cracks trap dirt.

- *Boiling.* Immerse everything in a pan of water and boil for 10 minutes. Keep the bottles in the sealed pan until you are ready to make them up. Regular boiling can shorten the lifespan of teats.
- *Steaming.* Electrically operated steam units sterilise effectively without chemicals and are large enough to hold a good quantity of bottles and accessories. The sterilisation cycle takes 10–12 minutes. It turns off automatically and can be re-used soon after. This is handy when you're in a hurry or discover you're one teat short. You can also use a vegetable steamer, but if you do, reserve it for bottle use only (not general cooking) and keep a close watch on it while it's on the heat (15 minutes) as the water will evaporate if left boiling for too long.
- *Chemical sterilisers.* Sterilising units use cold water and a chemical solution or soluble tablets. This sterilises in 30 minutes and items can be left soaking for up to 24 hours. When you are ready to make up the feeds, every part of the bottle kit needs to be rinsed well with previously boiled and cooled water.
- *Microwave.* Special sterilisers are available for use in microwaves, designed to avoid any 'cold spots'. Otherwise a microwave is not suitable for sterilising.
- *Dishwashers.* After cleaning your bottles and teats with a brush, you can run them through a dishwasher cycle that may be hot enough to sterilise them, and you'll need to make up the feeds as soon as the washing programme has finished. Check with the manufacturer regarding temperature settings and sterilisation.

Making up feeds using powdered milk formula

1. Boil the water and leave for a few minutes to cool slightly. Do not use water that has been boiled repeatedly as this increases its sodium content.
2. Wash and sterilise your bottles, teats and caps, and any jug you are using for mixing. Sterilising methods are listed above.
3. Wipe clean the area and wash your hands.
4. With the boiled water still hot (around 70°C/160°F) fill the sterilised bottle to the required level.
5. Using the measuring scoop provided, follow the instructions for mixing precisely and add the powder to the water in the bottle. Across the UK the standard measurement is 35ml (1fl oz) of water to one level scoop of powder. Using more than this will make your baby ill. To be sure you use a level scoop, use the spatula provided or a plastic knife (and keep them sterile).
6. Place the disc on the bottle, then the teat, then the lid, and shake it well so the formula dissolves.
7. Test the temperature of the milk by squeezing a few drops onto the inside of your wrist. If it feels hot rather than warm, cool it by standing it in cold water or holding it under a running tap.
8. If your baby drinks only half the milk in a bottle, do not give her the remainder later. Germs breed rapidly in warm milk and can cause digestive upset.
9. UNICEF guidelines recommend that you do not make up bottles in advance, since powdered milk is not sterile. If you are on the move, take freshly boiled water with you in a sealed flask, and make up the feed when you need it.
10. Never boil water or heat bottled milk in a microwave.

Water softeners and mains water

Do not use domestic softened water for your baby. Water softeners work by replacing hard insoluble calcium with sodium (from salt). Although the water is not salty to taste it will have higher than normal concentrations of sodium, which is dangerous for your baby's kidneys. The manufacturer of the water softener will have advised the installer to leave at least one tap out of the system, to deliver mains water. Mains water that has been put through a filter still needs to be boiled before you give it to your baby, at least until she begins to eat solids (and in every case if you are unsure of the safety of the tap water).

▧ TYPES OF FORMULA MILK

Cow's milk formula

Your baby requires specially processed milk. Raw pasteurised cow's milk, as delivered to your doorstep, is unsuitable without modification for children under one year of age. Almost all baby milk powders are made from cow's milk. 'First' milks are whey based and more easily digested when your baby is young. 'Second' or 'follow-on' milks are casein based and take longer to digest – these are suitable for your older baby. Different brands tend to contain the same, or very similar, components, but your baby may find some brands easier to digest than others and you may wish to exclude some ingredients if you have a special diet (vegetarian or kosher, for instance). For your first feeds, buy a small tin of baby milk powder until you feel confident that it is suitable. If you are switching from BREASTFEEDING, your baby's digestive system may take time to adjust to the formula. Never give your baby standard cow's milk, condensed milk or skimmed milk powder mixed with water. These contain too much salt and protein for your baby.

Many baby milk formulae can contain genetically modified (GM) products and these may not be labelled. If you want to avoid GM products, opt for organic formula. Until your baby is six months old, do not use 'follow-on' milk, whose constituents are not suitable for her digestive system.

Non cow's milk formula

A small number of babies show an adverse reaction to their formula and this may reflect an ALLERGY OR INTOLERANCE. If your baby develops DIARRHOEA, fails to gain weight or has a skin rash, take her to the doctor who will consider the possible causes.

Below six months of age the only alternatives recognised as nutritionally complete, and reducing the risk of an allergic response, are the cow's milk hydrolysates. Hydrolysates are partially digested cow's milk formula milks – and are generally lactose free. The cow's milk protein

has been broken down by a scientific process into the amino acids which make up the protein. As a result the milk is not recognised by a baby's immune system as a cow's milk formula, and the reaction that causes diarrhoea and general upset, which amounts to the symptoms of cow's milk intolerance, stops almost immediately. These special milk products have various trade names. The most frequently used one in the UK is Pepti, although Nutramigen is also available. These are designed to be safe and nutritionally complete, and are available only on prescription.

You may be advised to try formula based on modified soya, which can be bought in chemists and supermarkets or prescribed and may be used after six months of age. These milks are also lactose free. They are usually recommended if there is a history of allergy, but not as a preventive measure, as there is no scientific evidence that suggests soya-based milks prevent allergy occurring later, although they may well help reduce apparent cow's milk sensitive symptoms in some babies. Like cow's milk formula, soya formula requires no supplementation. Never give unmodified soya milk as it does not provide sufficient nourishment and the sodium content may be dangerously high. Soya-based formula feeds may contain an excess of plant oestrogens (phyto-oestrogens) and it is best to consult a paediatrician if you use soya formula milk exclusively.

Goat's milk infant formula is banned as a baby food for babies under one year in the UK and EU. It has not been proven to reduce allergies and contains insufficient iron, zinc, B6, B12 and folate. Older babies fed with goat's milk formula need to take supplements.

Anti reflux milks

There are several cow's milk-based formulas available which have a ready added thickener for babies who have problems with reflux (page 554). They are especially useful for the mild reflux baby, where the fuss of adding the antacid Gaviscon can be avoided.

Follow-on milks

Follow-on milks, which contain iron, are really only useful for babies of about one year of age who have extra nutritional needs, such as long-term lung problems, or other chronic illnesses, and who are unable to tolerate solid diets. If your baby has no special dietary needs, it is fine to give her pasteurised 'doorstep' cow's milk after one year of age.

Boundaries

See Parenting, boundaries.

Bow legs

See also Rickets.

Bow legs occur when the knees do not touch when the ankles are pressed together, either in a lying or standing position. Some degree of bow legs is quite normal for the first two years – almost all children have bow legs when they first learn to walk and will gradually lose the tendency. In the first year, then, it is unlikely that you will be worried about bow legs.

If you are concerned that the gap between your baby's knees is very pronounced, or the 'bow' effect only appears in one leg, check with your doctor or health visitor. True bow legs are caused by a bending and slight twisting of the shin bone that is actually part of the process of normal development of strong bones. Rarely, the bow may be the result of rickets, which is usually due to deficiency of vitamin D.

MASSAGE and cranial OSTEOPATHY can assist the natural processes that straighten the legs and can begin early. It is very rare for any specialist orthopaedic or surgical treatment to be required, other than in the most severe cases where expert advice is needed. If your child does require specialist treatment, osteopathy can still be very useful in conjunction with other therapies.

Breast lumps

A breast lump is very common during pregnancy and even more so during breastfeeding. Your greatest concern will probably be cancer, but this is extremely rare, occurring in just three in 10,000 pregnancies, and only 3 per cent of breast cancers are associated with pregnancy or milk production. A painful lump is more likely to be caused by a blocked milk duct (page 91). This

has a sharply defined edge and is easily diagnosed. If the swelling can be massaged away and/or an ultrasound scan detects milk inside the lump, this will confirm the diagnosis.

If you have lumpy breasts, this may be your body's unique reaction to hormones and the effect may increase during pregnancy.

Some women have extra accessory breast tissue in their armpit, called the axilla, that swells during pregnancy and breastfeeding. It is normal breast tissue and the swelling diminishes with time, usually within two weeks.

Action plan

Ask your doctor to examine any breast lumps and, if necessary, arrange an ultrasound scan to check the nature of the lump. The ultrasound is identical to the one used to scan your baby and it is safe (page 33).

Breast pain after birth

See Breastfeeding, difficulties, pain.

Breast pain in pregnancy

See also Breastfeeding, difficulties; Pain, mother.

During pregnancy hormonal changes cause your breasts to enlarge. They may feel full, heavy and harder than normal and tender to touch. If your breasts usually become very sensitive before a period, you are more likely to feel uncomfortable in pregnancy.

Action plan

- Wearing a supportive cotton bra during the day and a sports bra at night will help. Don't hesitate to increase your bra size as pregnancy progresses.
- Gentle massage may also be soothing: see the guidelines on page 83.
- Some women are nervous that pain indicates breast cancer. Most cancers are not painful but if you are concerned, ask your doctor to examine your breast. You may also be offered an ultrasound scan to check the painful area.
- If the pain makes you anxious, there may also

be underlying issues fuelling your anxiety – for some women breast pain is related to a fear of being a mum. You may want to seek emotional support.

Breastfeeding, advice

See also Breastfeeding, difficulties.

Breastfeeding gives your baby love, food, contact and security. Your breast milk is the best food for your baby and breastfeeding provides many rewards for you, too. In the mother–baby dyad where you and your baby are frequently together, you naturally tune in to him. Your baby leads the way and your body automatically gives him what he needs. Your 'bodymind' (page 73) picks up and responds to all your baby's subtle signals, including eye contact, smells and the pattern of your baby's suckling, as well as more obvious body movements and noises. For the majority of mums and babies, time together is all that is needed for feeding to be successful and enjoyable.

Feeding from birth for six months is optimal. Some mums and babies continue breastfeeding for one, two or more years. Others breastfeed for only a few weeks or months. Successful breastfeeding offers your baby – and your relationship – the best possible foundation so it is worth investing time and effort in it for as long as feels good. Breastfeeding is a two-way partnership with your baby. If either of you feels it is time for breastfeeding to end there are many other ways for your partnership to thrive.

Why breastfeeding is best

- Breastfeeding is nature's recipe for love and bonding. It encourages your body to produce hormones that help you fall in love with your baby, and your milk delivers love hormones (page 82) to your baby.
- Feeding your baby from your breast allows your body to continue to nourish your baby after birth, a natural part of your intimate relationship.
- Your milk has your smell and taste, which are familiar and reassuring for your baby.
- Your milk quenches your baby's thirst and hunger. Its calorie content changes to meet his needs from feed to feed, and within a single feed.

- Components in your breast milk help your baby's intestine develop optimally and absorb nutrients effectively.
- Antibodies in your breast milk protect your baby from infection.
- Breastfeeding reduces allergies and asthma.
- Breastfeeding assists the natural contraction of your uterus after pregnancy and helps postnatal weight loss in conjunction with good nutrition and exercise.
- As you allow your baby to feed as much or as little as he wants, he knows he is valued and his needs for love, food and contact are met. He feels safe.
- The action of feeding from your breast and constituents in your milk offer pain relief for your baby that is thought to be more powerful than morphine – useful if birth was painful or when your baby is unwell or teething.

Ten ways to make breastfeeding simple and enjoyable

1. Create quality time to be together, to allow your 'bodymind' to tune in to your baby – his pace is slower than yours. In-between feeds is as important as during feeds. Your daily dance also includes touching, talking and playing.
2. Feed on demand. Your baby knows when he is hungry and thirsty, and the volume and fat–liquid ratio of your milk will meet his needs when you allow him to guide you.
3. Nourish yourself with fluid, food, sleep and rest.
4. Be patient and allow your baby and yourself time to get used to feeding.
5. Ensure your baby latches on well and you are feeling comfortable and your body supported. Generally, babies are naturals and when positioning is good, feeding is easy and problems are much less likely to crop up.
6. Be prepared for a range of sensations – including pleasure and bliss, tingling and discomfort, and dreaminess and tearfulness.
7. Know that the 'let down', when milk comes to your nipples, can be painful.
8. Don't hesitate to seek advice if you are uncomfortable or if you are concerned your baby may not be getting enough.
9. Feel your feelings and go with your instincts. Sometimes doubts arise because of family

beliefs or peer pressure. It can be tough to feel confident if your mother or partner or friends are not supportive or if you had difficulties feeding when you were a baby.

10. Spend time with other like-minded breastfeeding mums and babies.

The following entries give further details to help you both settle into feeding, and address any difficulties that may arise. In addition, you may tap into one of the many resources for breastfeeding mothers, and if their advice feels good it will be useful for you. The wide selection includes La Leche League, Association for Breastfeeding Mothers, The Breastfeeding Network and NCT.

Colostrum and breast milk

When your baby is born, your breasts produce colostrum – a rich sweet liquid that boosts your baby's energy, quenches his thirst and helps him feel comfortable. It is a rich source of energy and love hormones and is loaded with protective antibodies and substances that aid digestion, as well as pain-relieving endorphins.

After a few days, colostrum is replaced by milk. This tastes different. Your milk contains love hormones and antibodies, as well as vitamins, minerals, fat and protein – everything your baby needs. The constituents of your milk continually change to accommodate your baby's needs.

You may hear people talk about 'fore milk' and 'hind milk'. This refers to the different types of milk that flow in a single feed. When your baby starts to suckle, your milk is thirst-quenching and fast flowing. Once your baby's thirst is quenched, the fat and protein content of your milk increases. When you and your baby breastfeed regularly and you are in close contact with one another, your bodies fall into synch and your breasts provide the very best nutrition, whether your baby is five days or five months old.

▇ BEGINNINGS

You can begin to breastfeed as soon as you feel up to it after the birth. You may bring your baby to your breast just minutes after he is born and he may suckle before the placenta is delivered.

He will probably nuzzle and move around as he tries to attach to you. It is amazing that even when less than half an hour old, a baby is able to wriggle up his mother's torso, locate the nipple by smell, and position himself. Your baby has a reflex to suckle and to feed, and a powerful drive to connect with you: the intimacy of breastfeeding in the safety of your arms is an extension of the intimacy and protection of the womb. He will turn towards your breast for comfort and for food when he needs to, and at other times will rest peacefully without sucking. Your baby's role in the breastfeeding partnership is one of leadership: as he gives you signals, your body will respond to him with a release of love hormones and a 'let-down reflex' as colostrum, and later milk, flows to your nipples.

If you plan to feed straight after birth but events don't make this possible – perhaps you or your baby need some extra care – there will still be huge benefits whenever you start to feed and you can enjoy these by setting the scene for calm time together. If you have a caesarean delivery, the medical team can help you get comfortable and begin feeding when you are in the recovery room.

Setting the scene

For your first feeds, if it is quiet and there is minimal disturbance, you and your baby will be able to focus on one another and connect. Your baby can focus clearly on your face when he is at your breast and his other senses, smell and touch, drive him to find and latch on to your nipple. Turn the lights down, switch off the television or radio and consider unplugging or switching off the phone. Choose a comfortable chair, or nestle in bed, and ensure that your position is not straining your body. Your baby will probably alternate between exploring your face and making eye contact with you, and closing his eyes, perhaps dozing or slipping into a state of bliss (this is one of your baby's states of consciousness which he frequently enters).

Your milk flow will be encouraged through regular and frequent feeding and lots of physical contact between feeds, preferably skin to skin. You may want to extend close contact throughout the day with kangaroo care (page 518) and in the bath, where you can rest together and feed safely.

In the early days and in the weeks that follow you may need to ask friends or family to help with daily tasks so you have time and space to relax with your baby and allow this pattern of guidance and response to gently fall into place.

Difficulty getting started

Some mum and baby partnerships take to breastfeeding easily. Others take time. When there is quality time, and you and your baby can relax together and you are rested and well nourished, feeding is likely to go well.

Most problems can be overcome with love and focus, good positioning, perseverance, patience and support. The most important thing is contact – being physically in touch with your baby is the key. Rarely, a baby may need time to recover from birth, if there have been difficulties, or there may be developmental issues (such as tongue tie, page 516) that make it difficult to feed.

For some mums there is an emotional element. When there is depression and anxiety breastfeeding difficulties are common. There is often a feeling of fear: Can I do it? Can my body really nourish my baby? Will it hurt? Will I look unattractive? Will my breasts droop? These issues can reduce confidence and the motivation to feed. They are part of the emotions of feeding that are discussed on page 87.

▩ CARING FOR YOUR BREASTS

When feeding goes well, your breasts will care for themselves. There's no need to clean your nipples except with water when you take a bath or shower. Your baby needs the natural bacteria carried on your skin to populate his bowel, help his digestion and boost his immune system, and loves the smell of you. Your breasts produce their own moisturising fluid.

You can help your breasts stay comfortable with a good bra, preferably made from cotton with thick shoulder straps and no wiring, and by keeping them dry and tending to any problems as soon as they arise. An important point to remember is to keep feeding – even if your breasts become sore – as this will help drain your breasts. If your milk builds up this is uncomfortable and may lead to blocked ducts and mastitis (pages 91 and 95).

Your breasts may leak before, between or after feeds. You can absorb this leakage with washable or disposable breast pads. Leakage varies from woman to woman. It's often most profuse in the early days, and diminishes after several weeks. Plastic-backed nipple shells are not recommended as they can stop air getting to the nipple and encourage the skin to crack, as do plastic-lined pads.

Massaging your breasts

You may want to massage from time to time to ease any discomfort that arises when you feed. Don't use any scented oils, and avoid massaging your nipples and areola (the brown area surrounding your nipple). A pure oil, such as almond, is good for your skin, but you may massage without oil if you prefer. The purpose is to soothe your breasts rather than encourage milk flow.

Begin at the periphery of your breast (covering the whole area) and massage gently towards your nipple. This mimics the direction of milk flow through the ducts. Focus on any sore patches. Use the palm of your hand and stroke your breast firmly but gently – you should not feel pain. Start at the top of your breast (12 o'clock) and massage towards your nipple. Then move on to the next segment (1 o'clock) and massage from the periphery towards the nipple. Go 'round the clock' like this so that each segment receives attention, and each stroke ends at the edge of the areola. You may find it easier to massage after warming your breast in the bath or shower.

▩ COMFORT AND POSITION

With a good position, your milk will flow freely, your baby won't tug on your nipple and make it sore, and he will find it easier to feed and to digest. How your baby latches on is very important for both of you.

Latching on

In an ideal position, your baby takes your nipple and the areola into his mouth. Your nipple needs to be at the back of your baby's mouth in the soft palate while his lower lip is folded back to cover the areola. In this position your baby does not suck directly on your nipple and instead creates a rhythmic pressure on your breast to stimulate milk flow. If your nipple is touching the roof of his mouth (his hard palate) this may make your nipples sore (page 97).

If it hurts
Though the sensation of milk coming in may be 'sharp' for around a minute, any pain beyond this signals a poor position. If you feel pain, ease your baby off by gently breaking his suction with your finger, reposition and try again.

If your baby's nose is blocked
If your baby's nose is blocked by your breast, do not press your breast away from his nose as this may plug a breast duct (page 91). Instead, take him off and reposition him.

If your breasts are swollen
Achieving a good latched-on position may be tricky when your milk replaces colostrum around the third day and your breasts enlarge. If your breasts are very swollen and your baby has difficulty getting a grip, try cupping your areola between your thumb and forefinger to make it protrude a little. You may need to soften the areola by expressing a little milk (page 89). Your breasts will settle down once your baby starts sucking and you both settle into a rhythm. If they become full and heavy, they may be engorged (page 92).

If your baby doesn't open wide
Some babies don't open their mouths wide enough to take in any more than the nipple. If this is the case, encourage your baby to open wider by stroking his cheek with your nipple or by squeezing your areola gently between your fingers to express a few drops of milk to tempt him. When your baby is quiet and alert, try to teach him to open wide by showing him your wide-open mouth: from birth he will enjoy mimicking you. You can also lightly squeeze the palm of his hand, as this may trigger the reflex to open his mouth. If you try to place him on your breast when he opens wide during crying, his tongue will be too far back in his mouth and he may find it hard to latch on. You may need to calm him before feeding.

If your baby just doesn't seem interested in feeding, and is not complaining, he may not be hungry. If he is not feeding well and he is upset, you may need extra support. We look at breast rejection and difficulty sucking on page 99.

Watch out - signs that your baby isn't latching on well

If your baby isn't latching on well, she may not be getting a full feed and there is a risk that problems could develop for you (like blocked ducts). The quickest remedy is to ease your baby off and reposition. Look out for these signs.
- Breastfeeding hurts.
- Your nipples take on a 'wedge' appearance.
- Your nipples are painful, stretched and may be cracked.
- Your breasts do not feel fully emptied after a feed. They may be engorged.
- Your baby's nose is blocked by your breast.
- Your baby gulps noisily or sucks very fast without falling into a steady rhythm.
- Your baby does not appear relaxed while suckling.
- Your baby seems hungry even after a long feed.
- Your baby is reluctant to end a feed, even after 40 minutes.
- Your baby is not gaining weight as you would expect.

Holding your baby

There is no right or best way to hold your baby – every mum–baby dyad does things differently, and most settle into a favourite position soon. Even so, remember to change position if one part of your breast is tender or inflamed because this will encourage the milk to flow freely and your skin to heal.

You will be most comfortable if you are well supported and relaxed.

- Sit in an upright chair and bring your baby to your breast, rather than leaning over to give your breast to your baby, and always ensure your back is well supported.
- Have your feet flat on the floor or raised on a small stool.
- If you get stiff or sore, focus on your posture and try yoga exercises, which can ease tension (page 571).
- If you are worried or upset, your body will feel tense and stiff; you may need to dispel your anxieties.
- Having low blood sugar or being dehydrated may cause you to feel tense, so ensure you eat and drink sufficiently.

Traditional position

Sit upright and hold your baby with his belly towards your belly with his face at one breast and his feet towards the other. You could use a pillow or two to bring him to breast height, or a V-shaped breastfeeding cushion. Support his back with your arm and be sure not to restrict his neck, so he can extend his head back and lead with his chin while coming onto your breast. Some mums like to use one hand to cup the breast. Place your baby so that your nipple is just above his upper lip and as he opens wide, guide him up onto your breast. You will soon find this becomes second nature to you.

Rugby hold position

This is a good position for beginners or to slow down your flow. Sit down, rest your baby on a pillow under the arm on the side you will be feeding from with his feet tucked by your side, pointing behind you, and his nose to your nipple. Cradle him close to your body, using your hand to hold his neck. Put your spare hand on your breast in a 'C' hold. Babies often latch themselves without much assistance in this position. Make sure he has at least as much of your areola in his mouth below the nipple as above it.

Lying down

Lie on the side you are going to feed from, with your baby's feet facing your waist. Prop yourself up on your elbow, with your supporting hand on his neck. When he is securely latched, slide your arm down flat so you are lying comfortably on your side.

If your flow is very fast

Try the rugby position with your baby sitting fairly upright. Alternatively, you can control a very fast flow by feeding with your baby on your tummy while you lie on your back so gravity is in his favour. When you're sitting up you can limit the flow by pressing and releasing on the areola with two fingers.

▨ DAILY RHYTHM

Twenty or 30 years ago, it was common for babies to be fed according to timetables set by the parents, usually every three or four hours, and sometimes strictly timed to the minute. Some parents still choose to do this but it is more appropriate for your baby to lead the way. He will let you know when he is hungry or thirsty and he will feel good when his needs are met.

It is preferable to think in terms of rhythm rather than routine. The rhythm will change, like a piece of music. If your baby eats at set times but spends a lot of time crying, he will be unhappy – probably the schedule isn't right for him at this time. If you are tired and anxious because your baby is constantly feeding, you will be unhappy. If so, maybe you can help your baby take a fuller feed or gently extend the periods between feeds by a few minutes at a time.

Whatever your rhythm, it will need to alter when there is illness, teething, dreams, growth spurts, and so on. Unfortunately, peer pressure can be powerful and it is common to feel inadequate if another mum or dad declares that their baby 'is always so predictable' or is 'already sleeping through the night'. A predictable rhythm suits some babies, but not others. Please remember it's important to do what's right for each person in your family.

Feeding on demand: following your baby's lead

Most babies initially ask for milk frequently. After a few weeks, many begin to feed at more widely spaced intervals. Your baby will have his own rhythm. If you are well nourished and rested, and your milk flows well, you will be giving him just what he needs: breastfeeding works on a supply-and-demand basis.

Enjoy offering your breast frequently. It is the perfect contact for you both. It may be difficult to do if it goes against the advice of your mother, midwife or friends, but your baby is your best guide. He knows when he is hungry and when he is full. By receiving milk when he asks for it, your baby will gain confidence, build trust in you, and find it easier to separate from you, and from breastfeeding, when he is ready to do so. It is not a rod for your back.

In the first week

Your baby, with a stomach the size of a walnut, needs to suckle little and often. A gap of around two or two-and-a-half hours between feeds is the average but some babies eat every hour or every four hours. Preferably, unless your baby has a long sleep, don't go longer than three hours between feeds. Breast milk is digested more quickly and efficiently than bottle milk, so if your baby is bottle-fed he may go longer.

It's reasonable to aim to feed for at least 20 minutes on one breast, but some babies feel full within 10 minutes, and others take up to 60 minutes. As long as your baby is gaining weight, the feeding time is irrelevant. Being in touch with you is an important part of each feed and the nutrition of breastfeeding comes from milk and from touch. Your baby may love to doze with your nipple in his mouth, even if he is not actively sucking.

Initially, your baby will probably feed at only one breast. At the next feed, offer the other. Many women use a ring, a ribbon or a brooch to mark which side to feed from.

From the second or third week

Your baby may now feed for longer, and rest longer between feeds. At some stage, your baby won't be satisfied after one breast. Offer him the second and let him suck as long as he likes. At the next feed, begin with this breast.

After a number of weeks

After four weeks, but perhaps sooner or later, your baby is likely to empty both breasts at each feed. If he nods off mid-feed, you can gently wake him by squeezing his hand, rubbing his feet or blowing on his cheek, and encourage him to take a full feed. You may find that undressing him helps. Breastfed babies cannot overeat, but eating enough will help your baby feel satisfied. When you begin to

recognise a pattern to his appetite, this will help you plan your days.

Feeding at night

See also Sleep, baby; Sleep, mother.

Your baby needs to feed often, and this includes during the night. Although some babies do 'sleep through' by 10–12 weeks, and a small number do so earlier, most are woken by the need for contact and/or a feed for several months.

Many parents are anxious about getting enough sleep. This is understandable, as having a new baby does alter your sleeping patterns and you will probably feel tired. Anxiety, however, may get in the way of good sleep. Many things can improve your quality of sleep – there are suggestions on pages 495–7. Please remember that your baby does not have the same sleep requirements as you, and his patterns will change. As a newborn, he will tend to go down for the 'night's' sleep around 10 or 11pm, and wake three to four hours later (page 490). Bedtime gradually gets earlier, and the gaps between feeds gradually get longer. Because you'll be waking when your baby does, sleeping during the day will help you catch up.

Many parents enjoy sleeping with their baby and mums and dads often discover that this makes feeding at night much less disruptive. Co-sleeping comfortably and safely is discussed on page 487. If you prefer not to co-sleep, consider having your baby in a basket next to your bed, or adding some width to your bed to make extra room for him next to you. He needs to feel close to you, especially during the first six months.

Growth spurts

Some babies have a 'growth spurt' (or an appetite spurt) every fourth day; others every fourth week. Just before he enters a spurt, your baby may seem more settled, demand less food and sleep longer. A day or two later, he'll ask for more food – letting him suck as frequently as he wants tells your breasts to produce more milk. When your supply increases to meet his demand, he may feed less frequently, as your milk will have changed to provide the calories he needs.

■ EMOTIONS AND FEELINGS

See also Emotions.

Baby

As your baby suckles at your breast, he has a deep connection with you – his mouth at your nipple, warm milk on his tongue, his nose sensing your aroma, his belly on yours, his hands pulsing at your skin. This is his world – the feel and smell of mum, thirst and hunger satisfied, and delicious milk. Breast milk is a pain-reliever and a pleasure-bringer, and its hormones and other chemical components can transmit powerful emotional messages to your baby (page 81). Sometimes you may feel him picking up on your feelings. Similarly, his moods affect you. Breastfeeding is a very powerful way for you to be there for your baby when he has intense feelings, as it offers safety and helps him feel loved and accepted.

Your baby has lots of feelings. He may show these by being relaxed or tense; he may suck gently and rhythmically or guzzle; his eyes may be open or closed; his palms clenched or open. Your baby does not think in words like you do but you may get a sense of how he feels while he is intimately connected with you during a feed. Among his 'seven big feelings' are the following.

Love and pleasure
* I feel blissful and happy.
* I have no fear, I am totally comfortable.
* I love the warmth, smell, sounds and taste of mum.
* How nice to be skin to skin.
* I feel safe and loved.
* Mmmm, this soothes my sore head.

Discomfort, anger, fear
* My tummy feels sore.
* I do not feel safe, I am frightened I will fall.
* Why is the milk not here yet?
* This milk tastes horrible today.

Bonding and separation anxiety
* I feel connected when I touch my mum's breast.
* I feel good and my mum is smiling at me.
* I feel good, dad is here too.
* Where's mum? We are separated. I feel abandoned. Ah, here she is. I feel loved ...

* I have lost the nipple. Oh no. Oh good, it is back.

If you would like to read more about your baby's emotional world, turn to page 206.

Father

Breastfeeding brings up many feelings for every father. You may be delighted that your baby is being nourished in the best way possible, and enjoy seeing your partner and baby together. There is lots of time between feeds to hold and love your baby. Many fathers love the intimacy and enjoy nourishing their partner with good food, drinks of water, respect and love. You may relish this.

Sometimes breastfeeding can be upsetting for fathers. This may be a general feeling for you, or may crop up from time to time. You may feel upset that your partner is tired, even exhausted, and your lover has disappeared. You may feel resentful or jealous that your baby is always top priority and you are neglected or rejected. You may also feel guilty as you recognise that you are upset and you know how much your baby needs to be mothered and your partner needs to mother. Like many men, you may need great reserves of patience – things do change with time and in the early days, although it's important that your needs are met, it is best for your baby if you do not let your needs overshadow his.

Some of your feelings have their roots in your past. You may re-experience feelings that you had when you were a baby feeding at your mother's breast, or from a bottle, which have been dormant in your unconscious until now, such as a longing to be close, fear of separation, pleasure, love, and perhaps anger. All your feelings are real and important, even though some may be easier to explain rationally than others and you may not consciously remember your babyhood. It's normal to feel positive as well as negative (page 237). It may sometimes seem as if you are like a baby and you may long for your partner to mother you with the devotion she is showing your baby. This is your inner baby surfacing. You may even be depressed. Watching your feelings rise and fall and talking and being supported by other people in your life will help you enjoy this time and remember it with pleasure in years to come.

Mother

You may feel intensely emotional during each feed – and, indeed, in-between. The primary emotion for women is often deep pleasure and love – a unique kind of bliss. The contact triggers love hormones to flow through your body and stimulates you to focus on your baby, so you may feel totally absorbed in him. Many women talk of the experience being physically and emotionally delightful, as fulfilling as an orgasm.

In addition to pleasure, feelings may include melancholy, anxiety and even anger. You may at times feel drained and overwhelmed by the amount your baby needs you to sit and feed him. It may make you feel depressed and not able to carry on.

The way you feel emotionally affects the hormones that stimulate your milk flow, your energy and confidence, and your body tension. Similarly, breastfeeding and the demands of mothering will impact your emotions. It is a two-way process and looking after yourself emotionally is an important part of sustaining a breastfeeding partnership that is fulfilling for your baby and for you.

Inner baby and outer baby

The smells of breastfeeding and the flow of feeding hormones, combined with the intimate connection between you and your baby, stimulate memories that have long been held dormant in your 'bodymind'. In the half-wakeful state of a quiet night-time feed it may sometimes seem as if you are like a baby. This is the energy of your inner baby surfacing, bringing with her the feelings from your past. For many women, this is a deeply emotional state – with few words to explain it. It is part of the magic of feeding and sometimes part of its challenge.

Simply being in your feelings is a powerful way to be open-hearted for yourself and your baby. Your baby will be very sensitive and may be lulled by your pleasure, or pick up tension if you feel upset, hurried or uncertain. If you do feel tense, you can reassure him and reduce tension if you take time to relax and if you are honest with him about the way you feel. Some feelings may be difficult to explain rationally but they are all part of your seven big feelings (page 208).

Feeling ambivalent?

Some mums can feel ambivalent about breastfeeding. This feeling may be present occasionally, frequently or all of the time. If any of the issues below ring true for you, it may be helpful to spend time with other breastfeeding mums or talk to your health visitor or lactation consultant. Remember that practical measures and having some emotional support may help you feel more comfortable to follow your preferences.

* You may not want to feed but feel you should because of your mum's views, or the influence of the media, friends, midwives, and so on. In this case, it is best to spend lots of time with your baby and decide what suits your partnership best – rather than striving to meet other people's expectations.
* Your friends may all want to bottle-feed and it's not easy being different.
* Your partner may not be supportive, and you may feel nervous about losing his affection if you persist with breastfeeding. Find time to talk and acknowledge that the breastfeeding period is only a small part of your long partnership together.
* You may worry your breasts will droop and your sexuality is being compromised. Again, appreciating the bigger picture may reduce your fears.
* You may be worried about sleeping enough, or spoiling your baby. Breastfeeding won't spoil your baby and there are many ways to get enough sleep.
* You may be worried that you need to eat more to make milk, and won't lose weight. In fact, with good nutrition (pages 253–65) breastfeeding may actually help weight loss.
* If you are concerned that your baby is not getting enough from you, rest assured that this is a common worry and usually unfounded. Your health visitor can assess your baby's weight gain (page 285).

Feeling blue?

Feeling a little down after the birth – the 'blues' – is common (page 219). Usually several factors are involved. Your personal response to feeding hormones, and/or difficulty feeding may be major elements, or some of many. If feeding is going well and you are feeling down for other reasons, your sadness or tears may be most intense when you breastfeed or when your breasts fill before a feed. You may begin to feel better if you take measures to improve your mood – probably with a combination of practical steps and by having emotional support.

You may be tempted to keep yourself busy to avoid the uncomfortable feelings, or you might want to stop breastfeeding. On a positive note, depressing feelings can have a constructive element and it may be useful to acknowledge them as guides. They may urge you to ask for support and make some changes that benefit you and your baby.

Some women choose to stop breastfeeding in an attempt to relieve tiredness, get more time to themselves, and avoid emotional highs and lows. This can make a positive difference for some women. When there are other causes of depression, stopping breastfeeding may give only temporary relief, or none at all, and there may be further sadness over lost intimacy. Do talk to someone if you are unsure what to do (overleaf). Other mums may be your best allies and supporters. Your GP or midwife can put you in touch with a breastfeeding counsellor. You could turn to a local or national support group, or visit a counsellor or psychotherapist. The suggestions on pages 208–9 outline simple steps towards feeling better.

▓ EXPRESSING MILK

During the first six to eight weeks, your baby will need all the milk you produce. This period is an important time when you and your baby form a mutual partnership where you learn to respond to one another, and it's an irreplaceable time for bonding. Your 'bodymind' takes this time to respond to your baby's demands and regulate your milk flow. It's not advisable to express milk until Week 8 or later. Occasionally, it is useful to express a little milk to release tension, to relieve pain or to stimulate your flow. For this you may choose to express by hand (below).

How often to express

After Week 8, if you wish your baby to have your milk while you are not around, keep expressing to a minimum as it's best to have the intimate contact of skin on skin during a feed. A minimum for you may be once a week or a fortnight, allowing someone else to feed your baby so you have longer to go out, or to rest. Alternatively it may be once a day. More than once a day may trigger a reduction in your milk supply.

Expressing with a breast pump

After Week 8, if you wish to express you may find it easiest and quickest with a breast pump. There are many breast pumps on the market. Ask a friend or your health visitor for a recommendation. You may need to try more than one before you find something that suits you. Without the stimulus of your baby sucking, your let-down reflex may be weak, with just a small amount of milk flowing. Having baby's smell on a blanket or babygro might help your milk to flow.

You may find it easier to express from one breast while you are feeding from the other (if your baby gets sufficient milk from one breast only) or to express when your baby has had enough at the end of a feed. If you are expressing while you are feeding, choose a time of day when your milk flow is strong (often this is the morning feed) and you think there's more than enough for your baby. If you're expressing regularly, your breasts will adapt most easily if you express at the same time each day. Always express into a sterilised container.

Because it is not the same as sucking, the amount you express is not a close match to the amount your baby drinks at a feed. As you express, continue until the heaviness in your breast subsides, or the flow drops. Expressing too much may over-stimulate your breasts, and this can lead to discomfort or mastitis.

Expressing by hand

Hand expressing may take patience and practice, yet it is worth it as it best mimics your baby's sucking and will maintain your milk supply better than breast pumps.
- Take your time and try a few times before you need the milk. If you rush, your urgency will almost surely interfere with milk flow.
- Expressing in a warm bath or shower is often easier, or using a warm cloth on your breast and gently stroking it towards the nipple before

beginning. It may help to have your baby with you, or something that smells of him.

- Wash your hands, place your thumb flat against the upper edge of your areola and cup the rest of your hand under your breast. Gently push your breast back against the chest wall, then gently squeeze your thumb and forefinger together without sliding them over your skin. Release the pressure on your fingers and then repeat, building into a rhythm. Let your milk flow into a sterilised bowl.
- Don't be rough – it shouldn't hurt. You may need to rub a pure oil (such as olive oil) on your breast (but not on your nipple).
- Remember your posture – sit at a table or stand over a high worktop so you don't have to stoop.

Expressed milk and safety
If you express milk to feed your baby later, it's important to keep it safe. Always use a cleaned, sterilised breast pump, and sterilise the bottles, teats, cup or spoon you use, and be aware of safe storage times:

Milk at room temperature	Keep for a maximum of six hours
Milk in fridge, 5–10°C	Keep for a maximum of three days
Milk in fridge, 0–4°C	Keep for a maximum of eight days (if temperature rises above 4°C after three days, use the milk within six hours or throw it away)
Milk in freezer –18°C or lower	Six months
Frozen, defrosted in fridge	12 hours
Frozen, defrosted at room temp	Use immediately

* This advice from Breastfeeding Network, 2007

Breast milk separates when it is refrigerated or frozen – a shake will blend it again. Your baby may drink the milk at room temperature, or enjoy it warm. Follow the guidelines for heating milk on page 78.

Giving expressed breast milk to your baby
The majority of mums who express feed the milk to their baby from a bottle (or another adult – often dad – does). Some prefer to use a cup with a small, soft spout – even young babies can take liquid like this. For very young babies, expressed milk may be given from a teaspoon, and if your baby is in a special care baby unit he can be tube-fed your milk. If you decide to use a bottle, there is advice for mixing breast and bottle on page 75.

▨ WHEN BREASTFEEDING ENDS
If you bottle-feed from birth, or when you stop breastfeeding, it can take a few days for milk production to stop, and this can be uncomfortable or painful. For your own comfort, and to ease your baby's transition, it is best not to stop suddenly. Cut down a feed or two a day so your breasts make less and less milk. This also reduces the risk of an excess build-up of milk and of mastitis (page 95). Wear a good bra with firm support and use pads if your breasts leak. If you need more support, try wrapping a towel or large cloth around your upper body so that extra pressure is applied to your breasts. If your breasts feel uncomfortably heavy and tight they may be engorged (page 92).

Stopping breastfeeding is often emotionally charged for mum and baby. Some mothers feel the time is right, and there is no sense of loss; others feel sad. There can also be relief, for example, if you feel more energised, enjoy extra freedom and perhaps a rise in libido. You may be angry if you feel you have been put under pressure to stop before you want to. You may feel guilty. The mixture of emotions may be confusing. The separation from your baby may be a significant part of any sadness or guilt, but you can still spend as much time as before with him. You will also be affected by hormonal changes – don't be surprised if you become weepy. If you feel overwhelmed, the advice in the emotions section (pages 206–25) may help.

Your baby may have chosen to stop feeding, and feel happy and confident to be weaned. Or he may be reluctant and angry. If he is upset, you can be there for him, with lots of time being close and with skin-to-skin contact, and tell him what is happening. If you are out at work during the day, sharing a bath and relaxing together in the evening may be a lovely way to stay intimate.

Breastfeeding, difficulties

Breastfeeding is a partnership between you and your baby. While you both have the instincts to breastfeed successfully, each of you will be learning. Your 'training' may be over within a day. Alternatively, you may take days or weeks and welcome professional support. Even after you feel settled there may be days when things don't go so well. The cause could be one of many problems, ranging from your baby being ill to you feeling unwell or tired.

When things don't feel right you may worry that you are not a good enough mother or your baby is reacting abnormally. It may help to remember that breastfeeding does not come easily for everyone, and some difficulties cannot be prevented. Most problems, however, are simple to overcome.

Action plan

If you are having difficulties, especially if you feel pain, it's important to take action straight away to prevent the problem getting worse, and ask for medical advice if you are at all worried. Whatever the problem, the golden rules are:

* Continue feeding and spend quality time in skin-to-skin contact with your baby.
* Remember that positioning is often the key to successful feeding (page 85).
* If you need assistance, your midwife or a breastfeeding counsellor or lactation advisor may help you.
* Care well for yourself, as this will help to maintain your energy and milk supply.

Treatments for specific problems are listed under the individual entries that follow.

Your feelings

When feeding is difficult, you may be emotionally upset and distraught; the difficulty may make you feel bad, or feeling low could be at the root of feeding problems. Feelings range from

ambivalence and depression (page 174) to anxiety and anger, which can interfere with comfort, milk flow, sleep and bonding. The action plan on page 208 may help you trust yourself and your baby and begin to work through any significant emotional issues.

▦ BLOCKED DUCTS

As milk flows to your nipples it passes through breast ducts. If a duct becomes blocked it swells, forms a lump and your breast may become inflamed. The swelling has a sharply defined edge and may get worse after a feed. If there is any doubt about diagnosis, the blockage may be confirmed by ultrasound scan.

Clearing a blockage and getting back to comfortable feeding is usually relatively straightforward, and it is important to act quickly. If a blockage persists there is a risk that bacteria from your skin may enter the duct, infect the trapped milk, and cause mastitis (page 95). Although mastitis can usually be treated and need not interfere with successful breastfeeding, it is very painful and increases the risk of a breast abscess (page 95).

You may be upset, and some women feel guilty that somehow they are not doing well enough. Please remember that although there are measures that reduce the risk of blocked ducts, the problem is not always preventable.

What happens

* Anything that restricts your milk flow can cause blocked ducts.
* Your baby may not be latching on well, and not drain your breast adequately. This is usually the main factor.
* You may favour a position that does not allow your baby to drain each segment of your breast equally. This may be because your nipple(s) are painful or cracked, or could reflect the position you tend to take that is most comfortable for you, or the side you hold your cup of tea on.
* There may be a build-up of milk because you are producing an excess in the early days, or your baby is sleeping longer at night, or you are working and missing feeds. The reservoir of undrained milk may thicken and block one or more milk ducts.

- If you are wearing a tight bra or clothing, or grasping your breast too tightly while feeding, this may constrict the opening of the duct.
- Nipple shields can stem the flow of milk.
- Very occasionally, a duct is anatomically narrow and blocks easily.

Action plan

Feeding your baby
- Keep feeding, and spend time skin to skin.
- Feed more frequently if you can. This will help to unblock milk ducts and clear any infective organisms.
- Check your position and ensure your baby latches on well.
- Use a different position each time you feed to help drain the affected area.

Caring for your breasts
If you feel lumpy or tender areas try gently warming your breast for 10 minutes with a warm compress (not hot) before feeding. This loosens dry milk in the ducts. You could try using a small amount of the aromatherapy oils frankincense, geranium or chamomile in the compress. Alternatively take a warm shower or a bath before a feed.

Breast massage (page 83) can help milk to flow before a feed and release excess after a feed. Be gentle but it will be uncomfortable till the blockage clears. Always massage gently from the periphery towards the nipple. You could use a natural oil (almond, grape seed or vitamin E) and try mixing it with frankincense, geranium or chamomile essential oils. Remember, though, that your baby is very sensitive to smell. If you do try oils, use them only after a feed and wash your breast with unscented soap afterwards. Some lactation consultants believe it is better to avoid using any oils – see what suits you and your baby.

If your breasts do not empty fully after a feed and a massage, you could use a breast pump. Do not strain your breasts – once the flow has slowed to a drip, stop pumping as too much can exacerbate the problem.

Homeopathy
You may take the most appropriate remedy (30c potency) once an hour for four hours. Then re-assess and take the most appropriate remedy (30c potency) every two hours for the next eight hours. If there is no improvement within 24 hours, seek professional advice. Your homeopath may advise you to take a high potency (200c) remedy.

- *Belladonna* (30c potency) is the first remedy to use when you feel very sensitive, particularly to light, noise, touch or being jarred, there is sudden swelling and sudden throbbing pain, with heat and redness around the blocked duct or red streaks running from the nipple to the circumference of your breast. You may have a fever.
- *Bryonia* if pain builds up slowly but you are still sensitive to movement, and your breast feels stony-hard and engorged, you feel dry and dehydrated, irritable and unsociable, better from applying firm pressure to your breast.
- *Phytollacca* if you have shooting pains radiating from your breasts into your armpits, find it unbearably painful to feed, feel hot and sweaty at night and have swollen glands, your breast is red and needs support.
- *Mercurius* if you have flu-like symptoms that are worse at night, you are very thirsty and sweaty and the blocked duct forms a distinct hard lump.
- *Pulsatilla* if your breasts are swollen, pain varies and you have a fever, feel weepy and need consolation. This remedy relieves emotional stress and the feeling of being overwhelmed. It may work to take a dose of *Pulsatilla* and follow it with another remedy to address your specific pain.

▥ ENGORGEMENT

Engorgement occurs if your breasts get too full with milk and become swollen. The main problem with engorgement is discomfort: your breasts may feel hard. Fortunately, it is not difficult to reduce the swelling and ease the normal flow of milk. Engorgement does not cause lumps, which are more likely to be due to blocked milk ducts (page 91).

What happens

Engorgement after birth
On the second or third day after birth, when your breasts begin to produce milk they may swell to up to three times their normal size. This is a good sign that your milk will soon be flowing freely. This swelling usually reduces within a few days.

Engorgement beyond the newborn period

Later, engorgement may continue, or begin for the first time, if your breasts are not drained completely.

* You may be producing an excess of milk (this will settle down in response to your baby's needs).
* You may be missing one or more feeds.
* Your baby may not be draining the milk completely.

If your breasts become very swollen, your nipples may become flat, and this makes it harder for your baby to latch on and drain your milk, see Action plan, below. If engorgement continues and the milk is not drained, there is a risk that your milk ducts may become blocked and mastitis (page 95) may develop.

Engorgement when you stop feeding

When breastfeeding comes to an end, you may stop gradually and so may not experience any swelling. If your breasts continue to produce milk, they may become swollen for a few days before reducing the milk supply because they are no longer being stimulated by your baby.

Action plan

Feeding

It will be painful to feed your baby but it will help if you continue so that she drains your breasts. You may need to encourage her to feed more frequently if she is not a demanding baby, particularly if she goes for longer than five hours without a feed. Pay close attention to her position so that she latches on well (page 83). In a few days your breasts will respond to her needs.

* If your nipples are flatter than usual, you can help them protrude by placing your thumb and forefinger above and below the nipple, and gently pressing inwards and then together. Once your baby is latched on, the pressure from her mouth should keep your nipple erect. Take care that your fingers do not obstruct her mouth and that her lips are on the areola – not on the nipple. Some techniques for inverted nipples (page 98) may also help.
* You could express some milk before a feed to reduce tension and allow your nipple to protrude.

Breast care

* A simple remedy for engorged breasts has been used for centuries. Keep cabbage leaves or a bowl of grated carrot in the fridge. Place one or other between your breast and bra for 10–20 minutes, every four hours. This can help to draw excess fluid away from your breast. Do not keep the cabbage or carrots on your skin for more than 20 minutes as this may cause cracks in your nipples. Research suggests that it's the coolness of the vegetable, rather than the vegetable itself, that has the greatest effect. A cold gel compress or a flannel may be similarly soothing for you.
* Gentle breast massage (page 83) encourages milk to flow to your nipple and drain away.
* A warm/hot flannel might help your milk flow. A hot shower may do the same.
* Check your breasts after each feed for lumps or tender areas. This will help you to attend to them early and prevent mastitis.
* If you have stopped feeding, follow the suggestions on page 90 to reduce soreness. It is best not to express your milk because this will stimulate more milk production. The discomfort usually settles in 48 hours. Some hospitals use bromocriptine, a drug that reduces prolactin hormone levels. This may cause nausea and, when the drug is stopped, breast milk production may recommence.

Homeopathy

You may choose the appropriate remedy in 30c potency and take it every two hours for eight hours. Then re-assess and take the most appropriate remedy (which may be the same as before) three times per day for another three days. Then re-assess the situation:

* *Belladonna* or *Bryonia*, often used to release milk blockage, are discussed under blocked ducts (page 91) and can also help engorgement.
* *Pulsatilla* if your breasts feel stretched, you feel weepy, want company and consolation, feel hot, hate stuffy rooms but aren't thirsty.
* *Lac Caninum*, which helps to regulate the milk supply, for swollen, lumpy breasts with pain moving from one side to the other but better for warmth and rest and when your breasts are supported.
* *Calc Carb* if your breasts are swollen but not red, with milk that looks bluish and

93

transparent, you have cold sweats and feel anxious and weak.

Aromatherapy

Peppermint and cypress oils are both helpful when used on a cool compress placed against your swollen breast(s) for 20 minutes every four hours. Remember your baby's sensitivity and do this after a feed and/or wash your breast before feeding.

▨ LOW MILK FLOW

Anxiety about having enough milk is very common, but in most cases milk flow is fine. Your baby is unique and may feed for short periods, or alternatively remain on your breast for up to an hour. You are unique too, and the sensation of your milk coming in may not be very strong. The time spent feeding or your own physical sensations aren't necessarily a reflection of milk flow. The best measure is your baby: if she is gaining weight, urinating regularly and seems content, these are signs that you are producing enough. If your breasts leak milk or it sprays out when the let-down reflex is active, you definitely have sufficient milk.

If your baby is not gaining weight adequately (page 559) your doctor or health visitor will help you consider the cause. It is important to have your baby checked closely in case there is an underlying problem. But in most instances the cause is low milk flow. The good news is that with attention to the way you care for yourself and your baby's feeding position and technique, your flow is likely to improve.

Action plan

The usual golden rules apply:
* Keep feeding and spend lots of quality time with your baby, preferably skin to skin. The more time touching, the greater the stimulus to your hormones and your milk flow.
* Take your lead from your baby, feeding her as often as she wants, and let her signal when she has had enough. If you regularly stop a feed before she shows you she is full, you may produce less milk than she needs. Your breasts respond to her sucking and need the stimulation to produce adequate quantities of milk.
* Remember to care for yourself (and let others support you).

There may be other factors:
* Your baby may feel full because she is retaining air. She may need help to burp so she can continue feeding and stimulate your breasts efficiently.
* If your baby is not demanding, she may not ask to be fed very often. She will need encouragement and you may need to feed frequently. If she tires easily and stops sucking after a few minutes, try to rouse her by undressing her before a feed, talking to her, or gently massaging her hands or feet. Over time, she is likely to suck for longer periods.
* If your baby is frail or premature or has abnormal development of the tongue and mouth, her sucking reflex may be ineffective. In order to keep your milk production going, you may have to stimulate your breasts using a pump to empty them at the end of each feed.
* If you are tense because you are in pain or you are stressed, anxious or upset, or you are reluctant to breastfeed, the let-down reflex may be hindered. Relaxing and feeling supported is likely to help.
* If you have returned to work and do not express while you are away, your milk flow may reduce through lack of stimulation or if you are not getting enough rest. You may need to re-evaluate your daily and weekly schedule.
* Occasionally, medical conditions are significant. These include low (and sometimes high) thyroid levels (page 514), and excessive blood loss in labour and birth (page 360). Once the underlying condition has been addressed, milk supply is likely to increase providing you feed frequently.
* Some medicines can restrict milk flow: the combined contraceptive pill for instance (page 154) is not advised during breastfeeding.

Supplementing with or switching to formula

You may be tempted to 'supplement' your baby's feeds with formula milk. This works for some people – often a bottle of formula last thing at night – but not for all. Sometimes feeding less means a reduced milk supply. You may prefer to begin by cancelling other commitments, trying homeopathy, attending to your diet and the amount of rest you are getting, and feeding your baby as often and for as long as she enjoys it – this will boost your supply. If, on balance, you would rather mix breast and bottle (page 75), it is useful to wait until your baby is four to five months old. Another option is to stop breastfeeding completely (page 90). This may be a challenging decision but if it makes both of you happier it may be best for your family.

Homeopathy

To increase your milk supply you may try *Urtica Urens* (6c potency) four times per day for three to five days and then re-assess. You may also take one of the following remedies three times a day for three days and re-assess:

- *Lac Defloratum* (30c) if you are feeling despondent and anti-social, feel better for rest and warmth and have a headache.
- *Pulsatilla* (30c) when your milk flow is scanty, thin or disappears, particularly if you feel weepy and vulnerable and want company and feel worse for being in a hot stuffy room, better for fresh air.
- *China* (30c) if you are exhausted. Taken morning and night for one week, *China* is a great pick-up remedy.

Aromatherapy

To stimulate milk production, try fennel, jasmine, lemongrass, clary sage or geranium, used when you massage or in a compress. Always mix the essential oil with a carrier oil (page 36). Massage your breasts gently after feeding so the oil will be fully absorbed when your baby next feeds. If it irritates, wash the oil off immediately. Fennel passes through to your milk and can settle your baby's digestion, but should not be used if you are epileptic. Avoid clary sage before sleep, as it causes vivid dreams, and do not use it if you have been drinking alcohol.

▓ MASTITIS AND ABSCESSES

Mastitis is an infection in the breast that usually follows blocked ducts (page 91), and it cannot always be prevented. It can be very unpleasant but usually responds well to treatment. In a tiny percentage of breastfeeding women, mastitis infection is severe and may progress into a breast abscess.

What happens

Bacteria are normally present on your skin. If they reach retained milk in a blocked milk duct, they may cause an infection and mastitis may develop. The infective bacteria are usually Staphylococcus. Rarely, mastitis develops without blocked ducts.

Signs of mastitis

- In the early stages, mastitis involves slight swelling and redness and a slight rise in your temperature. The redness and temperature rise distinguish it from breast engorgement.
- Your breast may be hot to touch.
- Your breast may feel lumpy and hard.
- With severe mastitis, your breasts will be very red and painful and you may have a high temperature and flu-like symptoms.

Susceptibility

Susceptibility to mastitis infection increases if your immunity is low – for instance if you are unwell, very tired or emotionally low, if you are not eating nutritiously, or if you smoke. You are more susceptible if your baby does not empty your breast. Having mastitis with one baby does not necessarily mean you'll get it a second time.

Abscesses

You may be offered an ultrasound scan, which can detect whether the mastitis is associated with an abscess. An abscess is a collection of pus that forms in the tissues. It is a more severe form of infection and occurs in the breast as a complication of mastitis, when some of the breast tissue is damaged. A breast abscess causes a very high temperature, severe flu-like symptoms, and a very red and extremely painful large lump in one breast. If you have taken antibiotics, the temperature, pain and redness may be less obvious.

Action plan

If you are getting recurrent mastitis, take professional advice and ask someone to help you establish a good position to ensure your baby is draining your breasts effectively. Poor drainage is almost always the initial trigger that leads to mastitis.

The advice for blocked ducts is very useful if you have mastitis (page 95). Caring for yourself (pages 121–4) is important too.

Unless you are in severe pain, do try to keep feeding. This helps to drain your breast and maintain your milk supply. Your baby has been exposed to the bacteria causing the infection since birth and will not be harmed. Expressing a little milk before a feed may make it easier for your baby to latch on and empty your breast. Please follow the advice on page 83 for establishing a good position. If the pain is too intense or the infection does not settle despite treatment, it may be necessary to stop breastfeeding.

Ensure your bra is not putting excess pressure on all or part of your breast.

Treating mastitis: medical care
Mastitis may make you feel very unwell but once treatment starts recovery is usually rapid. The following are the most commonly supplied drug treatments:

Ibuprofen
Mastitis may reduce within 48 hours in response to anti-inflammatory agents such as ibuprofen. You may take it if the mastitis is mild, your white blood cell count is normal (it rises if there is an infection) and your temperature is not very high. The dosage will be advised by your doctor or midwife. Ibuprofen is best taken after food to prevent the stomach becoming inflamed. Do not take ibuprofen if you have asthma, stomach ulcers or an allergy to aspirin.

Paracetamol
This can relieve pain and reduce a temperature and you may take this in the dosage advised by your doctor or midwife.

Antibiotics
If mastitis is severe or you have a fever that is rising and you feel sick or your nipples are cracked, or your white blood cell count is rising, or you have recurrent mastitis, an antibiotic is advisable. It is essential to continue to encourage your breast to empty completely to reduce the risk of an abscess forming.

If you are allergic to the usual antibiotics prescribed for mastitis, there are others you can take. The recommended antibiotics are believed to be safe for babies. A small amount of the

antibiotic appears in your milk and is passed on to your baby but it is very unusual for a baby to suffer side effects. The commonest effect is diarrhoea in the baby. It is best to complete the course to reduce the risk of the mastitis returning, unless advised to stop by your doctor or midwife. If you don't feel better after two days you may need to consult your doctor and change medication. If you take antibiotics you may choose to use complementary support, such as taking probiotics (see page 35).

Intravenous antibiotics
Rarely, when mastitis is severe, a hospital stay is advised so that antibiotics can be given intravenously (by vein). If this happens, your baby may be able to stay with you on the ward, and you may still be able to continue feeding her.

Antifungal drugs
Thrush (candida) infection in the milk ducts can lead to mastitis too. If mastitis does not improve on antibiotics, you may need antifungal treatment for candida (page 117).

Treating an abscess: medical care
An abscess needs to be treated with intensive intravenous antibiotic therapy, possibly in hospital. You may be upset that you cannot stay at home but babies are usually welcome to stay with their mums.

If the abscess does not respond to antibiotics within 24 hours, the pus will need to be drained. A small collection can be removed in the ultrasound room by using a needle with local anaesthesia. Larger collections are drained in the operating theatre under general anaesthetic. A soft plastic drain is then left in place for a day or two. Early drainage of pus is essential to protect your breast tissue and cure the infection.

Although some women elect to continue to feed on both breasts, many discontinue if they have had surgery. The operation site is uncomfortable (but not very painful) for a few days. With love and support from your friends and family you will find it easier to recover when you get home.

Homeopathy
For mastitis remedies, consult the symptom pictures listed for blocked ducts. If you require antibiotics, or surgery for an abscess, it is best to

consult a homeopath for individually prescribed treatment. The suggestions on page 34 may help support you while you take antibiotics.

■ NIPPLES, CRACKED

If your nipples become cracked, this may bring sharp, piercing pain at every feed. The cracks may bleed. They do not cause your baby harm, even though some blood may show up in her stools (page 447). Cracked nipples are more common in women with fair or sensitive skin, but seldom occur when latching on and positioning are good. Thrush (candida) can cause similar symptoms. Cracked nipples are much more common with a first baby, so don't be put off breastfeeding for your second.

What happens

If your baby does not latch on properly and takes your nipple instead of the areola into her mouth, there is a lot of pressure on your nipple from your baby's palate. While she sucks, she will draw blood to your nipple and the pressure of sucking and blood beneath the skin can cause small cracks.

Action plan

The only way to treat and prevent further cracks is to ensure your baby is well positioned and correctly latched on. The suggestions below will help to soothe your nipples, and they are likely to heal well if you care for them. Everyone is different: if one method doesn't work, try another. Whatever method you use, continue feeding, paying extra special attention to position and latching on. Changing your baby's position with each feed can help, as it alters the pressure on the skin of your nipples.

While attending to your feeding technique, it is important to treat the cracks because they are a route for infection and increase the risk of mastitis.

- Massage your nipple skin gently for a few minutes after a feed with a small amount of natural oil, and then expose your nipples to air for as long as you are comfortable to do so. A good mix is a ratio of one to nine: one part wheatgerm to nine parts almond oil, plus two

to three drops of calendula tincture in a 50ml bottle. Use a small amount so that your nipple does not become too moist. The oils do not heal the nipple, but are soothing. You might prefer to try a small amount of *calendula* or vitamin E cream. Sometimes expressed milk applied to the nipple after a feed and left to dry is very soothing.
- Wear a well-fitting natural cotton bra.
- Avoid waterproof lined breast pads or bras – they keep your skin wet and this can delay healing.
- Protect your nipples from being rubbed by coarse clothing and wash with water only – avoid soap and astringent wipes.
- Infection on the skin, particularly with candida (thrush), will prevent healing: it's important to tend to any infection.
- Using a cold cabbage leaf as recommended for engorgement (page 92) is useful, provided you also air your nipples to allow them to dry. Remove the cabbage leaves after 20 minutes to prevent the skin becoming soggy.
- Nipple shields are occasionally helpful as a temporary solution until the cracks heal, but need to be used carefully (and rarely as a first choice) in combination with airing your nipples. They are available from chemists or your midwife may supply them.
- If your nipples suddenly become red after months of feeding you may have a new infection of thrush. You'll be more susceptible if you have recently had antibiotics. One way to tell is to check your baby's tongue and her nappy area for signs (page 117). Thrush can be treated with specific antifungal tablets and creams, by exposure to sun and with homeopathy.

Homeopathy
You may take the most appropriate remedy (6c potency) three times a day for up to five days and then re-assess.
- *Castor Equi* if your nipples are cracked, sore and extremely sensitive and you cannot bear to have anything near them.
- *Graphites* if your nipples are cracked and blistered or bleeding.
- *Silica* if the cracks bleed and you have burning or splinter-like pains while feeding.
- You can also use a soothing application of 10 drops *Hypercal* tincture diluted in 250ml of

boiled, cooled water then dry your nipples and apply calendula cream or Rescue Remedy cream.

• If you have thrush, turn to pages 118–19 for remedy suggestions.

▦ NIPPLES, FLAT OR INVERTED

Some women have naturally flat or inverted nipples, but it is rare for this to interfere with feeding. You may need to spend lots of time as you get feeding established so you and your baby are comfortable. Occasionally it is useful to encourage the nipples to protrude in pregnancy. If your nipples are not naturally flat and become flat after you have started feeding, a likely cause is engorgement (page 92), which can be simply reduced.

Action plan

The key is to spend time with your baby, skin to skin. The hormones produced by your body in response to the touch of her skin stimulate your nipples and breasts. It is equally important to attend to latching on and your baby's position. You may respond to hands-on help from your midwife or breastfeeding counsellor.

• Breastfeed as soon as possible after the birth and at least every two to three hours to help your baby drain your breast fully and avoid engorgement.

• Hold your breast with your fingers underneath and thumb on top. Press and push back towards your chest and then press your fingers and thumb together lightly to elongate the areola and encourage your nipple to protrude.

• Gently massaging your areola to draw the nipple out may help – start very delicately while your nipple skin gets used to it. You can begin, gently, in pregnancy.

• Breast pump manufacturers sell a small plastic thimble-size device that fits over the nipple, can be worn under a bra, and has a small suction balloon to draw the nipple out. It needs to be attached for 10 minutes before a feed and can be reused. You can also use it in pregnancy to prepare your breast. Alternatively, try using a breast pump, which may draw out your nipples before feeding.

• There are breast shells designed for flat or inverted nipples to be worn for 30 minutes before a feed – they fit inside your bra. They are plastic with a hole through which the nipple can protrude, and a rounded dome cover. You can begin to wear these in pregnancy and if you use them after birth be sure to wash and sterilise them regularly to guard against infection. These are used less often than the plastic thimble.

▦ PAIN

Pain is a common problem in breastfeeding, especially when you are still learning the technique. The keys to reducing pain are almost always positioning and spending time with your baby skin to skin. This encourages successful feeding, and also promotes your body to produce pain-relieving substances. More specific measures will usually depend on the underlying cause:

Pain with swelling

As your breasts produce milk, they enlarge, and as your baby feeds, they reduce in size. Occasionally, they may feel painfully swollen.

• Within a day or two of the birth, your breasts are likely to feel uncomfortable. This is not serious: the swelling is a result of your milk coming in. It may be considerable until your baby establishes feeding and drains your milk efficiently. If you continue feeding, this discomfort passes within a few days.

• The swelling is called engorgement (page 92) and may also happen if your breasts produce more milk than your baby drinks. Feeding on demand helps your body to match your baby's rhythm and reduces the accumulation of milk.

• Your breasts may become painfully swollen when you stop breastfeeding before milk production stops. The tips on page 90 may help relieve discomfort.

Pain before a feed

Let-down pain may occur at the beginning of a feed as the small muscles in the wall of each milk duct contract and eject milk towards your nipple. It reduces as your baby feeds. After a few days, let-down pain usually diminishes but for a small minority of women it continues.

• For some women, let-down pain can be intense. If the pain is considerable, and to guard against excessive build-up of milk and the risks of engorgement (page 92), you can gently express a little milk before feeding your baby. This will also help to reduce excessive flow.

- Sometimes a candida (thrush) infection (page 117) can cause pain before a feed. Unfortunately the problem may be diagnosed as thrush when the real cause of pain is improper positioning. If you are unsure of a diagnosis, ask for a second opinion before starting any treatment.

Breast and muscle pain
Generalised breast, nipple or muscle pain is almost always down to positioning. If so, the remedy is to attend to your baby's position. Remember, if your breast is painful it is still important to keep feeding.

- Muscle pain can stem from the way you hold your baby while feeding or carrying her. Sometimes it is linked with underlying emotional tension (page 221). You may feel pain in the pectoral muscles on the front of your chest, behind your breast and into your shoulder and perhaps your neck. It may be confused with mastitis but your breast won't be red. You or your doctor can diagnose muscle pain by feeling the tender muscle. Gentle stretching and changing feeding position may ease the discomfort, and you may seek treatment from an osteopath (page 424).
- Blocked milk ducts cause pain with a hard lump in the breast. Pain arises from the pressure of the milk and inflammation of the surrounding tissues. It is important to drain the blockage (page 91) to reduce the risk of mastitis.
- Pain with redness and swelling may be a sign of mastitis, which needs prompt treatment (page 95).
- Cracked nipples (page 97) may occur if your feeding position is poor and your baby does not latch on properly.
- With your doctor's advice you may take paracetamol or ibuprofen (for doses see page 429).

If you have pain, try not to get downhearted. It may be encouraging to know that many women experience discomfort and it is usually temporary. Once you have targeted the cause and taken appropriate measures, you and your baby have a very good chance of settling back into a comfortable and rewarding feeding partnership.

▨ REJECTION BY BABY

Breastfeeding connects you and your baby, and is a vital source of nutrition. If your baby does not show any interest in feeding, it is important to consider possible reasons and to address them. You may be concerned that your baby is not well. You may even feel uncomfortable because you feel you are being rejected. Usually, these fears are groundless, the problem soon passes and these issues are resolved.

What happens

Breast rejection straight after birth
The majority of babies enjoy connecting with their mums and suckling at the breast very soon after birth – some within minutes, some within an hour or two. Some babies are less interested and do not turn to the breast for a feed for several hours.

- If your baby has swallowed amniotic fluid during birth, her full stomach may quell her appetite. She may be sleepy and calm, and not ask for milk.
- Much less commonly, the sucking reflex may be weak (usually this is due to prematurity, page 455).
- Your soft breasts are flexible and usually able to mould to the shape of your baby's mouth and the pattern of her sucking. Rarely, a developmental problem such as CLEFT LIP or TONGUE TIE interferes. If your baby is affected, specialist consultants will offer you support and advice to help you establish feeding or, alternatively, to express milk for your baby until treatment is completed and she can breastfeed.

Rejection after feeding is established
- If your baby is behaving unusually, cries, seems to be in pain or is quiet and withdrawn, these may be signs of illness or infection. She may have a small appetite, or feel too tired to suck.
- Discomfort from earache, teething pains or colic can reduce your baby's appetite, distract her, and it may be uncomfortable to suck or swallow.
- Taste and smell may put her off if you have eaten something unusual, washed with a new soap, or used a new perfume.
- Some babies react by withdrawing or going off their feeds when there is tension or conflict in the family.

- If you are stressed, your milk flow may be low. This may be frustrating for your baby.
- If you are feeling trapped or upset, your baby may sense this and find it difficult to enjoy the intimacy of feeding. This can be part of a cycle, as her rejection may perpetuate your feelings of not being good enough.
- You and your baby are in partnership and the connection of breastfeeding reflects the bond between you. Rejection, fear, uncertainty and anger may get in the way. Both you and your baby may have these feelings (page 210).

Action plan

Medical support

- If your baby seems unwell, consult your doctor.
- If your baby vomits after her feeds, particularly if this is projectile vomiting, consult your doctor (page 553).
- If your baby does not feed for six hours, it is important to prevent dehydration. She may take some water from a bottle or from a teaspoon or cup (the water must be boiled and then allowed to cool). Consult your doctor urgently if your baby is not taking fluids.

Being with your baby

- Being close to your baby will help the two of you to bond, and may create a calm and secure atmosphere for your baby to settle into a feed. You both need quality time. Plenty of body contact – preferably skin to skin – helps your baby feel secure, may increase her interest in your breast, and helps your breasts produce milk.
- When you feed, pay close attention to latching on and positioning so that you and your baby are comfortable, and your baby is stimulating your milk flow.
- You may want to relax together, maybe in the bath. As you both let go of tension, feeding may become easier.
- What you eat, your baby eats. She may be sensitive to one or more foods that irritate her stomach or bowel. If you identify something that upsets her she will feel much better when it is not present in your milk. She may have milk intolerance. If the sensitivity persists, she may connect feeding with discomfort and continue to reject your breast. Your midwife or doctor may help.

- If you are feeling anxious, tense or distanced from your baby, it is important to seek support and advice from friends, family and perhaps professionals. There are many ways to enhance bonding that may also improve your feeding partnership. These are explored on page 210.

If your baby rejects one breast

It may not be clear why your baby favours one breast over the other. It may be the shape of your nipple or the milk flow, or how comfortable it is for you. A pattern may begin very early on.

Your baby can be sufficiently nourished from one breast, but it is not optimal. You can try to resume feeding from the less-favoured breast by starting each feed there and by expressing milk regularly on that side. If this doesn't work, you may have uneven breasts for a time and will need to be careful not to develop mastitis (page 95) in the underused breast.

Your older baby

As your baby gets older, she may become distracted during a feed by everything that's going on around her. Creating a quieter space with less distraction may help her relax into feeding. Some babies stop showing an interest when they are ready to separate from the breast. By rejecting your breast, your baby may be saying she's had enough and is ready to become more independent. It may be time for breastfeeding to come to an end and if you stop (page 90) it is still important to create intimate time together, for example, in the bath, in bed, during bottle-feeding, etc.

▨ SWELLING

If your breasts swell, this may be part of the normal cycle of milk build-up before your baby drains your breasts at the next feed. If swelling does not pass, you may need to take measures to reduce engorgement (page 92). Swelling with acute pain and/or lumps may be a sign of blocked ducts (page 91) or mastitis (page 95).

Breath holding, baby

If your baby habitually takes a deep breath in, breathes out and fails to breathe in again for some time, you will naturally become concerned. It will not harm your baby but the persistent habit may be upsetting for the whole family. A common cause of breath holding is pain from acid reflux (page 554) and this can usually be simply treated. Other causes include feelings of anger or fear, which are natural and common for all babies (page 208).

Around 20 per cent of children show episodes of breath holding some time between the age of six months and four years, although, unusually, it may start earlier and go on later. There is often a history of breath holding in the family. Kangaroo baby care (page 518) reduces the incidence of breath holding.

What happens

Breath-holding episodes are self-limiting, each lasting just a few seconds, but this can feel like a lifetime for the adult who is watching. When your baby fails to breathe in, his lips and face will go red or blue. Depending on how long he holds his breath for, he may begin to breathe again normally, or faint. Fainting is a safety mechanism that relaxes the body and enables normal breathing to restart.

While unconscious, even for a few seconds, your baby may go stiff, and then twitch. This is a small fit, but the episode is so short there is no likelihood of brain damage. After a breath-holding episode, your baby will soon be bright and alert, whereas after a more serious fit, he is likely to be sleepy. Breath holding is not related to epilepsy, and is not a trigger for it.

A longer period without breathing may be more frightening and could be apnoea or, rarely, an apparent life-threatening event that is usually harmless but requires investigation.

Action plan

Medical care

- Ask your doctor if painful reflux or a hernia may be the cause. If so it can be treated.
- If your baby holds his breath as many as 5–10 times a day, every day, and each episode lasts more than a minute and does not seem to be related to a trigger, seek advice from your doctor or health visitor. Although it is probably a harmless habit, it is important to exclude the small possibility that it might be connected to a fit (seizure) disorder, or some abnormality of heart rhythm.
- If your child appears white or pale rather than red/blue there may be a more serious problem, suggestive of a possible fit, or heart rhythm or rate problem. This should be considered, particularly if an older or more mobile child falls to the ground, and must be investigated by a paediatrician.

Coping with, and preventing, breath holding

- Think about possible triggers and avoid them where possible.
- Remain calm while your baby holds his breath. If he is angry or afraid and you begin to shout or panic, this could increase his tension.
- Stay with your baby, who may be afraid of being alone.
- Distract or soothe your baby during crying episodes, as these may be one cause of breath holding.
- Skin-to-skin contact or contact with clothing is a very powerful way to reduce breath holding.
- Inform other people who care for your baby and let them know what you normally do.

Some infant psychologists propose that breath holding may be a way of getting attention. If you think this may be relevant, it's a good idea to talk to the rest of the family or other adults in your life and consider possible reasons for your baby wanting attention, and whether he is receiving quality time with you on a regular basis. A parenting class or your health visitor may offer useful advice and support.

Homeopathy

The following remedies may be helpful for breath-holding episodes. Give the remedy as soon as possible and again five minutes later. Use a soft 30c potency tablet that will dissolve quickly or can be rubbed onto the inside of your baby's cheek.

- *Arnica* if there has been injury or physical trauma.

- *Aconite* if there has been an emotional shock or your baby has been afraid.
- *Chamomilla* after a temper tantrum, anger or rage.

Breathing difficulties, baby

See also Foetal distress and asphyxia.

Most babies establish regular breathing within a few minutes of birth, during which time they are receiving a back-up supply of oxygen via the umbilical cord. A small percentage – around 2 per cent – have difficulty breathing. This is known as asphyxia (page 249), and rarely results in breathing difficulties beyond the first few minutes of birth. After birth, rapid breathing, noisy breathing, grunting or irregular breathing may occur, due to one of the causes listed in the following entries. A rare cause of breathing difficulties, often with oxygen deprivation that gives a baby a blue (cyanotic) appearance, is a HEART condition.

It is normal for a baby's breathing rhythm to fluctuate, depending on his state of wakefulness, and whether he feels relaxed or tense, peaceful or excited. Some studies show that babies who feel stressed show particularly marked variations in breathing rhythm, in part linked with stress hormones (page 310). Stress may arise for many reasons, including pain, fear, separation anxiety, the experience of incubation or special care, hunger or wind.

+ Red flag

If your baby stops breathing or has breathing difficulties, the first step is to assist his breathing:
- Use the ABC: ensure your baby's Airway is clear; check his Breathing; check his Circulation – this is a core aspect of first aid (page 4).
- You may need to carry out resuscitation (page 3).
- Call for help – dial 999. The medical team may be 15 minutes away.

Babies tend to breathe regularly when they are held, skin to skin, by their mother or another adult in whose arms they feel safe. Your baby's breathing will change depending on what is happening. He will also mirror you, and babies given prolonged skin-to-skin contact (page 517) have few variations in their breathing.

ABSENCE, APNOEA AND ALTE

If your baby stops breathing you will naturally become concerned and you may panic. It is actually quite common for the normal breathing pattern of a healthy full-term baby to be irregular, with pauses of up to 20 seconds between breaths, until the age of three months. If you see that your baby is not breathing, count to 20, and then gently rouse him if he has not started to breathe in that time. This will probably be enough to make him breathe normally again.

Apnoea
Cessation of breathing for an extended period followed by the resumption of normal breathing is known as apnoea and is more noticeable during sleep or when a baby has a chest infection. It occurs more often among premature babies, although by the time a premature baby leaves the special care unit, the episodes of apnoea will have stopped or reduced considerably. In rare cases, apnoea may be a symptom of an underlying cause that needs investigation or treatment, such as WHOOPING COUGH (pertussis) or seizures/FITS.

Apparent life-threatening event (ALTE)
If apnoea is prolonged, although terrifying, this will not result in your baby dying. As the oxygen levels in the brain fall, he will faint. This will cause him to relax, and his airway will relax too so he can breathe normally again. This may be called ALTE, or an apparent life-threatening event. It is extremely frightening for a parent or any other adult watching, especially if the baby's colour changes (to blue, white or perhaps very red-faced).

Some parents fear that their baby has died, but this is not the case. ALTE has previously been called 'near-miss SIDS' but this is not accurate because there is no association between this type of irregular breathing and sudden infant death. Between 1 and 6 per cent of babies are reported to have ALTE. The many possible causes can be investigated by specialists but usually nothing is found and the events stop.

+ Red flag

Seek urgent medical attention if your baby is breathing unusually noisily, coughing or wheezing, seems short of breath and especially if there is a blue colour to the skin. There is a small chance that your baby may have inhaled a small object, and be choking (page 6). If the medical team diagnose an infection, treatment can begin early.

Checks following ALTE

It is certainly better to be safe than sorry, and you do always need to report such an event. Every baby who has ALTE is investigated fully.

* Following the initial care, your baby will be admitted to hospital so that medical professionals can observe any more spells of breathing difficulty if they occur and listen to your baby's normal pattern of breathing.
* Your baby will be monitored for low blood oxygen levels with a tiny pad placed on his hand or foot (called a pulse oximeter) and will be tested for ANAEMIA and infections, including whooping cough. His heart rate may also be monitored and a chest X-ray or ultrasound scan carried out to check for heart disorders. Some causes of noisy breathing can lead to ALTE including gastro-oesophageal reflux (page 554).
* If your baby has reflux, or there is evidence of a fit, he may be given medication.
* You will be reassured and given advice about what to do if a similar event recurs.
* Most babies who have an ALTE have no breathing problems in the future. Some parents are advised to use an apnoea monitor for extra precaution.
* After ALTE, your baby will have follow-up assessments and any treatment required for an underlying cause.
* You may need reassurance and support to

reduce your anxiety of it happening again. If all the tests are negative then the event does not indicate that your baby is at any higher risk of sudden infant death.

▇ NOISY BREATHING

Noisy breathing (stridor) is more common in babies over one month of age. It may be due to several possible causes, which are, in order of commonness:

* A COUGH resulting from chest infection – this is the most common cause.
* Reflux onto the vocal cords (page 554), which accounts for about 75 per cent of all cases of noisy breathing.
* Asthma (page 36).
* Laryngomalacia or floppy larynx (page 104).
* An underlying heart condition, although this is very rare.
* Swallowing an object or choking, also very rare in young babies.

The best course of action is to seek medical attention as soon as possible to discover what is causing your baby to breathe noisily.

Medical diagnostic techniques

The doctor may examine your baby by listening to his breathing and looking at the larynx while the baby sits on your lap. It is most likely that there is no serious cause. If you or your doctor wish to investigate further, your baby may be given further tests, such as:

* A chest X-ray to inspect his heart, lungs and bones.
* A barium swallow, where your baby swallows a dye that shows up on X-rays. This is used to detect the reflux (page 554) or backflow of stomach contents up the oesophagus and into the lungs. Usually the diagnosis is made after your doctor has considered the background history, such as when and where your baby breathes noisily, for how long, and what makes it better or worse, and has examined your baby. X-rays are rarely used.
* A pH test for acid reflux may be carried out by a nurse or specialist paediatric gastroenterologist.
* An echocardiogram (an ultrasound examination of the heart) checks for any abnormality, and an

ECG checks the heart's electrical activity and rhythm.

- An examination of your baby's upper airway using a flexible fibre-optic viewing device (endoscope) placed in the nose may be carried out by a specialist in paediatric respiratory medicine.

Laryngomalacia (floppy larynx)

Laryngomalacia is floppiness of the larynx (voice box), which is part of the upper airway. It occurs in about 10 per cent of otherwise healthy children and shows up as noisy breathing, usually starting several weeks after birth. The noise is often high-pitched, may sound like grunting, and will get worse if your baby gets agitated or excited or has a cold. It tends to get better or disappear in sleep. A floppy larynx is not a serious condition and usually corrects itself by the age of 24 months, and often earlier.

The floppiness is caused by an excess of the normal flexibility in the cartilage rings that keep your baby's airway open – it is not caused by any structural weakness or muscle paralysis. It is frequently linked with gastro-oesophageal reflux (page 554), and may be aggravated by the reflux, which can be readily treated.

In fewer than 1 per cent of cases, it interferes with feeding, leading to failure to thrive (page 559). Less commonly, it leads to temporary difficulty with breathing, and rarely it is connected with an underlying condition. Thus if your baby shows symptoms a paediatrician may want to examine him. For instance, if your baby has large birthmarks there may be a need to look down his throat – an investigation called microlaryngobronchoscopy (MLB) – to check that the noisy breathing is not arising from a birthmark, or strawberry mark (page 52), in the larynx.

Medical care

Laryngomalacia usually corrects itself. However, if your baby is having difficulty feeding, or has had an apparent life-threatening event (ALTE, page 102), a doctor will want to investigate further. These will be similar to the investigations listed above, under medical diagnostic techniques (page 103).

In extremely rare cases, the condition is severe enough to need highly specialised surgery to stiffen the walls of the trachea (windpipe) and larynx.

■ RAPID BREATHING AND GRUNTING

See also Premature birth.

If your baby appears to be breathing very rapidly, the breathing is noisy or there is grunting, seek medical advice. The most likely cause is transient tachypnoea of the newborn (TTN), respiratory distress syndrome (RDS) or infection.

Transient tachypnoea of the newborn (TTN)

While a baby is in the womb, the lungs contain liquid produced by the cells lining the airway. In most cases this fluid is rapidly absorbed into the circulation once breathing begins. If there is a delay in the absorption of this fluid, it can inhibit airflow into the lungs, and the baby will need to breathe fast to overcome the resistance. This is TTN. The condition affects up to 5 per cent of healthy term babies, and is 20 times more common in babies born by CAESAREAN SECTION. TTN is rarely serious and the lung fluid is usually naturally absorbed into the circulation within a few hours, allowing the baby to breathe normally. TTN is, however, the most common cause for transfer to a special care baby unit (SCBU) where a baby can be given additional oxygen and/or antibiotic treatment in case there is an infection in the lungs.

If your baby has TTN, the course of action will be determined by the precise symptoms and the judgement of the midwife and doctor looking after you and your baby. In some hospitals, it is routine to begin antibiotic treatment early as the breathing difficulty may be a symptom of infection, particularly Group B Strep (GBS, page 269). An alternative approach is to delay treatment unless a baby has other signs of illness, such as floppiness or low blood sugar, since many babies who grunt immediately after birth are fine within a few hours. If breathing difficulty persists for more than four hours then antibiotics are always recommended, and blood cultures and ear swabs (using a small cotton pad to take a sample of fluid from the ear) will be taken to check for infection. Results take a minimum of 48 hours and if they are negative then antibiotics are stopped.

When breathing difficulties continue, a baby is typically transferred to a special care baby unit. Occasionally, the baby needs some type of respiratory support, usually oxygen. Additional respiratory support may be provided in the form of continuous positive airway pressure (CPAP). This is a small nose or face mask placed on the baby's face that delivers a current of air of sufficient pressure to help open up areas of the lungs so that more oxygen may enter the blood. Occasionally a ventilator may be required.

Respiratory distress syndrome (RDS)

During the last six to 10 weeks of pregnancy, a baby's lungs produce surfactant, a molecule that lowers the surface tension of the lining of the lungs to allow them to expand in air. If this surfactant is absent, usually when birth is premature but occasionally following asphyxia or if a baby is born at term and the mother has DIABETES, there will be difficulty breathing. This is respiratory distress syndrome (RDS). Elective caesarean section is also associated with a much higher risk of the baby developing surfactant dependent respiratory distress, although this is less likely if performed at 39 or 40 weeks. RDS requires special care (page 497).

Infection

In premature babies, or babies born after premature rupture of the membranes (that is, more then 18 hours before birth), or a long labour, there is a chance that infection from the mother's vagina may pass into the uterus and reach the lungs as the baby performs breathing movements. Newborn babies are sensitive to the GBS infection (page 269). In the rare case that a baby is infected with GBS before birth, early symptoms may include grunting and rapid breathing, and there is a chance that pneumonia may develop. Infection is treated by intensive intravenous antibiotics and a baby may require respiratory support, occasionally requiring some type of mechanical ventilation until the infection clears.

Breathing, mother

See also Labour and birth, mother, breathing.

Your breath is an incredibly powerful tool for health. Most people do not use the full capacity of their lungs and miss out on the energy of oxygen and the chance to fully expel toxic gases and to feel deeply relaxed. Breathing well is helpful for men, women and children, and your baby will show you just how natural and nourishing deep breathing can be. Awareness of your breath may help you relax, remain calm if you feel stressed and to 'refuel' when you are tired but do not have time to sleep. Breathing through contractions (page 362) or practising antenatally may be the first time you become aware of your breath.

Your breath is your ally when you have uncomfortable feelings. An automatic reaction to fear, anxiety, pain and anger is to take short shallow in-breaths. This increases tension and confusion. Breathing deeply, on the other hand, provides energy and allows time for you to override your body's conditioned responses and focus calmly on the present. Your out-breath offers you the gift of relaxation: it is difficult to remain uptight when you breathe out.

If you feel panicky or anxious your breathing will be fast and shallow. This is called hyperventilation. It is associated with feeling light-headed and faint, sometimes with chest tightness. Taking a moment to focus on your breathing – rather than the thing(s) that stress you – may greatly reduce your tension; and taking regular breaks in your day to do one or two minutes of deep breathing may reduce your general anxiety. Women who have panic attacks can reduce the anxiety by breathing deeply.

Tips for breathing deeply

- Let your diaphragm expand as you breathe in – like a balloon filling with air – and then contract as you breathe out. This action massages your internal organs: your diaphragm is a powerful muscle.
- Allowing your lungs to fully deflate as you exhale will help you inhale more deeply. As you practise, begin with awareness of the out-breath.

- Place your hands on your tummy below your belly button and feel the rise as you breathe in and the fall as you breathe out.
- Your baby is an excellent teacher. You will see his diaphragm rising and falling and his rhythm change depending on whether he's awake, asleep, calm, tense, hungry or feeding.
- Awareness increases with practice. A reasonable goal is not to be focused on your breath all the time but to develop the skill to tune in to your breath when you need to boost your energy, relax or face a challenge.

You may practise deep breathing at a yoga or antenatal class or at home. If you are keen to take it further there are numerous exercises, often with roots in YOGA, that energise and relax mind and body. In yoga, the postures are designed to allow deep and full breathing, a foundation for peace, meditation and a powerful flow of vital energy.

Breathlessness, mother

See also Asthma, mother.

Approximately 50 per cent of pregnant women feel breathless before Week 20 and even more by Week 40. Usually, this accompanies physical exertion but it may occur when you lie down.

What happens

If you are fit and have good cardiac function, the increased demands on your heart may pass unnoticed. Lying on your back or sitting or standing for a long time may bring on breathlessness because this reduces the return of blood to the heart. This might also make your blood pressure fall, giving a feeling of faintness. If you are anxious, you may be unaware that you are taking fast, shallow breaths (hyperventilating).

Breathlessness is usually nothing to worry about, but when it is sudden, severe or prolonged, or happens when you are relaxing, it may indicate ANAEMIA (low red blood-cell count), or, rarely, a HEART or lung problem. It may be due to asthma (page 38) or a chest infection (page 160), which will also cause coughing.

+ Red flag

On rare occasions a blood clot from a deep vein thrombosis (page 545) in the leg may travel to the lungs, causing a pulmonary embolus. The sudden onset of breathlessness with no apparent cause may be the first sign of this life-threatening condition, particularly if associated with chest pain and calf pain, although it can occur without pain. It needs urgent treatment.

Action plan

If there is an underlying physical cause for breathlessness, it may need treatment. Your blood haemoglobin levels may need to be checked to rule out anaemia. Otherwise, simple steps may help and when pregnancy is over, breathlessness will no longer be an issue.

Medical care

If breathlessness comes on suddenly or is severe consult your doctor urgently. If you have leg or chest pain, call an ambulance.

Diet and lifestyle

- Multivitamin and mineral supplements and good nutrition are generally helpful and may reduce anaemia.
- A graduated exercise programme will help, provided your heart and lungs are normal. Ask your doctor or a fitness trainer to advise you.
- Try altering posture by lying on your side and avoiding sitting and standing still for prolonged periods. Tightening and releasing your calf and leg muscles or your buttocks 10 or 15 times will help to pump blood to your heart. This will also help if you feel faint (page 71).
- If you are anxious or depressed (page 174) seek support to reduce hyperventilation. VISUALISATION may help you relax and YOGA will help you breathe deeply.

Homeopathy

You may take the most appropriate remedy (30c potency) three times per day for up to four days and then re-assess the situation.

- *Aconite* if breathlessness is accompanied by fear and palpitations, often with symptoms worse at night.
- *Arsenicum* if you feel weak yet restless, agitated and worried, are pale and perhaps feel worse around midnight.
- *Ipecac* when you also feel nauseous, chilly on the outside yet warm inside and worse after eating and at night.

Breech birth

See *Labour and birth, baby, position*.

Broken bones

See *Accidents and first aid, baby, broken bones and fractures*.

Bronchiolitis (RSV)

See also *Coughs and colds, baby*.

Bronchiolitis is a common viral infection that affects over 90 per cent of children by the age of two years. It is often caused by the respiratory syncitial virus (RSV), found in the air, but many other viruses cause similar illnesses. Babies are most susceptible in the first four weeks after birth. Premature babies or those suffering from congenital heart disease are more vulnerable.

What happens

Bronchiolitis starts with a cough, initially dry, with a tinny, metallic quality. After three or four days, or perhaps as long as a week, the cough becomes wetter, the baby develops a runny nose and may go off his feeds. The cough usually brings on wheezing (like asthma) and symptoms tend to worsen for up to five days before improving. Usually there is no fever. If your baby gets a temperature after about four days, this probably indicates that a bacterial infection has also developed in the bronchioles. The cough may linger for up to eight weeks, but if your baby is feeding and putting on weight you can rest assured the cough will stop.

Action plan

- In general no specific medicines are needed. Your doctor may advise you to give an asthma treatment, such as salbutamol as a syrup. This may help.
- If your baby has a fever (bacterial infection), bronchiolitis will take longer to get better and antibiotics may be needed for five days or more.

You may visit your homeopath after a medical diagnosis. Before your baby is nine months old it is not appropriate to home-prescribe.

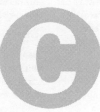

Caesarean section

Delivery by caesarean section ('C-section') is now the second most common operation performed on women, after episiotomy (page 369). In the UK over 20 per cent of babies are born by caesarean. In some countries the figure is 40 per cent.

A caesarean may be carried out because a medical need becomes apparent during pregnancy (called a planned caesarean) or in labour (emergency caesarean). Many women now choose to have a caesarean for reasons other than medical need (elective caesarean). A woman may prepare for a vaginal birth and not expect a caesarean, with the result that she is upset and shocked when the need arises. It is therefore a good idea to discuss the possibility with your partner so that you will be better prepared should you need the operation. Looking into the possibility will not increase your chances of needing a caesarean, but may increase your acceptance and reduce your fear should a caesarean become necessary. If a caesarean is likely, you might be able to visit the operating theatre and talk to an anaesthetist as well as your obstetrician and midwife.

Important questions to ask your hospital include their rate of caesarean delivery, their policy on elective caesareans, the type of anaesthetic used, whether your partner can stay with you in the operating theatre, postnatal care (including how soon you will be encouraged to hold and feed your baby after birth) and how long you may stay in hospital following the operation.

Elective caesarean section

Reasons for choosing a caesarean when there is no medical necessity are personal and diverse. The main desire is usually to avoid labour and vaginal delivery. For some women this may be motivated by a deep-seated fear of pain. This may follow a previous traumatic labour. Some doubt their physical ability, and worry about the wellbeing of their baby. Others shy away from vaginal birth because they are scarred by physical or sexual abuse (page 546). Vaginal prolapse (page 317) and incontinence are less common after a caesarean, although these only occur after a small minority of vaginal births.

Knowing that there is no need to give birth vaginally may have a positive effect and improve your physical and psychological wellbeing in pregnancy. Even so, the decision may not be easy. If you are afraid of giving birth but not certain you want a caesarean, your midwife or a counsellor may help you to identify and work through your fears. If you can talk with other women who have delivered vaginally and by caesarean, hearing their stories may help you to make a choice. If you are certain you want a caesarean even without medical indication, you will need to book into a hospital where this is possible.

The rights and wrongs of choosing to have a caesarean are not clear cut and opinions alter with increasing safety of the procedure. A caesarean is a major operation that carries some risks of complications, especially for the mother, is more expensive than a vaginal birth and has a longer recovery period. Therefore most healthcare professionals prefer to avoid the operation except where there is a clearly defined medical need. For some doctors, fear of litigation does play a part. Doctors are rarely sued for performing unnecessary caesareans but are sometimes sued for not carrying out a caesarean in time.

Most women now feel that the stigma attached to not delivering normally is disappearing, and the operation is no longer seen as a failure. Some parents feel that a caesarean birth deprives the baby of an important experience – a vaginal birth. The flood of hormones that follows a vaginal birth for the mother is less intense during and after a caesarean but bonding between mother and baby can still be intense if there is close skin-to-skin contact in the hours and weeks following birth.

The advice throughout this book encourages you to be actively involved in your antenatal health and care and in maintaining your energy during labour – by following it you may increase your chances of delivering vaginally.

Bear in mind, though, that many caesareans are a necessary intervention and can save the life of the mother or baby or significantly reduce the trauma that may occur in a vaginal birth. Not all caesareans can or should be avoided.

Emergency caesarean section

Emergency caesarean is sometimes performed because the mother's health is at risk. But the most common reason is to ensure the baby's safety. An emergency caesarean section may be needed after labour has started:
- If your labour is progressing slowly (see LABOUR AND BIRTH, MOTHER: PROGRESS, SLOW).
- If your baby moves into an awkward position (malpresentation).
- If your baby has foetal distress.
- If there is abnormal BLEEDING.
- If the umbilical cord (page 339) is compressed or prolapsed.
- When FORCEPS or VENTOUSE assistance for a vaginal delivery fails (see LABOUR AND BIRTH, MOTHER).
- With very high blood pressure that does not respond to medication.

In an emergency, the decision to operate is often taken quickly and events may seem out of your control. Yet for most couples the compensation is that the delivery is successful and mother and baby are well. It is usually easy to give a short explanation of the reasons for operating, even in an acute emergency, and a longer discussion may sometimes be possible. You may then want to discuss all the details with your doctor and/or midwife after the birth so you feel informed.

Planned caesarean section

The most common conditions that prompt a planned caesarean are:
- Your baby is too big to pass through your pelvis (page 368).
- Your baby is 'small for dates' (IUGR) or at high risk of FOETAL DISTRESS, so it is safer to be delivered by caesarean than to remain in the womb.
- Your baby is in an awkward POSITION (malpresentation) or is breech (see LABOUR AND BIRTH, BABY).
- You have had a previous operation on your uterus (the most common reason is surgery for FIBROIDS, but many women do have a normal birth after a fibroid operation).
- You are having triplets or TWINS, and the position of one baby is not optimal.
- Your placenta is low lying (PLACENTA PRAEVIA).
- You have severely high BLOOD PRESSURE (pre-eclampsia).

If you decide, in discussion with your midwife and obstetrician, that a caesarean section is the safest way for your baby to be delivered, you may feel relieved, or you may be disappointed that you won't deliver vaginally. Some women feel they are somehow to blame, or become angry with the medical team. You are likely to have weeks or months to go into your feelings and prepare yourself. It may help to remember that most of the events that necessitate a caesarean are not in your control and your baby has a major role to play.

Except where it is safer to deliver sooner, the operation is usually set for Week 38–9 to ensure your baby is fully developed and to reduce the risk of breathing problems associated with PREMATURE BIRTH. If labour begins spontaneously before this date, the operation can be done in early labour.

▦ EMOTIONS AND FEELINGS

See also Emotions.

Initially, most women and their partners feel joy and relief at having a wonderful baby. Postnatal euphoria is common, especially when the operation has gone well and mum has lots of time with her baby. For many people, the dominant feelings continue to be positive and there are few hindrances to enjoying their baby. Equally, euphoria can fade or pass if you become tired or if you have postnatal blues, as most women do (page 218). This is similar to the range of emotions that surface after a vaginal birth.

Following a caesarean, the blues may be intensified by the effects of anaesthesia, the frustration of being physically limited and the hormonal effects of your milk coming in, and if the incision feels uncomfortable. It may be useful to acknowledge this combined effect on your mood, and also that it should pass as your body recovers and you adjust to what is happening.

If you knew you were going to have a caesarean delivery, you will have had a chance to review your feelings. Even so, you may become weepy and upset as most mothers do at some point after birth. If the operation followed a long labour and/or was performed as an emergency, you may feel exhausted and numb, shocked and/or angry. Some parents ask why the operation was not performed sooner. Others feel the decision to operate was made too quickly and a vaginal birth might have been possible.

It is often easy to forget that a caesarean is usually performed for reasons dictated by the baby. Some women feel guilty that their baby has been denied the experience of a 'natural' birth, and many envy mothers who have given birth vaginally. These and other feelings can take months to surface. They cannot all be explained rationally but they are part of your 'bodymind' (pages 73–4) and are very important. As with any aspect of postnatal blues or depression, it is useful to give space to your emotions and seek support from your midwife and doctor, friends, family and your wider community.

▦ OPERATION DETAILS

In a caesarean section your baby is delivered within five to 10 minutes of the first incision being made. If you receive an epidural or spinal anaesthetic you can remain awake to greet your baby at birth. You may hold your baby while your abdomen is being stitched. A general anaesthetic may be used in an acute emergency or if you prefer to be asleep.

Preparing for surgery

Before surgery you will be asked to follow standard pre-operative precautions. You'll need to avoid food and drink for four to six hours beforehand to minimise the risk of vomiting during or after surgery, and you'll be given a tablet or liquid to neutralise the acid contents of your stomach. In an emergency caesarean in labour, you may already have had some food or drink before the decision to operate was taken. This may increase the risk if you have a general anaesthetic but with epidural anaesthesia there is little risk of inhaling stomach juices.

Into the operating theatre

You and your birth partner, if he or she is with you, will probably feel a mixture of excitement and anxiety. Operating theatres can be daunting. The brightly-lit room, sterile equipment and medical staff behind masks and gowns can be unsettling, particularly in an emergency. You will be escorted to the theatre by a midwife, and he or she will stay with you throughout the operation and talk you through each stage. The anaesthetist will be there on your arrival and will stay by your side until you are on your way back to the postnatal ward. Theatre nurses and doctors are usually good-humoured and very aware of the natural anxieties of expectant parents.

Before you enter the theatre you will be asked to sign a consent form. Most hospitals welcome the father-to-be or birth partner into the theatre if he or she chooses. Only in the rare instance that the caesarean section is an acute emergency will the birth partner be asked to leave. He or she may be welcomed back when the emergency is under control and the operation is in progress.

An intravenous drip is inserted into your arm to keep you fully hydrated and will remain until you are drinking normally, usually within 12 hours. The drip is also useful should you need extra fluids or medicines. A catheter tube is inserted into your urethra to drain urine from your bladder and reduce the risk of bladder injury during surgery. It will remain in place for 12–24 hours following the birth. Most women find these procedures only mildly uncomfortable, and once the drip and catheter are in place they seldom cause any discomfort.

Support stockings and an inflatable pump on your legs during surgery are used to prevent blood clots in your calves. Your abdomen will be shaved at the hairline to the level of the pubis. It is not necessary to remove all the pubic hair.

Homeopathy and aromatherapy before the operation

- *Aconite* (200c), one dose, if you are afraid or anxious. This is useful for your birth partner, too.
- *Hypericum* (30c) may be helpful if you are having an epidural.

If your caesarean is planned you could have a bath or a massage before going to hospital, scented with oils of neroli to help you relax, jasmine, to boost your confidence, or sandalwood to calm your nerves.

Anaesthesia

Most hospitals give an epidural. If you are already in labour, this will offer relief from contraction pains. During the operation it stops you feeling any pain but you may still feel touch and pressure. If you do feel any pain, the anaesthetist will increase the amount of anaesthetic you receive. It will not send you to sleep and can be left in place to give pain relief for 24 hours following the operation. Alternatively, your doctor may choose to administer a spinal anaesthetic (page 383). This works more quickly than an epidural but wears off more quickly – after six hours. Sometimes an epidural and spinal are combined. You may be able to request general anaesthetic, if you prefer.

A general anaesthetic is usually given in an emergency. You will be unconscious during the delivery but will usually be able to see and hold your baby within 30 minutes to one hour of birth. In the meantime, your baby will

appreciate being held by your birth partner. Skin-to-skin contact is most comforting.

The operation

In theatre you will not be able to see the operation because your abdomen will be screened by sterile drapes. Your partner may choose to watch or to remain close to your face. Your abdominal skin will be disinfected and the obstetrician will make a neat incision along the bikini line in a process that opens your abdomen and gently separates, but does not cut, the abdominal muscles to expose your uterus. The incision to open the muscular wall of the uterus is horizontal and in the lower segment of the uterus (lower uterine segment caesarean). This follows the natural line of your body and results in a stronger scar that is less likely to break in a subsequent labour.

The membranes of the amniotic sac surrounding your baby are then cut and the obstetrician will carefully deliver your baby. As your baby is delivered, the obstetrician may need to push on your abdomen to help the birth. Sometimes forceps are placed on the baby's head to aid the delivery. Once your baby has been delivered, the umbilical cord will be clamped and cut. Your baby will be quickly checked by the midwife or paediatrician. If she needs any help with breathing, oxygen will be given.

Meeting your baby

Then it will be time for you to see your baby. Your partner or midwife can hold your baby while you touch her and make eye contact. While you are meeting your baby for the first time, the obstetrician delivers the placenta, checks your uterus and begins to stitch the incision.

Many hospitals urge mothers to hold their babies against their skin as soon as possible and a midwife will probably guide you as you breastfeed for the first time, often while the operation is being completed. This is an opportunity for focusing on your baby and the positive aspects of the birth.

Stitching

Blood loss is kept to a minimum, but on average is greater than during vaginal birth.

After the placenta and the membranes have been delivered, special clamps are used to reduce bleeding. Repairing the uterus and abdominal wall can take up to 30 minutes because there are six separate layers to be stitched. The time and care taken are very worthwhile, as they guard against scar rupture in future pregnancies. Modern suture (stitching) material is very strong, and dissolves naturally within six weeks, so there is minimal risk of the wound being disrupted. The only suture you will be able to see is the line on the surface of your skin. The stitches here may be of the dissolving type or may need to be removed about five days following delivery (a quick and painless procedure).

After surgery

The stitched incision on your abdomen is protected with a dressing and vaginal bleeding is checked. You and your baby will be helped out of the operating area back to your room on a special trolley. The drip in your arm will be left in place and continue to provide fluid and nutrients as you recover. Your midwife will check frequently to ensure you are comfortable and you are not bleeding excessively. You will be offered an antibiotic to prevent infection and anticoagulants to prevent blood clots in the veins.

▒ RECOVERY AND POST-OPERATIVE PERIOD

As with any major operation, you will need time to recover physically. You will also go through the normal after effects of birth, including discharge of lochia (page 362), afterpain contractions and breast engorgement as your milk flows in. After a major life event and major surgery, it's important not to expect to do too much. The physical effects of the anaesthetic, the surgery and discomfort associated with healing may bring TIREDNESS and low energy, rocky emotions, tearfulness or anger. As each day passes you will feel a little stronger. Most women feel well enough to go home within four or five days.

Some women are surprised at how quickly they recover, both physically and emotionally, but others feel exhausted or depressed for weeks or months. (There is a range of recovery times following a vaginal birth, too.) While you may be eager to get back to 'normal life', remember that taking on too much too soon may drain your energy, leaving you tired and emotional, and this could slow your recovery and reduce your milk supply.

- The best advice is to listen to your body and rest if you feel tired or sore. Gradually do more until you are back to your normal self. Your doctor will give you a checkup at six weeks.
- The more time you spend with your baby, resting and sleeping in the early days, the better. If you find it difficult to be alone it may be easier if friends or family visit. Their company and practical help and your midwife's advice may reduce your anxiety about what you 'should' be doing and feeling.
- Take care how you lift heavy weights, including shopping, laundry and even your baby. Try to keep your back straight and bend your knees as you lift.
- Get out of bed without discomfort by rolling over with your knees together and turning from your shoulder, then swinging your feet onto the floor and sitting up.
- You need to avoid strenuous activity, including housework and vacuuming, for six weeks.
- Check with your doctor when it is safe for you to drive a car, and ask your insurance company for details of your cover. It is not necessary to wait for six weeks.
- You will be able to make love without interfering with healing as soon as you feel comfortable and in the mood. If you feel under pressure to make love before you are ready, the advice on page 470 may be useful.
- Remember your multivitamin and minerals and antioxidants. Your body will heal more effectively if it is given the right nutrients.

✚ Red flag

Please call your GP, your consultant or the hospital urgently:

- If you feel unwell, nauseous or feverish (temperature over 37.5°C/99.5°F).
- If your abdomen feels tender or swollen for longer than 24 hours.
- If the stitched area of your abdomen become red, swollen or painful after 24 hours. This may indicate infection and it is important that medical treatment begins promptly.

Pain and discomfort

Pain and discomfort are sharpest over the first few days. Your anaesthetist may leave your epidural in place for up to 24 hours so you can have a 'top-up' when you feel the need, or you may be given painkilling injections and long-acting suppositories. Let the midwives know if you feel uncomfortable so you can be relieved quickly. As your discomfort gradually reduces you can move on to milder painkillers. These may be needed for a week or two.

Many people are virtually pain-free in a few days. It is common, however, to feel sore on one or other side of the incision for several weeks. This arises from the internal stitches at the edge of the incision in the sheath that encloses the muscles of your abdominal wall. Moving and walking realigns the cut sheath and can help to ease the pain. Very rarely, a nerve may be trapped in a suture line, giving ongoing discomfort. Injecting the area with a local anaesthetic solution can numb the nerve.

You may have some back, neck or head pain arising from your posture and the strain on your body during the operation or as you lie in bed and care for your baby. For advice on reducing pain see page 431.

If your pain is still severe after two weeks it is advisable to have your doctor examine you.

Urine and bowels

The urinary catheter is removed within 24 hours, as soon as you are mobile. You may not have eaten in labour and for 12 or more hours after the operation so your bowels will be relatively empty. When you do begin to eat, bowel movements usually return within two or three days but CONSTIPATION is common (and painkillers tend to make this problem worse). Occasionally, glycerine suppositories and a high-fibre diet help. Lactulose or linseeds may also be beneficial (page 152).

Numbness

Sometimes the nerves to the skin around the incision are affected during the operation. The nerves usually recover within 18 months and numbness reduces.

Mobility

Within 12 hours, the midwives will support you as you sit up, get out of bed and take your first steps. Most women can sit up unaided within 24 hours. You may even be mobile before the woman in the next bed who had a vaginal delivery with forceps and an episiotomy.

If you feel faint or dizzy as you try to rise, try eating something to boost your blood sugar and ask for help to get up slowly. Women are nervous about getting up because they feel weak, and there is a common fear that the incision will open. Be reassured that modern sutures are very strong and will not break.

As soon as you feel well enough, walk around but do take things gently, and build up slowly. Moving as early as possible eases breathing, improves healing and reduces the risk of deep vein thrombosis. It is best to wear elastic stockings until you are completely mobile. Remember that you need your energy for feeding and for your own recovery, so while moving will lift your spirits and your energy, if you do too much it will be exhausting. Gradually increase the amount you do and cut back if pain is intense or if you feel tired.

Caring for your abdomen, wound and scar

The dressing on your wound may be removed the day after the operation.

* The wound need not be protected from water – in fact it's a good idea to take a daily bath or shower – but it is important to dry the incision site well afterwards.
* If your skin becomes red or the site of the incision remains very tender there may be an infection in the subcutaneous tissues. You will be given antibiotics routinely as a preventive measure but if an infection does develop a further course may be needed.
* Vitamin E oil on the wound and taking vitamin and mineral supplements and antioxidants (page 263) by mouth can promote healing and improve your skin condition. Healing cream is available from homeopathic pharmacies.

Homeopathy

After the operation, the following remedies are invaluable. You may take each remedy in the indicated potency, three times a day for five to seven days:

- *Arnica* (30c) is the main remedy for trauma – it reduces swelling, encourages healing, particularly at the site of the placenta, and controls bleeding.
- *Hypericum* (30c) works particularly on nerve trauma and is a specific remedy for use after an epidural.
- *Bellis Perennis* (30c) assists the healing of deep tissue and helps ease soreness.
- *Calendula* (30c) speeds up the healing of the scar both internally and externally.
- In addition, *Hypercal* tincture (10–15 drops in the bath) promotes healing.

If you become constipated, you may take *Nux Vomica* (30c) three times a day for two days (see other remedies on page 153).

If you feel emotionally sensitive, which is often the case if the caesarean was an emergency, or you feel a mixture of emotions – anger, resentment or even humiliation, for instance – take *Staphysagria* (200c) every two hours for the six hours following delivery.

Aromatherapy and other complementary care

Useful aromatherapy oils in a bath or a massage (perhaps on your feet, hands or face); include neroli, chamomile, sandalwood and lavender for relaxation. If you feel angry, guilty or upset, try frankincense, ylang ylang or rose. Acupuncture can offer effective pain relief and boost tissue healing.

Physiotherapy and osteopathy

Cranial osteopathy is useful to realign your body after pregnancy and the operation, and in response to any new strains. If you are troubled by pain, or you feel stiff and uncomfortable, physiotherapy may help. Mothers and babies alike may also benefit from osteopathic treatment (page 424). Whereas physiotherapy tends to be useful in the later stages of recovery, osteopathy is more effective as soon as possible after the birth.

Exercise

It is safe to begin gentle exercises in bed after two to four days and to walk at a gentle pace when you feel up to it, but you need to delay demanding exercise for six to 12 weeks. Tips for post-caesarean exercise are on page 229.

Feeding and baby care

You and your baby can begin to breastfeed soon after the delivery with some help from the midwives. Your main concern will probably be feeling strong enough to lift and hold your baby. Your midwife will help you find a comfortable position for feeding with the aid of pillows to help protect your scar, and your partner or another helper can give assistance if you need support once you are home. You may find lying on your side easiest until you are comfortable sitting up to feed. Kangaroo care (page 518) may make it easier for you and your baby.

In the first day or two, you may not be able to change your baby's nappy – your partner or a midwife can do this. You will soon be hands-on and provided the changing place is at waist height, this won't put pressure on your wound. Bending down to floor level comfortably will take at least a week or longer. Involve your partner and helpers as much as possible. They will enjoy being useful and can lift your baby and pass her to you for the first couple of weeks. When you have to lift, always bend your knees to protect your back and your scar from strain.

If you share a bath with your baby you'll initially need someone to hand your baby to you and take her from you when you've finished. If you can't get help, top and tail your baby for the first few days until you can move more easily. This involves a simple wash of face, hands and nappy area with a clean cloth or cotton wool dipped in warm water. For cleaning your baby's eyes and ears, use a fresh piece of cotton wool each time, and use water that has been previously boiled and has cooled.

Bonding with your baby

Meeting and bonding (page 210) with your baby is a powerful way to overcome any feelings of shock or disappointment you may have experienced. Many women feel a strong connection in pregnancy. If birth was difficult and either you or your baby is ill or irritable the process of bonding may take more time.

Sex

Your libido depends on how you feel. Most women wait four weeks or less but it may be longer until you feel comfortable and at ease. If you feel well it is not necessary to wait until after your four-to-six week check. (See also pages 474–5.)

REPEAT OR VBAC

The old saying 'once a caesarean always a caesarean' no longer applies. Between 60 and 80 per cent of women are able to give birth vaginally the next time.

Women are often nervous to have a vaginal birth after caesarean (VBAC) in case the scar in their uterus ruptures. This is extremely rare (less than 1 per cent after lower segment caesarean section) but may be very dangerous for mother and baby if it does occur. Very rarely, for technical reasons, the incision may be in the upper part of the uterus, where it may be weak and a repeat caesarean is usually recommended.

Vaginal birth after caesarean (VBAC)

- If the medical reason for having a caesarean previously does not arise in your current pregnancy, you have a good chance of a vaginal delivery (for example, if your first baby was a breech presentation but your second is head down).
- Even if the same problem recurs, such as your baby being large or in occipito posterior position (page 344) or your baby experiences foetal distress, a vaginal delivery is not automatically ruled out.
- If your first caesarean was planned a subsequent labour will be equivalent to a first birth.
- If you went through labour the first time and your cervix did dilate, even if you did not reach full dilation, the length of the second labour is usually shorter.
- In a subsequent labour, it is best to avoid medical induction of labour or oxytocin to stimulate your uterus. These medications may increase the risk of scar rupture. You will be closely monitored in labour and it may be routine in your hospital for a needle to be placed in an arm vein in case you require fluid replacement.
- If your labour is progressing normally then it is usually safe to continue but if it is prolonged or there is foetal distress, a repeat caesarean is the best option.
- If you have had two or more caesareans then it

is most likely you'll have a repeat operation. However, a vaginal birth may still be possible if your obstetrician agrees.

Timing a future pregnancy

Within a few months of the operation, your wound will have healed completely, so spacing the next baby will depend more on personal preferences and your financial and social circumstances. You may be advised to take time to recover physically and emotionally, and to wait nine months before conceiving again.

RISKS AND CONCERNS

As you prepare for a caesarean you will no doubt have a number of questions. Modern obstetric practice means the operation is a much safer procedure than it was 20 years ago, and complications are less common. Nevertheless, there are hazards and the recovery period is generally longer than that following a vaginal birth. It may be reassuring to know you are not alone as it is natural to feel afraid of surgery. If time allows, discuss your feelings with the birth team before surgery. The potential complications are listed below but it is unlikely you or your baby will experience them.

Risks for the mother
- Infection of the incision. You will be given antibiotics to guard against this.
- A scar. The scar will be in your pubic hair and will not be visible, even if you wear a bikini. Modern stitch materials are very strong so the scar will not open when you move or pick up your baby. Your abdominal muscles are pushed aside (not cut) during surgery and will recover in a few weeks. In a few women, sometimes after weeks, the scar thickens and this is called a keloid.
- Deep vein thrombosis. The risk of blood clots and pulmonary embolism (blood clot in the lung) is reduced if you wear elastic stockings and can become mobile as soon as possible. In many hospitals, anticoagulant drugs to thin the blood are given after caesarean, particularly to women with a previous history of thrombosis.
- Anaesthetic complications. The safest anaesthetic is an epidural (page 383). Under

general anaesthetic there is a small risk of inhalation of acid stomach juices into the lungs (Mendelson's syndrome). Restricting food and administering antacids before surgery largely prevent this and you will be closely monitored during the procedure.

- Excess bleeding. This may occur during the operation if there are large blood vessels supplying your uterus. Bleeding is reduced by careful operative technique and skill. Sometimes a BLOOD TRANSFUSION may be needed. Although severe bleeding is rare it can be life threatening.
- Bladder or bowel injury. This is rare. The bladder is gently pushed down before the uterus is opened, and the bowel is also protected.
- Late abdominal adhesions. These are bands of scar tissue involving the bowel, bladder or the uterus that may develop in a minority of women. They may cause abdominal pain, urinary symptoms and, rarely, bowel obstruction, necessitating further operations.
- Effect on breastfeeding. Where there is good support, the rate of breastfeeding is as high as after a vaginal birth. You may want to begin straightaway, even while you are being stitched.
- If expectations of a vaginal birth were high the disappointment of needing a caesarean may lead to post-natal depression.

Risks for the baby

A caesarean section is often performed because medical staff believe the baby may be at risk of trauma, or FOETAL DISTRESS with reduced oxygen supply. Caesarean delivery reduces these risks.

- Some obstetricians believe that hormones released during a vaginal birth may help a baby make the journey of birth and adapt to breathing in air, and a caesarean deprives a baby of this natural assistance. It is true that babies born by caesarean section are more likely to need help with breathing but this applies to a minority, unless a planned caesarean has been performed too soon and the baby is premature.
- Where caesarean section follows a long and difficult labour or an attempt at a forceps delivery, a baby may be irritable and shocked.
- If the caesarean has been carried out under

general anaesthetic, the baby may be sleepy but is likely to recover well within a few hours.
- In a PREMATURE BIRTH the baby is delicate and this presents a risk of injury as the baby is being delivered.

Possible effects on a baby

Depending on the reason for the caesarean your baby is likely to adjust to being born just as she would if born vaginally (page 331). In a planned or elective caesarean, physical birth trauma is less likely than if your baby is born vaginally with assistance from ventouse or forceps.

If the caesarean was prompted because your baby was having difficulty, she may need time to recover. The process depends on the situation and differs from baby to baby – some are very resilient and some are sensitive. A paediatrician may need to assist your baby if there was considerable foetal distress or if the birth was very premature and intense care may continue for some time.

The experience of birth is important but it is likely that the care your baby receives after birth is more important in helping her feel comfortable and in supporting a strong bond between you. Babies mirror their parents and if they feel welcomed and loved this will help them to recover well. Your baby will appreciate being held and talked to and may be soothed by skin-to-skin kangaroo care (page 518), MASSAGE or cranial OSTEOPATHY. Your baby is likely to yearn for contact with mum. A caesarean requires that you take time to rest and recover and this provides many opportunities for you and your baby to be together and explore one another.

Some psychologists believe a caesarean may affect a baby emotionally and hamper the relationship between mother and baby. These hypotheses are theoretical: babies' brains are able to adapt, and those born by caesarean section find little difficulty getting used to life outside the womb. Bonding usually happens easily, and can be encouraged with lots of skin-to-skin contact, frequent feeding and time together. If your baby seems detached, the advice on page 210 may be useful.

Candida (thrush), baby

See also Candida (thrush), mother; Skin, baby.

If your baby develops redness and white pustules in his mouth, it is most likely to be a thrush (candida) infection. This can make feeding uncomfortable and is a common cause of nappy rash. If he has oral thrush in the days after birth he may have contracted the infection from your vagina, and he may then pass it to your nipples, and a cycle of re-infection can set in. You may be aware of thrush in your vagina (page 118) and/or on your nipples. You both need to be treated at the same time. If you or your baby is receiving antibiotic treatment, the antibiotics can kill the good bacteria in the gut that normally keep candida in check, creating conditions for candida to thrive.

Action plan

- If your baby's nappy area is affected, you may be prescribed an anti-fungal cream: the same preparation is useful for babies and adults.
- In addition you may be prescribed hydrocortisone cream to use in small amounts, to reduce inflammation and pain.
- Your doctor may suggest using nystatin or imidazole medication.
- Homeopathy is often very effective (see below).
- Tea tree essential oil has anti-fungal properties. Just one drop in a baby bath is effective.
- Give your baby time without his nappy on, and change his nappy frequently. There are other tips for reducing nappy rash on page 418.
- To reduce the risk of further infection in yourself, follow the advice on pages 117–19.

Homeopathy

If your baby has candida in the nappy area and the mouth and is being breastfed, it is advisable for both of you to be treated at the same time. You may use the most appropriate remedy for him in 6c potency four-hourly for 24 hours, then re-assess. Either continue with the same remedy, or you may change to a more appropriate one, three times a day for up to three days and re-assess. Remedies for you are suggested on page 119.

- *Borax* if your baby salivates more than usual, his mouth is hot, breastfeeding seems painful, he dislikes downward motion and his nappy area looks red and itchy.
- *Natrum Mur* for oral and rectal thrush, with white patches on the tongue and gums and a persistent desire to feed, serious demeanour and a dislike of fuss or contact.
- *Merc Sol* when there is profuse salivation, perhaps smelly breath, the nappy area looks sweaty, moist and yellowish and there are small pimples.
- *Calc Carb* when there are white patches on the roof of the mouth, sour possetting (regurgitated milk), white spots in the nappy area and your baby is lethargic and obstinate.
- *Sulphur* when the nappy area is red, sore and itchy and is worse from heat or warmth of any kind; bathing in warm water may aggravate it.
- You may also use *Hypercal* tincture, 10 drops to 250ml (½ pint) of water, and bathe your baby with soaked cotton wool at every nappy change.
- *Calendula* cream is very soothing and may act as a good barrier cream applied to the nappy area.

Candida (thrush), mother

See also Candida (thrush), baby.

Candida is a yeast organism that inhabits the mouth, throat, intestines and genito-urinary tract of most humans. It is one of many organisms kept in balance by a properly functioning immune system. In the vagina it exists in balance with lactobacilli bacteria. If the number of friendly bacteria is decreased, candida transforms from yeast to a fungal form and starts to invade the body, causing a candidiasis infection (thrush). Nearly 75 per cent of women will have had at least one genital 'yeast infection' in their lifetime. It is an irritating infection and is usually self-limiting but can occasionally persist. Pregnancy makes you more susceptible. Treatment is usually straightforward and lifestyle measures can offer effective prevention. Candida can be passed from person to person, such as through sexual intercourse or to a baby at birth or when breastfeeding.

What happens

Candidiasis affects a wide variety of organ systems, and is particularly common in warm, moist areas, such as the vagina (leading to vulvovaginitis), the mouth (oral thrush), the eyes (conjunctivitis) and the rectum. It can also affect nipples and breast tissue during breastfeeding and may be associated with cracked nipples (page 97). In a person with a compromised immune system the internal organs may be infected and severe illness may result.

Candida organisms may multiply and trigger an infection for a number of reasons. These can include:

- Use of antibiotics, which destroy friendly as well as harmful bacteria.
- Pregnancy, because the hormones alter the acidity balance of the vagina and diet changes may increase sugar levels.
- A weakened immune system, for example if you are depressed, or have a rare immune system disorder.
- DIABETES or a diet high in sugar (page 261).

Symptoms

Redness is always a feature of candida infection. The main symptoms are:

- Itchiness and burning sensation in the infected areas. Other organisms may cause similar symptoms and a swab culture is useful to confirm the diagnosis.
- Oral thrush appears as one or more small white plaques in the mouth and on the tongue, and these are sometimes painful.
- Occasionally candida causes shallow painful ulcers in the mouth or vagina.
- On the insides of the thighs or under the arms or breasts it can produce painful general redness and white pustules.
- Inflammation of the genital area (vulvovaginitis) causes red labia and a white itchy discharge often described as 'cheesy'.
- Thrush deep in the breast can cause pain and redness.

Action plan

Thrush can be treated, often with a combination of dietary changes and medication. Treatment to reduce itchiness and consequent rubbing reduces the risk of a secondary infection in broken skin.

Diagnosis

Diagnosis can be made with a visual examination and confirmed with a swab test. In the case of vaginal or urethral thrush, a laboratory test will rule out a urinary tract infection that may also lead to a burning sensation. Ask your partner to be tested since candida can be passed through sexual contact.

Lifestyle and diet: prevention and cure

- Maintain cleanliness, especially after using the toilet. Always wipe from front to back as organisms from the bowel can be easily transferred to the vagina.
- Candida loves warmth and moisture. Wear loose cotton underwear, which allows air to circulate. Tight jeans increase the warmth.
- Reduce scented toiletries, which may irritate. You may be allergic to some types.
- Candida thrives on sugar and loves an acidic environment. Reduce refined and sugary foods, including fruit juices and colas, which are best avoided altogether.
- Try to cut out food that is fermented and contains yeast, including bread, wine and beer.
- Eat whole foods with plenty of immune-boosting, fungi-busting garlic, onions and olive oil. Kale, turnip and cabbage may inhibit fungal growth.
- Make sure you are getting enough vitamins A, B complex and C as well as the minerals zinc, iron and magnesium (but do not take an excess of vitamin A during pregnancy, see page 263).
- You could take probiotics in the form of lactobacillus (acidophilus) tablets or pessaries. These destroy the fungus and create a natural barrier to infection and are particularly useful if you need to take antibiotics.
- Eating 145ml (5fl oz) live yoghurt, which contains probiotics, per day can dramatically reduce the chance of a vaginal or bowel thrush infection. It is best eaten at the end of a meal when the acidity of the stomach is reduced by the food.
- Inserting yoghurt into the vagina during pregnancy and straight after birth is not recommended. A month or more after birth you could try inserting a few teaspoons of plain live yoghurt or lactobacillus pessaries before you go to bed until symptoms improve.

Medical care

If self-help measures fail, your doctor may prescribe medication. Some strains of fungal infection are resistant to standard drugs. With accurate diagnosis you will be able to target the treatment effectively. A swab test can identify the variant: Candida galabrata is more drug-resistant than the more common Candida albicans.

- You may be offered an antifungal pessary to insert into your vagina, together with ointment for applying to the vulva. Towards the end of pregnancy, treatment reduces the chance of infection being passed to your baby.
- Antifungal cream is useful for thrush on the skin including the nipples.
- Antifungal tablets are very effective but they are not recommended during pregnancy. Sometimes a prolonged course of medication is needed for recurrent thrush and eating changes improve the recovery rate.
- Nystatin is the original polyene antifungal remedy. It affects the cell wall of the fungal organism. You may take it by mouth after pregnancy and it can be given to a baby. It is also used for long term treatment of chronic candidiasis in adults.
- Gentian violet solution is messy but can cure resistant thrush in the mouth or the vagina. For oral thrush a mouth rinse with a very dilute hydrogen peroxide solution can be effective for adults (beware of burning from concentrated solutions).

Herbal treatments

- Calendula cream or tincture can ease itching.
- Echinacea, taken in tea form or as a tincture two to three times a day, is good for boosting the immune system of adults but should not be given to a baby. Take for a maximum of 15 days, then have a break of 15 days.
- A dilution of tea tree oil in the bath or, from Week 24, chamomile oil, may help.
- After the birth you could insert tea tree oil pessaries into your vagina. These often work well in combination with probiotic pessaries. It is best to take advice from your midwife or herbalist.

Homeopathy

The following are the most commonly used remedies. You may take the most appropriate remedy in the 30c potency three times per day for 48 hours and then re-assess the situation. If there is no change, consider a different remedy. If there is an improvement, continue with the same remedy three times per day for up to one week or consult your homeopath if there is no change.

- *Borax* for a discharge that is hot, burning, watery, like egg white and quite profuse. There is itching and sensitivity in your vagina, inflammation, and the strange sensation of hot water flowing down the thighs. You may feel worse from any downward motion or sudden noises, and better in cool conditions.
- *Sepia* for a thick, corrosive yellowish discharge with an offensive smell, a bearing down sensation, severe itching and vulval inflammation. You probably feel exhausted, irritable and emotionally stressed and all your symptoms are aggravated by any additional stress.
- *Calc Carb* if you have a milky, yellowish discharge that burns and is sour-smelling. There is vaginal itching, worse after urinating. You may feel chilly, anxious, exhausted and sluggish with sugar cravings or an increased appetite.
- *Arsenicum* for a burning, acrid, thin, clear-coloured discharge. Your vagina feels hot and the vulva is inflamed and burns, but there is no itching and all symptoms are relieved by warmth. You may be feeling anxious and restless but weak.
- *Natrum Mur* for burning, pain and itching. Your vagina feels dry despite having a white discharge resembling egg white. Emotionally you may feel despondent, preferring to be alone; you may have headaches, dizziness, backache, and digestive disturbances. You feel better for cool bathing and cool fresh air and worse in warm stuffy environments.
- *Kreosotum* for thrush with a burning, acrid, corrosive discharge and violent itching that has to be scratched leaving the area red, raw and very sore. The discharge can be profuse, milky or yellowish and fairly offensive – stains the underwear (smells like rye bread or unripe corn). You are likely to feel restless and irritable and weak.
- *Hypercal tincture* may help to alleviate symptoms – add 15–20 drops to the bath or 10–15 drops to 250ml (½ pint) water to pour over the area after going to the loo.

CHRONIC CANDIDIASIS

Many healthcare professionals acknowledge the existence of chronic candidiasis infection or candidiasis hypersensitivity syndrome, which is similar in nature to chronic fatigue. It leads to symptoms such as low energy, depression, absent-mindedness, headaches, skin problems and hyperactivity and recurrent vaginal thrush infections. Some people believe it may also be an underlying cause of persistent constipation, diarrhoea, flatulence, abdominal pain or urinary problems. The symptoms resemble complaints that may also be attributed to allergy or intolerance.

Chronic candidiasis is not universally accepted. The argument for its existence is based on the belief that candida and other related fungi multiply when other friendly bacteria are knocked out. If candida creates yeast and this happens repeatedly, the build-up can weaken the immune system, which may already be weakened if you have been on antibiotics, eat an excess of highly refined or processed food, have a diet high in sugar and fat, consume high levels of toxins in the form of nicotine, alcohol or drugs or do not exercise sufficiently. Once the immune system is weakened, you may also be more susceptible to developing adverse reactions to foods and chemicals, and to succumb to infections that would normally be easily conquered (such as the common cold).

If you believe you have candidiasis hypersensitivity syndrome, it is best to visit a nutritionist, homeopath or other qualified practitioner who will examine your lifestyle, diet and medical history. Holistic attention to lifestyle and diet may increase your general health, immunity and vitality, and may reduce the need for antibiotics in pregnancy and beyond. If you have chronic thrush, you may also be given anti-fungal medication. If it improves your vitality, it is worth it.

Caring for baby

See also Parenting.

Parenting is a journey and all parent–baby partnerships follow their own unique paths. Of all of these, the path that begins from the heart is the one that supports parents to care for their babies in the best possible way.

Love and parenting

Like all parents, you will learn on the job, both to do the practical things like nappy changing

and bathing, and to meet your baby's needs as you get to know her. Parenting from your heart will help you follow your gut feelings and tune into your baby, and follow your in-built drive to care for and nurture your baby (page 211). Your baby will let you know what she needs, and you will get more adept at understanding her as the days pass. Meeting her needs is an active way to express your love. And when your baby feels her needs being met, she is likely to feel secure and contented. The tips on page 208 give simple guidelines for doing this while also caring for yourself.

Your baby's needs are physical – to be with you, warm, fed and comforted – and emotional – to feel lovingly held, listened to, played with and supported when she is angry or upset. These will be easily and quickly fulfilled if you slow down to her pace and tune in, keep her close to you, and enjoy skin-to-skin contact. Please remember that caring for yourself will help you stay present for your baby, and is an equally important element of family life (page 121).

■ CONTENTED BABY

A contented baby feels comfortable and will show this with inquiring looks, a relaxed body and healthy expression through smiling, crying and body movements. She will entice you to bond with her.

Recipe for contentment

Your baby is most likely to feel contented when she has her basic needs met, for example:

* She feels loving touch and is held skin to skin.
* She is fed when hungry, supported to sleep when tired, and feels your joy as she explores and plays.
* She feels safe to express herself and her feelings are acknowledged.
* She feels accepted and listened to by the adults in her world.
* There is no threat of separation or being hurt.
* Family boundaries are fluid so that she feels held and safe but not restrained as her needs change from day to day.
* Any pain or illness is lovingly addressed.

Compliance and contentment

There is an important distinction between compliance and contentment. Babies are genetically primed to elicit love and care and learn how to please and receive attention from the people on whom they depend. The learning is not rational, but rapid brain development (page 273) begins to determine behavioural patterns from birth, if not earlier. Babies tend to naturally avoid doing things that upset or anger their care givers – because when adults are angry, upset or stressed, they are less able to be truly present and caring towards their babies.

When a baby learns that she is accepted whatever she does and whatever feelings she expresses, and frequently perceives joy and love in the faces of her parents and carers, she is likely to feel good. When she feels safe and her needs are met she is likely to continue freely expressing herself. Such a baby tends to be contented and also explorative and friendly. Some babies learn early that it is safer – less uncomfortable – to comply: which means suppressing or seldom expressing their needs. Suppressed children are often in a state of resignation and sometimes nervous or confused, and this state of mind may continue through life. Your baby is most likely to be contented when you are there for her, and when you are loving, caring and attentive. It is definitely okay to listen to her and to follow her lead (page 432).

▓ IF YOU'RE CONCERNED

If you are ever concerned, your instinct can help you support your baby and alert you to a problem, if there is one. Using your head will help you acquire practical information and make decisions in times of pressure. Even first-time parents have good hunches – so play your hunches – what have you got to lose?

When your baby has an unusual cry – particularly if it sounds pained and is high-pitched – or if she is unusually quiet or unresponsive, or seems to be in pain, you will automatically kick into action. Most caring parents have an innate sense of knowing when something may be wrong. By the same token, most parents know how to soothe their babies and when to seek advice.

If in doubt, just ask. It helps to think over your questions in advance so you are sure you have covered everything. You may need another adult with you for support and so that between you, you hear all the important facts, or to be with your baby while you talk to a professional. What matters is that you are listened to, and heard. You will possibly discover that what you are worried about is not at all serious. This is preferable to discovering that your baby needed professional attention and you did not act on your feelings.

Who to ask

In the UK, you may call or visit your midwife, your GP surgery or health visitor, and at any time of day or night can call NHS Direct (listed in the phone book) or if it is an emergency, call 999. You may have access to a paediatrician, or visit the emergency department of your local hospital. Meanwhile relatives and friends may be on hand or at the end of the phone. In addition there are sources of information on the web, as well as parent advisory and help lines.

Caring for you

Parenting is about being there for your baby, and you will do this best when you are also there for yourself. Caring for yourself is a top priority and it is always possible, even when you are full-on with your baby. There are many aspects. Some you can incorporate into your day without any forward planning, such as taking five minutes to sit calmly, breathe deeply and rejuvenate yourself. Others may need a bit of practical organisation, such as making sure you have good food in your cupboards and maybe someone to shop or cook for or with you. In many areas support is important: when you need professional or medical help, for instance, or so that you can take a bit of time out to chill, to exercise or to do whatever feels good.

The journey into parenthood is one of life's most remarkable transitions – a real roller-coaster ride. The events that occur at this time can be stressful. How you care for yourself and feel cared for has a huge impact on the way your ride feels, and the way your baby experiences life with you.

If you feel well cared for and have a strong support network and you and your baby are in good health, this is a great foundation for your baby and you to enjoy your love affair. If this is not the case and you feel stressed, overwhelmed or uncertain, this may reduce your enjoyment. Yet even difficult times present a great opportunity to consider and alter your situation.

▒ BASICS

Throughout this book we encourage you to care for yourself. There are of course many different ways you may do this. You can look up the entries that interest you (for example, eating, emotions, sex, sleep or receiving bad news). As a brief overview, it may be helpful to remember five basics that may boost your wellbeing:

1. Spend time with people who you love and who love you. Love is the key.
2. Accept and encourage support from others.
3. Eat well, exercise, rest and play.
4. Listen to your feelings – probably your most useful guides.
5. Keep an element of flexibility so you can assess and alter schedules as your and your family's needs change.

Your reality

You will 'learn on the job' and adapt each day. Most parents discover their instincts are strong. You may be surprised that tasks you thought would be difficult are actually simple and you become adept at juggling different aspects of your life and the needs of each person in your family. Some aspects might feel difficult or stuck – perhaps a relationship, issues with your baby or your feelings.

At times you may need considerable courage to trust and act on your personal truth, particularly if it is at odds with the expectations of your friends or your family of origin (page 207). Choosing to care for yourself and letting others care for you will help you to nourish your baby, yourself and your family. Your child learns from how you live your life.

Are you worth it?

Feeling cared for depends on many factors and there are at least two sides: how others care for you and how you feel when you are nurtured and

loved. Your experiences as a baby, and the attitudes in your family, affect the value you give yourself today and whether you feel comfortable when someone loves and supports you.

It is very common for adults, particularly mothers, to put their own needs last. While it is important to prioritise your baby's needs – for he is totally dependent on you – it is counterproductive to neglect yourself. When you are well cared for, you offer a strong, reliable and loving presence for your baby, and you will get more enjoyment from your roller-coaster ride.

If it does not come naturally to love and care for yourself, you may need to make a conscious effort to lower some of your defences and accept that it is okay to be nourished. You may be surprised that a few small changes begin to make a huge difference, and each small bit of love and care helps you feel more energetic, more confident and more loving. The people around you – including your baby – will probably flourish too.

▒ FRIENDSHIP AND SUPPORT

See also Childcare; Relationships.

Some people never find themselves short of company or help; some have a small group of family and friends; while others feel isolated. Whatever your situation, your community is potentially large: friends and family, colleagues or neighbours, midwives, health visitor or GP, other expectant parents or parents at antenatal and postnatal classes, local societies or courses, internet buddies and more.

In pregnancy, and particularly when your baby arrives and you are on your own at home with him, the days can seem long. It is common to miss being with other adults and being independent. Feeling upset, overtired, stressed or poorly nourished are all signs that you could benefit from practical help and companionship.

While it can take years to make good friends, it doesn't take long to extend your community, and early parenthood is a great time to meet new people. You may meet other parents at classes or groups. Many of the other people in a class may be in the same position as you and would value your friendship and support.

Feeling supported is not always about being with other people. Your mum or your oldest friend may not be on hand to change a nappy, but could be on the end of a telephone to encourage you and listen to the daily run-down of your baby's development.

You and your baby

It is obvious that your baby needs you in many different ways. It may be less obvious that your baby also supports you. In his own unique way, he is able to bring you joy and love and help you feel good. He is skilful in expressing himself and the more time you spend together, the more easily you will tend to his needs as they arise, with minimal stress. It is a positive thing to accept your baby's guidance but it is not appropriate to confide your sorrows, anxieties or anger in him. He is not a mini adult and cannot offer you what you need to be able to work through such feelings. Unwittingly, some adults do use their babies and children either as therapists or as bargaining chips in relationship disagreements. When there are disagreements between you and another adult, it is always more appropriate to make time to talk, away from your baby. The advice on page 462 may help you address conflict and avoid bringing adult issues into your relationship with your baby. It may sometimes be useful to try professional counselling or therapeutic support (page 162).

You and your partner

The ideal in any relationship is mutual support. The key foundations are love and acceptance, and sharing practical tasks in a way that suits your unique setup. When you are both there for one another and are able to express your needs this will enhance your relationship, allow each of you to feel cared for and help your baby feel loved and secure. If either of you does not feel cared for, it is important to express this (page 462). You can then make changes. If you are separated, respecting and assisting one another is no less important, although it is not always a reality.

Your extended family

Your family may be nearby and you may get on well and be there for one another. If, however, you come from a difficult or dysfunctional family, or you are far apart, you may have to manage on your own. If your relatives seem

intrusive or inconsiderate, it might be useful to arrange a time to talk honestly. The tips for active listening (page 462) may come in handy.

Your wider community

Beyond your family and friends your community already extends further, and has the potential to grow. Your healthcare team may be a useful resource and at local groups (such as antenatal clinics, baby massage, toddler groups) you may form friendships that last for decades.

Enroling help

Many people find it difficult to ask for help but there is no need to feel apologetic. Most people appreciate what it's like to have a baby and enjoy the rewards of giving and sharing. It is likely that your friends and family would prefer to know how you are truly feeling and to help you. Spending time together is usually mutually fulfilling and tends to improve relationships.

Enroling someone to help you without pressure for them to say 'yes' involves asking clearly, and accepting they may say 'no'. Even if you feel disappointed the seed may germinate – they may feel better about doing something for you later, or you may think of someone else who could help. This is different from being coercive or pressuring another person to say 'yes'.

When you are open to a 'no' your tone and body language convey this and you won't sound forceful. If you are coercive, the person may feel upset or obliged and may not do the task with a good heart. Feelings of resentment and pressure often build up most intensely in the closest relationships: you may need to alter the way you ask for help from your partner, your parents and your siblings. The energy of acceptance, sharing and freedom of choice is likely to improve your relationships and is great for your baby to experience and learn from.

■ TAKING STOCK

With a new baby your individual and family needs can change significantly each day or each week, and certainly from month to month. Assessing what's working and what isn't – maybe at the end of the month, when you feel pressurised or when life feels good and you want to remember the ingredients – is a useful way to keep a balance. You may want to follow this checklist, which reflects the five basic ingredients of caring for you. The questions here focus on you. You could extend them to your baby, your partner and your family.

1. Love
   —Who makes me feel loved?
   —How much time do I spend with friends?
   —How much quality time do I have with my baby?
   —How often do I enjoy intimate moments with my partner?
2. Support
   —When do I ask for support?
   —Do I get the help I need around the house?
   —Do I get the help I need to care for myself and my baby?
   —Is something worrying me about my baby's or my own health or behaviour?
   —Who can I ask for advice?
3. Looking after me
   —What time do I take to exercise and relax?
   —Is the way I'm eating making me feel good?
   —How much time do I devote to work?
   —Am I taking time to nourish my spirit?
4. Feelings and emotions
   —How much time do I take to listen to my feelings?
   —What makes me feel good?
   —Are some feelings troubling or persistent?
   —Would it help to talk to someone?
5. Being flexible
   —Do my days feel relaxed or stressful?
   —Are my expectations realistic?
   —Do I need to discuss an issue that is causing conflict or making me feel stuck or upset?
   —Does something need to shift to help me feel more content?

WHEN THINGS GET TOUGH

Sometimes things get tough, for whatever reason. It is really common for parents to feel overwhelmed, particularly if there is anxiety, tiredness or depression, or there are pressures from money, housing, family, and so on.

If you have the five basics (page 122) in place, you will have a good foundation. A practical measure may be to make a wall chart or create a page in your diary listing what works well for you – it's best to do this when things are going well. Your personal chart may show that one area is not working for you – and that's the one that needs attention – or it may help you adjust the balance when you need to. Then, if things get tough, you may refer to this as you take stock.

It is always helpful to consider your feelings. What is coming up for you? What might be triggering this feeling? As you find the answers, or through taking the time to be present for yourself, you may begin to feel less overwhelmed and more flexible and therefore more able to accept that an alternative is possible. This can happen even if you begin with no idea of what needs to change. Once your emotional energy alters – say from being overwhelmed to acceptance, or from being stuck to being open – a process of change has begun.

Carpal tunnel syndrome

See Hand pain and carpal tunnel syndrome.

Cerebral palsy

Cerebral palsy (CP) is a term that describes a range of abnormalities of movement, muscle tone and posture. About one in 400 babies is affected. It is more common in babies born prematurely and in complicated pregnancies, such as those where a baby's growth is restricted (IUGR) or if there has been severe FOETAL DISTRESS.

The cerebral palsies of childhood are linked by a common underlying cause – damage to the brain. The affected area in the brain is associated with muscle control and body movement. The damage often occurs in the womb long before birth but symptoms may begin after labour or even months after birth. The symptoms that become apparent depend on age because different areas of the brain are brought into use as a child grows.

In the last 10 years the frequency of cerebral palsy in babies born with a low birth weight and in premature babies has fallen by almost a third. Unfortunately cerebral palsies amongst the biggest group affected – full term babies – has not changed.

What happens

Cerebral palsy is related to damage to or poor development of the brain, usually during pregnancy, or much more rarely at delivery, and sometimes after birth. The cause is not always clear. Some possible causes are: maternal infection in early pregnancy; a difficult or PREMATURE BIRTH, perhaps associated with BREATHING DIFFICULTIES or bleeding within the baby's brain; a genetic disorder, or postnatal MENINGITIS.

In fewer than 2 per cent of babies with cerebral palsy can the cause be attributed exclusively to FOETAL DISTRESS AND ASPHYXIA and sub-optimal care in labour. Severe asphyxia and lack of oxygen may cause irreversible brain damage.

▥ DIAGNOSING CP

It is unusual for CP to be suspected before around six months of age, when failure to reach a milestone, such as head control, rolling or hand control, may become apparent. The only way to reliably detect the condition is by skilled examination of a baby at three- to six-month intervals from birth to about 30 months.

In the first three months

The only outward sign that a baby may have a cerebral palsy is irritability, difficulty settling after feeding, and erratic sleep and feeding patterns. However, the majority of babies who behave like this are not affected by CP.

Around three months of age

A baby with CP may feel stiff (hypertonic). Some babies seem floppy (hypotonic), but become stiff around six months of age, or may show some reflexes that would ordinarily disappear by this time.

Between six and 12 months

A parent may now notice delays in one or more areas of development, or a doctor may be the first to notice. For 85 per cent of babies who sit, roll or walk later than expected there is no underlying abnormality. A small proportion do have an abnormality of the nervous system, and may go on to be diagnosed with cerebral palsy.

By 12–15 months

A reliable diagnosis of cerebral palsy can now be made. There are some highly specialised brain scans, called PET (positron emission tomography) and MRI (magnetic resonance imaging) scans that can detect some of the abnormalities in the brain that give rise to the symptoms.

Action plan

If you have any worries you need to arrange to see your doctor or health visitor for a formal developmental assessment. You may be referred to a paediatrician and then to a paediatric neurologist (who specialises in brain conditions). A full examination of the nervous system will show signs of abnormality in reflexes and muscle tone and power.

The doctor may order a series of diagnostic tests that could include: electroencephalogram (EEG) to record the brain's electrical activity, MRI, PET and computerised tomography (CT) scans; vision and hearing tests and blood genetic testing (page 266). These tests are usually diagnostic but may give normal results when there is obvious cerebral palsy. Many parents find the lack of an explanation of their child's problem very difficult to accept.

The diagnosis of cerebral palsy is very stressful and counselling and support will be an important aspect of care for your baby, for you and for your family. Friends, family, neighbours and local groups may be lifelines for you.

Treatment

There are no cures for cerebral palsy, but there are treatments that can minimise the effects. These may be a mixture of physical therapies, complementary therapies and some drug treatments. Specific treatment will need to meet your child's needs, depending on her condition, and tolerance for medications, procedures and therapies.

Treatment focuses on minimising problems and maximising your child's capabilities. Your child will need support from a number of specialists: they may include paediatrician, nurse, social worker, orthopaedic surgeon (to treat muscles and bones), neurologist, ophthalmologist (to treat eye problems), dentist and a rehabilitation team for physiotherapy, massage, occupational and speech therapy.

In school, specialist teachers, support assistance and sign language specialists may be part of your child's care team. Ideally, these specialists will communicate and work together; in practice you may need to take a central role in liaising between specialists and organising many aspects of your child's care.

Medical care

Your child may need physiotherapy and positioning aids to assist sitting, lying or standing, or braces and splints to prevent deformity and to provide support or protection. She may need medications to help control seizures or to decrease spasticity in the muscles, given by mouth or as an injection. Surgical interventions may be used to manage orthopaedic problems. Nutritional support is another essential part of medical care, particularly if your baby finds it difficult to feed and later to chew and swallow solids.

Emotional and social care

The huge emotional impact of discovering your child has CP may be extreme in the first instance or it may not hit home for several months.

Special social and educational support will help your child enjoy her potential and take an active role in her family and community. This is usually centred in the home and may include complementary care from nurses and a rehabilitation team. The pressure on parents and any other children in the family is considerable with the demands of what may be 24-hour care, and with the emotional frustrations of the child with CP who feels limited in what she can do. Relationship break-up is very common when parents are struggling and it is usually critical to have support, and counselling can be extremely helpful. You will also need practical help so you can get some rest, and this may be offered to you as part of a family care programme. Attending group meetings with other families affected by cerebral palsy could provide a chance to be with people who can encourage you. This also provides an extended community where your

child may find role models as she grows, such as wheelchair users who excel in sport, and people using communication aids who are active in work and in the community.

Children with very severe forms of cerebral palsy often have their needs best met in a special needs educational environment with specially trained carers. This presents its own challenges to families.

■ TYPES OF CP

There are three types of cerebral palsy, depending on which parts of the brain are affected. Many people with cerebral palsy have a combination of two or more types. The effects vary from one person to another and early in life it may be difficult to define the type or predict the effect in later life.

- Spastic cerebral palsy (over 50 per cent) predominantly results in stiffness of the muscles.
- Athetoid cerebral palsy (affects 20 per cent of people with CP) involves involuntary movements that cannot be controlled.
- Ataxic cerebral palsy (30 per cent) affects control of the body in space and balance.

Spastic cerebral palsy

Spastic cerebral palsy is the type associated with the earliest damage to the developing neonatal brain – from about 10–28 weeks. It causes stiff muscles and a decreased range of movement in the joints, so someone with spastic cerebral palsy has to put in a lot of effort to walk or move. Hemiplegia is where one side of the body is affected; if both legs are affected it is diplegia; and if both arms and both legs are equally affected it is quadriplegia. Quadriplegic or bilateral (both sides, upper and lower limbs) spastic cerebral palsy is the type most usually associated with prematurity.

Athetoid cerebral palsy

Athetoid cerebral palsy causes involuntary movements, because the muscles rapidly change from floppy to tense out of the person's control. Speech can be hard to understand because of the difficulty controlling the tongue, breathing and vocal cords. Hearing problems are also common.

This can arise as a result of asphyxia during or after birth called hypoxic ischaemic encephalopathy, also known as HIE (page 301), and is the type associated with brain damage due to meningitis in the newborn period.

Ataxic cerebral palsy

People with ataxic cerebral palsy have difficulty with balance and may have poor spatial awareness, finding it difficult to judge their position relative to objects around them. Most people with ataxic cerebral palsy can walk but they are unsteady. They may also have shaky hand movements and jerky speech. This is the type least likely to be related to factors around birth and appears to be largely genetically determined.

Associated problems

Other difficulties and medical conditions are more likely in people with cerebral palsy. These include: constipation; urinary incontinence; epilepsy; sleeping problems; difficulty with speech, chewing and swallowing, visual perception and learning.

Cervical erosion and cancer

See also Bleeding, mother, during pregnancy.

The cervix is the neck of the uterus. It includes the opening through which a baby passes during a vaginal birth. During pregnancy, the cervix becomes soft and engorged with additional blood vessels. It has an inner lining of delicate, red, mucous (mucus-producing) cells and as it enlarges the opening may 'pout' and reveal the inner lining. This is known as an erosion, even though the cervix is not literally damaged or eroded. It affects most women at some time in their life and rarely produces symptoms. If the cervix has torn during a previous birth the appearance will be more obvious.

Sometimes this pouting produces a clear vaginal discharge. Occasionally erosion leads to bleeding from prominent cervical blood vessels, and this may be stimulated by intercourse, particularly in late pregnancy. The blood is usually bright red and not profuse.

Action plan

If you bleed it is important to report it to your doctor because blood loss may indicate an underlying condition that needs immediate medical attention. The doctor may carry out an internal examination to check your cervix visually.

If the bleeding is originating from the cervix, you will be advised to refrain from penetrative sex until the bleeding has been absent for at least a week. There is no risk to your pregnancy, nor does the bleeding indicate cervical incompetence (see below).

There is no treatment for an erosion in pregnancy unless there is an associated infection that causes the cervix to bleed more easily. An infection may respond to antibiotics and can be diagnosed on a vaginal swab test.

Cancer of the cervix

Cancer is extremely rare in pregnancy. When it occurs it may cause intermittent bleeding throughout pregnancy. Your doctor will see an irregular bleeding area when you are examined. It is possible to do a colposcopy examination to visualise the cervix more accurately during pregnancy, but this is rarely needed. You may be offered a cervical smear at your first antenatal visit or after delivery at your six-week check-up with your doctor.

Cervical incompetence

Cervical incompetence (weakness) occurs when the cervix opens early as the growing pregnancy exerts pressure. The cervix is, in effect, a valve mechanism consisting of smooth muscle and connective tissue.

This mechanism keeps the cervix closed during pregnancy but not completely sealed as there is room for mucus and fluid to leave the uterus. In the last few weeks of pregnancy, the cervix gradually softens so that it will open easily during labour. These changes are called effacement or ripening.

Cervical incompetence occurs in around 1 per cent of pregnancies and is believed to be responsible for 25 per cent of miscarriages during the second trimester (months four, five and six). Most miscarriages are not caused by a problem in the cervix.

What happens

Incompetence is most commonly caused when a woman has undergone laser treatment or cone biopsy surgery to the cervix for the removal of pre-cancerous cells. It may also result from excessive stretching of the muscle during a termination of pregnancy or a dilation and curettage (D&C) operation (page 412).

Very rarely it is caused by tearing in a previous vaginal birth. In some women, there may be no obvious cause. Some people are genetically prone to the weakness, and it may be linked with a heart-shaped (bicornute) uterus.

An incompetent cervix is usually discovered after a miscarriage later than Week 12. This process will often occur without pain or vaginal bleeding until the miscarriage begins. A vaginal examination or ultrasound scan during a subsequent pregnancy will check the length and dilation (widening) of the cervical opening to show whether it has ripened and dilated early.

Action plan

If an incompetent cervix has been suspected and early dilation is diagnosed, in a subsequent pregnancy a stitch called a cervical cerclage can be inserted some time between Weeks 12 and 16 to hold your cervix closed for the remainder of the pregnancy. This is done after an ultrasound scan has confirmed your baby is developing normally. It is a simple procedure carried out in hospital under a light 15-minute anaesthetic. A stitch is placed around the muscle of the cervix like a purse string. A vaginal swab will exclude an infection while the stitch is in place. Antibiotics may be given to guard against infection.

After a few days of rest, women usually feel fine and can continue normal activity although it is common to feel menstrual-type discomfort until the cervix settles into the new shape. You can have sex as normal when the discomfort has stopped.

The stitch is left in place until Week 36, when the main risks of early birth are over. It will then be removed by cutting the thread during a vaginal examination in the clinic. This is a simple and painless process with no need for an anaesthetic. Usually labour begins within two to four hours as the cervix ripens, but it may be sooner.

If labour begins before Week 36 the stitch will need to be removed. This is simply done by cutting it during a vaginal examination. If you have a vaginal discharge with or without blood, leakage of amniotic fluid or painful contractions of the uterus, you will need to go to hospital immediately to ensure that you are not in early labour.

Chickenpox

See also Shingles in pregnancy.

Chickenpox (varicella zoster) is universal. Many children become infected and 90 per cent of pregnant women are immune following a childhood infection. Very few adults get chickenpox, but it presents risks to the babies of the small number of pregnant women who do become infected.

What happens

Chickenpox is highly infectious, and is characterised by an itchy rash that develops into fluid-filled blisters. A fever may begin before the rash appears. The extent of the rash varies from person to person. Every part of the body can be involved. There may be pain in the abdomen if the bowel is involved, joint pain if the limbs are involved, and headaches if the brain is involved.

Chickenpox is transmitted by airborne droplets, usually through the breath, coughs and sneezes, and symptoms begin to show between 10 and 20 days after an 'incubation period'. Someone with chickenpox is infectious from 48 hours before the blisters appear until they crust over in around five days.

If you are immune, you pass antibodies to your baby, giving him 'passive immunity'. The immunity from pregnancy alone may persist for about six months after birth, and can be prolonged by breastfeeding. If you have not had the infection, you cannot passively immunise your baby. Most babies under one year who develop chickenpox have a very mild infection with few spots.

Chickenpox within a few weeks of birth

(neonatal chickenpox) is very rare. When it does occur it requires intensive treatment. Later in the first year, your baby may come into contact with the infection and develop symptoms, although if you are breastfeeding he may be protected by your antibodies. The illness is typically uncomfortable but seldom serious beyond the newborn period.

▓ BABY, BIRTH–21 DAYS

Babies born to mothers who have developed chickenpox within five days of birth are at risk of developing neonatal chickenpox. It is extremely rare, but does carry a risk of severe complications. Fortunately, the severity of the infection can usually be lessened if a baby is treated promptly after birth with an injection of varicella-zoster immuno globulin (VZIG). Following treatment, the illness is usually mild. If serious symptoms develop, despite VZIG treatment, antiviral drugs (such as acyclovir) can help.

▓ BABY, FIRST YEAR

If your baby is infected, your role is to ensure he feels safe and comfortable, remembering that he may be in pain and frightened and upset by the itching. Let others know your baby is infected. It's important to let any pregnant women know so that they can avoid contact if there is any doubt about their immunity. Some of your friends may want to come round with their own children to expose them to the virus.

Occasionally, chickenpox causes a form of conjunctivitis in which tiny spots affect the inside of the eyelids. These may rupture to produce minute ulcers. If lots of ulcers develop there is a risk of damage to the cornea (the front surface of the eye). In the vast majority of children with chickenpox, the eyes are not involved. If pus-filled spots or ulcers do appear, take your baby to see your doctor. Simple treatment, such as eye ointments, can be used to stop bacterial infection and irritation developing.

Medical care

- Soothing creams such as calamine reduce itching.
- If your baby has a fever, infant paracetamol in doses as directed on the bottle (page 430) will

help. This will also reduce any headache or joint pains your baby may feel.

General comfort

- Your baby may be very distressed. Do what you can to be there for him and arrange for another adult to be around to devote themselves entirely to cuddling and comforting your baby when you are taking a break, or if you cannot stay for some reason.
- Scratch mitts are useful – they will prevent your baby scratching his blisters. Scratching may cause open sores that are vulnerable to infection and may scar.
- Your baby may be more comfortable completely covered up, with socks, mitts and a hat, or he may prefer to be naked.
- Some babies like to be bathed in lukewarm water.
- Hanging porridge oats in a pop sock or pair of tights beneath the bath taps as you run the water makes the bath more soothing (almost creamy) and is a tested traditional remedy.

Homeopathy

Homeopathic remedies may be extremely helpful in alleviating itching and speeding up the duration of the infection. If you know your baby has been in contact with the infection before a rash is obvious but seems unwell, you may give the most appropriate remedy (30c potency), three hourly for the first 12 hours.

- *Aconite* if he develops a fever and seems anxious.
- *Belladonna* before the rash develops if symptoms appear with a very high fever (more intense than for *Aconite*), flushed skin and dilated pupils.

Once your baby has a rash, you may give the most appropriate remedy three times per day (30c potency). You may need to change remedies as the pattern of symptoms changes. If you are in any doubt, consult your homeopath.

- *Pulsatilla* if he has a low-grade fever, is clingy, weepy and intolerant to heat, has a runny nose and shows no thirst.
- *Rhus Tox* when the rash is very itchy, making your baby restless, worse at night and if he is worse when cold.
- *Ant Tart* if the rash looks bluish and is slow to develop into blisters, and is accompanied by a

loose rattly cough with lots of phlegm and a coated tongue.

* *Hypercal* tincture in the bath – add 10–15 drops to bath water – or add 10 drops to 250ml (½ pint) of boiled, cooled water and drizzle onto uncomfortable or itchy spots.

■ MOTHER, PREGNANCY

Infection with chickenpox in pregnancy is rare, affecting around one in 2,000 women.

What happens

If you are not immune to chickenpox and come into contact with the disease, you may get infected. Infection can produce a particularly severe illness in pregnancy with pneumonia and encephalitis (inflammation of the brain). It is more severe in women who smoke, have a compromised immune system (for example, through HIV infection) or take corticosteroids. If you have had chickenpox in the past there is no risk of you becoming re-infected if you are in contact with the disease. Contact does not carry a risk of you developing shingles (page 476).

Early pregnancy risk to baby

Miscarriage risk is not increased. In the very unlikely event that you become infected in the first 28 weeks of pregnancy, this poses a small risk of your baby developing foetal varicella syndrome (affecting roughly 2 per cent of the babies of mothers who are infected in early pregnancy). It is very rare after 20 weeks and by 28 weeks the risk disappears. The syndrome involves a group of birth defects that can include scars, defects of muscle and bone, malformed and paralysed limbs, a smaller-than-normal head, blindness, fits and mental retardation.

Late pregnancy risk to baby

If you contract chickenpox and develop a rash after 28 weeks, there is no risk to your baby, unless you have the rash within five days of birth. In that case your child has a 25–50 per cent risk of becoming infected and developing neonatal chickenpox (page 129), with a rash five to 10 days after birth.

If you develop the chickenpox rash within seven days of your baby's birth, you have probably been producing antibodies for up to 21 days prior to the spots appearing, so your baby will have received some passive protection by the time he is born. This may protect him fully or reduce the severity of symptoms if he becomes infected. Breastfeeding will help raise your baby's immunity.

Action plan

Immunisation

If you have not had chickenpox, or are unsure of your immune status, a simple blood test can confirm whether you are immune, giving a result in two days. You can be immunised before pregnancy with two doses of the vaccine. You must wait one month after the second dose before conceiving. This is a precaution, but women who have been inadvertently immunised during pregnancy have not had infected babies.

Contact

If you are not immune, any contact with an infected person puts you at risk. The infection may be passed on if you live in the same house as that person (90 per cent chance of infection), or meet face to face indoors for five minutes or outdoors for 15 minutes.

It is best to avoid contact, and to inform your doctor if you are concerned or if a rash develops. If you are not immune you may be advised to receive varicella-zoster immune globulin (VZIG) by injection as soon as possible. This helps to prevent chickenpox, or at least lessen its severity, and is effective when given up to 10 days following contact. It is not yet known whether VZIG given in pregnancy helps to protect a foetus from infection.

Early pregnancy treatment

If you are infected in pregnancy and your symptoms are severe you may need to be admitted to hospital. An antiviral (Acyclovir) is the medication of choice that can be used if you are more than 20 weeks pregnant and are treated within 24 hours of the onset of the rash. Before Week 20, however, no drug is recommended as there is a potential for drug-induced harm to the baby. The risk of harm is believed to be the same as the risk of chickenpox-induced harm. However, in some circumstances zoster-immunoglobulin, a blood product, is recommended to offer protection for the baby.

Between Weeks 14 and 20, your baby has a 0.5–2 per cent risk of being infected. You will need to discuss the implications with your specialist. You may choose to have extra monitoring. Amniocentesis is not accurate as there may be varicella virus in the amniotic fluid without any physical effect on your baby. Any physical effect can take over four weeks to be evident on ultrasound scan, and some effects (such as to the eyes) will not be apparent on a scan.

Late pregnancy treatment

If you become infected in late pregnancy when your baby is due, the best course of action is for the birth to be delayed for as long as possible by avoiding induction of labour. This reduces the risks to your baby. In the extremely rare event that birth cannot be delayed, your baby will need treatment in the form of both immunoglobulin and antiviral treatment (page 129). Chickenpox in the first week of life is very dangerous for a baby.

Child protection and abuse

See also Violence and abuse, mother.

The majority of children are very much wanted and loved. Many, however, suffer from abuse in its widest sense. A small number are victims of physical or sexual abuse. Abuse is a very sensitive subject. For everyone involved, a great deal of support is needed. This is particularly true for a baby whose reaction to abuse, whether physical or emotional, may involve feelings of pain, trauma, fear and confusion, and possibly physical injury. Children from violent families often grow up feeling anxious and depressed, and find it difficult to get on with other people. If abuse is recognised and support is available soon enough, adult behaviour can change, a child can begin to heal and to develop trust, and close and loving relationships may develop.

The risk of a child being physically abused is highest before the age of two years, and even newborn babies may be victims. If a mother is abused (page 546) her baby also suffers. Emotional abuse is also significant and more common than physical abuse. Often this begins

with neglect or denial of a baby's needs and feelings. A baby may also feel abused if his parents or siblings consistently speak to him with hurtful or demeaning language or an unpleasant tone of voice.

Within families a history of abuse or neglect may pass through generations, and as a result family structures emerge where children may be more prone to abuse. The risk of abuse is greater for a child when a carer who is not related by blood becomes part of the family, such as step parents and cohabiting partners. Father–child bonding is incredibly valuable: fathers are five times less likely to abuse if they are close to their babies from birth.

What happens

Your baby is the most vulnerable member of your family. The adults around him create his environment and control many of the events, conversations and actions that he experiences, and he looks to adults for emotional comfort, reassurance and love.

Family patterns

Unfortunately patterns of behaviour tend to be repeated and the way an adult felt as a baby – perhaps neglected, excessively controlled, afraid or depressed, or exposed to anger or violence – may affect the way that person parents. The repetition of 'family of origin' patterns usually happens completely unconsciously. On a positive note, there is always a potential for change (page 207) and with support many people who suffered as children can be helped and can then offer their own children a positive start.

Abuse in pregnancy

It is normal to feel anxious or ambivalent in the face of a huge life change. Pregnancy is the commonest time for men to begin physically abusing their partner (page 546), perhaps with numerous effects for the baby. Among mothers, feelings of anxiety or depression may reinforce some potentially harmful behaviours such as continuing to smoke or take DRUGS. In the womb, a baby cannot give informed consent to consumption of alcohol, cigarettes or drugs, and in some countries this is seen as a form of abuse. Abuse in the womb may also come about through denial of nutritional needs, for instance when there is anorexia (page 200).

Emotional abuse and neglect

Babies have a rich emotional life and a range of feelings in reaction to each experience. The relationships formed in early life may be reassuring and fun, and feel safe. If a baby's emotions and needs go unnoticed or are neglected, this is a form of emotional abuse. If family life or relationships are stressful, your baby may be at the receiving end of angry, frustrated or anxious behaviour. Jealousy may be a factor, more common among men who see their baby as an intrusion or a threat, and rivalry may occur with siblings. Angry feelings are common but the important thing is the balance. If a baby feels more anger than love he may feel hurt and afraid. He may cry more and some parents or grandparents may react by becoming angry or distanced.

When a child is left in isolation beyond the normal periods associated with sleep and rest, this is the equivalent of solitary confinement. In some families it may be considered acceptable to leave a baby alone for long periods, either in a separate room, or in a play pen, or in the same room as the adults but left out of the action (for example, in a car seat in the corner). If he is ignored or deprived of contact and stimulation, this is emotional abuse. Babies need contact, love and stimulation to develop and thrive. It is well known that babies need to be held and touched and too little touch may be very upsetting. Sometimes abuse takes the form of feeding a baby too infrequently.

Physical abuse

Hitting is never appropriate. It is intensely frightening and confusing for a baby. Babies who are exposed to physical violence may learn to equate being loved and cared for with being submissive or feeling pain or fear. It may also be physically harmful. Even a small amount of force may cause serious injury. Shaking is another way parents may react to CRYING or vent their anger, and can cause severe long-term damage. It is highly inappropriate. More severe forms of abuse include deliberate physical harm and sexual abuse. The effect of physical harm is combined with the emotional impact, and reflects the type and frequency of injury. At worst it may lead to brain damage, developmental abnormalities or even death. The motivation for an adult to harm a baby is always linked with the adult's own feelings (often these are rage or helplessness), and is never the baby's fault.

Effects on a baby

Your baby's experiences form a foundation for his self-esteem, his understanding of relationships, and his outlook on life (page 206). Feeling insecure because of abuse may make him withdrawn, nervous and easily upset or hyperactive and challenging. High levels of stress hormones may disrupt his sleep and appetite and may also reduce immunity. Some babies cope by surrounding themselves with an emotionally protective layer almost like a second emotional skin. If a baby has felt any abuse, either in pregnancy or after birth, the effect depends on what has happened, his personality, and how he is welcomed and cared for in pregnancy and after birth.

- He may find it difficult to bond with mum and dad, and to interact with other children and adults. He may not be able to trust others. It is well known that exposure to violence in the early years can affect the way the brain develops and a person's capacity to love and be loved.
- He may cry a lot, have colicky symptoms, and have difficulty sleeping.
- Some abused babies fail to gain sufficient weight.
- He may smile later than expected, and infrequently. He may even be depressed.
- He may be slow to reach developmental milestones, such as playing, and exploring and speaking. Later he may find it difficult to pay attention or to concentrate.
- He may act aggressively.
- He may be quiet and withdrawn.
- He may be nervous.
- He may have obvious physical injuries.
- He may have a series of illnesses.
- Later in life he may experience a higher incidence of social difficulties and addictions.

Action plan

There may be a number of measures that can prevent abuse. Repair, too, is possible in a loving and secure relationship.

Supporting yourself before and after birth

The best cure for abuse is prevention. If you personally feel threatened, the initial step may be to address this. There is advice on page 548. You may want to hold out, in the hope that things will get better. This might happen, but in the majority of families if the situation is already bad it is likely to worsen. Support and practical help now make a huge difference.

You may need assistance to address other stressful issues in your life. Having support may boost your confidence to stand up for your baby and for yourself. It might be appropriate for you or someone else who will be caring for your baby to seek active treatment for anxiety or depression or counselling for relationship conflicts. If you were emotionally or physically abused as a child, one of the most useful steps may be to seek counselling or psychotherapy (page 162).

Being there for your baby

Before the birth, your baby can feel whether he is wanted and secure. After the birth his behaviour reflects his unique personality and the care he receives. If he is met with love and acceptance and his needs are met, he may feel safe and enjoy the pleasure of bonding, play and exploration.

Subtle abuse, such as spending little time with your baby or neglecting to touch him and talk to him, may be relatively easily resolved with insight into what he needs (page 206) and perhaps some guidance. Seeing your child as an individual who does not plan to be difficult or destructive may alter your view and your behaviour. Your health visitor or GP may help you get in touch with individuals, local groups and useful organisations and you may soon begin to trust yourself and feel at ease with your baby.

Child protection in action

It is not always easy to admit to abuse, or to ask for help: abuse can be very well hidden. If you are in need of help, contact a healthcare professional, social worker or a confidential parent help line; they are able to direct you to immediate support.

Healthcare and educational professionals are trained to notice signs that suggest a need to investigate for the possibility of child protection-related issues, and to notice behaviour in the adults responsible for the care of the infant that may indicate depression or emotional difficulties. Any child under the age of one year who needs hospital treatment for bone fractures or bruises will usually be referred to a child health specialist as a matter of precaution.

There is a child protection team in each county or borough and all follow national guidelines regarding steps to be taken should abuse be suspected or reported. The team may consist of a range of child specialists including health, educational, social work and police child protection officers. If this happens, usually a meeting is held with the parents or carers. The team is there to help families overcome difficulties, preferably in the family home to begin with.

The priorities of child protection workers are the early recognition of risk factors and then working with the family to prevent injury, neglect or emotional harm. Any actions taken are always, at least in the first instance, in the interest of the child. Usually this means working closely with a family or carer, with opportunities for supervised parenting, attendance at parent groups, and supplementary support for a mother, child and father, when present. Families often find the close monitoring distressing, particularly if they do not feel it is justified; but the intention is always to prioritise the child.

There may be input from a specialist healthcare worker or a social worker. Sometimes parents are offered parenting skill classes, a drug and alcohol team may be involved, as may be specialised child psychologists and psychiatrists and similar specialists for parents. Even financial benefits may be needed to help families get out of stressful situations that may result in children being abused.

Rarely, children will be removed from their families, but only if all other types of resolution have been shown not to work or if a court decides it is the right course of action. Even then, major efforts are made to reconstitute families wherever possible, but usually with strict advice as to attendance at support groups, regular health checks and other related support. To permanently separate children from their families is always seen as a last resort, or only one to be used in an urgent situation.

If a situation improves and a baby is given love, support and encouragement, positive experiences may replace feelings of upset and hurt. Support for parents and the wider family to help them change in such a way that they are able to protect their child is the aim of all the professionals involved in this work.

Sadly, even though there are thousands of 'happy endings' every year, there are still occasions where families cannot or will not change, and their children remain at risk, or go on to be further damaged. This is rare.

Childcare

Finding care that is right for your baby may take you into a maze of waiting lists, contracts and compromises. As you explore the field, you and your baby may both feel separation anxiety (page 220) and will show your own reactions to this. Where childcare suits you both, the predominant feelings are trust and contentment. When childcare isn't suitable, your baby may complain or become upset, and it can be a nightmare. You need to pay attention and acknowledge the warning signs, and they are simple: your baby is unhappy, and you feel uncomfortable.

▓ THE RIGHT CARER

Your baby needs to feel safe and loved. She will benefit most when the adult(s) she is with focus on her, understand her requests and meet her needs. These priorities rank more highly than the carer's qualifications. It may take time and courage to find a happy balance.

The carer will be more effective when you are clear about your expectations. You can outline these when you meet for an interview. At the same time you'll learn about his or her expectations. Remember that your intuition about whether he or she is open, honest and loving is usually a very reliable guide.

It is essential to regularly assess the way the relationship is working. Make time before you leave and when you come back to catch up. It is best to book a chat after the first week and at intervals after that. If something serious crops up arrange to talk very soon.

Interviewing a potential carer

With a list of questions you'll be sure you don't miss out anything important. The points below might help you and could be used to form a contract if you need to draw one up.

The carer's childhood
* Ask about her experience as a child.
* Ask about how her family functioned.
* Ask about her feelings about the needs of tiny babies.

The carer's approach
* Discuss her ideas about being there for your baby.
* Does she enjoying playing with and entertaining children, can she sing or play an instrument, is she happy to go swimming with your baby?
* If you're leaving your baby away from home, find out about sleeping arrangements and spaces for play.
* Discuss her approach to food and breastfeeding and what kind of food she considers 'healthy'.
* Ask her about safety, how she minimises risks and what she would do in an emergency.
* Find out her view on discipline for babies and young children.
* Ask if she is planning to do any further training or if she would consider this if you asked. For instance, you could spend time together with a nutritional therapist.

The carer's background
* Ask about her qualifications and experience.
* Ask why she left her last job.
* Have a look at references and follow them up.
* Ensure she has first aid qualifications.
* Find out if she has a driver's licence and whether she has a car of her own.
* Does she have any allergies (for instance to your pets) or dietary needs that may affect her work?
* Ask if she smokes or drinks alcohol during the day.

Finances and conditions
* Discuss pay (including tax issues), holidays, overtime and sickness.
* Find out if the carer has insurance.

- Are there limits on the length of time she can work for your family?
- Discuss an acceptable period of notice if either of you want to terminate.

Setting ground rules

It is preferable to have rules written down. Try to be as clear as possible about your wishes, your baby's rhythm and expectations, and the days and times you require care. You can do this without being dictatorial. A few guidelines will allow your carer to be spontaneous and loving with your baby within a comfortable framework.

- Be clear about the carer's duties and whether these include housework.
- Be clear about hours of work and holiday times.
- Discuss important issues such as smoking, alcohol, food and sleeping times.
- Give contact details for you and your partner, with backup contacts, such as grandparents, friends, neighbours, doctor.
- List things to do if your baby's unwell or there's an emergency.
- Provide a communication book for the carer to make a record of each day.
- List contacts to help in case of domestic emergencies, such as plumbing, electricity, car breakdown.
- Arrange a date to assess how things are going.

Your options

You'll get details of childminders, maternity nurses, nannies, nurseries and crèches from your local health visitor or Children's Information Service, or from advertisements in local and national publications. Most professional carers are women. You will have your own preferences and your baby will show her likes and dislikes very clearly. You may need to try more than one approach, or interview a number of people, before you find something that feels right.

Maternity nurses

A maternity nurse is a qualified nanny trained to care for newborn babies. She will take over the care of your baby when you want, and bring her to you for breastfeeding. Most maternity nurses aim to get a baby into a 'routine' and sleeping through the night from an early age;

many are not mothers themselves. You may prefer to offer infant-led care and follow your baby's rhythm.

Mother's helps and doulas

A mother's help may do a variety of domestic duties to leave you free to rest and care for your baby. A mother's help may be a regular part of your life for years.

A DOULA fulfils a similar role with a greater emphasis on baby care and feeding, and some doulas begin to help women before and during birth. The main qualification is to be friendly and caring, offering emotional support and practical help and advice wherever she can. Most doulas are mothers.

Nannies

Nannies will care for your baby in your home and may live with you or come to your house for agreed hours. Nannies vary widely in the qualifications they hold, the amounts they charge, the services they offer and the treatment they expect. You could explore the possibility of sharing a nanny with another family to reduce costs.

Au pairs

Au pairs are young people who come to the UK to stay with a family and help with childcare while getting a taste of another culture and learning English. Their working conditions are regulated and they expect a minimum weekly payment as well as accommodation, meals and involvement in family life. What your au pair does in her spare time is up to her.

Because they are young and may be away from home for the first time many au pairs need emotional support, and this may involve a considerable amount of mothering from you. Your au pair won't necessarily be trained in childcare. It's common for au pairs to move on after around a year.

Childminders

A childminder uses her own home as a mini crèche. Childminders usually have their own children, many are flexible regarding hours and most are less expensive than nannies. Every childminder is required by law to register with the local authority and must attend a pre-registration course run by the local Social

Services Department. Disadvantages may be the absence of care through school holidays or cancellation at short notice if there's a contagious illness in the house.

Nursery or crèche

In a nursery or crèche your baby will be cared for along with a group of other children and babies by a team of qualified nursery nurses and people undergoing training. The great bonus is the social interaction and the resources and space that are seldom available at a childminder's or in your own home. One of the greatest disadvantages is the high rate of infection from common childhood illness and, if the ratio isn't optimal, the potential for your child's needs to go unmet. A good guide of standard is the frequency of staff turnover. Most nurseries offer a degree of flexibility around hours. Some don't take children below the age of two. All nurseries must be registered with the local authority and are thoroughly inspected each year.

Grandparents or other relatives

There's a very special bond between many children and their grandparents. Grandparents have often grown in patience with the passing years and take unrestrained pleasure in playing with their grandchildren.

If one of your parents has offered to look after your baby, and you get on well and share similar values, it may be a perfect arrangement whether or not you give payment. Some people find it hard to be straight about their preferences with their own parents and using them for regular care is not a suitable option.

Making ends meet

You may be entitled to financial assistance towards childcare: visit your local Social Services office, ask at a Citizens' Advice Bureau or investigate child tax credits. If you are a single parent, you may be able to get some assistance while you train or look for work. Your baby may also be eligible for a place in a community nursery operated and subsidised by your local authority. About one in 10 employers offer assistance with childcare through an allowance or voucher scheme or with subsidies.

▨ YOUR BABY'S HAPPINESS

When you have chosen childcare your baby will need to settle in and make a gradual separation from you. She will appreciate you being with the carer and will take her lead from you, by watching how you relate to the other person. If she feels your confidence and trust, she is more likely to be relaxed. It is useful to spend time with your baby at the nursery or with the carer on several days for increasing amounts of time. When you feel ready, leave your baby for a few minutes and you can then leave her for longer. Tell her you are going and you are coming back: even if she doesn't understand your words she'll understand your tone of voice. If your workplace and carer are flexible, you may be able to build up the hours you spend apart over a week or two.

Your baby may cry when you leave – this is normal separation anxiety (page 220). It may take her time to calm down: wait outside the door before going. If she does not cry, do not take it personally: it is probably a good sign that she feels secure. Most babies adapt well to change and enjoy going to nursery or spending time with a childminder or nanny.

If your baby does not adapt well

* Look at how you feel. Are you ready to separate from your baby?
* Consider your true feelings about the childcarer(s) – do you feel relaxed and confident?
* Consider whether the environment suits your baby. An extrovert child may thrive in a crèche, while an introvert may prefer personal care.
* Have courage. If you feel that the arrangement is not right, you will need to try alternatives.
* If you're concerned that your baby cries excessively when you leave, or she seems despondent or unhappy when you return, talk to her carer. This may be a signal of approaching illness. Alternatively, your baby may not be happy; some babies are more dependent on their mums than others and take a long time to settle.
* Look at the possibility that your baby is being mistreated (page 132). This is rare but very significant. Trust your intuition and ask other parents about their children's behaviour. Be

observant and notice cuts, scratches and bruises.

Handing your baby over to someone else can be heart wrenching and it's common to have anxieties: Will she be happy? Will she miss me? Will she be angry with me? Will she love the carer more than she loves me? Rest assured that babies are never confused about who their parents are. Your baby has enough love for both you and her carer. Although it may be hard at first, it helps to welcome and encourage the carer's love because if there is fondness between them – and a friendship between you and the carer – you'll find it easier to trust that everything is going well. The carer will become an important person in your child's life and may have many positive influences on your child and your family.

Chlamydia

Chlamydia trachomatis is the most common sexually transmitted disease in the USA and Europe. It can infect the penis, vagina, cervix, anus, urethra or eye. It usually gives no symptoms but its presence can have serious health consequences, particularly for women. Most significantly, it can lead to ectopic pregnancy or infertility. If infection is present in pregnancy, a baby may be infected and could develop eye infections or pneumonia as a result. Fortunately, once the infection is diagnosed, treatment is usually successful.

What happens

In women, the infection usually begins in the vagina and cervix. It can spread to the fallopian tubes or ovaries and even cause pelvic inflammatory disease. More commonly, it can scar and block the fallopian tubes, raising the risk of ectopic pregnancy and infertility. In pregnancy, it may cause spontaneous rupture of the membranes (or 'preterm rupture of membranes', page 391), leading to premature birth. After birth it can lead to infections of the uterus and pelvis.

Of infected women, 85 per cent show no signs. If symptoms are present, they begin five to 10 days after infection and may include bleeding or pain, fever, pain on urination or a yellowish vaginal discharge that may have a foul odour. These are similar to symptoms of gonorrhoea. Chlamydia can also infect the rectum, giving painful bowel movements. Around 40 per cent of infected men show symptoms, including discharge from the penis, burning while urinating or tender testicles. In this case female partners should be tested, too.

Between 20 and 50 per cent of babies born to infected mothers become infected. Chlamydia is the leading cause of neonatal conjunctivitis. In rare cases, this may cause blindness, but if chlamydia is identified as the cause, appropriate antibiotic treatment is usually effective. An infected baby may also develop chlamydia pneumonia, perhaps three to six weeks after birth. This usually responds to appropriate antibiotic treatment.

Action plan

Tests for chlamydia are not always recommended but if you have pelvic symptoms or your sexual partner shows symptoms it is worth asking for a diagnostic test. In some hospitals all women are tested.

Diagnosis
Special DNA culture tests on swabs taken from the penis, cervix, urethra or anus, as well as urine samples, give clear information. Your doctor may take a sample of a cervical discharge (like having a cervical smear).

Medical care
Chlamydia is easy to treat, and you and your partner need to be treated at the same time with antibiotics that kill the bacteria. If you are not pregnant you may be offered azithromycin to be taken in one dose, or doxycycline to take for seven days. Erythromycin is often prescribed for pregnant women and other people who cannot take doxycycline. It is also used to treat babies with eye infections or pneumonia caused by chlamydia. Your doctor will help you decide which is the best treatment.

Your baby
A baby who is exposed to *Chlamydia trachomatis* in the birth canal during delivery may develop a conjunctivitis eye infection or pneumonia. It is very rare for infection to occur after caesarean delivery.

If your baby develops chlamydia, conjunctivitis symptoms usually develop within 10 days of birth and tend to include discharge in one or both eyes and swollen eyelids. The recommended treatment is frequent use of erythromycin or tetracycline antibiotic eye ointment for about five days, with oral erythromycin for about 21 days. The oral treatment is recommended to target infection in other tissues.

Symptoms of pneumonia, including a cough that gets steadily worse and lung congestion, tend to develop within three to six weeks of birth. This may also be treated successfully with antibiotics.

There appear to be no long-term complications of chlamydia infection, providing initial treatment has been effective. Up to 20 per cent of babies require a second course of oral antibiotics.

Cholestasis

Cholestasis is a condition unique to pregnancy in which the flow of bile in the mother's liver is reduced. The main symptom of cholestasis is severe itching without a rash, usually beginning after Week 30, but sometimes sooner. The itch is often most intense on the palms of the hands and soles of the feet, and can be worse at night. It is not the same as normal skin itchiness associated with pregnancy, which commonly affects the breasts and abdomen where the skin is stretched and there is often an associated rash.

Cholestasis is more common in some countries (Sweden and Chile) and for women of Indian and Pakistani origin. There may be a genetic predisposition with a family history. In Europe cholestasis affects 2 per cent of pregnancies. With careful attention to the timing of birth, cholestasis is unlikely to have any ill effects on your baby and your symptoms will disappear soon after the birth. If you have cholestasis, there is a 60 per cent likelihood of recurrence in subsequent pregnancies.

What happens

Although the causes of cholestasis are unclear, it is known that the hormone oestrogen, produced by the placenta, interferes with the transport of bile salts. Itching (also called pruritis) may be caused by bile salts being deposited in the skin.

Urine may be darker and stools lighter, and you may have intolerance to fatty foods but in most instances mild cholestasis does not affect the urine and stools. Very rarely, cholestasis leads to jaundice (yellowing of the skin). As jaundice is a symptom of many other disorders, including gallstones and HEPATITIS, it always needs to be investigated.

Lower levels of bile also affect your body's ability to absorb vitamin K, the vitamin responsible for assisting blood clotting, and this may make BLEEDING after birth more likely in mother and baby. Your vitamin K levels return to normal within a few days of birth.

If you have cholestasis, your baby may be affected. When the levels of liver function tests and bile salts are very high there may be an increased risk of your baby passing meconium (page 447) before birth, FOETAL DISTRESS in labour and a doubled risk of PREMATURE BIRTH. Most importantly, there is a slightly increased risk of intrauterine death (page 399) before the onset of labour, which rises after 37 weeks. The actual level of risk is not known and has been exaggerated in the past. It is minimally greater than if you did not have cholestasis.

Action plan

If you are experiencing itching on your hands, feet, limbs and trunk but don't have a rash then your liver function will be tested by analysing a blood sample.

Diagnosis

The main diagnostic test for cholestasis shows a rise in bile salt levels in the blood. Elevated bile salts may be accompanied by alterations apparent in other liver function tests, most commonly the transaminases (ALT, AST), transferase and bilirubin. Each woman has her own unique pattern of results. Yours will be interpreted by your obstetrician to confirm a diagnosis. Blood tests are useful to exclude hepatitis and pre-existing liver disease and to monitor the severity of the cholestasis. The liver function test levels alter as pregnancy progresses and every hospital needs to be aware of the normal ranges in pregnancy so that treatments are not missed or done incorrectly.

An ultrasound scan of your liver checks for gallstones that may also reduce the flow of bile and cause itching. Gallstones are rare in pregnancy and they are usually not treated until after the birth. In the very rare event of a gallstone blocking the bile duct, the blockage may be relieved by means of endoscopic ('keyhole') surgery via your stomach.

Medical care

It may be difficult to treat cholestasis.
* Adenosyl methionine and ursodeoxycholic acid are medications that may ease the itching and liver function abnormalities. Symptoms may be relieved in 24–48 hours. Further research is being conducted to see if this treatment is safe and effective to improve the outcome for mother and baby.
* Cholestyramine binds bile acids but it is not effective in pregnancy cholestasis.
* Dexamethazone has not been proven to improve outcome.
* If cholestasis is severe you will be given vitamin K weekly, by mouth, to improve blood clotting, beginning after Week 30.

Food and eating

Attention to your diet, plus supplements to ensure adequate intake of vitamins, minerals and fatty acids, help to reduce the work your liver needs to do.
* Drink 2–3 litres (4–6 pints) of water a day. Stick to a mainly vegetarian diet with a reduction in dairy products and cheese and wheat and fatty foods and an increase in whole grain rice, barley, millet and buckwheat; and vegetables and fruits eaten raw or lightly cooked and eaten immediately.
* It may help to eat sesame and pumpkin seeds. Linseed soaked overnight in water can be added to food or drunk on its own.
* Cholestasis may be associated with a deficiency in the mineral selenium, which can be remedied with supplements.
* Avoid alcohol, and saturated fats – in fried foods and fatty meats, for example.

Soothing remedies to relieve itching
* Try to avoid getting too hot.
* Apply soothing lotions or creams such as

calamine, diprobase or aqueous lotion to the skin. A light chamomile-based cream may help, too. Itching may sometimes respond to antihistamines prescribed by a doctor.
* Take time to relax and rest during the day. Thinking that your baby may be at risk – although the risk is slight – is likely to make you anxious, and the itching may interfere with sleep.

Homeopathy

To alleviate symptoms of itching you may try the most appropriate of the following remedies in 6c potency, morning and night for up to one week and then re-assess.
* *Dolichos* where there is no visible eruption despite the maddening intensity of itching, the more you scratch, the worse the itch, and it is worse from warmth and at night.
* *Arsenicum* for a ticklish, crawling itch that burns after scratching, the skin becomes dry and rough and can bleed from excessive scratching. You feel anxious, restless and chilly and worse at night, especially after midnight.
* *Sulphur* for itching when the skin feels red, hot and burns after scratching, and is worse from any contact with water and in bed.

Liver support remedies such as *Chelidonium* and *Lycopodium* may be useful but need to be prescribed by a qualified homeopath.

Birth

The timing of birth will be decided by your symptoms and the results of bile salt and liver function tests. Ultrasound is less useful as an indicator of the optimal time of birth and any potential risks to your baby from cholestasis.
* Birth is usually planned for after Week 37 or 38 if the liver function levels remain elevated, because the risk of unexpected foetal death may rise beyond this time, and at this stage of pregnancy risks associated with premature birth have reduced.
* In severe cases with highly abnormal liver function tests and maternal jaundice, birth may be advised before Week 37, but this is extremely uncommon.
* Unless there are other indications for a caesarean section, birth is usually stimulated by induction of labour. Your baby will be monitored during labour as there may be a slightly increased risk of foetal distress.

After the birth

Provided your baby has been born safely, cholestasis in pregnancy will have no long-term physical effects on you or your baby. It is recommended that your baby has a vitamin K injection at birth (page 63) to prevent the slightly increased risk of vitamin K deficiency-associated bleeding linked with cholestasis.

Cholestasis does not cause lasting liver damage. Symptoms quickly disappear after the birth and you will soon forget the itchiness that was a constant presence for months.

You will need to repeat the liver function tests four weeks after the birth to ensure your liver is back to normal. Your medical team may advise you to be rescanned if you have gallstones. It will be best not to use an oestrogen pill as a method of contraception. There is an increased risk of cholestasis for other members of your family.

Chorionic villus sampling (CVS)

See Amniocentesis and CVS.

Circumcision

World-wide, around 20 per cent of men are circumcised. Circumcision has become extremely controversial, other than for religious and very rarely surgical reasons, and is no longer recommended by paediatricians as a routine procedure. The main religious groups for whom circumcision remains an important ritual are Jews and Muslims.

The foreskin produces antibodies, antibacterial and antiviral proteins and pheromones, and is designed by nature to be an internal organ like the vagina. Circumcision does not promote hygiene or prevent or reduce the incidence of urinary tract infection, cancer of the penis or the cervix later in life or sexually transmitted diseases. A typical western medical circumcision results in the loss of many of the erogenous sexual nerves and affects sexual pleasure, which is enhanced by the foreskin's gliding action.

Under normal conditions, a baby's foreskin is attached to the underlying glans of the penis and it does not start to retract naturally until three years of age at the earliest. Any attempt to retract or remove it causes pain and distress. Phimosis is a condition in which the foreskin of the penis is abnormally non-retractable. It occurs in less than 2 per cent of boys and it can often be treated by the simple application of a steroid cream. If this fails, a circumcision is advised. If, at birth, there is a suggestion of hypospadias (page 439), where the urinary opening is not at the tip of the penis, circumcision needs to be put on hold because the skin of the foreskin may be needed for reconstructive surgery.

In 1999, the American Academy of Pediatrics stated, 'In circumstances in which … the procedure is not essential to the child's current wellbeing, parents should determine what is in the best interest of the child. If a decision for circumcision is made, procedural analgesia should be provided.' Similar advice is offered by the Royal College of Paediatrics in the UK. In the past 20 years the rate of circumcision in the USA has dropped from 90 per cent to 60 per cent.

HIV and circumcision

Recent studies in Africa have shown that circumcision reduces the risk of contracting HIV by 70 per cent. One possible explanation is linked to laboratory studies which found that the foreskin is rich in white blood cells, which are favoured targets of HIV, the virus that causes AIDS. The absence of the foreskin may reduce infection through this route.

What happens

If you decide to have your baby boy circumcised there is no best way. All methods will be painful for him and distressing for you while his pain continues to upset him. However circumcision is carried out, almost all babies cry, particularly when being restrained by an adult or on a plastic board with Velcro straps. Newborn babies perceive pain as intensely as, or more intensely than, older children and adults. It is preferable to use a local anaesthetic cream or injection. The anaesthetic numbs the outer skin of the penis but the glans of the penis is not numbed and your baby will feel the foreskin being separated.

A sugary or alcohol-based drink does seem to reduce pain perception.

Ritual Jewish circumcision is traditionally done at eight days and does not usually use anaesthetic. It is done by a surgeon or a *mohel* (Jewish religious officer) who may not necessarily be a doctor. In the ritual form of circumcision the foreskin is separated from the underlying head of the penis then drawn forward and a protective shield is then slid across it before it is cut off. A similar method is used in some hospitals. Some doctors deliberately provoke erections in order to judge the 'cut-off line'.

An alternative method is to use a 'plastibell' device like a plastic bell. After the foreskin is separated the device is placed over the head of the penis and the foreskin drawn over the bell. A tie is tightened around the base of the bell to cut off the blood supply to the foreskin. After three to seven days the bell and attached foreskin drop off, leaving the tissue to heal. The pain caused is probably less severe than the pain of a ritual circumcision but because the bell is in place for a number of days pain may last longer.

Action plan: post-circumcision care

After circumcision by any method there may be two or three days of discomfort, usually associated with pain on passing urine. Frequent breastfeeding and cuddling and regular small doses of paracetamol will comfort your baby. If pain continues beyond the third day, get in touch with the *mohel* or surgeon.

After surgical removal of the foreskin, the penis is wrapped in gauze. It helps to keep the gauze moist and cover its inner surface with Vaseline to prevent it adhering to the wound. The gauze will appear bloody at first, but this usually dries up quickly. In most cases the circumcision site heals quickly because there is such a good blood supply to the penis. The gauze can be safely soaked off after three or four days. It is safe to bathe your baby 24 hours after the circumcision. No change in the type of nappies or the frequency with which they are changed is necessary, and no other special precautions are required.

Following circumcision the penis may appear swollen for at least two weeks. This is not unusual, and is due to the healing process. The pink head of the penis, the glans, will be visible.

Possible complications

The risks associated with circumcision are kept to a minimum by ensuring that the procedure is carried out by someone experienced in the procedure. Infections can be avoided by regularly changing the dressings. Complications with plastibell are less common.

Excessive bleeding is dangerous and if it continues for more than one hour after the procedure let the surgeon know immediately. He or she may come back or recommend you apply further dressings. If the bleeding is excessive it is essential to go to hospital for medical care, and rarely a blood transfusion may be needed. A tiny number of babies have an inherited bleeding disorder (page 56).

If bleeding begins after 48 hours, the site has become infected. You will see redness and swelling around the line of separation and your baby will be distressed and feverish. This is very rare and requires treatment with antibiotics. Your GP may refer you to a paediatrician.

If excessive skin has been removed, then erections may be painful – all boy babies get erections, usually when the bladder is full and presses on the veins at the base of the penis. Excessive removal of skin may also lead to the penis developing a curve because the tissue on the inner surface of the penis is shorter than the erect length of the penis. This is called a chordee (page 439) and may require surgery.

The majority of babies recover from circumcision in a few days and show few long-term effects. A significant minority, approximately 25 per cent, have redness and pain for longer than a week, are upset and do not feed or sleep well. The psychological trauma of a surgical operation without adequate analgesia may have a long-term emotional effect on a minority of babies similar to POST TRAUMATIC STRESS.

Homeopathy

Before circumcision you may be calmer if you take one dose of *Aconite* (200c potency) 30 minutes before the operation. For your baby, one 30c dose may help. Bach flower rescue remedy is often helpful: two to three drops for you and one drop for your baby immediately before circumcision. After circumcision, *Arnica*, *Hypericum*, *Calendula* and *Staphysagria* are the most beneficial remedies to use.

- *Arnica* may be used for trauma and to reduce swelling and inflammation.
- *Hypericum* works on the nerves.
- *Calendula* heals the wound.
- *Staphysagria* assists healing of the wound and deals with the emotional side of this procedure.

All of these remedies may be given in 30c potency morning and night for up to five days. You may also use 10 drops of Hypercal tincture in the bath for five days to assist healing. If you are in any doubt, consult your homeopath.

Cleft lip and palate

One in every 800 children in the UK is born with a cleft – an incomplete join – in the lip or the roof of the mouth (palate). During early pregnancy, separate areas of the face develop individually and then join together. If some parts do not join properly the result is a cleft, meaning 'split' or 'separation'. A child born with a separation in the upper lip has a cleft lip. A similar birth defect in the roof of the mouth is called a cleft palate. Since the lip and the palate develop separately, it is possible for a child to have a cleft lip, a cleft palate or both, and the severity of the cleft can vary.

What happens

With a cleft lip there is an opening in the upper lip between the mouth and nose. It looks as though there is a split in the lip. It can range from a slight notch to complete separation in one or both sides of the lip extending up and into the nose. A cleft in the gum may occur in association with a cleft lip.

The back of the palate (towards the throat) is called the soft palate and the front (towards the lips) is known as the hard palate. A cleft palate can range from a split in the soft palate at the back of the mouth to an almost complete separation of the roof of the mouth between the soft and hard palate. Sometimes a baby with a cleft palate may have a small lower jaw and difficulty with breathing. This condition is called Pierre Robin Sequence.

Babies with a cleft lip alone do not usually have any feeding difficulties and breast- or bottle-feeding is possible. However, a newborn baby with a cleft palate may need extra help if the cleft interferes with the creation of a vacuum needed for sucking. When this happens, bottle-feeding is usually more successful than breastfeeding. Special bottles and teats are available from the Cleft Lip and Palate Association (CLAPA).

The most common problems associated with cleft lip and palate are slow feeding and taking in too much air while feeding. This may lead to painful wind or COLIC and bringing up milk through the nose.

Action plan

A baby born with a cleft is contacted by a member of the Cleft Palate team, either from the local hospital or from a regional centre, usually within 24 hours of diagnosis. If the condition has been diagnosed or suspected from ultrasound findings during pregnancy, you may have already met the team. A Cleft Team might include a plastic surgeon, a paediatrician, a dentist, a speech specialist, a hearing specialist, an ear-nose-and-throat specialist, a nurse, and a genetic counsellor. Your baby may need plastic surgery to repair the opening and help to overcome problems with feeding and teething, hearing, speech, and psychological development.

To correct a cleft, surgery is usually done when the child is about 10 weeks old, with closure of the lip carried out first of all. However, repairing a cleft palate involves more extensive surgery and is usually done at nine to 18 months old, when he is better able to tolerate surgery. Children with a cleft palate are particularly prone to ear infections because the cleft can interfere with the functioning of the middle ear. The ear-nose-and-throat surgeon may recommend that a small plastic ventilation tube (grommet) be inserted in the eardrum to permit proper drainage and air circulation. The initial surgery to repair a cleft lip or palate is only the beginning of a process that may involve further operations as well as developmental support for your child. Additional surgery may be recommended when your child is older to refine the shape and function of the lip, nose, gums and palate.

Many affected children become self-conscious, and love, acceptance and encouragement from the parents are extremely important for self-esteem. Parents also require emotional support and may need ongoing emotional support and therapy.

Club foot

Club foot (*talipes equinus*) occurs where the sole of the foot is turned in and the four smaller toes sweep across towards the big toe. If you hold and support your baby in a standing position, the outer edge of the sole will touch the floor first. There are variable degrees of club foot. The mildest, positional talipes, is caused by the baby's position in the womb and corrects itself after birth. More serious club foot is probably caused by muscle imbalances or an underlying nerve disorder. This often runs in families. Overall about one in 300 babies is affected, and it is more common among boys, but very few need surgical treatment. Club foot is not painful. In very rare instances the club foot is due to CEREBRAL PALSY, usually beginning in pregnancy, and will be found with other abnormalities of posture and muscle tone.

If your baby has significant club foot it will cause problems when he tries to stand or walk. He may compensate by walking on the sides of his feet or on the tips of his toes, leading to abnormal patterns of muscle development, and his walking may be clumsy. With appropriate treatment most children who begin life with club foot lead a completely normal life with no limitation to walking, sports or other activities.

Action plan

Most commonly, club foot is mild and corrects itself. Physiotherapy, massage or just gentle stretching advised by a children's physiotherapist or masseur or osteopath can help speed up the process.

If club foot is due to an underlying nerve or muscle imbalance and gentle stretching does not correct the problem, you will need to see a specialist paediatric orthopaedic surgeon (child's bone and joint doctor). Severe club foot is often detected on ultrasound scan in mid-pregnancy enabling planning for specialist treatment after the birth. It does not affect labour.

- Some club foot conditions can be treated successfully with the non-surgical Ponseti

Method. Here, the foot is gently massaged and manipulated to stretch the contracted tissues and achieve nearer-normal alignment of muscle and bone. A plaster cast is applied to maintain the correction. Treatment is best begun in the first week after birth. After approximately seven days, the muscles and ligaments will stretch enough to make further correction possible. The cast is then removed and the foot massaged and manipulated again before reapplying the cast. This is repeated at intervals for approximately six weeks or until adequate correction has been achieved. Many babies who require correction need minor surgery to release their Achilles tendon (tenotomy) before the application of the final plaster cast. This is performed under local anaesthesia with a very thin scalpel. The tendon will heal and reattach within two to three weeks.
- If the club foot is more severe, surgical operations may need to be performed over months or years to achieve the best functional and cosmetic result.
- Botox injection is used in some cases to relax the muscles that cause club foot and so avoid surgery.
- Only if the club foot is part of a very severe condition, usually with other skeletal and spine problems, will a baby have a permanent walking disability.

▇ METATARSUS ADDUCTUS

Metatarsus adductus is another foot problem present at birth. It is just as common as club foot but sometimes overlooked. The foot is often shaped like the letter 'C' with the big toe pointing in and facing the other foot. This is treated by a physiotherapist, orthopaedic surgeon or podiatrist by stretching the foot and then reshaping it using plaster casts.

Cold sores

See Herpes.

Colds

See Coughs and colds, baby; Coughs and colds, mother.

Colic

See also Constipation, baby; Crying; Diarrhoea, baby.

Colic is the term applied by generations of parents to the symptoms of inconsolable crying (or even screaming) and apparent severe tummy pain. It is experienced by many babies at some time in the first six months after birth. If your baby is 'colicky' she may seem very stressed and agitated and be difficult to console. It's common for parents to suspect that something is desperately wrong. Usually, there is no serious underlying problem, yet colic puts pressure on the whole family.

Often an attack begins in late afternoon and continues without a break or in fits and starts through the evening and into the night, but it can appear at any time of day. Colic may prevent your baby and you from sleeping. This can trigger a cycle of colic attacks because sleep deprivation aggravates the situation.

Most colic starts by two months of age, although some babies develop it later, and it can continue for up to three months (hence the term 'three-month colic'). By six months, most colicky babies are more settled. Premature babies may follow the same time scale with symptoms starting after the baby reaches term.

What happens

Colic seems to occur when the muscle wall of the baby's intestine contracts excessively and for prolonged periods. To your baby, it may feel like severe discomfort or the pain of trapped wind. You can recognise the signs if usual efforts at comforting fail and the symptoms recur each day or every few days. Babies with colic often draw up their knees or hold their legs straight and rigid, and the abdomen is usually tense and hard. Colicky babies do not sleep during an attack, and may even wake with the episodes, usually at around the same time each day/night.

A prize awaits the person who discovers the cause and treatment of colic. Little scientific research exists even to guess at the causes or why some treatments work. Each baby is unique. You may notice that, if you are breastfeeding, some foods you eat aggravate your baby; or she gets colic if she does not suck long enough to

benefit from hind milk or swallows air as she feeds (because of a poor position, page 83). If you are bottle-feeding, the problem may be due to an intolerance to the formula milk, unsuitable teats or incorrect positioning during a feed.

Some people believe that colic happens because babies need to get used to digesting; others that it is an emotional reaction to a stressful birth or to stress in the family after birth. Reflux (page 554) and food ALLERGY OR INTOLERANCE can cause discomfort and are commonly mistaken for colic. Sometimes constipation or mild diarrhoea, or both, accompany colic, particularly if a baby has a food intolerance. Constipation or diarrhoea can give symptoms that may be mistaken for colic but disappear once the causes have been treated. Only occasionally colic may be a forerunner of irritable bowel syndrome (page 326) if it is caused by a food intolerance.

Very rarely, a bowel disorder, such as HERNIA, may give colic, but other symptoms are usually more prominent. If your baby has colic but is otherwise thriving, a serious cause is extremely unlikely.

Action plan

Crying and stress brought on by colic can exacerbate it, so wherever possible it will help if you can tackle it, first by eliminating the cause (if known), and then by easing your baby's pain when an attack occurs. If your baby has attacks at a certain time of day there are a number of things you can do about two hours before to ease an attack (although you may not eliminate it). Remember that every baby is different: remedies one family swears by may not suit another. Don't try every remedy at once – take it step by step.

Being with your baby

Spend time with your baby, holding her close, preferably skin to skin. This is the key. Among the many advantages of skin-to-skin contact are regulation of your baby's body rhythms and reduction of stress hormones (which can contribute to tummy pain and digestive sensitivity). You will also grow more finely in tune with her and more effectively meet her needs when they arise. If this helps you establish a more suitable feeding pattern, or eases your baby's anxiety, the results may be stunning.

Keeping contact as your foundation, there are many other things that may help:

- A warm bath may help release tension around your baby's abdomen and bowel. You may bathe together.
- Gentle MASSAGE may help and you can do this at any time while your baby and you are relaxed. Gentle abdominal massage, with pressure no greater than the weight of your own hand, may be soothing. Use gentle clockwise motions. A pure carrier oil (page 36) is useful to ease the sensation and ensure you don't put too much pressure on this sensitive area.
- A gentle leg massage can soothe, finishing with a cycling motion of the legs, which helps the stomach muscles move and puts gentle pressure on the intestines, encouraging the motion of faeces towards the rectum.
- Think about yourself – if you're breastfeeding, might your baby be sensitive to one or more foods you eat? How is your energy? Might your milk supply be dipping in the evening? Try to maintain a regular and nourishing diet. If you rush or miss your lunch, resulting breast milk quality may make your baby irritable at around 5pm.
- Give your baby lots of time playing and lying on her tummy.
- Colicky babies often love to be carried in a position known as 'tiger in the tree'. Lie your baby with her head resting on the crook of your arm and looking outwards, and her body resting along your forearm. You can use your other hand to gently massage her belly.

During an attack

- Stay with your baby. She may be afraid, upset, angry and in pain and needs your support while she has intense feelings. If you need a break, ask another adult to hold and soothe her while you rest.
- Try the classic tiger in the tree position (above). Movement may help her too – in your arms as you walk or while she rests in the pram. Some babies settle in the car but remember that it is best for your baby, when settled, to be lying on her back (rather than in a car seat) and try to avoid using the car as a pacifier too frequently.
- Do not massage during an attack when your baby is screaming.
- Distractions and cuddling and your soothing voice may be comforting.

- A drop of water or cooled mild chamomile tea or water with dill may be calming. If none of these work, try using gripe water, Infacol or Colic Drops. These are over-the-counter preparations that are safe and may be effective.
- Your baby may cry without a break or cry off and on as you try a number of different comforting techniques. She will eventually calm down. Ear plugs may help you cope.

After an attack

Let your baby rest peacefully. She will be exhausted but she may be hungry and need to feed. Having close body contact, preferably skin to skin, will reassure her and may reduce further attacks. You need to rest as well.

Complementary care and feeding tips

- Cranial osteopathy (page 424) and massage are powerful techniques that can release tension in your baby's intestinal wall.
- Try to feed your baby before she gets really hungry and worked up. In the early months she may need frequent feeds throughout the day.
- Take time to feed while you are both relaxed. Check your baby's position. Ensure she eats enough and is winded well. Expressing a little breast milk at the beginning of a feed may reduce air swallowing.
- Changing formula or using different water to make up the milk, or using a different style of bottle or teat, may help. A pre-sterilised bag inserted into the bottle contracts as your baby feeds and can minimise air swallowing.
- Your baby may be sensitive or have an allergy or intolerance to her milk or to what you consume that passes into breast milk. Try identifying problem foods and discuss them with a nutritionist, midwife or health visitor. Food and drinks that produce lots of gas are orange juice, vegetables, especially onions and cabbage, fruit such as apples and plums, spicy food and products with caffeine. Each baby is different and trial and error is the only way forward.
- Cow's milk intolerance is frequently given as the cause. Excluding it from your diet if you are breastfeeding may help. Remember that all artificial milks are based on cow's milk, unless specified. Substituting a goat's-milk-based formula is no longer recommended under one year and soya-based milks are not recommended under six months.

Medical care

If colic is severe, ask your doctor or health visitor for advice and to examine your baby to exclude an underlying reflux or bowel or food intolerance problem. There are prescription and over-the-counter treatments, but no single drug therapy has proved to be consistently successful. If your baby is below six months old, don't give her anything without consulting your doctor.

- Alcohol used to be part of all colic preparations, but this is no longer the case. Other active ingredients are usually sugar, which has been shown to have a pain-relieving effect in babies, and drugs that act on the smooth muscle of the bowel, reducing spasm and relieving pain.
- Alcohol is not recommended for you or your baby. Never give any alcoholic drink, however small, to your baby.
- Gripe water has been around for many years but it is usually not very effective for severe colic.
- Antacid medications sometimes help. Medicines to increase the motility of the bowel may sometimes be recommended but must be taken only on prescription from a doctor.
- Some doctors prescribe preparations such as the tranquilliser promethazine hydrochloride (Phenergan) in prescribed doses.

Homeopathy

Finding the right remedy to alleviate colic may be quite tricky as symptoms are often changeable, yet it is worth persisting. Homeopathy is useful in combination with the suggestions above. In an acute attack, you may use 30c potency every hour for up to three hours, then re-assess and choose the remedy that best suits the new symptoms. With less acute colic, you may give the most appropriate remedy (30c) three times a day, preferably before a feed, for two to three days, and then re-assess.

- *Chamomilla* for a colicky baby who is frantic, irritable, bloated with wind and has a hard abdomen, kicks and draws up her legs, may produce green, watery stools and is only relieved by being carried around or being undressed.
- *Colocynth* if your baby is writhing in pain and draws her legs in to her abdomen, is restless,

shows sudden signs of pain and seems better if she is leaning against something or her abdomen is massaged.
- *Nux Vomica* if you are breastfeeding and have eaten spicy food or drunk a lot of coffee, and your baby is woken by pain and distressed when straining to pass a stool.
- *Dioscorea* when pain is centred around the navel and is better when your baby stretches her legs out and arches her back.
- *Mag Phos* acts like an anti-spasmodic and helps if pain occurs sporadically with great windiness and reduces with warmth, massage and firm pressure.
- *Lycopodium* if pain is worse with pressure around the abdomen and from 4–8pm and perhaps if wind is linked with you eating too much fibre (such as wholewheat, cabbage, beans, etc.)

If you are in any doubt, consult your homeopath.

Caring for yourself

At times you will feel down, tired and anxious. Colic can be very stressful and you may be disappointed that things aren't as rosy or easy as you had hoped. Many parents feel embarrassed and some take the colic attacks as a sign that they are not good enough. Please remember that there are many possible reasons and many are not in your control. Make sure you care for yourself (pages 121–4) and take stock of the way you are there for yourself and for your baby, during the colic attacks and at other times (page 145). Try practical solutions and remember to seek support: if you have existing anxieties or DEPRESSION they may worsen when things are tough.

If you feel at the end of your tether and angry towards your baby, take heart that countless other parents have felt that way. If you feel an urge to hurt your child, it is essential to seek help from your friends, family or your doctor. Babies grow out of colic and the ordeal will come to an end. You may know other parents who have had a colicky baby and can talk about it with the clarity of hindsight – they may have reassuring stories that the colic was simple to reduce, that it didn't last long, and/or that once colicky attacks finish, the peace is miraculous.

Complementary therapies

See also Acupuncture; Aromatherapy; 'Bodymind'; Healing; Herbal medicine; Homeopathy; Massage; Nutritional therapy; Osteopathy; Reflexology.

Complementary therapies recognise 'bodymind' (the union between body and mind) – and treatment is designed to improve both aspects of your wellbeing. Complementary medicine encourages a process of healing that comes from within, aided by the therapist's guidance and treatment. It can also encourage your baby's wellbeing in the womb and enhance the bond between you. Complementary treatments may help to address and relieve your current symptoms and at the same time boost your strength, confidence and enjoyment on your own personal journey. Many ailments may be treated with a complementary approach, and throughout this book there are suggestions where appropriate. Babies and children can benefit from the combination of orthodox and complementary medicine, especially for symptoms that have high nuisance value, such as snuffly nose or recurrent skin rash, but no effective orthodox treatment, or where there are a range of treatment options.

When you visit a complementary therapist he or she will form a picture of you and where you are in your life. The relationship between you and a therapist is often the most influential factor in the success of your treatment. It is important to ensure that any practitioner you visit is qualified and experienced, and you feel safe and supported by that person. The various therapies on offer are increasingly widely researched and monitored, and there are numerous certifications and training programmes available. Ongoing studies and research improve safety and success rates.

▓ INTEGRATED HEALTHCARE

The term 'complementary' means that these therapies work with orthodox medicine to enhance the effectiveness of the treatment you receive from mainstream healthcare workers. They can also provide support in areas such as relaxation and emotional wellbeing.

When to seek medical support

Complementary therapies must be augmented by conventional drug therapy when there is an emergency or when the condition being treated does not respond. It is best to consult a medical practitioner in the following situations:

- If symptoms do not respond to the measures you have tried.
- If symptoms become worse.
- If there is a persistent high fever that reaches or climbs above 38°C (100.4°F) or if there are signs of severe infection, such as pain or pus formation.
- If there are signs of drowsiness, disorientation, confusion or a sudden loss of vision or there is loss of consciousness or fitting.
- If there is a severe headache with neck stiffness and light sensitivity.
- If there are severe pains that persist anywhere in the body.
- If there is severe loss of fluids and dehydration as a result of vomiting and/or diarrhoea.
- If there are respiratory and breathing difficulties.
- If there are signs of a severe allergic reaction.
- If there is excessive bleeding.
- If your baby has a rash.

There is now more freedom to combine complementary care with orthodox medical treatment. This is 'integrated healthcare'. You may, for instance, use homeopathy one day and require an epidural anaesthetic in labour the following day. Many people feel that integration offers the most wholesome support for body, mind and spirit of mother, baby, father and family.

In obstetric and antenatal care, integration is becoming much more widespread. Many midwives and an increasing number of obstetricians, for example, train in therapies such as acupuncture and homeopathy. Pioneering birthing centres offer a holistic integrated approach resting on the safety and technology of modern obstetric care.

Over the centuries there have been many approaches to healthcare. Not every approach suits every person, and often using a mixture of options brings the best results. The number of people using complementary therapies in the UK has risen exponentially this century.

Congenital abnormalities

See also Antenatal tests; Genes and genetics.

Any condition or variation from the normal, however small, that is present from birth is called a 'congenital' (born with) abnormality. These occur in around one in 10 babies and are usually of no significance. Occasionally they may be more serious. Many of the major congenital abnormalities can be cured or significantly improved with treatment but some do result in the baby having a disability. Around two thirds of major abnormalities are suspected or diagnosed during pregnancy, and as antenatal screening becomes more sophisticated, the number is increasing. However, even with the best and most detailed tests some conditions may not be detected. Specific abnormalities are covered separately within this guide.

What happens

Congenital abnormalities may occur because of:
- *Chromosomal abnormality* with a defect in one of the 46 chromosomes that occur in every cell of the body.
- *Gene abnormality* where the chromosomes look normal but one of the genes present on the 46 chromosomes does not function optimally (page 266). Most genetic abnormalities are inherited from one or both parents, but sometimes they occur for the first time in a child as a result of a new genetic mutation.
- *Developmental abnormality*, where there is abnormal formation of the body during

embryonic development. The reason behind abnormal development is often not understood – the process from single cell embryo to multi-billion cell baby is extremely complex.

▦ DEALING WITH A DIAGNOSIS

If your medical team suspects your baby has a congenital abnormality, the range of emotions that follows may be overwhelming, confusing and difficult to cope with. Fortunately, in many cases, further tests prove there is no underlying problem. Medical research is constantly striving to improve the accuracy of prenatal screening tests to minimise the distress caused by false positive results.

Sometimes the diagnosis is confirmed. Parents are often overpowered by feelings such as hopelessness, guilt, anger, pain and denial and there may be a strong sense of grief and loss. These feelings are discussed on page 45, where you will also find suggestions for practical and emotional support.

For some abnormalities that may cause significant problems parents opt for termination of pregnancy. For many anomalies treatment plans can be made to ease a condition or correct it after birth. There are some conditions that cannot be treated and these may not become evident until after birth. Whatever degree of severity, and whatever your social and financial situation, ongoing support and contact with caring professionals, support groups and other families who are similarly affected will be invaluable.

▦ PREVENTING CONGENITAL ABNORMALITIES

The majority of anomalies are not preventable and occur by chance. As molecular biology and pre- and postnatal testing improves, the accuracy of predicting and diagnosing congenital abnormalities becomes more reliable. Now all the genes of the human genome are fully mapped it may be possible to predict in advance of becoming pregnant whether your family is susceptible. In the future, gene therapy could become increasingly available and may even begin before birth.

Action plan

Some abnormalities are preventable:

Nutrition

The importance of optimal nutrition and achieving a balance of vitamins and minerals is discussed on pages 263–5. The best-known benefit is the prevention of neural tube defects (anencephaly and spina bifida) with nutritional supplements containing folic acid, a B vitamin. In addition it is likely that the optimal balance of the other vitamins and minerals may reduce the incidence of other congenital abnormalities.

Medication

A number of medications may cause congenital abnormalities. These include drugs to treat epilepsy, chemotherapy for cancer, some acne treatments and warfarin to thin the blood. If you have a medical problem that requires medication it is best to discuss treatment before conception and to change to the safest medication (page 407).

Alcohol

It is now advised to avoid alcohol throughout pregnancy – there is no safe level (page 190).

Recreational drugs

There are a number of street DRUGS that may cause congenital abnormalities.

Industrial hazards

Workers in some industries exposed to radiation or chemicals may be at increased risk (page 303).

Inherited genetic disorders

There are conditions of a genetic nature that are passed on in families. The best-known are CYSTIC FIBROSIS, sickle cell anaemia and thalassaemia (page 476) and TAY-SACHS DISEASE. If there is a family history then the advice of a genetic counsellor is very helpful to assess the risks. It may be possible to provide diagnosis using IVF before the embryo is implanted in the uterus. During pregnancy or after birth diagnostic tests allow you to plan treatment.

Congenital dislocation of the hip (CDH)

See Hips, congenital dislocation.

Conjunctivitis

See Eye infection and swelling, baby.

Constipation, baby

See also Colic; Poo, baby.

Constipation occurs when stools become firmer and harder and are not passed regularly enough, and the passing of the motion is uncomfortable. There is a wide variation in the frequency of stools among babies. It is normal for a baby to have a bowel movement as often as several times a day, or as seldom as once a week if breastfed. In very rare cases, and only if entirely breastfed, there can be up to two weeks between bowel movements. If your baby is constipated she may be uncomfortable and seem very upset. There may be bloating in her lower abdomen, and you may notice that she strains to pass a stool. Her stools will be harder than normal and she may have colic pains caused by the build-up of faeces and gas and the stretching of the intestine walls. She may cry when she eats, or refuse to eat.

Constipation is rarely a problem for an exclusively breastfed baby. The usual time for constipation to become a problem with BREASTFEEDING is when solids are introduced. It is common among bottle-fed babies as formula milk is less easily digested than breast milk. Most bottle-fed babies need to have daily bowel movements to avoid constipation.

If you think your baby is constipated, look at the possible causes and rest assured that, except in very rare circumstances, it presents no long-term problems.

Emotions

Constipation may cause you and your baby considerable emotional distress: the focus on bowel activities may affect you all. Social taboos and family cultures sometimes lend meaning to frequency and type of bowel movements and you and your partner may have strong views that affect the way you respond to the issue, and how often you talk about it. If you have your own personal anxieties around food, these could influence the situation. Some people see faeces as dirty, which is not the way a baby sees it, and

149

worry that being constipated retains toxins, although this is contrary to the medical view.

Even when small, your baby may pick up on your concerns or stress. It may be helpful to talk to your health visitor or to spend time with a nutritional therapist and consider the family's eating habits, as well as your baby's current constipation. There may be other issues, not associated with food, that are causing stress and might be a contributory factor, since hormones connected with anxiety and stress (page 310) have an effect on the intestines. Sometimes parents believe their baby's constipation reflects inadequate parenting skills. This is one of many possible sources of parental guilt (page 213) and it is seldom appropriate to make the link with you being 'good enough'. It is likely that once the cause of your baby's constipation is clear, small changes will help to relieve the problem. Being there for your baby and helping her in the best way you can is most certainly good enough.

What happens

Food (milk) passes through the small bowel and into the large bowel where much of the liquid is absorbed and the stool becomes firmer. It then travels to the rectum, where it is stored, and is expelled by reflex action. If passage through the large bowel is slow or the food contains little liquid, too much water will be drawn out of the stool, which then becomes hard and is difficult to pass. If passing a motion is difficult or painful, your baby may be reluctant and faeces may build up in the bowel. This can happen even when your baby is very young and pain overrides the expulsion reflex.

Your young baby

Unusual causes of newborn constipation, such as disorders of the digestive system (below), often lead to other symptoms such as vomiting and severe abdominal distension.

Your weaned baby

When you have weaned your baby on to solid food, the frequency of her bowel movements and the consistency and appearance of stools depend on what she eats. Gradually, your baby will develop an awareness of the presence of stools in her rectum and her reflexes diminish, so stools are passed less frequently. If she passes less than

one stool every other day and shows disturbed behaviour, such as drawing up the knees, squirming and crying, and these signs persist, then constipation is becoming a problem.

If your baby has an illness and drinks less than usual, her stools will reduce in frequency and will become harder and more difficult to pass. This temporarily leads to constipation, and usually gets better after the illness has passed and eating habits are back to normal. Occasionally, passing hard motions results in cracks (anal fissures) that are painful and constipation becomes more persistent. ALLERGY or intolerance to milk and other foods, including coeliac disease, may cause constipation. Behaviour concerning the potty is also significant – although a baby cannot control her bowels before the age of one year, if potty use is aggressively encouraged early, babies can become upset and constipated.

Action plan

After the birth your midwife will check to ensure your baby is able to pass stools and there is no obstruction. Later, if you are concerned, your doctor or health visitor can check for constipation. Accumulated faeces in the large bowel can be felt by lightly touching the abdomen. Steps to reduce constipation are usually straightforward.

Milk and fluids

* You can give your baby extra fluids. If you are breastfeeding, give more feeds. If you are BOTTLE-FEEDING, give extra bottles of boiled, cooled water.
* If your baby drinks formula milk, check you are mixing the powder with enough water (page 74). You may talk to your doctor about switching to a different brand.
* If your baby is over six weeks old, soak a handful of prunes in boiled water overnight and give the juice to her, either on a spoon or in a bottle.

Solid foods

* Once your baby is weaned, a good balanced diet (page 557) with variety and sufficient fluid can help prevent constipation. If your baby becomes constipated, take a look at how and what she eats.

- A small increase in fibre will help give the stools bulk and assist their movement through the large bowel. Try porridge and purées made from fruits or vegetables with skins on. Prune purée is good. It is important to avoid wheat bran and granary breads, which may be recommended sources of fibre for adults but in a baby can cause further constipation and colicky pains.
- Cut down on foods that are commonly linked with constipation, such as rice and bananas, and introduce your baby to a variety of vegetables and fruits.
- Be aware of food allergy and intolerance (page 14), especially formula milk protein, and wheat.

Relieving discomfort
- If your baby is relaxed and enjoys it, MASSAGE her abdomen gently (page 145). You can move on to a leg massage, finishing with a cycling motion, which will help the stomach muscles move and puts gentle pressure on the intestines, encouraging the motion of faeces towards the rectum.
- A warm bath with massage may help release tension around the anus and bowel and encourage a stool to pass.
- When you wash your baby's bottom, apply some nappy cream or Vaseline around the outside of the anus – this will help it stretch as a hard stool passes and may prevent painful cracking.
- Do not put anything inside the anus in an attempt to stimulate a bowel movement – it may cause both physical and psychological damage.

Medical care
If the suggestions above are not working, your doctor may encourage you to pay close attention to your baby's diet and fluid intake. If the doctor believes the condition may respond to treatment he or she may recommend some of the following, all of which are regularly used in babies of three months and older.
- Usual treatments are by mouth, such as: lactulose, to soften the motions, and senokot or specially prepared syrup of figs or prune juice, to stimulate the bowel to empty. Senokot syrup is only available on prescription (granules and tablets are not suitable for young children). Usually a combination of softeners and stimulants is required.

- In general, the less attention you and others place on your baby's motions and on her anus, the better. This is because excessive focus on this usually aggravates anxiety. It might even start a process of association that may lead to phobia and anal fixation complexes. If your doctor examines your baby's anus, let your baby know in advance and talk to her and reassure her during the process.
- Rarely, suppositories such as glycerine are used, although for a very constipated baby there may be no other option, at least at the start of treatment.
- Very infrequently, enemas may be useful if other treatments are not working.

Homeopathy
As well as looking at possible underlying causes such as allergy or intolerance, the following remedies may be useful when constipation is not an ongoing problem. Consult your homeopath who may advise giving the most appropriate remedy (30c potency) three times per day for two to three days and then re-assess. For persistent constipation it is best to seek advice for constitutional treatment from your homeopath.
- *Alumina* if there is difficulty even though stools are soft, your baby may be lethargic and feels better passing a stool upright. It is useful if your baby has just started formula milk.
- *Nux Vomica* for a tense and irritable baby who has a persistent urge to pass a stool but does not produce or passes only very small amounts.
- *Bryonia* for a baby who is very thirsty, doesn't pass a stool and has no urge to, and finally produces a hard, dry and dark stool with difficulty.
- *Silica* if stools are partly expelled then slip back again, there is stomach cramping, and slow weight gain may be a constitutional feature.

Possible associated problems
If your baby appears to be constipated and is not gaining weight or shows any other unusual symptoms such as a distended abdomen or vomiting, seek the advice of a doctor. The bowel may be blocked and obstructed.

Chronic constipation
This is constipation that lasts for more than three months in older babies, with or without episodes of what is called spurious DIARRHOEA

(spurious because the underlying problem is constipation). The diarrhoea results because the large bowel does not absorb water from the liquid stools entering from the small bowel. Firm hard motions remain in the large bowel, causing constipation. This may result in overfilling of the large bowel, which leads occasionally to dilation or lengthening of the large bowel. This is called megacolon, and as a result emptying of the bowel is difficult. However this is all reversible with expert treatment and advice. Once the constipated child or adult has developed the complication of megacolon the treatment required to deal with the problem is long term, over two or three years in some instances of severe constipation.

Cystic fibrosis

This genetic disorder is a rare cause of constipation and bowel obstruction in the newborn period. The constipation is due to thick and sticky stools, a condition called meconium ileus. Usually this can be treated by special enemas to clear out the thick motion but CYSTIC FIBROSIS itself is a long-term problem for affected children.

Food intolerance and coeliac disease

These more commonly occur in older babies after weaning. In a younger baby, constipation may be one of the symptoms of cow's milk allergy (page 19) and most formula feeds are based on cow's milk.

Hirschsprung disease

This rare condition affects about one in 4,500 babies and arises when the nerve supply to the bowel does not develop normally. It is diagnosed by a barium enema X-ray and a biopsy (tissue sample) of the bowel. The condition is suspected if no motion is passed within 72 hours of birth, or there is passage of a hard pellet of meconium, called a meconium plug. An operation may be needed to remove the affected piece of bowel. In breastfed infants the motions are very soft and the operation may sometimes be put off for months.

Obstructions

These are rare and are most often diagnosed when there is vomiting (often bile stained) associated with abdominal distension and constipation. In this case, a baby may become ill and needs urgent diagnosis and treatment. Some obstructions may be detected during pregnancy ultrasound scans. Obstruction may arise from intestinal atresia (narrowing and blockage of the intestine); intestinal malrotation, where the bowel twists and surgical treatment relieves the blockage; or intussusception, where the bowel folds in on itself and there is also diarrhoea and bleeding (page 61). Rarely, the passage of motions is obstructed by an imperforate anus, where the rectum and anus are narrowed or not correctly linked to the intestine. This is diagnosed by examining the anus and needs surgical treatment.

Constipation, mother

Constipation is a relatively common problem in pregnancy. Whether you are constipated depends in part on the normal frequency of your bowel movements and whether the problem is affecting your quality of life. Many people think it's necessary to go to the toilet at least once a day. Yet the range among healthy people is much wider – between three visits a day and once every three days. Constipation usually involves passing unusually hard stools or inability to pass stools for many days.

If you feel constipated you may be reassured by a visit to your doctor, who will want to rule out other possible causes. For example, if constipation is accompanied by symptoms such as abdominal bloating or pain, or alternates with DIARRHOEA, you may have symptoms of an IRRITABLE BOWEL. If you are reluctant to pass stools because of pain or bleeding there is a chance that you could have PILES or an anal fissure.

After the birth, as your hormones change, constipation may disappear, particularly if you have made beneficial changes to your diet.

What happens

Some pregnancy hormones relax the smooth muscle in the wall of the intestine, reducing muscle tone and slowing activity throughout the bowel. This may bring on atonic constipation (related to muscle tone).

The other common type of constipation is spastic constipation, where the muscles go into spasm. This may be due to:

- Feeling anxious or stressed. Stress hormones may cause the wall of your intestine to go into spasm, which impedes bowel movement. In addition, stress may cause you to change your eating and drinking patterns.
- Intolerance or allergy after eating certain foods (often wheat and dairy).
- Excessive SMOKING.
- Over use of laxatives – even in the past – may have affected your colon so that it relies on this stimulation to contract.
- Spastic constipation may alternate with diarrhoea as part of irritable bowel syndrome.

After birth, a temporary feeling of constipation is common. Many women are nervous about opening their bowels when the general area is sore. There is no danger of causing damage to – or of breaking – stitches, however, and once you have passed the first stool you will feel relieved. It is completely normal to wait for up to three days after birth before visiting the toilet.

Action plan

You can usually treat and prevent constipation by following a diet that is high in fibre (roughage) and ensuring you drink plenty of fluids. Follow the nutritional advice set out on page 253 to give your body the fuel, minerals, vitamins and fibre it needs for your digestive system to work well. In addition, some of the suggestions below may help you.

Water

Drink at least 2 litres (4 pints) of water a day to ease your bowel movements by keeping stools soft. Try chamomile, lemon balm, peppermint and ginger teas, but don't drink too much after 6 or 7pm to avoid night-time visits to the loo.

Fibre

Fibre is the part of foods of plant origin that the body cannot digest. It readily absorbs water to bulk out waste matter and so assist its passage through the lower bowel. If digested food is not moved along quickly enough, your bowel will reabsorb fluid, making the stool hard and compacted and more difficult to expel.

- Begin with a gradual increase in fibre, perhaps a bowl of oats a day, or a handful of seeds (such as linseeds), or some extra raw or steamed vegetables.
- You may want to cut down on wheat, or change from white bread and pasta to wholemeal, which has a higher fibre content. Note that bran is derived from wheat and it may increase constipation if you are intolerant. This includes wheat-based bran breakfast cereals. Some people choose to stop wheat completely and instead opt for rice, millet or oats.
- Your digestion may take two or three weeks to adjust to the increase in fibre and you may experience abdominal cramps or excessive flatulence in the meantime. Try cutting back on the amount of fibre in your diet and then gradually increasing it until you find the optimum level for you.

Laxatives

Laxatives encourage the passing of stools. It is preferable to avoid laxative drugs and enemas that stimulate the bowel wall in pregnancy, unless your doctor has prescribed them for you.

- Whole linseeds are safe and effective. Try 1 tablespoon sprinkled into food or added to a glass of warm water once or twice a day. It may take two weeks for you to feel the effect.
- Thyme added to your cooking could also improve digestion.
- An alternative is a bulk laxative, such as lactulose, which works like bran by absorbing water into the stool and increasing bulk and intestinal movement. It is available without prescription and can be safely taken twice a day.

Watching for allergy and intolerance

You might want to note your reactions to what you eat and avoid any foods linked with allergy or intolerance.

- Note that if you are wheat intolerant, extra bran may make the constipation worse.
- Intolerance to milk (lactose intolerance) is common (page 20).

Supplements and iron

- It may help to change your iron supplement to an elemental iron preparation for easier absorption.
- Reduce your intake to one tablet every one or two days. Take iron one hour before a high-fibre

meal with a glass of juice or vitamin C supplement as this aids absorption.

Homeopathy
You may take the appropriate remedy (30c potency) three times per day for three days and then re-assess:

- *Nux Vomica* if you have a persistent urge to pass a stool though none is produced, have fullness in the rectum, feel stressed and have persistent dull headaches.
- *Bryonia* for constipation with no urge to pass a stool, when stools are hard, dry and dark, you feel irritable, and worse in warm stuffy environments, and very thirsty.
- *Sepia* if you have shooting pains up the rectum with lots of straining, pass large, hard stools and feel full and heavy in the abdomen with a dragging sensation.
- *Lycopodium* if you feel bloated and flatulent, strain to pass hard stools yet feel you have not emptied your bowels, cannot bear tight clothes and the constipation may be a result of feeling emotionally upset or away from home.
- *Alumina* when it is difficult to pass even soft stools, you need to strain, there is cutting pain and even bleeding; you feel better for eating a high-fibre diet and warm food and drink.

Exercise and aromatherapy
- In most cases, exercise and yoga stretches aid digestion and encourage circulation, stimulating bowel movements. Try walking, swimming or any other activity that is safe during pregnancy.
- Massage your abdomen in a clockwise direction. From Week 24 it is safe to use an oil containing lemon and black pepper.

Contraception

Your fertility will return after birth and although breastfeeding can have the effect of reducing or completely suppressing ovulation it is not a failsafe mechanism for avoiding pregnancy. Many women who do not breastfeed are surprised when they become pregnant within weeks of birth. Sometimes the surprise comes even when the previous conception was assisted medically. Unless you're hoping to become pregnant right away, you need a reliable method of birth control – even if you are breastfeeding.

Your postnatal check is a good time to ask your doctor about the options or your local family health clinic can advise you.

The following are the principal methods of contraception currently available.

Barrier methods
- Condoms (plus spermicide) can be highly effective but unless you are meticulous in your technique this method can fail. The condom must be worn before penetration and the man must withdraw as soon as possible after ejaculation, before he loses his erection. After the birth, if your vagina is sensitive, the condom can be uncomfortable and the spermicide might cause irritation. Some couples believe that pausing to put on a condom can take some of the spontaneity out of lovemaking.
- Diaphragm and spermicide, like condoms, can affect the spontaneity of lovemaking, although it can be in place earlier and left for longer. If you have used one before you may need to be refitted for a bigger size after birth.
- IUS (intra-uterine system) with hormones is highly effective. It can be inserted at your postnatal check, from six weeks after the birth. The hormonal release reduces your womb's receptivity to a fertilised egg. A benefit is reduced menstrual pain and bleeding. Possible disadvantages include irregular bleeding that can take weeks to settle, cessation of periods, lethargic mood and discomfort on insertion. Some types can be left in for five years.
- IUD (coil) without hormones is only slightly less effective than the hormonal form. For some women it increases the duration of bleeding and pain with periods, and increases the risk of infection and ectopic pregnancy (page 202).

The contraceptive pill and other hormonal methods
- There are two main types of contraceptive pill – combined oestrogen and progesterone and progesterone-only. While you're breastfeeding, use the progesterone-only pill. Oestrogen in the combined pill reduces milk flow. You can begin the combined pill after feeding stops. It is worth discussing the pros and cons with your doctor and seeing what suits you, as each woman's physical and emotional reaction to the extra hormones is unique.

- Implants and injections. Depot progesterone is inserted under the skin or injected into a muscle where it is released slowly over three months, to suppress ovulation. This method may be preferred by those who worry they might forget to take the pill. Side effects include irregular periods and this may last for months after the contraceptive effect is said to wear off. It may cause weight gain and premenstrual symptoms.

Other methods
- Natural birth control (also known as the rhythm method) involves learning to recognise the signs that indicate the days when you can conceive and avoiding penetrative sex then or using barrier contraception. This method can be very effective but requires practice and, ideally, guidance. You will need several menstrual cycles to pass to be sure of your own unique pattern, and it is possible to conceive before your first period after the birth.
- Sterilisation (vasectomy for men and tubal ligation for women) should be regarded as a permanent choice to stop fertility and you will need to discuss this option carefully.

Pregnancy with a coil in place
Although the protection of a copper-containing coil (IUD) is high, roughly 3 per cent of coil users do become pregnant. When this happens, the coil is usually not removed and pregnancy usually progresses without problems, but there is a higher chance of an ectopic pregnancy, or a miscarriage. It is important to have an early ultrasound scan at six to eight weeks to confirm all is well. There is also a higher chance of bleeding from irritation by the coil in the first half of pregnancy, but this usually settles down.

Provided there is not an ectopic pregnancy or a miscarriage, a coil does not present a risk to your baby's development, nor can it pierce the amniotic sac. Unusually, if the string is visible, a coil may be removed after week eight because some doctors believe this reduces infection entering the uterus. It is much more common for the coil to be left in place. After your baby is born the coil will be born with the placenta.

The newer progesterone IUS (opposite) has a very low pregnancy rate of under one in 1,000. There is currently no data indicating a possible effect of progesterone on a developing baby. If you conceive using IUS, consult your doctor for advice.

Cordocentesis

See Amniocentesis and CVS.

Coughs and colds, baby

See also Asthma and wheezing, baby; Blocked nose, baby.

Coughing is a protective reflex designed to stop milk, mucus and other fluids from entering the airway. It is also the mechanism for expelling excess mucus or fluid. A cough is an extremely common symptom. It is usually caused by – or follows – a viral infection or cold, which a baby gets on average seven times a year. For some children a runny nose may last all winter. Some children produce a lot of catarrh and others have a persistent cough, particularly at night. If your baby shows these symptoms but seems happy, do not worry. Most coughs and colds are self-limiting. Only if your baby has BREATHING DIFFICULTIES or a very high FEVER do you need to call for urgent attention.

What happens
The cough reflex clears the air passages of the excess mucus which the lining of the lungs produces to clear an infection, and keeps the passages clear to allow oxygen into the lungs. Coughs and colds may bring on one or more symptoms:
- A runny nose, or a blocked nose.
- A dry cough, that does not produce sputum (mucus from the lungs and saliva).
- A wet cough, producing sputum.
- When the airways are blocked or inflamed, a baby younger than 12 months will breathe more quickly because before this age he cannot breathe more deeply.
- Your baby may become upset, and may be more tired and irritable than normal if the cough or a blocked nose is disrupting his sleep.
- Your baby may go off his food.
- Her breathing may be a little noisy.
- Continuous coughing may trigger vomiting.
- Green, brown or bloody sputum is usually caused by an infection.

155

■ CAUSES

The majority of coughs and colds in babies are caused by a virus. These infections are self-limiting and are fought off by the baby's own immune system. Usually viral infections pass in three to four days and any fever tends to resolve within 36 hours. Antibiotics will not clear a viral infection but will usually treat a bacterial infection, especially one that sets in following a cold or flu. It is not always easy to tell a viral from a bacterial infection. Other causes of coughs include asthma and reflux.

Viral infection

Although all babies get viral infections, some are more susceptible than others. The most significant factor that determines this is a baby's immune system. The antibodies your baby receives from you in pregnancy disappear after four months. After birth he begins to build up his own antibodies and his immune system matures in response to the antibodies passed to him in your breast milk and the infectious organisms he encounters in the environment.

Babies born prematurely are generally more prone to viral infection, possibly because their immune system is immature. In addition, they are less likely to be breastfed. Regular exposure to viruses is also an important aspect. Babies cared for in a large group or with older children have more frequent coughs and colds. Babies who are undernourished, for example because they have a chronic illness, are also more susceptible to infection. Passive SMOKING can increase both the incidence of viral infections and their severity because it makes the immune system less effective.

Viral infections include:
* The common cold.
* Bronchiolitis (page 107).
* Croup (page 164).
* Pneumonia (page 446).

Bacterial infection

Bacteria are one possible cause of respiratory infections. They may complicate a viral illness because the virus weakens the body's immune system and airborne bacteria can then more easily invade the lining of the airway. Bacterial infections tend to follow a viral infection and can cause persistent fever and listlessness, poor feeding, rapid breathing and a wet or moist-sounding cough. At this stage, medical advice and antibiotics are needed. Bacterial infections include the now uncommon pertussis (page 568).

Asthma

Asthma is characterised by wheezing and coughing. The small airways, the bronchioles, are inflamed and narrow and also produce excess mucus. As a result, the air passages become constricted, causing the characteristic wheezing sound of asthma during breathing. The cough is usually worse at night. It may occur without a preceding cold and may last for weeks. The symptoms are usually triggered by a viral infection of the lungs but for a few children an allergy can trigger the same symptoms. Asthma is covered in more detail on page 36.

Reflux

Coughing may be a symptom of reflux (page 554), where your baby's stomach contents flow back up into the oesophagus involuntarily, and this stimulates the cough reflex to prevent the stomach contents entering the lungs. Coughs and colds temporarily worsen the reflux but some coughs are due to reflux alone, in which case treating reflux may eliminate the coughing altogether.

Immune deficiency states

Immune deficiency states are very rare, and diagnosed after frequent and severe infections, usually with protracted DIARRHOEA and failure to thrive (page 559). The very small number of babies who have an immune system deficiency may benefit from long-term use of antibiotics under supervision of a specialist paediatrician. The genetic disease CYSTIC FIBROSIS can also cause coughing, but usually there are other clues, such as poor weight gain, diarrhoea and recurrent respiratory infections.

Treatment and care

The key to treating a cough or cold and relieving your baby's symptoms is to treat the cause. Possible causes are outlined below.

+ Red flag

An indication that the cough may be part of a more serious problem, perhaps bronchiolitis infection (page 107), is that your child may not be able to drink his normal amount of milk, or pulls off your breast increasingly. If your baby refuses milk for two or more consecutive feeds it is best to ask for professional advice.

Take your baby to your doctor or local children's emergency department immediately if any of the following occur:

- Rapid, wheezy or laboured breathing, blue lips, grunting while breathing, inability to feed or talk.
- Fever (above 39.5°C/99.5°F over eight weeks of age or 38 °C/100.4°F below eight weeks).
- Coughing to the point of vomiting, inability to sleep due to persistent cough, coughing up blood.
- Excessive sleepiness, refusal to eat or drink, drooling with difficulty swallowing.

See your doctor if your baby remains feverish or stops feeding for more than 24 hours, or appears lethargic and more sleepy than usual or if a cough or wheeze persists for longer than five days.

Making your baby comfortable

- Continue feeding to give your baby comfort and nutrition. You may need to feed little and often, particularly if your baby has a blocked nose.
- He may breathe more easily if you dissolve a drop of eucalyptus/albus oil in some hot water or a vaporiser and place it in the room at night. Before three months, use vapour rub on his vest rather than on his skin. Humidifiers and vaporisers increase humidity in the air. This may soften the mucus and help clear a cough and is particularly useful if your baby has sensitive (irritable) airways following a viral infection. Cold-mist vaporisers give off cool air and avoid the risk of scalding with hot water.
- To reduce night coughing prop the head of your baby's cot up at night by 5cm (2in). This will help mucus drain away from the nasal passages. During the day, your baby may prefer to be upright – a papoose or sling could make this easier.
- Outdoors cold air can trigger coughing if the airways are sensitive. This is not harmful but can be upsetting for your baby. Being outside is preferable to being cooped up indoors, so wrap your baby up well when you go out.

Medical care

- If your baby has a fever or raised temperature give the treatments described on page 240. Paracetamol suspension in the right dosage for a baby (page 429) helps to reduce temperature and relieve pain. Keep your baby cool to help lower his temperature.
- The cough is useful to clear infection so don't give your baby cough mixture (cough suppressant) unless directed by a doctor or other relevant healthcare worker or your baby is unable to sleep because of coughing, or is coughing to the point of vomiting.
- Nasal decongestants may help. The best drops are salt water or saline drops, available over the counter or on prescription. These moisten and release mucus blockage and reduce swelling. Do not make them up yourself as the concentration of salt must be exact.
- Decongestant drops containing medication to shrink the lining of the nasal passages must be obtained on prescription from your doctor. They are only suitable for babies aged over six to nine months. They are used for a maximum of two days because of the increased risk of swelling if used for longer. If your baby has a blocked nose lasting months, your GP or an ear-nose-and-throat specialist may consider a short course of corticosteroid decongestants.
- The vast majority of colds are viral and will not respond to antibiotics. However, a cough can sometimes be caused by an opportunistic bacterial infection, in which case a prescribed antibiotic is likely to bring rapid improvement.

• Treatments for the individual infections are covered in the following entries.

Massage and aromatherapy

In addition to any other treatments your baby is receiving, you can ease congestion with MASSAGE. Only try these techniques when your baby is calm and for a few minutes. If your baby starts to cry, stop immediately.

• Facial massage. Rest your baby on your thighs, facing you as you sit with your knees raised. Press gently with one finger of each hand and trace the outline of the cheek bones from the top of the nose, down the sides, downwards and outwards. This helps to open the nostrils. Practise on yourself first until you have mastered the technique.

• Chest massage. Lie your baby on his back across your knees, with the head and trunk leaning back over the side of your lap. Pat the centre of his chest lightly with cupped hands. You can use a massage oil scented with lavender, myrrh and frankincense. After massaging the chest, turn your baby over so that he lies across your lap on his belly, and gently pat his back with your cupped hands. This helps to expel mucus by compressing the lungs and bronchial tubes. If your baby is very congested, he may vomit.

• Aromatherapy oils can help your baby's breathing when they are heated in oil so their scent fills the room. Try eucalyptus citrodora, eucalyptus radiata, pine and lavender.

Homeopathy

Mainstream medicine may be effective in offering superficial relief (for example, pain relief or cough suppressants), but responding to the underlying causes and body constitution that may make a cough or cold linger or make an individual baby particularly susceptible may require other approaches. Homeopathy plays an important role here. There is a wide range of homeopathic remedies that suit coughs and colds. Some work very quickly and over time you will learn which remedies your baby responds to well. One of the great advantages of using homeopathy for colds is that when treatment starts early – as soon as you suspect your baby is becoming unwell – it may greatly reduce the severity and duration of the illness. If you are in any doubt, consult your homeopath.

Colds

You may give the most appropriate remedy (30c potency) three to four times a day for a few days and then re-assess. If your baby has recurrent colds, constitutional treatment under the care of a fully qualified homeopath would be most beneficial.

• *Aconite* is the remedy of first resort for a cold that starts suddenly. Given promptly, it may shorten the illness. Also good for a cold that develops after exposure to dry, cold, windy weather, is worse at night, with lots of sneezing, and perhaps a dry croupy cough, possibly a fever, restlessness and anxiety. *Aconite* works best in the early stages of a cold. After 24 hours the pattern of symptoms may have changed, requiring one of the following remedies:

• *Arsenicum* for colds that appear gradually and then affect the chest, leading to wheezing, with a watery acrid nasal discharge that reddens the skin, making your baby thirsty for sips and worse at night. There may be accompanying DIARRHOEA, anxiety and chilliness.

• *Natrum Mur* for recurrent colds or colds that follow emotional upset in the family (such as bereavement), with lots of sneezing in the morning, watery eyes, dry cracked lips, and profuse, watery nasal discharge that becomes thick and white.

• *Pulsatilla* for sniffles in the newborn accompanied by a lot of crying, and for recurrent colds or end stages of a cold with thick yellow–green mucus (often from the left nostril) with symptoms worse from lying down. There may be some clinginess and whining and, significantly, no thirst.

• *Euphrasia* for colds with accompanying eye symptoms, streaming from the eyes with tears that seem to sting, swollen eyes sensitive to light, nasal discharge that is bland and profuse, but non-irritating, and there may be an accompanying cough.

• For colds that linger with thick persistent mucus you may try a combination remedy to alleviate congestion and drain the mucus: *KaliBich*, *Pulsatilla* and *Hydrastis* in a low 6c potency given twice a day for up to one week.

Coughs

There are numerous remedies that can be used and subtle differences between them, so it is important to be observant. You may give the most appropriate remedy in 30c potency three times per day for two to three days and then re-assess. Your baby's pattern of symptoms may change several times in the case of a lingering cough. If your baby has recurrent coughs, constitutional treatment (taking a remedy over a longer term to address underlying susceptibility) under the care of a homeopath would be preferable.

Dry coughs:
* *Aconite* for a dry, irritating, croupy cough with sudden onset, when there is anxiety and restlessness and your baby is woken by the coughing. The condition is much worse at night.
* *Arsenicum* for coughing that's worse around midnight and in the early hours, with a dry wheezy cough, intense restlessness and anxiety, perhaps with diarrhoea. The baby may feel better for sipping at intervals and for being upright.
* *Ferrum Phos* when symptoms aren't intense and a cough follows a cold, is worse after eating and first thing in the morning, dry, hacking and hoarse, and lingering.
* *Spongia* for a barking, croupy cough with hoarseness that may wake your baby in a panic in the earlier part of the night and your baby feels better if coughing in an upright position. *Spongia* helps to open the bronchioles.
* *Phosphorous* for a dry, hard, ticklish cough that's worse for lying down but your baby still seems happy, sociable and retains a good appetite.

Loose, productive coughs:
* *Pulsatilla* for a cough that is loose in the morning and throughout the day, but tends to become much tighter in the evening and at night, is productive with lots of thick yellow–green mucus, worse from lying down and in a warm stuffy environment and where there is little thirst but your baby is weepy, clingy and miserable.
* *Hepar Sulph* for a loose, deep rattly cough accompanied by thick yellow mucus, the baby tends to sound croupy and croaky at night and his mood is irritable.
* *Antimonium Tart* for a loose rattling cough when it's difficult to cough up mucus, the baby is better for sitting up but may be drowsy, weak and sweaty with a slightly blue tinge around his mouth.

Spasmodic coughs:
* *Drosera* helps a violent, tickly cough that often comes in bouts, ending in retching, choking, even vomiting, it is worse after midnight and the early hours and after lying down and eating or drinking.

Croup
There are some specific remedies that can bring a rapid response for babies and children with croup (page 164).

▓ PREVENTION
There is, unfortunately, no way you can guarantee that your baby will not catch a minor cold. You may be able to strengthen your baby's immunity though, which may help avoid some infections and hasten recovery.
* Breastfeeding strengthens your baby's immune system.
* The feeling of being loved, safe and content also helps to heighten your baby's immunity.
* Homeopathy can be effective (page 305), with a constitutional remedy (that strengthens your baby's constitution and addresses any underlying susceptibilities) suggested by a registered homeopath.
* ACUPUNCTURE and HERBAL MEDICINE prescribed from a qualified practitioner can help, too.
* Avoid exposing your baby to cigarette smoke, which irritates the airways and weakens the immune system response.
* If environmental pollution is an issue, reducing your baby's exposure may help.
* Many traditional ideas that pass down from generation to generation have not been scientifically confirmed but it doesn't mean they are wrong. While vulnerability to infection is not influenced by cold winds, draughts, too little clothing, going to bed with wet hair or wearing too many clothes, for a baby who is susceptible these may be significant.
* Stuffy rooms and poor air circulation may contribute, particularly if you and your baby are in contact with an infected person. Fresh air is good for your baby as long as he is warm enough.
* If your baby has an ALLERGY, breastfeeding and reducing contact with known allergens will reduce the risk of asthma.
* Echinacea in herbal form is a tonic used by adults. It is not suitable for children under the age of three years.

Coughs and colds, mother

See also Asthma, mother; Breathlessness, mother.

During pregnancy you are providing oxygen both for yourself and your baby and, like every woman, you will unconsciously alter the way you breathe. As pregnancy advances and your uterus grows, your lung capacity is reduced. Sometimes this extra challenge for the respiratory system leads to breathlessness and increases susceptibility to coughs and colds, and chest infections such as bronchitis, or means that a minor chest infection lingers. It can also worsen symptoms in asthma sufferers.

What happens

A chest infection may begin as a common cold, usually caused by a virus picked up through close contact. It might linger because you cannot breathe so deeply, particularly in late pregnancy, and coughing will be less effective in clearing your chest. Infection may increase the sensitivity of the lining of your respiratory tract and deep breathing may irritate it, causing coughing. This 'irritable airway' may continue for weeks. If you get a chest infection and also suffer from asthma there is no risk to your baby unless your asthma becomes very severe. Intense coughing may lead to pain in the muscles between your ribs or on your abdomen. Occasionally, sinusitis develops following a cold. This is an infection of the mucus membranes lining the sinuses, and typically causes pain around the eyes and the front of the head.

Action plan

If you catch a cold or have an irritating cough, the priority is to look after yourself.

Medical care
- Antibiotics do not treat viral illness and the majority of coughs/colds are viral. However, antibiotics may be given to treat a secondary bacterial infection, which is common following a viral illness such as cold or flu. Many are safe during pregnancy.
- If you wish to take painkillers you can use paracetamol in moderation (dosage recommendations are on page 408). Remember that cold and flu remedy drinks powders contain paracetamol, so take care not to overdose.
- You can safely take proprietary over-the-counter cough remedies in the second half of pregnancy, in moderation. Many contain paracetamol or aspirin so be sure not to take too much. Codeine linctus is also safe, in moderation, up to four times a day.
- If you have a long-standing cough and irritable airways your doctor may advise a combination of antibiotics, antispasmodics and steroids to reduce the cough, clear the infection and reduce related asthma. You may be able to reduce the discomfort of coughing by inhaling an infusion of eucalyptus or with physiotherapy.
- If you have a persistent cough that does not respond to treatment, a chest X-ray taken while your baby is screened with a lead apron can check for underlying causes, such as tuberculosis, which is very rare. It is uncommon to need an X-ray during pregnancy, however.

Lifestyle and diet
- Drink plenty of water to avoid dehydration and prevent mucus congestion. Keep up your daily intake of vitamins and minerals. If you are taking vitamin C to combat colds, don't exceed 3 g (3,000 mg) per day.
- Hot water with a dash of lemon and honey may help. Honey soothes the throat and lemon fights infection. Garlic and onions, cooked or raw, are known for their decongestant properties. Eat fresh vegetables – raw or steamed, preferably with their skins on – and citrus fruits.
- When you feel up to it, aerobic exercise, perhaps a brisk walk, encourages deeper breathing and will help to clear your airways. Walking in the fresh air is particularly useful if your sinuses are blocked.
- Rest helps your body recuperate.
- If you smoke try to give up – it increases the risk of chest infection.
- Inhalation of steam may help to clear your chest. Lean over a basin of hot water and drape a towel over your head. Alternatively run a hot shower in a small bathroom.
- Some YOGA postures help to open the chest and give the lungs more room to breathe, and may relieve discomfort.

Aromatherapy and homeopathy

- You can use an oil in conjunction with steam, or in your bath or with MASSAGE (head massages can really help). Lemon is beneficial at any time, and after Week 24 you can try eucalyptus (particularly good for clearing stuffiness), tea tree, lavender or chamomile.
- Homeopathy may be very effective and address subtle differences in symptoms. The suggestions for your baby's coughs and colds (page 158) may apply to you as well. Alternatively, you may try the most appropriate of the following remedies (30c), three times per day for two days and then re-assess. Continue if the symptoms are improving. If your symptoms change, switch to the most appropriate remedy and re-assess after two days.

Colds

- *Bryonia* for colds that progress gradually, with dry lips, skin, throat and constant thirst and you feel irritable and prefer to be quiet and left alone. It is also for colds that linger in the nose, affecting the head and throat, and then travel quickly down to the chest.
- *Allium Cepa* for a streaming cold, profuse, watery nasal discharge that burns the nose and top lip, streaming watery eyes with bland, non-irritating tears, lots of sneezing and a tickling cough. Conditions may be worse when lying down and being in a warm room and improve in fresh air.
- *Hepar Sulph* for well-established colds with thick yellow mucus. Glands may be swollen with a sore throat and you may feel very chilly and over-sensitive. Temperamentally, you may feel irritable, impatient and snappy, worse at night from any physical exertion, and better from wrapping up warmly.
- *Nux Vomica* for colds brought on by over-work, lack of sleep or over-indulging. Characteristically, the nose runs during the day but is completely blocked at night, there is lots of sneezing and an inability to get warm. Your mood may be irritable, impatient, driven and touchy.
- *Nat Mur* for colds in which a continual streaming, runny nose alternates with blockage and congestion. Nasal discharge is either clear or like thick egg white, there is profuse sneezing with watery eyes, and a feeling of dryness, particularly of the lips. It is often accompanied by cold sores. You may feel worse as a result of

loud noise, having to make an effort or sympathy, and better from fresh air and being quiet and private.

Dry Coughs

- *Bryonia* for a dry, irritating cough, usually triggered by a tickle in the throat, coughing with a splitting headache and stitch-like pains in the chest. Breathing in deeply may lead to further coughing, made worse by bending forward and movement. It may be improved by remaining still and applying pressure to the chest.
- *Causticum* for a dry, burning, hollow cough with pain felt all the way down the throat into the chest. Mucus may feel embedded in the chest so that you can't cough it up. You may feel worse for lying down and better for sips of cold water.

Loose productive coughs

- *Ipecac* for a loose, rattling cough, often accompanied by nausea, a sensation of congestion and mucus in the chest. It is worse from extreme temperatures and better in the fresh air and while resting.

Spasmodic coughs

- *Ignatia* for a tickling, hollow, spasmodic cough. You may find the more you cough the more you need to cough. There may be a lump in your throat, accompanied by sighing. It may be made worse by yawning, emotional events and the cold, and better by warmth and eating.

Sinusitis

For recurrent or chronic sinusitis it is always advisable to see a qualified homeopath who will work with you to strengthen your constitution. For a sudden attack, you may take the most appropriate of the following remedies (30c potency) four times per day for two days and then re-assess. Either continue with the same remedy three times per day if you feel you are making good progress or you may try another remedy if it better reflects your new symptoms.

Kali Bich (Number 1 remedy) for sinusitis after a cold with thick, stringy mucus – usually yellow–green – when there is pressure and congestion, particularly at the bridge of the nose and under the cheek bones, pain in spots over the eyebrows, loss of smell with violent sneezing, you feel worse when bending forward, after sleeping and from cold weather, and better from warmth and pressure to the affected area.

Hepar Sulph for sinusitis with thick yellow–green mucus that smells, you are sneezing, your nose is very congested, there is aching at the root of your nose and your face feels sore and achey even when lightly touched, your mood is decidedly irritable and snappy, and you feel worse for cold, at night and from touch, and better for warmth and wrapping up.

Mercurius for sinusitis with thick yellow–green mucus that is offensive, your mouth feels coated and your breath smells, you have a metallic taste in your mouth, pain extends from sinuses to teeth, nosebleeds may occur at night, you may have swollen glands, feel chilly, sweaty and drained, and feel worse at night and from temperature changes.

Pulsatilla for sinusitis that follows a lingering cold, when nasal congestion is worse at night followed by a runny nose in the morning, pain is felt in the sinuses, you want company and sympathy, and feel worse from a hot stuffy environment and better for fresh air.

Hydrastis for sinusitis with a watery, burning discharge that becomes a thicker white/yellow, there is a sensation of a constant drip and constant blowing of the nose, severe frontal sinus headache, and you feel worse from cold, windy weather and better from rest and pressure.

Counselling and psychotherapy

See also Emotions.

If you feel emotionally upset, angry, anxious or depressed you may benefit from professional help. It is difficult to help yourself out of uncomfortable feelings or an unfulfilling life or relationship without the support of someone else. The difficulty is greatest if you have an anxiety or depression disorder. Supportive therapy can be particularly helpful if you need medication, especially when setbacks occur.

Every individual counsellor and psychotherapist takes a unique approach that stems from his or her training, experience and personality. Broadly speaking, counselling tends to focus on your present feelings and anxieties and

practical options for change, while psychotherapy takes you more deeply into your unconscious and your memories and feelings to enable you to change old patterns. Both processes may take you through events in your past and deepen your insight into your feelings and behaviour.

Whoever you visit, establishing a trusting relationship is an important step. You will be encouraged to explore difficult and sometimes painful emotions. If, in therapy, something 'clicks' and you come to a realisation that had previously eluded you, it has been worthwhile. Your goals will be personal and may include a quest for balance, a desire to boost self-esteem, or a need to improve one or more relationships.

Counselling and psychotherapy are available for individuals, couples, families or groups. Some therapists use one way of working. Others draw on more than one technique. Your choice will depend on what is available in your area and the advice you get from your medical team and from your social group. It's a good idea to ask a range of questions at your first meeting. These might include asking about the therapist's:

- training and experience;
- personal views on family systems and family of origin (see page 207);
- choice of techniques, such as hypnosis, art therapy, visualisation or regression; and
- flexibility regarding meeting times and contact between meetings.

Your choice will probably depend most heavily on whether you feel comfortable with the therapist rather than on any 'defined' approach.

Counselling
This is an umbrella term for support that provides space for you to talk about and work through confronting issues such as anxiety or fear connected with birth or illness, medical care and treatment choices, your relationship with your baby's father, confidence and assertiveness. You may seek counselling regarding practical issues such as BREASTFEEDING and family boundaries (page 432).

Psychoanalysis and psychodynamic psychotherapy
Based on Freudian theory, these techniques look at early life events that were traumatic but are not consciously remembered. The aim is to

resolve past issues and learn to approach conflicts without resorting to old patterns that are no longer helpful.

Analytical psychology

This considers the memories and emotions stored in your unconscious mind that affect your feelings, actions and relationship choices. It is linked to Jung's theories.

Behavioural and cognitive psychotherapy

This looks at the associations between your thoughts, feelings, behaviour and lifestyle and family/social environment, and encourages you to focus on what is happening 'here and now' as a way of altering unhelpful behaviour patterns.

Experiential constructivist therapies

These look at the way you interpret experiences and create a story around them. It is based on the belief that an old story may still influence your actions and choices even though it is not relevant to events today. This method constructs a model for seeing things in a different light. Neurolinguistic programming (NLP) is one of the best-known approaches.

Family, couple, sexual and systemic therapies

These aim to look into patterns of belief and the roles and behaviours that become established in relationships, and then to build new and more fulfilling patterns.

Humanistic and integrative psychotherapy

This includes different psychotherapy approaches that consider a person's body, feelings, mind and spirit. The relationship between therapist and client is a vehicle for experience, growth and change.

Hypno-psychotherapy

This uses hypnosis to bring about a state of relaxation that allows a shift in awareness. During hypnosis, the therapist can tap into your deeper levels of consciousness and draw attention to new possibilities and different patterns of behaviour and emotions.

The 'success' of therapy tends to be progressive, and it may take some time for you to feel the results, particularly if you need to address a number of issues. Many counsellors and psychotherapists work from the premise that

when emotional issues are brought into conscious awareness, this is a catalyst for change. Similarly, working with the subconscious triggers change in your inner world and the way you experience life.

In the process of therapy you may become increasingly skilful at identifying and trusting your feelings, and valuing their guidance as you accept what is currently happening and when you want to influence the direction of your journey through life.

Couples

See Relationships.

Cracked nipples

See Breastfeeding, difficulties.

Cradle cap

Greasy, yellow or brown scaly patches of skin on the scalp, and sometimes in the nappy area, usually signify cradle cap. It is very common in babies from around six weeks after birth. It is not irritating and is only temporary. Sometimes a thick scaly or crusty layer may cover the whole scalp, with the scales becoming flaky over time and rubbing off easily. It may affect other areas of the body such as the back of the ears, the shoulders and the nappy area, particularly around the genitals.

There are simple treatments to reduce the scales, even though the condition usually clears up naturally over anything from a few weeks to 12 months. Occasionally it persists for longer.

Cradle cap is also known as infantile seborrhoeic dermatitis or nappy psoriasis (but is not actually a form of psoriasis, a chronic skin disease that is extremely rare in babies).

What happens

Cradle cap is not caused by infection, allergy or poor hygiene and the actual cause is not known. It may be linked with sebaceous (grease and sweat) glands in the skin of newborn babies, which can be overactive due to the effect of the mother's hormones still in the baby's circulation. The glands release a greasy substance that makes old skin cells attach to the scalp as they dry and fall off. There may be a relationship with naturally occurring yeasts (fungi) in the skin. No particular baby is more at risk than any other.

The condition may recur in puberty. A different form of dermatitis, atopic dermatitis (infantile eczema), often develops as the cradle cap is improving. Eczema generally continues for several years and is itchy (page 204). Cradle cap is not itchy.

Action plan

- The first line of treatment is to wash your baby's hair and scalp with natural mild baby shampoo. As you dry her hair, rub gently with a towel to remove some scales. Soft brushing can also gently remove some scales.
- A light covering of any natural vegetable or seed oil can help, too. Avoid olive oil as this encourages proliferation of a yeast called malassezia which may be part of the cause of cradle cap.
- If the cradle cap doesn't improve with frequent washing or if the rash spreads to other areas and red or inflamed areas cause irritation, your doctor may prescribe a medicated shampoo containing an antifungal and a weak hydrocortisone (corticosteroid) cream. Weak steroids have minimal effects in the doses used if use is limited to once daily.
- An antifungal cream is sometimes used but only in the most severe cases which have not improved with gentle treatments.

Homeopathy
You may try the most appropriate homeopathic remedy in 6c potency, three times per day for three days and then re-assess.
- *Graphites* when the scalp is encrusted and weepy, the hair matted and it may be smelly.
- *Lycopodium* if the scalp is dry and scaly with a brownish tinge, but not infected and the condition tends to spread to the eyebrows (looks like dandruff). There may be cracks behind the ears.
- *Sulphur* if the scalp is dry and itchy, your baby is irritated, hot and bothered, and all symptoms are worse from heat of any kind.

- *Calc Carb* for crusty, sour-smelling cradle cap in chubby babies who tend to sweat easily around their head.

Cravings

See Food and eating, mother.

Croup

See also Breathing difficulties, baby; Coughs and colds, baby.

There are few things more frightening than the sound of your baby gasping for air and making a hollow, rasping noise, like the barking of a seal. This is the classical sign of croup, a frightening but rarely serious infection. Croup is a respiratory infection, usually due to a virus, that leads to inflammation of the bronchi (lung airways), trachea (windpipe) and larynx (voice box). It usually lasts from three to seven days and is generally worse at night. It is most common between the ages of three months and three years, after which time the airways have enlarged sufficiently, so breathing is less hampered if there is another infection.

What happens

As a result of a viral infection, cells in the lungs, voice box and windpipe react by secreting mucus that narrows these air passages. The secretions dry and thicken, making it even more difficult for your baby to breathe.

Action plan

What you can do:
- Try not to panic: remaining calm will lessen your child's anxiety. Hold your baby – he may begin to breathe more easily if relaxed.
- Take your child to the bathroom and close the door. Turn on the hot water to fill the room with steam. Do not put your child in the shower. Hold him in your arms while you sit on the toilet or a chair (not on the floor – steam rises and collects in the upper part of the bathroom).

Calling your doctor and medical care

During a croup attack it is a good idea to keep in touch with your baby's doctor. Urgent medical attention is necessary if your baby shows the following warning signs:

- He is struggling to breathe in or out and the breathing is noisy, even while calm, especially when breathing in.
- The front of the chest appears to cave in towards the backbone while breathing in and there is a crowing noise as air passes through the air passages. This often occurs in the middle of the night, when the air is coolest.
- Your baby is restless, cannot sleep or is too breathless to feed.
- Croup-like symptoms, together with drooling and pushing out the lower jaw on breathing, may all be signs of a throat infection called epiglottitis. Your baby will also appear quite unwell, with a high fever and may get very frightened. Epliglottitis is a very rare but dangerous condition that always needs hospital treatment.
- Your doctor may prescribe oral or inhaled corticosteroid medication, which can reduce the severity of symptoms, but your baby may need hospital treatment. Antibiotics are rarely required, but may be given if it is thought there is a bacterial infection.

If your baby is gasping for air, remember there is a possibility that he could be choking. Check the airway and if you believe your baby is choking you must act quickly (page 6).

- Open the window to let in cool air. This helps to create more steam. Allow at least 15 minutes for the steam to ease the symptoms. If the symptoms continue and this doesn't ease your baby's breathing, it is time to seek emergency care.
- If your baby begins to breathe more easily and is ready to go back to sleep, use a vaporiser in his room.
- Crying is a good sign – if your baby is crying you know he is able to breathe.
- A drink of boiled, cooled water may help.
- Feed your baby as usual, or let him suck for comfort.

Homeopathy

If the attack seems mild, you may try homeopathic remedies – if it is severe or you are concerned, ensure that your baby is seen by a medical doctor.

Aconite (30c) is usually the best remedy to give when croup begins, and again half an hour later. Then you may choose the most appropriate remedy below (30c potency) to give every two hours for three doses. If there is improvement, you may continue with the most appropriate remedy three times a day for three days. If there is no improvement, seek medical advice.

- *Aconite* if your baby goes to bed fit and well and wakes suddenly with a hoarse, dry cough, usually around midnight, he makes noises and coughs on breathing out, is very frightened and restless and may have a fever.
- *Hepar Sulph* if your baby is irritable with a hollow, croupy cough with rattling, thick, persistent mucus that makes him gag, a feeling of chilliness and coughing that is worse in the morning, evening and the earlier part of the night.
- *Spongia* for a suffocating, dry, harsh cough that sounds like a saw going through dry wood, and laboured breathing with gasping, he looks very fearful and is much worse from breathing in.

Crying

See also Caring for baby.

Your baby's voice is unique to her and your body will respond to her cry above any other baby's, within hours of birth. You will often know instinctively just how to respond. This instinct is strongest when you spend lots of time in contact with your baby. It is completely normal for your baby to cry as she expresses her feelings (page 208) and asks for her needs to be met. Some babies are mellow and seldom cry for long, while others are very vocal. There may be days when you wonder if the crying will ever stop.

Why does your baby cry?

* Crying is communication. All babies cry. Your baby may need something, or may be expressing her feelings. Your baby may need to be held.
* Crying can indicate illness. If your baby is in severe pain her cry is likely to be shrill and your instinctive response will be a gut feeling that drives you to act. Sometimes crying from illness is weak and feeble.
* Hunger is a common reason for crying and you will soon understand your baby's hunger cries.
* She may be uncomfortable from digestion and indigestion. She may cry before moving her bowels or because she needs to bring up wind. COLIC is a potent cause of crying.
* Your baby may be too hot or too cold, have a dirty nappy, or wet clothes from dribbling or milk.
* If you are unhappy, worried or irritable or there's tension in the family, your baby may mirror this with her own upset.
* She may cry if she is tired but not relaxed enough to sleep.
* She may yearn to explore – maybe a different location, a change: she is naturally curious and explorative.
* Crying can release pent up energy; your baby may hold tension from her position and experience in the womb; from birth; or from something that happened yesterday or today.
* The time of day may be relevant – babies are often unsettled in the evening and the reasons vary (such as hunger, tiredness, picking up mum's fatigue).
* She may be feeling pain from growing teeth (page 509).

What happens

Your baby's cry can speed up your heart rate, set off hormones that make you feel protective, and may bring milk to your nipples. These reactions are just right: your baby is dependent on you and by crying she is asking to get her needs met.

In time, you will begin to recognise different cries. Your baby is capable of covering a staggering five octaves in pitch (that's half a piano) and has many different patterns. If she's bored, for instance, she may cry intermittently, pausing as she waits to see if you're taking note. Learning her language will be an ongoing process. Although it may be difficult at times, try to relax and let go of your own tension so you can feel your instincts and be objective.

+ Red flag

If you're worried, watch the clock – what may seem like an hour may only be five minutes. If you think your baby is sick, call your doctor or health visitor and ask for medical advice. If your gut reaction is fear or panic act quickly and find help.

Any change in your baby's 'normal' crying, either duration or pitch, may alert you. If she doesn't settle and there are other signs such as refusing or not finishing feeds, changes in colour or frequency of bowel motions, then play your hunches and seek advice.

Action plan

Sometimes you may be able to soothe your baby quickly. At other times it may take longer, depending on the reason and your baby's mood. Many babies who are constantly close to their mothers cry very little. Mum is in tune with them, and their needs are met quickly. In this case, providing your baby is not in pain from an underlying medical problem, it is likely that she will not cry for long.

* Spend time with your baby. You may enjoy carrying her with you during the day (preferably skin to skin).
* Consider the common practical reasons – hunger, too hot/cold, boredom as listed above – and take action where you feel it's appropriate.
* If your baby has pain, BREASTFEEDING will often help.

- Your baby may need help to relax and get to sleep.
- If she is not hungry, her nappy is clean and she has been winded, and you don't think she is in pain, the best thing may be to listen as you hold her, 'There now, have a good cry, let it all out. I hear you.' She will not understand the words but she will hear your tone and feel lovingly held.
- She may be calmed if you walk with her, dance or sing, and hold her in a certain way. 'Tiger in the tree' pose (page 145) suits many babies.
- MASSAGE and gentle physical play might help. If your baby has a 'crying time' try to pre-empt it. This is discussed in detail in colic (page 144). This needs to suit her and is best begun after you have soothed her in your arms.
- Music, the sound of water or the washing machine may be calming, or your baby may relax in a bath with you, or in bed with a familiar blanket or an item of your clothing.
- Quality time is important. Your baby can sense when you are not emotionally present even though you are physically with her. She may become calm when you focus on her and let go of your tension.

If your baby cries a lot

Some babies do cry a lot – perhaps as much as six hours a day – and in this case it may be useful to ask for a medical opinion or seek support to help you care for yourself and your baby as well as possible. It can be disheartening but have faith that crying is likely to diminish as your baby grows older.

- Excessive crying may be due to a medical problem or colic – seek advice, and consider COMPLEMENTARY THERAPIES. Massage and cranial osteopathy may help.
- It may be useful to resolve conflict if there is arguing or tension in your house (page 461)
- Your baby may find the world unsettling and need to be introduced to new objects and people gradually with the feeling of being emotionally and physically held and protected.

If your baby seems unhappy and resists your efforts to calm her down, you might feel rejected and frustrated. If you know you are doing your best to meet your baby's needs,

that there is nothing physically wrong, and if you've tried everything you can think of but nothing's worked, it's time to take care of *yourself* so that you don't become overwhelmed. When you begin to feel refreshed and calmer, your baby may mirror this. Remember that you do play an important role: it is important to care for yourself (page 121) and your baby equally.

- Put your baby down safely, walk out of the room and take a short break. Your baby will be okay for a few minutes; although it is preferable to arrange for another loving adult to stay with her.
- Accept as much help as you can, and try to meet other parents regularly. You may find tips and support from a local baby clinic or mother–baby group, your GP, health visitor or paediatrician or a local or national support group.
- Try not to stay in: being isolated is worse than being embarrassed. Everyone knows that it's natural for babies to cry.
- Hearing your baby's cries may bring up memories stored in your unconscious mind from when you were a tiny baby, and this can add to your stress. It may help to talk to a friend or a counsellor.
- If your partner is not supportive it may be because he finds it difficult and overwhelming. Being honest about what's happening for you both may help you support one another well, and give your baby security. Active listening can be very helpful (page 462).
- Phone a friend or relative, your health visitor, GP or the CRY-SIS help line.

▓ EVENING FRETTING

Although not every baby has fretful times in the evening, most do, and few parents know why. Your baby is likely to have an hour or two (or three, or four) when she cries almost non-stop and wants to do little else except suck at your breast or her bottle and doze in your arms. This may last for the first week or for as long as five or six weeks.

The general advice for soothing your baby and caring for yourself if she cries a lot applies at any time of day. When your baby's crying time arrives it helps to go with it. Find a comfortable position – lying down is perfect if she wants to feed – and use the time to relax. Try soothing music and turn the lights low. Accepting that your baby needs to be comforted and probably needs to feed will help minimise stress for you, whereas trying to stop her crying and get on with other things will almost certainly be exhausting and ineffective.

A few pointers may help in the evening:

- She may be crying because your milk supply has dipped: a nutritious lunch and afternoon snack and a short nap may improve your supply and make a big difference to your baby's evening.
- Your baby may be extra hungry, and a long feeding session may precede a long stretch of sleep.
- Some babies have colic (see page 144), and this often comes on in the evening.
- The evening may be your most difficult time – if you are tired, frustrated, want a break or feel stressed, your baby may mirror this, and it may affect your milk flow.
- Your baby might find the busy life of the bright, wide world overwhelming and by the end of the day want to be held and fed calmly. You could try bathing, massaging and/or feeding your baby half an hour before her regular crying time in a softly lit, quiet room.
- Sometimes your baby may have pent up energy and feel better after a kick about, a bath or massage.
- If your partner is out at work he may come home with fresh energy and be just the person to play with and soothe your baby while you take a break.
- If you are on your own with your baby, arranging for a friend or relative to pop in for an hour or two may be similarly helpful.

While difficult evenings persist, get to sleep as soon as your baby finally drops off. Put the answerphone on and don't worry about the washing up. In several weeks, this stage will almost certainly have passed.

▥ LEAVING YOUR BABY TO CRY

Being left alone to cry is not okay for a baby. It can be intensely frightening and deeply upsetting. It is not always possible to stop your baby's crying but it is preferable to be with her and let her cry in the safety of your arms. Crying is her language and you don't always need to 'fix' something for her.

In the late 20th century there was a prevailing opinion that tending to a crying baby instantly was a sure route to having a spoilt child. This view is being ousted as attitudes are changing and babies are being respected as sensitive, feeling people. There is also scientific research indicating that a baby cries less if she learns that her cries are answered promptly. When you tune into your baby you will notice she communicates in many ways other than crying. Science also shows that babies whose cries are repeatedly ignored may indeed cry less but only because they are too tired to continue, and in time they learn that it is not worth crying: a response known as 'protest despair'.

Babies under six months of age do not cry because they are naughty, and they cannot be spoilt. The development of the brain at this age means it is impossible to think and plan ahead. Nor can young babies learn to wait or to fit in with others' needs: they only express their needs. In the early months your baby has the reflex to cry and as she gets older she will be more able to over-ride this.

Your response helps your baby learn how to ask for support in the big wide world. Her brain development is rapid and she experiments and discovers how to use her voice effectively. If she regularly gets an appropriate response she knows she is understood. If the opposite occurs and her cries are repeatedly ignored she may feel misunderstood, doubt her voice and find it difficult to trust others. She may then cry more, or become passive, with subdued and undemanding behaviour.

- As a rule of thumb, do not leave your baby to cry.
- Whenever possible, let her cry in your arms. Sometimes she may prefer to have her own space – stay with her with the reassuring touch of your finger in her hand or your hand gently resting on her body.
- Your baby learns from repeated or particularly intense experiences. Leaving her for a couple of minutes very occasionally may not be deeply upsetting. In reality it may take this time for you to get to her if she has been sleeping in another room.
- At night your baby may surface from deep sleep and cry gently for a short period and then drop back to sleep. Follow your instincts and if you sense that she needs reassurance, be there for

her; otherwise she may go back to sleep best if there is no interruption. The technique known as 'go in often never pick up' works for some babies. For others being disturbed makes it more difficult to settle back to sleep, and others need touch to feel safe enough to go back to sleep. See what suits your baby. For 'controlled crying' as part of sleep training, see page 489.

OLDER BABY

Your baby's expression of her feelings and needs will alter as the weeks and months pass. Typically, babies seem 'settled' between four and 12 weeks after birth and tend to cry less; in part this reflects the parent's increased confidence as well. There may, however, be days when crying persists.

- Crying may still signal illness, fear and the need for loving care.
- She may complain if she's not getting enough attention or is not being acknowledged and made part of your conversations.
- Your baby has a growing urge to explore physically and may object if she can't touch or taste something – if it's dangerous, replacing it with something safe may satisfy her curiosity.
- She likes to chat in her own developing language.
- When she begins to eat solid food she might have discomfort from digestion or be more thirsty.
- She may cry through frustration of not being understood. From around eight to nine months babies are able to learn simple sign language and this can be fun for all the family. There are books and DVDs with simple guidance.
- There may be triggers, such as the time of day, a thing, a person, a place, or a position you hold her in. Make some notes and consider asking for an objective view.
- Some babies have more than the usual dose of energy and cry less when they are stimulated.
- Some babies don't like sudden changes and if something is different – perhaps you've gone to work, introduced a new carer or redecorated – give extra comfort and see if things improve.

Separation anxiety

Around six to eight months after the birth, your baby begins to realise that she is a separate individual. Before this, she has the sense that you

and she are one. Crying and clinginess in months six, seven, eight and nine, and sometimes beyond, can be expression of anxiety about being separate and maybe feeling alone. This is one of your baby's big feelings (page 208).

She may need lots of contact and reassurance as she tries on the new feeling of independence and discovers whether it feels safe. The transition to independence takes years and even as adults we still need companionship and loving relationships, and separation anxiety continues to be a source of distress.

PARENTS' REACTIONS

Almost all parents find dealing with crying a challenge, and it is often coupled with sleep deprivation, which tends to reduce reserves of patience and stamina. Crying can stimulate all kinds of feelings, and can be very draining. If you think you cannot cope, you will certainly not be the first person to feel this. It is an indication that you need extra support so you can meet the practical demands of parenting and have the energy to nurture yourself and your baby.

- Use your network of support to ease the pressure on you, for help at home, to allow you undisturbed time with your baby as well as some time out.
- You may be able to soothe you and your baby at the same time: try bathing together with some lavender oil, or play music and dance. Try to anticipate the times of day your baby feels calm.
- Be honest. You may be surprised how relieving it is to say to your baby how you feel: '*I feel frustrated and tired, but it is not your fault. I am here for you. Please don't worry about me, I have the support I need and there is nothing you need to do.*' For you both this is more positive than saying, '*Shut up! I can't take any more crying.*'
- Even if you feel upset and tired, simply being with your baby may be enough as you let go and dwell in the moment. You are tuned to mirror one another. Breathing with her while she's relaxed can be very calming. There will also be times when it's best for you to take a break while another adult stays with your baby.
- Earplugs may help to turn down the volume to a level that does not upset you.
- If days pass and things don't get better, call your health visitor or doctor and let them know how you are feeling. You may find crying

169

depressing and there are many ways of alleviating the stress (page 176).

* When you and your baby are together your moods and energy affect one another. If you are upset, anxious or angry it is best to find support from another adult so you do not project these feelings onto your baby.

Is your inner baby crying?

The sound of your baby crying activates areas of your brain and body that have been quiet since your babyhood, and this brings up memories and emotions that may have lain dormant for decades. If you are aware that this happens it is interesting to relate your childhood to your feelings now. Chat to your parents about how you were at that age. Talking to your partner, a friend or a counsellor may help you distinguish between your feelings and your baby's feelings. It may then be easier to remain calm and soothing.

Cystic fibrosis

See also Congenital abnormalities.

Cystic fibrosis (CF) is an inherited condition that leads to thickened mucus, which can block the airways and lead to lung infections. It also affects the digestive system. It has a large impact on daily life and can be debilitating. Today, life expectancy for those with CF is 31 years, on average, but it is constantly improving. About one in 2,500 babies born in the UK have the disease.

What happens

The defective CF gene causes a protein called the cystic fibrosis transmembrane regulator to function abnormally. The flow of water and salts in and out of the body's cells is altered, creating thick mucus. In the lungs, this blocks the airways and can cause infection and cysts to develop. In the digestive system it is difficult to digest fats, proteins and the fat-soluble vitamins A, D, E and K.

Babies with CF usually show bowel and chest symptoms within the first year. Some may have an obstructed bowel from birth, and a smaller number suffer from constipation and rectal

problems. Some children do not show any symptoms until later in life.

Testing for CF

The likelihood of inheriting the disease is discussed together with antenatal tests for CF on page 30. Not all sufferers are identified in pregnancy but from 2007 all babies in the UK have been tested as part of the heel prick test, which is routine at six to eight days after birth. The older 'sweat' test analyses the content of salt in sweat on your baby's skin. The salt content is high in affected children. This test, which can be performed from the second month, is being phased out.

Action plan

The problems associated with cystic fibrosis can be reduced if the condition is diagnosed early. Caring for a baby with CF involves careful control of diet, including vitamin supplements, physiotherapy to remove sticky mucus, and the regular use of antibiotics and physiotherapy to reduce infection in the lungs. A baby with CF is cared for by a specialist medical team. The parents play a critically important part in treating and supporting their child. Loving commitment can be stressful for everyone in the face of fear for the baby and concerns for future babies and the practical and emotional challenges are usually considerable (page 45).

At present there is no cure. However, ongoing research holds the possibility that gene replacement will become a future reality. Until then the goals of treatment are to ease the symptoms and slow the progress of the disease.

Cystitis and urinary tract infections, mother

See also Trichomoniasis; Urine, blood and stones, mother; Vaginal discharge.

The urinary tract consists of the kidneys, the ureters (the tubes connecting each kidney with the bladder), the bladder itself and the urethra (the tube through which urine passes out of the body). Urinary tract infections affect up to

10 per cent of women. Infection usually enters the urethra and spreads to the bladder, where it is called cystitis (bladder inflammation) and causes an increased need to urinate as well as a burning sensation as the bladder empties.

In a very small number of women, infection may extend via the ureters to the kidneys, where it is called pyelonephritis and causes symptoms of FEVER and abdominal pain, usually in addition to bladder symptoms. Occasionally, urine may contain bacteria without causing symptoms. This is called bacteriuria. It may not lead to cystitis, but women with bacteriuria are predisposed to cystitis. Bacteriuria is also associated with vaginal infections (page 541) and slightly increases the risk of PREMATURE BIRTH.

What happens

Women are more prone to urinary infection because the female urethra is shorter than the male's. Urinary infection is also more likely during pregnancy because the tone (tension) in the muscle of the bladder wall and the ureter, taking urine to the bladder from the kidney, relaxes, and slows the flow of urine so bacteria have longer to multiply. This increases the risk that bacteria from the bowel or vagina may enter the bladder. Flow may slow further as the pressure the uterus places on the bladder increases. After the birth, cystitis may occur after bruising following a CAESAREAN delivery or when a catheter has been used. If there has been vaginal prolapse (abnormal downward displacement, page 317), this increases the risk of infection.

Irritable bladder

An irritable bladder may cause symptoms similar to a urinary infection but the urine does not contain organisms. There is usually a history of the condition prior to pregnancy but the urine must be cultured (page 534) to exclude an infection. Kidney stones may also cause urinary blockage with resultant kidney pain or infection.

Action plan

Medical care

If you have bladder or kidney pain, you need to visit a doctor – there is more urgency if you have a fever.

- Your doctor will ask you to take a mid-stream urine sample. You do this by holding the labia apart and catching a small amount as the urine flows. It can be tested in your doctor's surgery but for an accurate diagnosis the urine is cultured in a laboratory to identify the organism(s) and so determine which antibiotic(s) to use.
- Infection needs to be treated with antibiotics. After treatment you will be offered another urine analysis to check that all the bacteria have been eliminated. Women with recurrent urinary infections may require a long-term course of antibiotics.
- You may be offered an ultrasound scan if you have lower back pain to check whether your ureter is excessively dilated (widened), which usually indicates a pregnancy effect or, rarely, a stone. Most stones pass into the bladder and operations to remove them are usually deferred until after birth.
- Infection caused by vaginal prolapse diminishes when the condition is treated.

Diet and lifestyle

- After passing urine, take extra care to wipe yourself from front to back to reduce the chance of transferring organisms from the anus or vagina to the urethra and bladder.
- Drink plenty of water to flush the bladder and the ureter, preferably before 6pm so the need to pee doesn't disturb your sleep.
- Onions, garlic and chives help to prevent the growth of harmful bacteria. Barley water (without sugar) can soothe urinary infections.
- For cystitis, unsweetened cranberry juice is a proven remedy – drink a glass three or four times a day. This helps prevent harmful organisms sticking to the bladder wall, so they are more easily flushed out. Don't drink the sugared variety, which may increase your susceptibility to CANDIDA (thrush), and can cause weight gain.

Homeopathy

If you have a fever, severe kidney pain or blood in the urine, you will need a medical examination and opinion. For recurrent bouts of cystitis it is advisable to consult a qualified homeopath, who may recommend *Berberis*, a bladder support remedy, in low potency. For an isolated attack of cystitis, you may take a suitable remedy (30c potency), every two hours for eight hours and then re-assess the situation. If there is no improvement please consult a qualified homeopath or see your GP.

- *Cantharis* if the burning pain is too severe to ignore, there is a cutting, sharp or scalding pain before, during and – worst of all – after urination, you constantly want to urinate, you feel as if your bladder can't empty and only small amounts of urine are passed, you have lower back pain and feel irritable and worse for moving.
- *Arsenicum* for cystitis accompanied by anxiety, restlessness and chilliness and a feeling that your bladder is not emptying well, with nausea and diarrhoea. You feel better for warmth.
- *Apis* for fluid retention and extreme sensitivity to heat with irritability and restlessness, a constant desire to urinate, a scalding sensation when urinating and improvement with cool air and cold compresses.
- *Staphysagria* after catheterisation, intervention during labour or pain after sexual intercourse, lingering burning pain after urinating and urine is passed drop by drop, you are easily angered or offended, and feel better from warmth and resting.

Aromatherapy and acupuncture

Sandalwood and patchouli, added to the bath or on a compress, can soothe. After Week 24 of pregnancy you can try lavender and chamomile. ACUPUNCTURE can bring relief.

Cytomegalovirus (CMV)

Cytomegalovirus (CMV) is a common viral infection that usually causes no symptoms. It is most common in young children and 50 per cent of adults have been infected. Past infections have no significant effect in pregnancy, but if you become infected for the first time when you are pregnant there is a chance that you may pass the infection to your baby. Fewer than 1 per cent of women get the infection for the first time in pregnancy, and of these only a small minority pass the infection to their babies. Rarely, this may cause serious illness and lasting disabilities and, very rarely, CMV can be fatal.

Infected adults occasionally develop a flu-like illness, which can include a sore throat, fever, aching limbs and fatigue. For people with

disorders of the immune system such as HIV, CMV can cause serious illness.

What happens

CMV is a member of the herpes virus family and can be passed on through contact with infected body fluids, such as saliva, urine, blood and mucus and during sex. It can be transmitted from mother to foetus during pregnancy, or during birth or in breast milk, but babies infected after birth rarely develop serious problems from the virus.

Roughly, one third of women who have a first infection in pregnancy pass the infection on to their babies, and 10 to 15 per cent of these babies develop serious illnesses. If you have been infected more than three months before conception, the risk of your baby becoming infected is extremely low. The antibodies in your circulation will prevent your baby from being infected.

Congenital CMV

Of the very few babies with congenital (present at birth) CMV, the vast majority (about 90 per cent) show no symptoms at birth. Most remain unaffected. Within one or two years of birth, however, around 10–15 per cent show signs of one or more neurological abnormalities such as mental retardation, learning disabilities, hearing or vision loss. Congenital CMV infection is a leading cause of hearing loss in children. Uncommonly there are early signs that may include unexplained low birth weight, small head size in relation to the body (microcephaly), liver enlargement, pneumonia, rash at birth, anaemia or hearing loss. These may indicate other causes: CMV infection can be diagnosed within three weeks of birth by identifying the virus in body fluids.

Action plan

Routine testing for CMV in pregnancy is not undertaken in the UK. If you develop CMV symptoms or you request a test, your doctor may recommend two or more blood tests to look for rising levels of the antibodies that emerge with CMV infection. IgM antibodies are the first to be produced in response to an infection, followed by IgG antibodies, which provide long-term protection against future infection and confer protection on your baby. Therefore, a recent infection is apparent if the IgM antibodies are increased whereas if IgG antibodies are present this indicates an old infection, and so is not dangerous for your baby.

If you are diagnosed with CMV in pregnancy, your baby can be tested for infection using AMNIOCENTESIS. The results are 80 per cent reliable, although even if your baby is shown to be infected, there is no way of telling how severe the infection is, or what effects it may have. The advice of an obstetrician specialising in infections may be extremely helpful while you consider the possibilities, bearing in mind that roughly a third of women pass the infection on, and only 10–15 per cent of babies exposed to the infection are seriously affected. You are likely to be offered detailed ultrasound scans to check for brain abnormalities or other potential effects of CMV.

Treating congenital CMV
At present, there is no treatment that can halt or reverse the effects of congenital CMV. However, doctors are investigating whether a new antiviral drug called ganciclovir, which is used to treat adults with AIDS who have CMV-related eye infections, may help babies with congenital CMV. This is a highly specialised and potentially toxic treatment, which must be supervised by a specialist in paediatric infectious disease.

Prevention
Although most people contract and develop antibodies to CMV before adulthood, there are preventive measures. These may be particularly important if your work involves children or healthcare:

* Wash your hands thoroughly after any contact with the saliva and urine of young children, and carefully dispose of nappies, tissues and other potentially contaminated items.
* Avoid drinking from glasses children have been using – in some day-care centres, as many as 70 per cent of children between the ages of one and three may be excreting the virus.

You may want to request a CMV test. If the antibodies present in your blood show that you have been previously – but not recently – infected, there is little need to worry.

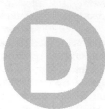

Dad

See Father.

Dehydration, baby

See Diarrhoea, baby.

Depression and anxiety, pre- and postnatal

See also Emotions, sadness and happiness.

Depression, often with anxiety, is common during pregnancy. When postnatal depression occurs, it is often well established in pregnancy, peaking around Week 32. Unfortunately, many affected women (and even more affected men, who are less frequently seen by health visitors and doctors) do not receive support, either because they are not correctly diagnosed or because they do not seek help.

If depression lingers without treatment and support, there could be many consequences for you and your baby. It may be daunting to read about the possible effects but acknowledging the reality may inspire you to seek help. Feeling depressed is not your 'fault' and there are many ways to relieve it. The course of depression is variable: a bout may pass within days but if it is severe or is not addressed, an episode may last months. With treatment most people recover sooner.

If you think you may be at risk, it is wise to draw on your network of friends and family and team of midwives, doctors and health visitors. With trusted support, perhaps including psychotherapy (page 162), you may be able to minimise feelings of upset and enjoy many positive aspects of being with your baby and making the transition into parenthood. You may also need medication.

■ CAUSES AND SYMPTOMS

There is no single cause of depression. Hormones in pregnancy and after the birth play an important role for many women, but they are only part of the picture. You have your unique reaction to changing hormones and your underlying personality and life circumstances are key. If you have had depression in the past you will be more susceptible now. If you have a family history of depression this may increase the risk for you, but it is useful to remember that experiences are often more influential than genetic predisposition. Even severe depression in the past need not be repeated if your life is less stressful now and you feel well supported. By the same token, people who have no history of anxiety or depression can become overwhelmed by the practical reality of parenting, or by feelings that surface from the past, such as previous miscarriage or loss, or unresolved emotions from childhood (page 207). Your baby will make a very significant contribution and depression may be increased if your baby is ill or difficult to care for. For some people having a baby of the wrong gender can trigger great disappointment. Sometimes anxiety sets in as a cycle (page 311).

Some families have a genetic tendency to abnormal neurotransmitter chemicals and hormones in the brain. Depression or anxiety may arise from an imbalance in three neurotransmitters – serotonin, noradrenaline and dopamine – and in this case often responds well to medication.

Depending on your family and cultural background it may be easier to admit to feeling anxious or having physical symptoms than it is to admit to feeling depressed. Some people experience physical problems including pain, tiredness and infections that are outward manifestations of depression.

If you have been depressed with a previous baby

If you became depressed in a previous pregnancy or after a previous baby and you now feel more positive and better supported, you may not experience the problem again. If your circumstances are similar or if you are anxious about depression recurring, consider talking to your GP, midwife or health visitor, and to a therapist such as a homeopath or counsellor. Having support and an objective assessment may help you make appropriate plans to reduce the intensity of your emotions this time round. If depression was severe in the first pregnancy and you notice the condition reappearing, you may wish to try medication. The options are covered on page 176.

Post traumatic stress

If you have experienced a terrifying event, perhaps concerning you or your baby, or something that happened before you became pregnant, you may be at risk of post traumatic stress. This is an anxiety state that also involves depression and is covered in more detail on page 448.

Symptoms

One of the most disabling symptoms is that it 'saps the will'. Depression typically involves a number of other symptoms, which vary from person to person. Every mother and father has some of the symptoms listed below. Whether they constitute depression depends on their degree and whether there are more bad days than good days.

* Feeling anxious, frequently or constantly. One of the signs is excessive concern that you or your baby have an undetected health problem. Anxiety symptoms occur in 80 per cent of people with depression.
* Feeling inadequate, sensitive, tired with poor concentration, suddenly overwhelmed by feelings of helplessness and unable to stop yourself from weeping.
* Feeling out of control and frightened by the responsibility of parenting. Some people describe the feeling as close to madness.
* Feeling irritable and angry, and that life is not fair.
* Avoiding other people.
* Lacking energy and enthusiasm, having difficulty with daily tasks, with a desire to do nothing else but sleep but you do not sleep well, even when exhausted.
* Not being interested in your baby.
* Loss of appetite or eating in excess.
* A series of aches, pains and illnesses.
* Using alcohol or other drugs for distraction from reality.
* An extreme form of depression may lead to thoughts of hopelessness and suicide.

Possible impacts of depression on your baby

Depression will have an impact on your physical health, your happiness and the attention you pay to your baby. Your behaviour may range from ignoring your baby and neglecting her needs to frequently chastising and shouting at her. Your baby may be resilient and may be minimally demanding, or her behaviour may challenge you. Babies can also be depressed and this may show with difficult or withdrawn behaviour (page 48). In pregnancy, when extremely high levels of stress hormones are passed to a baby they trigger emotionally stressful feelings.

Babies of mothers who suffer from depression are more likely to have BREASTFEEDING problems, to sleep poorly and to cry more – all of which tend to compound a mother's depression.

Other potential impacts could include conflict in your relationships and difficulties at work or with financial and household management, and any of these stresses will affect the level of security and comfort your baby experiences. Sometimes depression can be

175

associated with violence and other forms of abuse (pages 131 and 546).

■ PUERPERAL PSYCHOSIS

The very rare but most intense and dangerous form of depression is a psychosis where you become out of touch with reality. The psychosis may be mainly depressive and alternate with euphoria (mania). This is a bipolar disorder, also known as manic depression, and is usually present before conception. Other psychoses, such as schizophrenia, may also flare up during or after pregnancy.

■ SUPPORT AND TREATMENT

If you have a significant number of symptoms, you may be inspired that change is possible – looking at depression as an illness that can be treated helps a lot of people feel less daunted by the prospect of moving on.

Ideally, it is best to address depression before birth if it is already present. After birth, early and effective treatment may transform a difficult experience of parenting into one of acceptance and shared joy.

Taking the first step – seeking support – may be a great leap of courage if you feel at fault or guilty. This applies particularly if your family does not believe in acknowledging depression and finding emotional help; or if you have always set yourself very high standards and think you are failing.

Support may begin with practical help, for example, so that you can have more sleep, quality time with your baby, exercise, and eat nutritiously. This can make a huge difference, and for many people when the practical aspect of life gets easier, the emotional difficulties are less overwhelming.

Even though difficult feelings can reduce when life is less stressful, usually the emotional pain or conflict remains beneath the surface and it is helpful to explore this. The action plan for being in touch with your feelings on page 208 gives advice to support you as well as your baby. The majority of people find it hard to be compassionate towards themselves, particularly if depression is intense, and feel much clearer and more hopeful with professional support. You may

seek medication if that's appropriate in your case, or psychotherapy (page 162) and/or other complementary therapies (page 222).

Medical care

Your health visitor or doctor may offer extra visits at your home or in the surgery or suggest counselling or therapy if they suspect you may be suffering from anxiety or depression. Your GP may offer to put you in touch with someone else who has had similar experiences. If you are depressed after birth, a postnatal support group could give valuable support and companionship. If you have an emotional disorder that is extremely disruptive to your life, your doctor may suggest medication, or recommend a consultation with a psychiatrist who may prescribe medication.

Medication may bring immediate relief. It can help with panic attacks, anxiety symptoms, depression, obsessive behaviour, violent and anti-social behaviours, and psychosis. In the short term, medication can reduce symptoms and may help you approach the source of your upset.

Sometimes drugs alone can achieve good results, but this is usually not the case. For instance, medication may put a stop to obsessive behaviour rituals but such behaviour usually rests on a basis of feelings of anger, victimisation or guilt, and the influence of these feelings may only be reduced with therapy. It is preferable to have loving support and counselling or therapy at the same time.

Medication for emotional disorders does not come in a single form. If your doctor or therapist believes medication may help you, it is best to find the most suitable drug.

Antidepressants and anti-anxiety medications

An antidepressant boosts the level of neurotransmitters important in fighting depression. Each of the major classes of antidepressants – monoamine oxidase inhibitors (MAOIs), tricyclics, and serotonin re-uptake inhibitors (SSRIs) – affects brain systems in a different way. Some of the newest SSRI drugs, including prozac, have relatively few side effects but have not been licensed for use in pregnancy.

The decision regarding drugs needs to be

taken by you and your doctor, weighing up the pros and cons. Antenatal and postnatal depression can, for some women, carry a greater risk of harm to their baby and family life than the risk associated with antidepressant drugs. If there is a likelihood of withdrawal symptoms it will be important for you to feel supported when you decide to stop taking the medication.

Until recently, benzodiazepines were the primary medications for anxiety. They are, however, extremely addictive and are not suitable in pregnancy and during breastfeeding. Newborn babies may have drug withdrawal symptoms if the drug has been taken in pregnancy (page 192). A bipolar disorder with severe underlying depression may require long-term medication, often involving lithium.

Progesterone
Progesterone in the form of injections or pessaries (capsules inserted vaginally) has been claimed to reduce the severity of postnatal depression, although some obstetricians are sceptical about this. If you have a previous history of depression or severe pre-menstrual tension, some doctors advise progesterone on a daily basis immediately after the birth to prevent a rapid withdrawal of the hormone as the placenta is born. It may help with postnatal mood swings.

Development, baby

See Growth and development, baby.

Diabetes

Diabetes mellitus is a disorder that causes abnormally raised blood sugar (glucose) levels. Insulin is a hormone produced by the pancreas that assists the transfer of glucose from the bloodstream into body tissues such as the muscles and liver. In diabetes, the pancreas produces insufficient or no insulin and/or the tissues are resistant to the insulin that is produced. Pregnancy can worsen existing diabetes and also cause it to appear for the first time. Diabetes that occurs for the first time in pregnancy is called gestational diabetes.

If you already have diabetes, you need to plan pregnancy carefully. Babies of diabetic mothers are at higher risk of CONGENITAL ABNORMALITIES and pregnancy and birth-related complications. These risks can be greatly reduced when blood sugar levels are controlled before and after conception through lifestyle measures – especially by healthy EATING, vitamin and mineral supplements and regular EXERCISE – and with medication where necessary. There is a wide range of blood glucose monitoring kits that enable people with diabetes to check their blood sugar levels regularly and adjust food intake and medication accordingly.

What happens

There are three types of diabetes mellitus: gestational diabetes, type II diabetes (the most common type), and type I diabetes.

Gestational diabetes begins in pregnancy, most commonly around Weeks 20–4 and usually disappears after birth. Hormones made by the placenta have a blocking effect on insulin. This is known as insulin resistance and in gestational diabetes the pancreas does not produce enough additional insulin to overcome the resistance. The risks of gestational diabetes rise with obesity, a family history of diabetes or if a previous pregnancy was associated with an excess of AMNIOTIC FLUID, a LARGE BABY or a stillbirth. If you had gestational diabetes during one pregnancy you are more likely to develop it in a subsequent pregnancy. Gestational diabetes can be regarded as a form of type II diabetes (see below). Around 50 per cent of women who have gestational diabetes develop type II diabetes within 15 years.

Type II diabetes is also known as non-insulin dependent diabetes (and formerly adult-onset diabetes) and affects 90 per cent of people with diabetes. It occurs when the pancreas produces insufficient insulin and/or the tissues are resistant to the insulin that is produced. It is often associated with being overweight and can sometimes be controlled by following a healthy diet and taking regular exercise. In many cases people with type II diabetes require oral medication and a small number of affected people may also need to take insulin.

Type I diabetes is also known as insulin-dependent diabetes (and formerly juvenile-onset diabetes) and occurs when the number of insulin-producing cells in the pancreas is reduced. People with type I diabetes need to take insulin daily for life in addition to paying strict attention to following a healthy diet and taking regular exercise.

Implications for your baby in pregnancy

If blood sugar levels are well controlled, the risks to babies of diabetic mothers now are only marginally higher than in a non-diabetic pregnancy. The rare complications are mainly related to poor blood sugar control:

- *Hypoglycaemia.* If blood sugar falls too low it can make you feel weak, confused and sweaty. Intense hypoglycaemia can be dangerous for you and your baby because glucose is an essential fuel for brain and body.
- *Birth defects.* Gestational and type II diabetes generally do not cause birth defects. The incidence of congenital abnormalities is proportional to the control of blood sugar and any vitamin or mineral deficiencies in the mother.
- *An excess of amniotic fluid* may cause PREMATURE BIRTH or encourage your baby to take an awkward position for birth. Amniotic fluid levels are related to blood sugar levels.
- *Excessive foetal growth.* If high levels of blood sugar cross the placenta, your baby's endocrine system responds by producing insulin and growth factors that stimulate organ growth and fat deposition. Large babies are more vulnerable during birth and may need to be delivered by CAESAREAN SECTION.
- In rare cases, severe uncontrolled diabetes can lead to stillbirth (page 501).

Implications for your baby after birth

Whether or not complications occur after the birth – and if so, how severe – will depend on how well blood sugar was controlled during pregnancy. Many babies of diabetic mothers do not have any difficulties. Where complications occur, they may include the following:

- BREATHING DIFFICULTIES may develop because the lungs tend to lack surfactant, the substance that allows the air passages to expand at birth.
- If your blood sugar levels have been high, your baby will have produced an excess of insulin to break down glucose. He will not have diabetes but will produce an excess of insulin for 5–10

days after birth. The excess insulin may cause very low blood sugar levels (hypoglycaemia). In a mild form this will leave your baby irritable, with jerky movements and behaving in an unsettled way. A prolonged fall in blood glucose may cause neurological damage because the brain needs sugar. Blood calcium and magnesium levels may also fall in the days after birth. Your baby will be monitored and frequent feeding usually prevents these complications.

- Your baby may have high levels of haemoglobin in his blood and has a slightly higher chance of developing neonatal JAUNDICE.
- In the long term a baby of a diabetic mother is at slight increased risk of developing gestational or type II diabetes.

Implications for you

Whatever type of diabetes you may have, the risk of complications can be greatly minimised by tight control of blood glucose levels and by strict attention to lifestyle and nutrition, with medication where necessary.

- If blood sugar falls too low it can make you feel weak, confused and sweaty (hypoglycaemia or a 'hypo'). This is most likely if insufficient carbohydrate has been consumed to match the insulin or medication you have taken. People with diabetes are advised to carry a source of carbohydrate with them and to eat it when they recognise the symptoms of a 'hypo'.
- There is a higher chance of contracting CANDIDA (thrush) infection in the vagina or breast or a urinary tract infection. This may increase insulin resistance.
- Pre-eclampsia and elevated BLOOD PRESSURE is more likely and will need ongoing monitoring, and treatment if necessary.
- Diabetes makes you more susceptible to excess WEIGHT gain, and this will increase blood sugar levels and make diabetes difficult to control. Likewise, excessive weight gain may stimulate gestational diabetes in susceptible women.
- Long-term complications of poorly controlled diabetes include increased risk of heart disease, stroke, kidney disease, blindness and nerve damage.
- Having diabetes can be emotionally demanding and people with the condition benefit greatly from the ongoing support of their family as well as their medical team.

Action plan

If you have type I or type II diabetes, or develop gestational diabetes, the key to a healthy pregnancy and to giving birth to a healthy baby is to maintain your blood sugar levels in the normal range and to eat and exercise well.

Diagnosing gestational diabetes

Often there are no symptoms and diabetes is detected from a routine blood or urine test. If you are having symptoms, these may include excessive thirst and/or urination, fatigue, genital itching and thrush, blurred vision and abnormal weight loss. If a blood or urine test shows abnormally high glucose levels, further blood tests of glucose tolerance may be carried out to confirm the diagnosis. In some hospitals a blood sugar test is taken two hours after a sugary drink to screen for gestational diabetes. This is carried out around Weeks 24–32 because the condition may not be evident earlier. If the test is positive, a full glucose tolerance test will be taken by measuring blood sugar levels half hourly after a glucose drink. If the levels are elevated then a diagnosis of gestational diabetes will be made, and you will be closely monitored. Treatment, as appropriate for you, may also begin.

Medical care

You will need frequent medical checks and assistance to keep your blood sugar levels well controlled. If your hospital has the facility, you can attend a pregnancy diabetic clinic staffed by expert midwives, nutritionists, obstetricians and endocrinologists (hormone specialists).

- Your blood may be analysed for levels of glycosylated haemoglobin. This is a chemical change to the haemoglobin in your blood caused by elevated blood sugar levels. It gives an indication of the level of glucose in your blood over the previous few weeks and helps your medical team assess how well your blood sugar is being controlled.
- The team may carry out other screening tests to check for possible long-term effects, such as to the blood vessels in the retina, the nerves in your feet and hands, and your heart, liver and kidney function.
- If you are nauseous and are VOMITING, treatment to replace fluid, minerals and food is important to maintain your blood sugar levels.

- The wellbeing of your baby will be closely monitored by clinical examination and ultrasound scans, as for HIGH-RISK PREGNANCY.

Monitoring your own blood sugar level and ketones

- You will be shown how to monitor your own blood sugar levels to help you keep your blood sugar under control. Urine sugar levels are often unreliable, especially in pregnancy.
- If you have type I diabetes you may be asked to give a urine sample in order to check your urine for ketones. Ketones are by-products caused by the breakdown of fat in the absence of glucose. Small amounts are produced naturally during any fast – including overnight – and in people who do not have diabetes the ketones are harmless. But in type I diabetics especially, high ketone levels can indicate an inadequate eating pattern or insufficent insulin. Excess ketones lead to acidosis (an increase in the acidity levels in your blood) which may be harmful to a mother and her baby in pregnancy.

Eating

What and how you eat is crucial to reduce symptoms and reduce or exclude complications. Establishing and sticking to a balanced diet is the best way to keep your blood sugar levels normal. You may take advice from a nutritionist or a specialist midwife, and use the principles laid out in the eating entry. Planning in advance is a good way to avoid skipping meals, and is particularly useful if you're feeling tired and can't be bothered to cook.

- Eating slow-burning carbohydrates every three to four hours – including healthy snacks between meals – helps keep blood sugar levels stable, avoiding hypoglycaemia (abnormally low blood glucose levels).
- Foods with low glycaemic index scores (page 261) are best for maintaining normal blood glucose levels.
- Current advice is to ensure that one third of the meal contains vegetables and fruit – or half the meal if you are overweight. It is important to eat fruit, but do limit your intake to two pieces a day. It is recommended that another third of the meal contains slow-burning carbohydrates (with a low glycaemic index score) such as whole grains, granary or wholemeal bread and pasta, brown rice, beans and pulses. The fibre

in these foods helps slow down the release of glucose and keeps blood sugar levels from rising too high. The recommended contents of the final third of a meal are protein and fats.

- Protein acts to stabilise blood sugar. You can get enough if you have beans, eggs, fish or meat in at least two meals of the day.
- Unsaturated fats and essential fatty acids are useful in moderate quantities but it is crucial to keep saturated fats (found in meats, cheese and cream, for example) to a minimum because a diet high in fat causes insulin to act less efficiently and may contribute to being overweight and increase the risk of heart disease.
- It is extremely important to limit sugar-based foods and drinks because these cause a rapid rise in blood sugar levels. In particular, limit fizzy drinks, sweets and chocolates and avoid fruit juice.
- You need to limit your salt intake because having diabetes makes you more susceptible to high BLOOD PRESSURE and pre-eclampsia.
- Your blood sugar levels may drop during the night. A late-night snack providing protein and complex carbohydrates can guard against this. For example, try brown rice and chicken, a small baked potato with a bean salad, or a sandwich with poached fish. The starch stabilises blood sugar levels in the early night and the long-acting protein will stabilise them later on.
- Taking a multivitamin and mineral supplement formulated for pregnancy as well as an omega-3 essential fatty acid supplement (such as fish oils) helps to improve foetal growth and control your blood sugar.

Weight gain

Weight gain and diabetic control go hand in hand. Too much body fat produces an insulin-resistant effect. Optimal weight gain for you depends on your weight before pregnancy and it is best to talk to your medical team or dietician. Diabetic women are advised to return to pre-pregnancy weight within four months after birth. If you have gestational diabetes, maintaining an appropriate weight may reduce the risk of developing type II diabetes in later life. There is more on weight during and after pregnancy on pages 564–8.

Exercise and rest

Regular exercise helps to make your muscles and tissues more responsive to insulin and so helps maintain normal blood glucose levels. Exercise may also help to reduce your cravings for sweets, but remember not to overdo it: resting is also important.

If you are taking insulin you will need to monitor your blood glucose levels more often. Exercise lowers blood sugar levels, as does insulin, and the combination may lead to hypoglycaemia. When you exercise it is important to take a sugary snack with you and you may be advised to monitor your blood sugar levels before, after and – if necessary – during your exercise sessions.

Birth

- If your baby is not too large and your diabetes is controlled, you may safely await the onset of labour.
- If sugar levels are not controlled, it may be best for your baby to be born between Weeks 36 and 40. The exact timing will depend on your baby's condition.
- During labour it is important to control blood sugar levels by having snacks or using an intravenous drip. Your insulin requirements may alter.
- If you give birth vaginally your baby will be closely monitored for FOETAL DISTRESS and your doctor will be aware that if your baby is large there may be potential difficulties (see page 396).
- On balance, a caesarean section is more likely if you have diabetes, but well-controlled gestational diabetes is not in itself a reason for a caesarean birth.

After the birth

Your body's insulin requirements drop rapidly as placental hormones decrease. If you are taking insulin, you need to decrease the dose. You need to monitor your blood sugar levels, food intake and insulin doses closely to prevent dramatic falls in blood sugar levels (hypoglycaemia). This is particularly important if you are not eating much while you recover after a caesarean.

If you had gestational diabetes, continue with a nutritious diet and closely spaced meals and take vitamin and mineral supplements. This will keep your energy high, improve the flow of breast milk, and reduce long-term complications. Women who develop gestational diabetes are at increased risk of developing type II diabetes so it is important to eat well and to have your blood sugar level checked annually.

Your baby

Feeding your baby early and frequently will keep his blood sugar levels normal. BREASTFEEDING may contribute to your postnatal weight loss, and could reduce your baby's chances of developing diabetes in later life.

Your baby's breathing will be monitored for a few hours after birth and he will be checked for jaundice in the days that follow. His blood sugar levels will be monitored for the first few days to check for HYPOGLYCAEMIA. This is done with a simple heel prick.

Diarrhoea, baby

See also Poo, baby.

It is quite normal for a baby to pass several stools a day, or just one in several days, and if your baby is breastfed his stools may be loose and runny. Diarrhoea is a sudden increase in the amount of stools, and the stools are looser or more watery than usual. The main concern is that if diarrhoea persists it may lead to dehydration.

What happens

Most mild episodes of diarrhoea last for less than 24 hours and pass without any treatment. Broadly speaking:

* *Mild* diarrhoea involves three or four loose but small motions in 24 hours. If your baby does this and is happy and drinking well, there's no cause for concern.
* *Moderate* diarrhoea involves five to six loose stools in 24 hours that are of medium volume.
* *Severe* diarrhoea is when there are eight or more watery stools that are so profuse that they leak out of the nappy and soil the clothes.

Diarrhoea can occur in any age baby. The normal loose frequent motions of a breastfed baby (page 447) are often confused with diarrhoea. If your baby appears well then the loose poo is unlikely to be significant, even if it does look just like diarrhoea.

Dehydration

It is common for health professionals and parents to overestimate the degree of dehydration and the minimum amount of fluid a baby needs. Most babies with an episode of diarrhoea do not become significantly dehydrated, and cope well as long as they have a regular (page 182) intake of fluid.

Dehydration may, however, accompany diarrhoea, because your baby is passing more fluid than usual. The extent reflects the severity of the diarrhoea. If your baby is also losing fluid from VOMITING or sweating from a fever or the room temperature is high, this will increase the risks of dehydration. A younger baby will more easily become dehydrated as other body systems for regulating water are immature.

Signs of *mild dehydration* include dry lips, although the inside of the mouth remains moist, and your baby will babble and play for short periods. There will be less urine. With adequate fluid intake and as diarrhoea reduces, mild dehydration usually passes.

Severe dehydration makes the lips and mouth dry and brings on listlessness and there is no urine for eight or more hours. Your baby may stop producing tears when he cries and his skin may appear pale or blotchy. Because your baby feels weak, he may suck feebly or refuse to drink. In addition, the fontanelle (soft spot on top of the head) may appear slightly sunken.

Causes

Diarrhoea may be due to any one of a number of causes. If due to an infection, your baby is contagious for a couple of days before the onset of diarrhoea and while diarrhoea persists. Sometimes diarrhoea is a reaction to antibiotics given for other reasons.

Gastroenteritis infection and food poisoning

Most cases of diarrhoea result from gastro-enteritis, which is caused by a viral infection that affects the lining of the gut and may also cause VOMITING. Other symptoms may include FEVER, stomach ache and generally feeling unwell. Gastroenteritis may last for a week or longer, and may appear to get better and then flare up again.

If there is blood or mucus in the stools, the infection may stem from bacterial food poisoning. This brings on diarrhoea and often vomiting within one to six hours of consuming the food, together with abdominal cramps. The symptoms improve within eight to 24 hours. Food poisoning is often caused by a bacterium called *Staphylococcus aureus* that contaminates food left at room temperature, particularly dairy and meat products. In some cases, parasites cause the infection, usually from contaminated water.

Escherichia coli (*E. coli*), a bacterium found especially in undercooked meats, can cause bloody diarrhoea and requires immediate treatment, perhaps in hospital, because it may result in a severe illness involving other organ systems, especially the kidneys and liver.

Diet and food intolerance

Diarrhoea can occur if your baby drinks too much fruit juice or has an ALLERGY OR INTOLERANCE. Milk intolerance (page 20) and coeliac disease (page 20) may cause diarrhoea. If the stools appear to be a strange colour, for instance very red or orange, this may reflect what your baby has been eating (such as red juice or cordial, carrots, yams). Remember that stewed fruits may increase diarrhoea.

Bowel disorders

- Stools that look like redcurrant jelly may signify intussusception, a rare condition where the bowel folds inside itself and needs surgical correction (page 61).
- Chronic constipation may be associated with episodes of spurious diarrhoea, usually after solids are introduced. This is a surprisingly common problem and accounts for one of the most frequent reasons for consulting a GP or being referred for specialist treatments. The diarrhoea results from the inability of the heavily loaded large bowel to absorb water from the liquid stools entering from the small bowel. As a result the liquid stool passes through the large bowel unchanged, and there is still constipation.
- CYSTIC FIBROSIS is a rare cause of diarrhoea. The stool is sticky and the child is usually failing to thrive, and may have respiratory symptoms.

Action plan

If your baby has diarrhoea, the most important step is to prevent dehydration. You may also need to treat a sore bottom and nappy rash (page 418). Medication is rarely necessary. Remember your hygiene: wash your hands after you have been to the toilet, after each nappy change and before and after handling food. Keep your baby's hands clean too.

+ Red flag

If your baby seems very dehydrated call your doctor immediately – severe cases need hospital treatment. The medical diagnosis for severe dehydration is a loss of at least 15 per cent of body weight since the illness began. For a very small number of babies, dehydration may lead to shock if fluid replacement has not been started within 24 hours or the fluid loss is unusually severe. Fluids to provide lost salt and sugar can be given in hospital but you must never give additional sugar or salt alone as they may cause harm.

Rehydration solutions can help. They are powders to be mixed with boiled, cooled water that can be bought over the counter in chemists. They contain a balanced mixture of electrolytes (such as mineral salts), which replace those lost in the diarrhoea. The pack gives guidelines for dosage but check with your doctor or health visitor if you are uncertain. If your baby doesn't want to drink, or is vomiting fluid, continue to offer him sips of rehydration solution frequently – even as little as a teaspoon at a time will help. Do not make your own solution of sugar and salt and do not use a rehydration solution alone for longer than 24 hours without consulting your doctor. If the vomiting has settled, and it usually does within 24 hours, then switch back to milk.

Give your baby fluids

In most cases, dehydration is not severe and medical care isn't necessary.

- If you are breastfeeding, encourage your baby to feed frequently, and let him suck whenever he shows an interest. If he is feeling unwell he may suck only for short periods. This is fine. For moderate diarrhoea there is no need to give your baby a rehydration solution (below) if he is taking his feeds.
- If you are bottle-feeding and your baby is less than six months old, stop formula milk feeds for 24 hours. Give boiled, cooled water frequently or preferably use an oral rehydration solution (above). If vomiting stops, even if diarrhoea persists, reintroduce the milk feed after 24 hours. If he is over six months old, 12 hours without a milk feed may be sufficient.
- Avoid fruit juices or sugary drinks as these can prolong or aggravate diarrhoea because of their high sugar content and do not contain the right balance of salts to correct losses of salt in diarrhoea.
- If your baby is not keeping any fluid down, see your doctor or go to a hospital casualty department. Take your baby's Parent Health record with you – the doctor or health visitor can estimate weight loss, and thus the extent of dehydration, by comparing his weight with a recent reading.

Medical care

Usually blood and stool tests are not taken, as there is rarely a need to treat other than with fluid replacement. Occasionally, a test may be recommended to determine whether the cause is viral or bacterial, but even if it is bacterial, antibiotics are rarely used. If medical care is needed, the principal aim is to replace excess fluid loss, and to keep up with your baby's daily requirements of fluid. For a small number of babies a short hospital stay is required.

If your baby has a fever you may give medication to bring down the temperature in doses appropriate for his age (page 429). This may also relieve any pain from stomach cramps.

Reintroducing solids for your weaned baby

- When your baby feels like eating and his stools have become semi solid, begin with easily digestible foods such as bananas, rice cereal, apples and white toast (BRAT diet).
- Avoid dairy products because while he has diarrhoea he may be susceptible to developing an intolerance to milk. Sucrose and lactose

intolerance (page 20) can occur after diarrhoea as a temporary phenomenon.
- If he doesn't feel like eating, do not worry, as long as he is drinking well. You will know that he is well hydrated if his nappies are regularly wet with urine.

Homeopathy

For mild diarrhoea (that may be accompanied by vomiting) you may give the appropriate remedy (30c potency) hourly for four hours, then every two hours for six hours, and re-assess. With improvement, you may give the remedy three times a day for two days. If symptoms change, you may try an alternative remedy. If your baby's diarrhoea is severe or has lasted more than 24 hours, or there is any sign of dehydration, consult your doctor.

- *Arsenicum* when there is chilliness, restlessness, exhaustion and anxiety, possibly with vomiting, very watery stools that burn the skin around the bottom. The cause may be spoiled fruit or food.
- *Podophyllum* for explosive stools the consistency of batter (often greenish), accompanied by gurgling and rumbling in the abdomen, and the stools are smelly and gushing. Your baby may be teething.
- *Chamomilla* when diarrhoea accompanies teething, is greenish and your baby is irritable, his mood changes and he will not be put down.
- *Pulsatilla* when stools are changeable and there is vomiting after eating rich food, your baby is whiny and clingy and not thirsty.
- *Phosphorous* for exhausting diarrhoea that is painless but profuse, there is an urge to drink but fluid is vomited, or if diarrhoea occurs after a shock and is accompanied by anxiety, although your baby seems good-humoured.
- *Sulphur* for watery, frothy diarrhoea, worse on waking, and a red, sore anus.

■ RECOVERY

After a mild bout of diarrhoea, it may take your baby two or three days to get his energy back, although his stools may continue to be watery for up to two weeks. There is a small chance that the loose stools are resulting from an allergy or intolerance, but it is more likely that the bowel is simply taking time to recover.

It is important to have your baby's weight monitored regularly. If he is not gaining adequately, your doctor can advise on treating the underlying cause(s) of his failure to thrive (page 559).

If diarrhoea persists

If you are breastfeeding your baby, it might be useful to take dairy products, especially bottled cow's milk, out of your diet for a day or two. This sometimes reduces the diarrhoea by reducing the amount of cow's milk protein (page 19), passing to your baby. If the diarrhoea settles it is probably fine to reintroduce the cow's milk into your diet.

Bottle-fed infants need a different strategy. Although the persistent diarrhoea usually settles of its own accord in two weeks, it sometimes continues, with poor weight gain. In this situation, your doctor may suggest you switch to a soya formula or lactose-free formula, or prescribe a formula designed for babies with diarrhoea. If your baby isn't gaining weight, you may be advised to switch formulas within four weeks. When your baby recovers, you may return to the usual formula. Many parents find waiting difficult and need emotional support while doing so.

Diarrhoea, mother

See also Heartburn and indigestion; Irritable Bowel Syndrome (IBS), mother.

If your stools become loose and watery and you have three or more motions a day, you may have diarrhoea, particularly if they contain mucus. Typically, diarrhoea is self-limiting but if it persists or is severe it is important to visit your doctor.

What happens

- *Being pregnant.* In some women bowel movements become more frequent during pregnancy because of altered eating and drinking habits or the intestine or colon's reaction to hormonal changes.
- *Infection.* Diarrhoea may be due to a viral or bacterial infection (gastroenteritis or food poisoning). In pregnancy this has no direct effect on your baby but may lead to dehydration. If it continues for more than three

days, it is worth seeking medical advice. In the case of a severe infection, you may also have nausea and vomiting or a fever and will need medical treatment.

- *Diet.* Diarrhoea may arise from a sudden change in diet. For instance, it takes time for your intestine to adapt to an increase in fibre or to supplements, particularly iron. You can assess this by stopping the supplements and seeing if the diarrhoea lessens and then altering the type of supplement. You may need to reduce the fibre in your diet and you might notice a difference if you take your supplement before a main meal.
- *Allergy or intolerance.* If diarrhoea persists for weeks, it may be due to an ALLERGY OR INTOLERANCE. You may need to note what you eat and how your body reacts, and then cut down on any suspicious food. Wheat and milk intolerance is common and so avoiding them may be very effective.
- *Pre-labour.* Diarrhoea is a common symptom of pre-labour when hormones released to stimulate the uterus also stimulate the intestinal walls to contract.

Diarrhoea may be a symptom of irritable bowel syndrome (often alternating with CONSTIPATION), usually accompanied by abdominal bloating or pain, or more rarely of bowel disease (page 320).

Action plan

Eating and drinking

- Drink to replace lost fluid and electrolytes. Rehydration powders and sports drinks for runners available from pharmacists replace depleted electrolyte reserves. Light soups also contain electrolytes. If you cannot tolerate these, it is important simply to drink any fluid that appeals but avoid fizzy drinks or sweet cordials.
- After 24 hours, if you feel like eating, choose bananas for their high potassium content, and/or plain white rice and white toast – their low-fibre content will not irritate your bowel.
- After 48 hours, introduce gentle, fat-free foods such as soups, boiled potatoes, cooked vegetables and egg.
- When symptoms subside, gradually return to your normal diet. Avoid milk and other dairy

products until you feel fully recovered but do try bio-yoghurt to replace normal bowel bacteria (or alternatively take probiotic supplements).

- If diarrhoea is an ongoing problem, it is important to maintain adequate nutrition for you and your baby. You may need mineral supplements so that you feel well and to avoid the risk of developing iron-deficiency anaemia.

Medical care
- Opiate derivatives such as loperamide and diphenoxylate are found in a number of branded drugs and may be prescribed if diarrhoea is severe and you need treatment. Although they are not licensed for use in pregnancy, your baby is not likely to be affected by them if they are taken on a short-term basis.
- Codeine phosphate is also an opiate and is safe in pregnancy and can be prescribed by your doctor.
- If diarrhoea is present in late pregnancy, your doctor or midwife may want to examine you as labour may have begun.

+ Red flag

If diarrhoea is severe and you are dehydrated or notice blood in your stools you need to be examined immediately by your doctor.

If diarrhoea persists, your doctor may carry out further tests, including a stool culture to check for infection or chronic bowel disorders such as inflammatory bowel disease (ulcerative colitis or Crohn's disease).

Homeopathy
You may choose the appropriate remedy for your symptoms, and take it in 30c potency three times a day for three days unless there is no change within 24 hours, in which case you will need to re-assess. If diarrhoea becomes severe it is best to contact your doctor.
- *Arsenicum* for diarrhoea accompanied by chilliness, restlessness and anxiety, burning pains in the abdomen and a desire for sips of

warm drinks. Arsenicum is the classic remedy for food poisoning arising from fruit or meat.
- *Podophyllum* for painless but profuse diarrhoea with sudden motions accompanied by gurgling and rumbling, and you feel weak and drained.
- *Sulphur* for watery, sour-smelling diarrhoea that drives you out of bed in the morning and makes your anus sore, red and burning.
- *Carbo Veg* for diarrhoea with extreme flatulence, abdominal pain and cramping with faintness and breathlessness. This is the usual remedy following food poisoning from chicken or fish.
- *Lycopodium* if you are anxious and your motions are accompanied by lots of wind. This remedy is usually chosen following poisoning from shellfish.
- *Veratrum Alb* for diarrhoea with colic and cutting pains, weakness and cold sweats (but no anxiety, as with *Arsenicum*), stools are watery and odourless and you crave ice-cold drinks.
- After a bout of acute diarrhoea, particularly as you have lost fluids, you may take *China* (30c) morning and night for up to one week – this will act as a mental and physical pick-up.

Aromatherapy
Essential oil of tangerine added to the bath or mixed with carrier oil and used for massage may help. From Week 24 of pregnancy you can use chamomile oil.

Diet

See *Eating difficulties, mother; Food and eating, mother.*

Dilatation and curettage (D&C)

This procedure may be needed if the placenta is retained in your uterus after birth (page 362); or in the event of a MISCARRIAGE.

Discipline

See *Parenting, discipline.*

Disproportion in labour

See Labour and birth, mother, disproportion (tight fit).

Doulas (paramana doulas)

A 'paramana doula' is a woman whose role is to be with another woman during labour and birth and who has attended a training course on fulfilling this role. The Greek word 'doula' means 'handmaiden' or 'servant'. It was originally used on its own but the connotations of 'servant' urged the doula community, led by French obstetrician Michel Odent and doula Lilliana Lammers, to add the term 'paramana', which means 'with mother'.

Most women who train as doulas are themselves mothers. The training does not equip a doula to play the role of a midwife or medical specialist, but does provide insight into methods that can ease labour, and information on the physiology of labour and birth, normal process, pain relief, and signs that extra help may be needed for mother or baby. The background knowledge is important yet the emphasis for a doula is to provide mothering and companionship (rather than nursing) to a mother.

The benefits of having a trusted female companion are widely known. This can shorten labour, reduce the pain, and reduce the need for intervention (including caesarean), improve enjoyment and relaxation for mums, dads and babies, and assist in creating conditions conducive to BREASTFEEDING and bonding. It was once common for women in labour to be joined and supported by their mothers, sisters or other women in the community who had themselves given birth. A doula fulfils this role in modern society. Doulas are more commonly invited to attend home births, but may also join mothers in hospital.

What happens

If you wish to have a doula with you, it is important to meet her in advance of the birth. If you are planning a home birth it is helpful for her to come to you, so the environment will be familiar on the day. During labour and birth, she will be present alongside your midwife and any doctors who attend to you. Her commitment to you will be to stay with you, providing continuity of care, even if midwives or doctors change. She may be quiet and unobtrusive. She may be hands-on and involved with decisions – if that is what you need – and she will support your partner if he is with you.

An important part of a doula's role is to help mother and baby have undisturbed time together immediately after birth, to meet, to touch, smell and explore one another, and to breastfeed. Some doulas offer postnatal support and you may invite help for a few hours at a time in the days or weeks after birth so you can rest, bond and feed your baby.

Doulas may advertise their services locally or you may use the internet to find a doula in your area. A doula charges by the hour or by the birth, and some offer reduced rates or complimentary services.

Down's syndrome (trisomy 21)

See also Antenatal tests.

Chromosomes usually occur as pairs. The term 'trisomy' describes the abnormal situation in which there are three chromosomes of a particular type. If a baby is born with three of the number 21 chromosome she has a condition called trisomy 21, better known as Down's syndrome.

The extra chromosome leads to specific facial and bodily features, including low-set ears, a relatively large tongue, a small round face, a flattened back to the head, almond-shaped eyes that slant upward and small hands with a single palmar crease (rather than two). Muscle tone is also reduced, which makes a baby floppy. Hearing and vision development may be delayed, affecting language development, and there may be associated heart problems and CONGENITAL ABNORMALITIES of the digestive system. There may be significant reduction in mental development.

Generally, Down's syndrome results in developmental delay in all areas, but most particularly in speech and language. Emotional development is also specifically affected. When growing up, and into adolescence and adult life, some Down's syndrome children may be more vulnerable due to differences in the way they express their emotions and read other people's emotional clues. Nonetheless children with Down's syndrome will experience the same range of emotional needs and expression, some perhaps more enthusiastically and with reduced inhibition then others. With the right support and encouragement, young people with Down's syndrome can lead the same emotionally fulfilling and happy lives as the majority of other young people.

The expected lifespan for a person with Down's syndrome is about 55 years, although this is very variable and the condition increases susceptibility to diseases such as leukaemia and thyroid disease, as well as early-onset Alzheimer's.

What happens

Some 95 per cent of Down's syndrome cases result from trisomy 21. Occasionally, though, extra chromosome 21 is attached to another chromosome; this is called translocation Down's syndrome (4 per cent of cases). This is the only form of Down's syndrome that can sometimes be inherited from a parent, although a parent may show no signs of the defect. More rarely, in 1–2 per cent of cases, mosaic Down's syndrome occurs when there is an error in cell division after fertilisation and a person has some cells with an extra chromosome 21 and others with the normal number.

Action plan

Screening in pregnancy

Integrated screening for Down's syndrome is now a standard part of antenatal testing, using the 12-week (nuchal) ultrasound scan and a blood test (page 31). If these screening tests suggest a risk of Down's syndrome that is greater than 1 in 250 you will be offered an AMNIOCENTESIS or CVS, which enables your baby's chromosomes to be analysed, to give an accurate result. If you have had a previously affected baby or you are over 35 years old, you may choose amniocentesis without prior screening.

Many parents choose not to have the screening tests. If the screening result is positive you will be faced with a difficult decision. You will need support as you find out how having a

child with Down's syndrome might affect your family and about options for care. You may consider terminating pregnancy.

Screening after birth

If at birth your baby shows signs of Down's syndrome, your medical team will advise analysing chromosome 21 from a sample of your baby's blood. Awaiting the results is an anxious time and you will need support from your antenatal team, your friends and family. Whatever your feelings, it is likely to be beneficial for your baby to be lovingly held and attended to. This may be hard if you are nervous. You may wish to speak to other parents who have a child with Down's syndrome, or contact your local Down's syndrome support group: a member of the midwifery or support team in hospital may help you gather contact details.

Treatment and care

No specific treatment is available for babies with Down's syndrome, but your baby will be thoroughly examined to ensure she has no other physical problems. The best treatment is to receive love, attention and care and to be welcomed as part of the family. She will have a strong personality. The degree of learning difficulty often reflects the support a child receives, and early educational opportunities and loving encouragement will maximise her potential.

Your baby will need regular medical follow-up, usually given by a local community paediatrician who has a special interest in the condition. It is best to treat any hearing or visual problems before they hinder language development. About 10 per cent of babies with Down's syndrome are born with heart or intestinal malformations that may require surgery. They are also at increased risk of leukaemia, thyroid problems, hearing difficulties and chest infections, and you and your specialist paediatrician will be observant for any significant symptoms.

What is the risk of having another child with Down's syndrome?

In general the risk is age-related (page 30) and for women under 40 after having one child with Down's syndrome, the chance of having another baby with Down's syndrome is 1 per cent. After the age of 40 the risk rises. A geneticist and genetic counsellor (page 267) will be able to outline the chances of Down's recurring in your unique case.

Drinking

See Drugs, alcohol; Food and eating, mother.

Drugs

See also Medications.

Usually women who become pregnant are keen to avoid recreational drugs, knowing that they present health risks for them and their babies. But for some, stopping is not easy, not only because addictions are hard to kick, but because underlying emotions that contribute to the need for relief can be difficult to address. The advice in this section is addressed to women but applies to men as well. Although men do not carry their baby through pregnancy or breastfeed, the effect of drug use on their health and behaviour may have a profound impact on their family and children.

Pregnancy is an opportunity to give up drug use once and for all. If you give up during pregnancy, you may make a commitment to stop permanently.

What happens

The most widely used drugs are nicotine (cigarettes) and alcohol, and both threaten adult health and the health of a baby in the womb. Recreational drugs such as cocaine and amphetamines also carry risks. Medications are usually prescribed when the risks of a condition needing treatment are greater than any risk associated with the medication; but in some cases medicines such as valium can be addictive and/or threaten pregnancy or the health of a baby. Many babies and children inhale secondary smoke (passive smoking). When drug use has negative effects on mum or dad, young children often feel the effects on their emotions and their ability to form trusting relationships.

Antenatal care

Unfortunately, women with addictions often feel that the midwives and obstetricians caring for them have a flimsy grasp of the issues. Some mothers do not seek antenatal care, often because they feel guilty or worry they will not receive sympathetic treatment. Those who do confide in a medical team usually discover that such fears are unfounded, and receive support that continues after birth. In many hospitals there are specialist midwives to help with addiction issues that include alcohol and smoking, and when a team knows about drug use they are able to take the necessary care measures to reduce the risks to the baby.

Implications for a baby

The effect of drugs on a baby is directly proportional to the amount taken during pregnancy and will be combined with any adverse effects from other drugs, poor diet, inadequate or excessive exercise and high levels of physical and emotional stress. When drug use involves sharing implements there is a higher risk of infection, particularly with needles that can spread diseases such as HEPATITIS B and C and HIV. Many babies exposed to significant drug intake in the womb show withdrawal symptoms after birth (page 192) and reduced performance at school age.

Your feelings

When you become pregnant, there may be an internal battle between your desire to continue a drug and your wish to do the best for your baby. You may be afraid of feelings that could surface if you stop and it may seem easier to continue taking the drug than to feel vulnerable and afraid. If you have good intentions but it proves difficult to stop you may be angry with yourself or with the drug, or with people who you feel have made you do it; you may also feel guilty. Guilt and anger can both be defence mechanisms – they protect you from feeling pain and they hinder change. Everyone who gives up goes through these feelings.

Acknowledging your feelings may be the first step towards seeking a way out. You could keep a daily diary of your feelings around consumption. This will increase your awareness and help you look at practical ways to change. Most people find it easier to accept and express their feelings with a loving, supportive and non-judgemental person. A specialist midwife or a counsellor may offer you this chance.

◼ ACTION FOR QUITTING

The best thing to do is to stop drug consumption. The less you consume, the smaller the potential effect on your baby, and the better your own health. No matter how long you have been taking a drug, quitting will benefit your health. Remember, it will get easier as time goes by.

When you are pregnant, you do not have the luxury of time to phase out consumption. Stopping requires effort and commitment and you are more likely to be able to stop when you feel supported by other people. The steps outlined below may be useful. If drug use continues, it is best to let your medical team know so they can help you in the best interests of safety for you and your baby.

1. Consider getting help.
2. If your partner smokes or takes drugs, ask him to stop with you.
3. Set the quit date and stick to it. Don't have even one puff, one pill, one sip, one snort …
4.. If you smoke, get rid of all cigarettes and ashtrays. Do not hold or light cigarettes for anybody else. For any other drug, keep it out of your life and don't offer to buy, carry, hide or prepare it for anyone else.
5. Avoid the people, times and places where you used to use the drug. You may need to change your work environment if you typically smoke/drink/use at or after work. You could switch coffee to a fruit smoothie.
6. If you've tried before without success and you are still unable to quit, talk to your doctor or midwife or counsellor about useful medications. There are often risks associated with these, and it's important to weigh up the pros and cons for you personally.
7. Eat well including taking supplements (vitamins and minerals and omega essential fatty acids). Vitamin and mineral deficiencies are common in people who smoke, drink or take drugs and you may find that when your nutrition improves, your cravings fall.
8. Exercise, and try doing something active when the urge hits.
9. Explore ways of relaxing, such as meditation, YOGA and deep breathing (page 105).
10. Hypnotherapy, ACUPUNCTURE and homeopathy are among therapies that do help many people.

Withdrawal and relief

One of the key commitments for successfully giving up is to 'be in your feelings' and accept the discomfort of being upset or angry or afraid, restless, jittery or uncomfortable from physical symptoms of withdrawal. In the short term this can be very difficult, and you will need lots of support. In the long run you may feel stronger and more in touch with yourself.

Medical care

Your doctor can advise you about the type of drug you are using and safer alternatives for you and your baby. Nicotine replacement therapy doubles the quit rate for smoking but during pregnancy patches may be damaging for your baby, as are replacement drugs for opiates.

Support groups

Stopping drug use often requires medical support and emotional counselling or therapy. A quitting or support group may provide an environment where you are supported as you acknowledge and attempt to shake off your addiction. There are many options, including Alcoholics Anonymous and Narcotics Anonymous.

Homeopathy

Several remedies may reduce physical cravings and also help the emotional feelings associated with giving up. If you visit your homeopath, you will be prescribed specific remedies to suit your addiction, your resolve, your lifestyle and your individual symptoms. Broadly speaking, the following may be useful, and should be taken with further guidance from a qualified homeopath:

- For diminishing alcoholic cravings and to ease the accompanying emotional state of nervousness, indecision and tearfulness, *Quercus* may be used daily in a low potency (6x) over a period of time.

In addition, under the guidance of your homeopath, you may take the most appropriate remedy in a 6c potency morning and evening for up to two weeks and re-assess.

- *Nux Vomica* is a detox remedy for alcohol as well as drugs and may address the effects of withdrawal such as shaking, twitching, trembling and irritability.

- *Sulphur* is a detox remedy, particularly when energy and moods fluctuate.
- *Arsenicum* may deal with the effects of long-term alcohol use and general toxicity from drug use, and for someone who is usually chilly, pale and emaciated with extreme anxiety, restlessness and guilt.
- *Avena Sativa* calms the nervous system in cases of drug addiction where there is chronic insomnia, fatigue, poor concentration, palpitations and headaches.

Craving and slipping up

Most people slip up from time to time. Try to accept your addiction, acknowledge you gave in to your urges, and re-commit to keeping away from the drug. To make things easier, try not to rationalise – 'I have given up for a while and a small dose will make no difference.' This is not true because addictive drugs work on a physical level and your body will crave the drug if you take it again.

Try not to be upset when you feel a strong urge to smoke/drink/take your drug. Use deep-breathing techniques (page 105) and acknowledge your physical and emotional feelings. It may take weeks or months for your cravings to pass but they eventually do diminish.

ALCOHOL

'Can I drink while I'm pregnant?' is a very common question. The safest option for your baby is that you avoid alcohol in pregnancy as it may harm your unborn child. You may also want to avoid alcohol for a few months before conceiving. You may decide it's okay to drink a glass of wine or beer occasionally. The final choice is up to you. As more is being learnt about babies' sensitivities to environmental toxins such as alcohol and tobacco smoke in the womb, the advice from medical bodies such as the Royal College of Physicians, the Royal College of Paediatrics and Child Health, and the World Health Organization is that it is safest to steer clear of alcohol altogether while you are pregnant. If you are in the habit of drinking regularly and/or large amounts you may need support and encouragement to help you cut down (page 189).

What happens

Alcohol is a central nervous system depressant that affects nearly every organ in the human body. And because it acts on the pleasure centres of the brain, one of its effects may be to make you feel low and depressed. Drinking, especially heavy drinking over a period of time, can contribute to a number of serious problems, including muscle, brain and heart disease, malnutrition, and digestive and liver problems. While you are pregnant the main focus regarding alcohol may be on the potential effects for your baby (below), but it is worth bearing in mind that alcohol use may have wider effects for your physical and emotional health, and within your relationships. If alcohol use is chronic it may also have an impact on your work situation and family income. After birth when parents are under the influence of alcohol (or suffering from hangovers) this inevitably affects the attention a baby receives, and also has an impact on the family.

A unit of alcohol is equivalent to: half a pint of medium-strength beer (4% alcohol by volume, ABV); or a 125ml glass of wine (12% ABV); or a 25ml measure of spirits (40% ABV).

The 'recommended' maximum number of alcohol units per man/woman each day/week changes as new information about the effects comes to light. When you are pregnant the recommended intake for women is zero units – it is best not to drink. At other times if you do drink it's important to remember that the alcohol content of drinks can vary (for example, beers commonly range from 3–8% ABV, but can be higher) and to be aware of the effect alcohol has on you. Everyone reacts differently.

Alcohol in pregnancy

In pregnancy, alcohol easily crosses the placenta to reach a baby. Inside the womb a baby suffers the effects of alcohol with an intensity reflecting the amount mum drinks. A baby's liver has a very limited capacity for breaking down alcohol and eliminating toxins. Alcohol interferes with the baby's ability to obtain sufficient oxygen and nourishment for normal cell development, and for normal maturation of the central nervous system and this may hamper development of major organs, including the brain.

The potential effect increases with the amount consumed. A baby is probably more vulnerable in early pregnancy. Bingeing probably has a more intense effect than the same amount of alcohol taken over a few days. Many women drink after conception but before they are aware they are pregnant without apparent ill effects to the baby. The risk of damage increases with the amount consumed and the regularity of drinking.

If a baby has suffered long-term effects from alcohol, these may become evident in his behaviour and appearance, either immediately after birth, or some time in the pre-school years. Babies of mothers who drank more than two units a day during pregnancy are more likely to be restless or hyperactive and to have difficulties with speech and concentration. This can be more noticeable in boys, who may show more signs of stress throughout childhood. The effects of alcohol exposure may be more marked if a mother also smokes, consumes a lot of caffeinated drinks and lacks essential nutrients in her diet. There are two recognised degrees of symptoms: foetal alcohol effect (FAE) and FOETAL ALCOHOL SYNDROME (FAS).

Action plan

If you drink occasionally, as soon as you know you are pregnant, cut down or stop, whichever feels right to you. If this is difficult, you may need to replace your normal drink with something else that's equally tasty: a fruit drink or non-alcoholic wine or alcohol-free beer with food. If you drink to relax, try something else to help you wind down – a bath, a good read, a phone call to a friend, maybe a MASSAGE, meditation or deep-breathing exercises. If you use alcohol as a pick-me-up, altering your diet and focusing on good foods (page 253) may provide an alternative. Altering your taste in pregnancy may remain beneficial for years to come.

If you are a heavy drinker and giving up is a challenge, the guidance for overcoming addiction on page 189 may be helpful. Being honest about an addiction is the first step, and it is worth finding support as you face practical and emotional issues that underpin your habit. Confidential help may be available locally and there are telephone and internet organisations you can contact.

Foetal alcohol syndrome

Foetal alcohol syndrome (FAS) is a range of mental and physical characteristics resulting from exposure to alcohol in the womb. Cell development of a baby during pregnancy is affected by excess of alcohol, and significant impact may result in developmental delay, learning difficulties, impaired growth, abnormal functioning of the central nervous system, physical abnormalities of the face, and behavioural difficulties emerging in toddler, pre-school and childhood years. Poor school performance, attention deficit disorder (ADD) and hyperactivity are all more common in children affected by alcohol exposure. At least one in 750 babies born in the UK each year has signs of FAS, although the true number may be higher and FAS may be a leading cause of learning difficulties later in life.

The facial features of FAS are relatively easy to recognise, and include a head with a small circumference (microcephaly), low-set ears, thin upper lip, small chin, short upturned nose and smaller-than-usual eye openings. Some of these effects may be visible on ultrasound scans after 20 weeks of pregnancy. From birth, a baby may also show signs of alcohol withdrawal (overleaf) and symptoms may persist for months. The severity of the effect reflects the amount of alcohol a mother consumes and the duration of consumption. A related condition, foetal alcohol effect (FAE), results in a less severe set of the same symptoms.

Because no amount of alcohol is proven safe, the best prevention is to stop drinking immediately you suspect pregnancy. Foetal alcohol syndrome is 100 per cent preventable if the mother avoids alcohol during pregnancy. There is no way of reversing the physical damage; effects on behaviour may be reduced with loving and attentive care throughout childhood but any neurological damage may still have long-term consequences.

Support and treatment

Mothers whose babies show the effects of alcohol in pregnancy are often battling with an addiction and a number of practical and emotional difficulties. The greatest difficulties for their babies are usually social and emotional, reflecting the effects of alcohol and the family environment. The best way to tackle any problems and provide the best possible quality of life for a baby is for the parents and wider family to be supported and guided out of addiction and into a more positive way of living. This can be a difficult journey (page 189) needing ongoing support and advice from social services and other organisations. Many babies and children in an unsupportive or damaging social environment do require social services support, and sometimes fostering and adoption.

Babies and children with alcohol-related physical damage often need developmental follow-up and, possibly, long-term treatment with good medical and dental care, regular visual and hearing checks, and glasses or hearing aids if these are required. Heart abnormalities (page 288) may require surgery.

For many behavioural difficulties expert psychiatric, psychotherapeutic or psychological support, perhaps with appropriate medicines, can help. Involving the parents and children together is usually the most effective approach. For children with educational difficulties classroom support and statements are useful. Some children benefit from special school programmes.

■ NEONATAL ABSTINENCE SYNDROME

Neonatal abstinence syndrome (NAS) is the term used when a baby experiences withdrawal symptoms from drugs. The commonest drug for which withdrawal is a problem is nicotine (opposite). Some drugs are more likely to cause NAS. Opiates such as heroin and methadone cause withdrawal in over half of the babies exposed. This may occur with cocaine, too, but this drug causes more symptoms due to its effects on development in the womb. Amphetamines, barbiturates, caffeine, narcotics (heroin, morphine, methadone, dihydrocodeine) and benzodiazepines (temazepam) can also cause intense withdrawal. Foetal alcohol syndrome refers to withdrawal symptoms following alcohol use in pregnancy.

If your baby is exposed to a drug, addiction begins in the womb and dependence continues after birth. When the drug is no longer available, his central nervous system becomes over-stimulated. The symptoms of withdrawal vary depending on the drug and the quantity used, and whether your baby has been born prematurely. They may begin 24 hours after birth or not until 10 days or even later, and could last for months. Problems tend to result from the combined effect of drug exposure in pregnancy and withdrawal after birth.

Symptoms

If your baby is suffering from withdrawal he may be hard to soothe. The most common symptoms of NAS are:
- tremors (trembling),
- irritability (excessive and high-pitched crying),
- sleep problems,
- hyperactive reflexes,
- fits/seizures,
- stuffy nose and sneezing,
- poor feeding and suck,
- vomiting and/or diarrhoea,
- sweating and unstable temperature.

Treatment

Skin-to-skin contact is usually very helpful, and your baby may feel rested and secure when he is swaddled. Medical treatment will be directed by your paediatrician and your baby will benefit from gentle loving care and touch. If you do not feel able to give this, particularly if you are struggling with an addiction yourself, having another adult carer is important for your baby. Some babies may need to be admitted to a special care unit for treatment. Homeopathy offers support and needs to be prescribed on an individual basis.

The long-term effects of NAS reflect the degree of exposure in the womb and the drug used, as well as withdrawal treatment. Exposure in the womb does present a risk of life-long symptoms such as inattentiveness and poor language skills, and drug addiction in adolescence or adulthood tends to be more common. Sudden infant death syndrome is also much more frequently encountered in this vulnerable group of infants (page 503). Your baby's environment and the love, support and nutrition he receives from you and other carers, particularly in the first two years, heavily influence the long-term outlook. Practical and emotional support for you individually or as a family may keep the potential negative effects of drug exposure and NAS to a minimum.

■ RECREATIONAL DRUGS

Recreational drugs can have potential risks for you and your baby and are best avoided. There are details of the implications and motivations behind drug use, together with tips for quitting, on page 189. The list below outlines the more common recreational drugs.

The most significant regularly used drugs are alcohol and nicotine. Both can have implications if consumed in pregnancy, and are covered separately (pages 190 and below).

Amphetamine (speed)

This drug can have a very intense effect on your baby. It causes severe constriction of your blood vessels and reduces oxygen for your unborn baby. It increases the risk of placental abruption (page 444), PREMATURE BIRTH, intrauterine growth restriction (IUGR) and stillbirth. It also suppresses your appetite, potentially reducing nutrition for your baby.

Caffeine

Caffeine intake has been linked with an increased risk of MISCARRIAGE and small babies (IUGR). In addition, when you consume caffeine in tea, coffee, colas, energy drinks or chocolate, your baby feels the same effects as you do and if you consume high quantities your baby may experience withdrawal after birth. During the second half of pregnancy, caffeine is cleared very slowly from your body and this is the time to reduce the intake substantially.

Cannabis/marijuana

This is the most common recreational drug used by pregnant women. Usually it is mixed with nicotine before being smoked, and nicotine increases the risks. Consumed alone, cannabis may be linked to IUGR and other effects on your baby. Many forms of cannabis are now regarded as being as hazardous for mother and baby as amphetamine, cocaine and heroin and alcohol.

Cocaine and crack

These constrict blood vessels, reducing oxygen flow to your baby, and have a major effect on brain and body development in the womb. The effects may be worse than heroin. Cocaine suppresses appetite so you may not provide adequate nutrition for your unborn baby. Regular use carries a high chance of congenital abnormality of the heart, intestine, brain or limbs (35 per cent) and of IUGR (30 per cent). There is also risk of miscarriage, placental abruption and stillbirth, and of premature birth because cocaine stimulates uterine contractions. Where brain growth has been affected there may be slow mental development for life. It may also be connected with sudden infant death syndrome (page 503).

Heroin and methadone (opiates)

These cross the placenta and increase the risk of death in-utero and premature birth. There may be slow mental development for life. A baby's withdrawal symptoms can be severe, often coming on a few days after birth and lasting weeks (opposite).

■ SMOKING

The risks of smoking to adults and to unborn and young babies are widely known, but nicotine is extremely addictive and 25 per cent of adults in the UK smoke cigarettes. Smoking is a common reason for a pregnancy to be high-risk, and maternal smoking remains the largest cause of premature birth, low birth weight (IUGR), disability and death. It has also been linked with an increased risk of late miscarriage and placental abruption (page 444). Although it is a difficult habit to break, the effects associated with smoking are preventable if you stop: pregnancy may provide a strong motivation to quit.

What happens

Everyone knows that smoking can permanently damage health, and in pregnancy, every inhalation reduces the blood flowing to your baby. Smoking in pregnancy and passive smoking after birth can have significant long-term effects on your baby. The negative effects of smoking are markedly increased if you drink alcohol or you do not have an adequate intake of calories, vitamins and minerals and essential fatty acids.

The effect of smoking on you and your baby

is directly related to the number of cigarettes you smoke and how deeply you inhale to get the nicotine effect. Passive smoking where you or your baby inhale other people's smoke by being in the same room also carries risks.

In pregnancy

In pregnancy, smoking causes spasm of your arteries supplying the placenta with oxygen and this reduces the blood flow to your baby. The nicotine and carbon monoxide you inhale reach your baby and further diminish nutrients and oxygen. This may have intense effects on your baby. Nicotine consumption can affect mental development in later life and predispose a child to take up smoking.

After birth

Smoking in pregnancy, and if you continue after birth, puts your baby at higher risk of sudden infant death (page 503) and COLIC, ASTHMA, flu, COUGHS and bronchitis, with each infection or illness lasting longer than average. This also applies to babies who inhale secondary smoke (passive smoking) from other smokers in the home. The odds of developing asthma are twice as high among children whose mothers smoke more than 10 cigarettes a day. Intellectual development may also be reduced, as there may be a noticeable effect on growth and on achievement at school, years after birth. Exposure to cigarette smoke in infancy is also linked with a greater likelihood that your child will become a smoker himself – an addiction before birth can prove hard to shrug. If you smoke very heavily in pregnancy, your newborn baby may suffer from neonatal abstinence syndrome (page 192) as he withdraws from the drug.

If your baby is being exposed to smoke, this carries all the risks associated with actively smoking. The more smoke in the atmosphere, the greater the risk. It is always better to keep your house a smoke-free zone and avoid taking your baby into smoky atmospheres. If you smoke, your baby ingests nicotine in your breast milk.

Action plan

Nicotine is one of the hardest drug habits to kick – it is a highly addictive substance yet it is more socially acceptable than many other drugs (although this is changing). The advice for

quitting on page 189 may help you stop, and it might be useful to join a local or national group. Acupuncture and hypnotherapy are thought to be very effective. You may need a great deal of support and will power. Even after years some ex-smokers still feel tempted. Remember, it is possible to stop and it is always worth it.

Dummies

Opinion has been divided over dummies for many years. Some parents give a dummy to their children from birth, while others are adamant that dummies won't feature at all. The usual parental concerns are:

• Will giving my baby a dummy make my life harder?
• Is a dummy good for my baby?

Your baby's need to suck

Your baby will not ask for a dummy – she doesn't know such a thing exists – but she has a strong reflex to suck and the action is familiar from sucking her hands and fingers in the womb. She may enjoy sucking and ask frequently for your breast, both for food and comfort. Sucking eases discomfort in her head, ears or mouth. It is also important for normal mouth development, and if your baby has a high narrow palate she may be more inclined to suck.

Sucking a dummy doesn't give your baby the sense of intimacy and loving touch she gets from skin-to-skin contact at your breast. Nor does it have the same benefits for your baby's head and jaw. It may be a useful complement to BREASTFEEDING, however, especially if your baby loves to suck and does not get satisfaction from her fingers.

Possible consequences for your baby

It is important to have a dummy sterilised regularly, otherwise there is a risk of picking up an infection. Whether sucking a dummy (or fingers or thumbs) has any other negative, long-term effects depends on each individual. For one baby, sucking may help to correct a postural imbalance or improve the rhythmic flow of cranial fluids, assist the development of nasal breathing and the pattern of tongue movements in a beneficial way. This baby will probably suck whatever she can. A baby may also develop the habit of sucking or chewing when she is upset. Self-soothing through sucking is a good skill to develop.

Excessive sucking may eventually alter the position of teeth and the growth and development of the jaw. Possible results include a reduced nasal airway space, which can lead to or aggravate breathing difficulties and may be linked with tonsil or adenoid problems in childhood, and with sleep disruption in adulthood.

If you are at all concerned, it is worth visiting a dentist who can advise you about your unique child. On balance, the advice may be that in terms of your baby's teeth and jaw development it's okay to suck now, but best to wean her off the dummy, thumb or finger by the age of four or five.

Using a dummy for peace and quiet

If sucking on a dummy helps your baby settle, this may also provide some peace and quiet for you. This can be a huge relief if your baby cries a lot. You may choose not to have a dummy from birth, but decide to introduce a dummy later on. Some babies have a dummy from time to time, almost like a plaything, or it may be a way to break the dependence on the breast or bottle each night to get off to sleep.

A dummy isn't always the best route to contentment. Your baby cries for many different reasons (page 166) and there may be times when a dummy gives temporary respite but does not satisfy her needs, for example, to feed, play, communicate or relieve pain. Although a dummy cannot 'plug' a baby into silence – your baby will still cry or shout when she has a powerful need to communicate – it may sometimes work like comfort food, soothing and distracting from true needs. Using a dummy inappropriately may send the message that her needs are not important. In the long run, it may even make things more difficult for you. For example, it may give temporary calm when she wakes from hunger at night, but this may be followed by angry screaming that makes it difficult for her to settle for a feed when the dummy no longer placates her.

Only you and your baby can judge whether her needs are being met. To make an informed choice, it is best to keenly observe your baby and your own reactions to her behaviour. Often the need for a dummy rests with the parents rather than with the baby. Using a dummy may quieten your baby's expression of her feelings (page 207), and you may feel less discomfort in response to her CRYING or frequent demands for contact. If you suspect you may be avoiding your own uncomfortable feelings, or your baby's pressing needs, the suggestions on page 208 may help you remain present for your baby and for yourself, whatever she is expressing.

Weaning off the dummy

Sometimes dependence could present difficulties, for example, if you lose the dummy or have to give it to your baby in the middle of the night. Weaning off the dummy may require considerable patience, although some babies stop of their own accord with little fuss. If you want to reduce dependence, begin during the day. You may be able to encourage your baby to suck her hands or fingers instead. She may object, but the transition may be over within five days. It is up to you both to see how it goes.

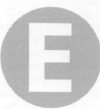

Ear infection and pain, baby

Ear pain, which may or may not be caused by ear infection, can make your baby very distressed. Ear infections are one of the most common reasons children see a doctor. Only rarely do they have serious consequences.

What happens

Ear pain may be part of an ear infection, and if so, your baby may have a high temperature, be restless, tug at or hit her ears, have a runny nose or a cough, shake her head and seem reluctant to suck. This group of symptoms may relate to other causes of discomfort, such as teething or a common cold (page 155). If hearing (page 286) seems to be affected, the cause may be glue ear (page 198). The only way to diagnose ear infection is to have your child's ear checked by a doctor.

Pain in or around the ear could be due to:
- An infection in the middle ear cavity (otitis media) when the middle ear is filled with mucus and pus. If tension builds up it may rupture the eardrum (below) and the ear will ooze some blood-streaked pus.
- A blockage in the Eustachian tube leading from the middle ear to the back of the nose. This causes a pressure build-up and pain behind the eardrum. It is similar to the pain that many people experience during a flight.
- Teething or a toothache or gum problem where pain travels to the ear.
- An infection in the external ear canal – otitis externa – also known as 'swimmer's ear'.

- A scratched ear canal or pain from a foreign object in the ear (such as a bead, stone or insect). This is rare under one year of age.
- Extremely rarely, an underlying meningitis infection may cause ear pain, also with fever, stiffened neck, and a rash that does not fade when a glass is pressed on to the skin.

Ear wax

Ear wax keeps the ear canals clean. It is a sticky substance that coats the ear canal and traps any dirt or foreign objects. The wax accumulates and works its way out towards the outer ear. If wax gets wet, it expands and may gently touch the eardrum and hinder its movement. This is why water in the ear seems to affect hearing and balance. As the wax dries under the influence of body heat, hearing returns to normal.

The only reason that wax may need to be removed from a baby's ear is so that the eardrum can be looked at during a medical examination. It is not done to improve hearing. It is dangerous to poke around in a baby's ear, and cotton-wool buds are only appropriate to use for cleaning the outside, never the inside of the ear.

Ruptured eardrum

If your baby has had symptoms of ear pain and a white or yellow pus-like fluid, possibly streaked with blood, drains from the ear canal, the cause may be perforated eardrum resulting from a middle ear infection. The perforation results in relief of the pressure on the sensitive middle ear structures and the infection drains out and resolves. The eardrum may heal in a few days with no trace of a scar and totally normal function. Occasionally, the eardrum may scar and reduce hearing. During this time some specialists recommend no swimming, as the healing eardrum should be kept dry.

The ability of the eardrum to heal without complication led many doctors in the past to use a tiny knife to slit the eardrum to relieve pressure and pain. This cured the infection and the bacteria involved could be identified from a culture. The practice is being re-introduced increasingly in modern medicine because of concerns regarding antibiotic resistance of the bacteria that cause middle ear infections, although this is still uncommon. Usual practice is to observe for 48 hours and to give antibiotics only if high temperature has not lowered.

Action plan

It is not always easy to know whether a baby actually has ear pain. If your baby seems uncomfortable, soothe her, offer drinks and you may give infant paracetamol (page 429) to reduce the pain and high temperature. Visit your GP if symptoms are severe or last longer than three or four days.

Medical care

* A small minority of doctors advocate treating all ear infections with antibiotics since there is a very small risk that an infection may worsen and infect bone surrounding the middle ear, or even the tissues surrounding the brain (meningitis).
* Most doctors believe no treatment aside from pain control is required for the first three days because 85 per cent of infections clear by themselves and many are caused by viruses (which do not respond to antibiotics). Avoiding them in the initial stages prevents the unnecessary use of antibiotics for most children.

Diet

The mucus-producing effect of cow's milk is so well known that many parents and paediatricians remove cow's milk from the diet of a baby or infant who is prone to chronic ear infections. Substitution of a cow's milk-based formula for either a cow's milk-based hydrolysed formula, or, in older children, a soya-based formula can be a very effective, and relatively simple, treatment. If the child is weaned then avoiding cow's milk-based solids, often with a dietician's advice, will help. About 30 per cent of children with ear infections have an allergy or intolerance and in most cases the allergen is cow's milk. Reactions include nasal congestion and sore throat, and when the passages become blocked and irritated, ear infection often follows. A very high proportion of children with chronic ear pain improve when cow's milk is taken out of their diet. If you breastfeed your baby, she will be at a far smaller risk of developing ear problems. Your breast milk will have a protective effect.

Complementary care

Many people feel alternatives to conventional medicine have significantly helped their children, particularly when there have been several ear infections and no improvement, despite orthodox medical treatment. These include homeopathy, herbal medicine, craniosacral osteopathy and acupuncture.

Homeopathy

Homeopathy may be a highly effective treatment for acute ear infections and ongoing ear problems, and may address numerous symptoms that may be linked with ear pain. Even if an ear infection is self-limiting, homeopathy may help to relieve symptoms and boost recovery.

When pain comes on suddenly or is acute, treatment is most effective if begun early with the most appropriate remedy (30c potency) hourly for four hours before re-assessing. The symptoms may change, and then a different remedy will be more suitable. Once the acute stage is passed, you may give the most appropriate remedy three times a day for two or three days. If your baby has chronic pain or recurrent episodes, it would be advisable to ask your homeopath for a constitutional remedy that would deal with the underlying susceptibility to ear infections, and for advice on treatment during the acute stage.

* *Aconite* at the onset of earache with sudden symptoms, possibly around midnight when your baby screams in pain, is hot, frantic, anxious and restless and may have a dry cough and NASAL CONGESTION.
* *Belladonna* for sudden onset, high fever, a flushed, hot face and head, perhaps dilated pupils and glazed eyes, the affected ear looks red – usually the right side – and your baby is worse for light and movement.

- *Chamomilla* for earache that accompanies teething where the ears look red, one cheek is red and the other pale, your baby is irritable, alternating from temper tantrums to miserable weeping, wants something and then refuses it, hates being examined and feels better for being carried.
- *Pulsatilla* for ear pain, perhaps worse on the left, swollen glands, nasal congestion with thick yellowish mucus, when your baby is clingy, weepy, whiney, feels worse in a warm stuffy environment and in the evenings. This is an excellent remedy for lingering ear problems.
- *Hepar Sulph* at the established stage of an ear infection if there are few distinguishing characteristics or if your baby's ears are extremely sensitive. Your baby is irritable, reluctant to be touched, feeling cold and clearly in considerable pain.
- *Mercurius* for recurrent ear infections where ear pain tends to be accompanied by a sore throat, swollen lymph nodes (glands) and bad breath and profuse sweating at night, excess salivation. The ear may produce a gluey, pussy, yellow/green, smelly discharge.

▇ GLUE EAR

Glue ear (also known as chronic secretory otitis media) is a condition in which thick sticky fluid collects in the middle ear, causing impaired hearing or temporary hearing loss. It affects up to 20 per cent of children and can lead to ear pain and may develop into acute otitis media. Glue ear usually occurs between the ages of two and five years, but can affect babies, particularly those who are prone to ALLERGY, have a CLEFT PALATE or live with adults who smoke.

What happens

Hearing loss is the most common symptom of glue ear, because sound waves are not conducted properly through the blockage. Without early detection and treatment this could lead to a delay in speech development. Normally, each ear is ventilated by a Eustachian tube, a channel running from the middle ear to the back of the nose. If the tube is blocked or fails to function, fluid can accumulate. If your baby develops a viral infection with a cold, it may spread to the ear – as nose, throat and ear are close together. Young

children are more susceptible than adults because the Eustachian tube is smaller and so is more easily blocked, and their adenoids (lymph tissue at the back of the nose where the Eustachian tubes open) are more likely to become enlarged.

Action plan

Diagnosis
Your doctor may conduct a number of tests.
- Audiometry measures hearing across a range of frequencies and there are special techniques for babies.
- Otoscopy involves looking at the eardrum with a hand-held instrument to look for bubbles of trapped fluid. It is also possible to check the pressure in the eardrum.
- Tympanometry assesses how the eardrum moves in response to sound, but it does not directly measure hearing. It is a useful test even in babies under one year old.

Treatment
Glue ear requires treatment in only around 10 per cent of cases. Of the remainder, around 50 per cent of cases get better on their own within three months, 25 per cent within six months, and 15 per cent within 12 months. If your child has frequent earache or may be at risk of developing speech problems, she may benefit from treatment. Some doctors advise a period of three months to watch for improvement before considering surgical treatment.

Surgical treatment for persistent glue ear is the insertion of grommets (in one or both ears). These are tiny tubes that are inserted into the eardrum to allow air to pass freely between the middle ear and the outside, and so equalise the pressure. First, a small incision is made in the eardrum to release most of the fluid and relieve the pressure and then the grommet is inserted. The operation is performed under a general anaesthetic as a day-case, and afterwards most children have near-normal hearing. The change can be quite dramatic. Many children who need grommets have enlarged adenoids too, so they may benefit if the adenoids are surgically removal (adenoidectomy) at the same time.

The grommets are usually kept in place for three to 12 months, after which they fall out or are removed. If they remain in place for too long this could lead to permanent perforation of the eardrum. The eardrum usually heals quickly after grommets have been removed. If they fall out prematurely or glue ear recurs, your child may need to have them reinserted. It is fine to swim with grommets but diving, when she is older, is not advised as the pressure may force water into the middle ear.

Other treatments

- Some experts advocate a long course of antibiotics (two to four weeks or more). This may treat the infection but does not necessarily avoid the need for grommets, especially if both ears are affected. Corticosteroids do not help.
- Some ear-nose-and-throat specialists recommend decongestant medicines containing pseudoephedrine. These are sometimes effective, although they can have side effects and the blockage can be worse when the drug effect wears off.
- If there is no improvement in hearing from inserting grommets hearing aids might be considered – usually if the hearing is so reduced that language development is delayed.

Homeopathy

The following remedies are commonly used to treat glue ear. You may choose an appropriate remedy to give in 6c potency morning and evening for one week and re-assess. In most cases, however, it would be more beneficial to consult your homeopath, who can recommend a treatment that suits your child's specific symptoms:

- *Kali Mur* for chronic catarrh with pain, hearing loss and swollen lymph nodes ('lymph glands').
- *Hydrastis* to encourage drainage of fluid when mucus is thick, yellow and stringy.
- *Mercurius* if your child has glue ear and is congested, with enlarged adenoids and/or tonsils, smelly breath and mouth breathing.

Ear piercing

If you wish to have your baby's ears pierced, it is worth considering the safety issues and the small risk of infection. With these in mind, it is better to wait until the age of four. Sharing this 'developmental milestone' with your child later might be more enjoyable.

- Minimise the infection risk by ensuring all equipment is sterile, keeping the initial ear posts in for about six weeks, cleaning the ear by rubbing it with alcohol daily, and making sure the clasp is not too tight.
- If the ear becomes red, pus forms around the site, or a fever occurs, contact your doctor. The first step in treatment is to remove the earring and allow the hole to heal.
- Sometimes a scar or keloid leaves a bump at the piercing site. If you have a family history of keloid formation, it is probably best to delay/avoid piercing.
- Contact dermatitis (allergy) may occur if your child has a metal allergy. Using gold or hypo-allergenic stainless steel posts may help to avoid this problem.
- Younger children tend to play with earrings and breathing in an earring is the most concerning danger related to piercing. Use studs or earrings that lie flush against the skin – hoops or hanging rings increase the risk of harm.

Ear shapes

Some babies are born with unusually shaped ears. Sometimes the shape is a result of pressure in the womb or during birth, or it may be genetic (and perhaps referred to as 'the family ear'). Usually the shape is of no consequence, either because it naturally becomes less pronounced or is simply part of individual appearance, and nothing needs to be done. However, there are times when treatment is sought or recommended. After birth, your baby's ear shape may alter if her head always rests on the same side as she sleeps.

The commonest reasons to seek help are minor changes, such as ears that seem to stick out more than is usual, a condition called 'bat ear'. Other ear shapes that may be regarded as in need of treatment include folded or lop ears, where the ear is folded down on itself, usually from pressure in the womb. Sometimes the outer rim of the ear is kinked, or cupped, or the outer folds seem to start well into the scalp, and the ear appears partly hidden, a condition called cryptotia.

All these are considered normal variants, and whether treatment is sought or not depends on the severity of the condition and parental preference.

Action plan

A recent innovation, the 'ear buddy', has proved to be an effective way of bringing about a significant correction without surgery. The ear buddy is a plastic-coated spring that, when worn continuously from within three months of birth, can quickly and effectively restore ear shape. It can be used in older children, and even in adults, but the treatment takes longer.

In some cases, plastic surgery is more appropriate. If this is an option for your baby, the best age for the operation is around one year old. The precise timing will be determined by your wishes, the advice of the surgeon, and the opinion of the anaesthetist. Usually surgery is complete before the child starts school.

Very rarely, there are conditions where an ear is absent, or severely malformed, with the malformation including the ear canal and middle ear. When this happens, expert genetic advice in addition to a plastic surgical opinion is important.

Eating difficulties, mother

See also Emotions; Food and eating, mother; Weight, mother.

Many women of all ages feel uncomfortable about their weight or body image and have pre-existing eating difficulties before conception. Pregnancy and parenthood will affect your relationship with food. It may be an opportunity for positive change, or it may intensify your habits. Pregnancy is a common time for excess weight gain to begin.

Some people move from one eating difficulty to another. For many people, greater awareness of the physical and emotional issues, combined with loving support, facilitates positive change. For a small minority, an eating difficulty is severe and it may be very difficult to change.

Implications in pregnancy and beyond

Being over- or underweight means you are not as healthy or energetic as you could be. You may also compromise your baby's nutrition in the womb. The risks are most serious if you were underweight and poorly nourished before conception. The emotional element may make it harder for you to enjoy a close relationship with your baby and your partner and to celebrate your skills as a parent.

What lies behind an eating disorder?

Many factors can contribute to eating disorders.

- Abnormal levels of brain chemicals may be linked with anxiety, perfectionism, and obsessive-compulsive thoughts and behaviours reflected in eating.
- Eating difficulties are often an expression of emotional dissatisfaction and low self-esteem (page 72).
- The roots of food issues can often be traced back to teenage experiences and the earliest encounters with food in infancy (page 258). New feelings about yourself and your body arising in parenthood may be very significant.
- An eating difficulty may be a sign of DEPRESSION.
- An eating disorder may be associated with alcohol or DRUG abuse, particularly with bulimia. Sometimes the addiction may be to laxatives, enemas and appetite suppressants, all of which carry risks in pregnancy.

ANOREXIA

Anorexia involves severe weight loss and is defined as being below 85 per cent of the expected weight for height and being afraid of gaining weight. The BMI (body mass index, page 564) is usually below 18. Despite the low weight, most anorexic women feel fat. Severe anorexia is life-threatening and professional help is essential.

Many anorexia healthcare specialists recommend delaying pregnancy until the illness is in remission. But because severe anorexia greatly reduces the chance of conception, this is an issue for only a very small number of women. The majority of anorexic women who successfully treat their eating disorder regain their ability to conceive.

When anorexia and pregnancy coincide, the risks to pregnancy are considerable. This eating disorder poses the most serious threat to pregnancy, particularly when present before conception. It can lead to maternal ANAEMIA, exhaustion and DEPRESSION. It may inhibit a baby's growth and development because of insufficient weight, poor nutrition, and vitamin and mineral deficiencies. Other risks for a baby include MISCARRIAGE, CONGENITAL ABNORMALITIES, INTRAUTERINE GROWTH RESTRICTION and PREMATURE BIRTH. The risks increase if laxatives and emetics are used. After the birth, exhaustion and depression often continue, although if you are able to breastfeed you may feel good about nourishing your child.

■ BULIMIA NERVOSA

Bulimia nervosa is defined as a pattern of eating excessively and purging by self-induced vomiting or enemas or the use of diet pills, laxatives and diuretics. Bulimia is becoming increasingly common and it can alternate with anorexia.

Occasional vomiting does not damage your health. Vomiting frequently may cause inflammation of your oesophagus (food pipe), tooth decay and gum disease. Frequent vomiting depletes your tissues of water, vitamins and minerals, causing abnormal heart rhythms and muscle spasms. If bulimia alternates with excessive weight gain, this will carry its own risks (page 566).

Most women with bulimia have a normal pregnancy and birth, although there may be discomfort from heartburn and abdominal pain, and dehydration symptoms such as weakness, fatigue and headaches. There is also a high risk of depression. Bulimia also increases the risk of miscarriage and premature birth. Laxatives and purgatives may also affect a baby in the womb and pass to a baby in breast milk.

■ COMPULSIVE OVEREATING (BINGE EATING)

Compulsive overeating (binge eating) is an 'addiction' to food. Very often the compulsion to binge reflects a deep need to be loved. Binge eating may occur in fits and starts when you are faced with difficulties and you feel stressed or it may be your way of life. People who overeat tend to be overweight but some control their weight gain by vomiting, over-exercising or taking laxatives. Pregnancy may

herald the onset of binge eating and it may be masked by normal weight gain or excused as a craving. Binge eating may be most intense after the birth if you are feeling lonely or isolated.

Action plan

Pregnancy brings an urgent need to attend to an eating problem and may be a catalyst for acknowledging some difficult emotions. Many women are taken by surprise that they have an eating disorder, particularly if it begins in pregnancy. The closer you are to a normal body weight, the safer it is for you and your baby.

It is very difficult to step out of destructive eating patterns without help. The first step is to confide in your friends and tell your medical team – this is the best way to be effectively supported. You may feel guilty, but your behaviour towards food and many of your persistent emotions have roots in your early life experiences, when you were too young to reason or to exercise control. With other people's encouragement, you may find it gradually easier to be loving and gentle with yourself as you explore your habits, and try out new ways of being around food. You will be able to try, stumble, fall back into a pattern and emerge again.

If the issue is severe, your doctor or midwife may recommend emotional support and therapy with an experienced professional. The process can be enormously helpful. As you look at your in-built responses to situations, your family background, your anxieties and self-image, you begin a recovery process. It may take considerable time for your habits and feelings to change, so patience is essential.

Medical and complementary care

* Not all eating disorders need medical care although in pregnancy regular meetings with your midwife may be an encouraging source of friendly and helpful advice.
* If your eating patterns are linked with depression you may benefit from professional support (page 176).
* If you have been using enemas or laxatives, ask your doctor for advice because they are dangerous in pregnancy. Try to reduce use and

to substitute natural foods such as linseeds to help your bowel movements. It may take up to three weeks for your body to respond.

- Many alternative therapies, including hypnotherapy, can be helpful. It is important to consult practitioners who are experienced in dealing with eating disorders.

Eating and weight control

Maintaining a healthy weight gain in pregnancy and an appropriate weight after birth will be easier if there is someone you can turn to who acknowledges your progress and helps you accept times when you are unable to reach your goal.

- You may use the general nutrition advice on pages 253–65.
- If you build up skills to maintain healthy eating during pregnancy, you will find it easier to continue these after birth.
- If you recognise the triggers for your eating habit, try to eliminate them.
- If you tend to buy binge food while out, it may be helpful to limit the time you have alone or the amount of money you carry.
- If you cannot give up vomiting or purging, try to delay it until your body has digested some of the food you have eaten.
- If you tend to binge after eating a normal meal, try washing up immediately and throw away all leftovers. This will keep you busy for those difficult first minutes after eating. If your mum found it impossible to throw out leftovers, or you were pressurised never to waste anything, you may find this challenging. Give it a go and see what happens.

Practical and lifestyle issues

The most important step is to let other people know how you're feeling and about the factors that trigger your habit. People who love and care for you will be pleased to help. The practical tips on page 123 may be relevant.

With your baby, after the birth

Your eating disorder might surface strongly after the birth when physical and emotional demands increase and you are caring for your baby day and night.

- It is important to continue with the strategies that helped you in pregnancy (such as appropriate EXERCISE, visiting a counsellor).

- You will find it easier to cope with your baby and with your own feelings if you have practical help.
- Try to take time to be with your baby and let yourself love and feel loved.
- Many women find BREASTFEEDING an important part of the recovery process.
- Your baby may be your best teacher, showing you how to recognise hunger signals and to stop eating when you feel full.
- At night when you are up with your baby and it is quiet you will need a lot of self-control if you feel an urge coming on, either to binge, purge or starve yourself.
- You may find VISUALISATIONS help you to relax.

If you slip back into a destructive pattern

If you do slip up, try to view the incident as a learning experience. A slip doesn't have to lead to a relapse, and a relapse doesn't have to lead to total collapse. Ask yourself what was happening that caused you to resort to a familiar coping device. Remember, it is okay to slip up and you can commit to trying again. Don't forget the support network around you.

Eating, mother

See Food and eating, mother.

Ectopic pregnancy

In an ectopic pregnancy, the fertilised egg implants outside the uterus, usually in one of the fallopian tubes. As the embryo develops, the placenta burrows through the thin walls of the tube and there is bleeding into the pelvis and abdominal cavity. The bleeding may be intense and cause severe pain and shock. This is a life-threatening emergency.

An ectopic pregnancy occurs in 1 per cent of pregnancies, but the rate is rising with fertility treatment. Other than in exceptionally rare circumstances, where the placenta implants outside the uterus in the pelvic cavity (in an extra-uterine pregnancy), the baby cannot survive.

Discovering that you have an ectopic pregnancy can be harrowing. Most women need continuing support as they absorb the news and choose the best course of action. Both expectant parents may go through a period of grief, sadness and mourning, often mixed with a sense of relief that the condition was detected and treated.

Pain

Almost every ectopic pregnancy is accompanied by pain, usually beginning from the affected fallopian tube and felt on one side of the lower abdomen. It may last for hours and stop and start as blood is released and reabsorbed. If bleeding is profuse, pain will spread and get much worse.

✚ Red flag

Shock

Losing blood from your circulation into your abdomen may induce shock. Symptoms may include weakness, light-headedness and shivering. If this happens, the situation is a life-threatening emergency requiring medical attention: call an ambulance.

Bleeding

Menstrual periods may stop with an ectopic pregnancy but occasionally bleeding occurs at the expected time. The menstrual bleed may be heavier and more prolonged than usual because the lining of the uterus is thickened by the pregnancy hormones released by the ectopic. Bleeding may be irregular and may raise concern about a threatened MISCARRIAGE.

Minimal symptoms

Symptoms may be minimal at first. If you have pain or spotting, a scan at Weeks 6 to 8 may reveal the ectopic pregnancy before it ruptures, causing internal bleeding. If the pregnancy receives too little blood in your fallopian tube, it will be absorbed. Modern ultrasound scans show that ectopic pregnancies can and do occur without causing symptoms.

Causes

Some ectopic pregnancies occur without any apparent reason. Certain conditions can increase

the risk, although it is important to remember that ectopic pregnancy is still unlikely. Risk factors include:

- Previous infection with scarring of the fallopian tube, usually caused by chlamydia.
- Previous surgery to the fallopian tube, with scarring (this includes a previous ectopic pregnancy).
- Becoming pregnant when an intrauterine contraceptive device (IUD) is in place, or while using the progesterone-only mini pill. These may affect the rate the ovum travels in the tube.
- With in-vitro fertilisation (IVF) and intrauterine insemination (IUI), the incidence of ectopic pregnancy is 4 per cent.
- Women over 35 years of age are at slightly increased risk.

Action plan

An ectopic pregnancy is a serious and potentially life-threatening condition that is best treated by early diagnosis and either 'conservative' or operative care. If you have pelvic pain, feel faint or suspect an ectopic pregnancy because of irregular bleeding or a positive pregnancy test, contact your doctor immediately.

Diagnosis

- The ectopic pregnancy can be visualised during an internal ultrasound scan using a probe placed in your vagina. An internal vaginal examination is not accurate.
- In the first 14 days after your first missed period, the ectopic pregnancy is small and may be difficult to see on a scan. The scan may need to be repeated the following week.
- Your GP or specialist can request an urgent blood pregnancy test detecting human chorionic gonadotrophin (HCG) levels. In a normal pregnancy, the HCG levels double every three or four days. A slower rise indicates pregnancy failure, either an ectopic pregnancy or an impending miscarriage. If HCG is not detected on the blood test an ectopic pregnancy is unlikely and your pain is from another cause, possibly from the area where you ovulated and released an egg this cycle.

Conservative care

If the ectopic pregnancy is seen to be small on an ultrasound scan (detected before Week 8) and the levels of HCG are low and rising slowly, the placenta may stop functioning. When this happens, the ectopic pregnancy will be absorbed by your body and there will be no need for an operation. This is 'conservative care'.

- If your hospital has the facilities, it is safe to observe progress with follow-up scans and HCG blood tests every two or three days. The scans show the pregnancy sac getting smaller but it may take up to 10 weeks to disappear and be reabsorbed.
- When conservative treatment is an option, you will have a higher chance of conceiving again and less likelihood of an ectopic pregnancy occurring in the future. Against this, there is the disadvantage of uncertainty as you wait to see whether surgery is needed.
- Many women prefer conservative care when it is an option, even though the waiting period can be emotionally difficult and pregnancy hormones remain in your system until the ectopic pregnancy is completely reabsorbed.
- It is possible to speed up natural absorption by injecting a powerful cytotoxic drug (methotrexate, used for the treatment of cancer) that travels through your bloodstream and destroys the foetal and placental cells. The drug is not used very often because it does have potential side effects.

Operative care

An ectopic pregnancy with internal bleeding must be removed during an operation. Modern techniques are minimally invasive. A laparoscopy operation is performed under general anaesthetic. In this procedure a tiny camera is inserted through your umbilicus into your abdomen to visualise the fallopian tubes and ovaries, and the pregnancy. If the tube appears to be damaged it may be removed together with the ectopic pregnancy, because it is likely to cause another ectopic pregnancy. If it appears unharmed it can be opened and the ectopic pregnancy teased out, so the tube is preserved. There is an increased chance of another ectopic pregnancy if the tube is left in place, and some women choose to have the tube removed, even if it appears normal, as long as the other tube can function. The laparoscopy operation usually leads to full recovery within a few weeks.

If the ectopic pregnancy is large (detected after Weeks 8 to 10), the operation needs to be a full laparotomy, which involves an incision in your abdomen. The fallopian tube will be removed. The operation requires a longer recovery time and is similar, in this respect, to a CAESAREAN SECTION.

If you have lost a large amount of blood then either a BLOOD TRANSFUSION during surgery or using vitamins and iron afterwards will prevent anaemia and aid your recovery.

A future pregnancy

- The fertility rates after an ectopic pregnancy are over 60 per cent, with a higher rate of conception among women who had conservative treatment (without surgery). Vitamin and mineral supplements may aid conception.
- If the tube has been removed, you may have to wait longer to conceive until you ovulate on the correct side.
- The chance of another ectopic pregnancy occurring is 4–5 per cent and it is highest in women who undergo IVF treatment or where the other tube is scarred.
- If you plan to use contraception, avoid an IUD or a progesterone-only mini pill.
- If you become pregnant again, have an ultrasound scan as early as possible, using a vaginal probe to visualise the pregnancy and to confirm where the placenta is implanted.

Eczema, baby

Eczema is an inflammation of the skin with itching, swelling, redness, or a burning sensation. It is referred to as the itch that rashes, rather then the rash that itches. Reddened spots, scales, crusts or blisters may be present, either alone or in combination, commonly on the trunk and limbs.

If your baby has eczema she will be uncomfortable when it flares up. It may also be difficult for you because eczema can be unsightly and feels scaly and strange. This is far from the image of a 'perfect' baby with velvety skin. With effective treatment, the severity and extent of the eczema can be reduced. You cannot avoid developing eczema, it is a matter of genetics; all you can do is delay it – by exclusive breastfeeding – or reduce the severity and extent, as well as the duration of the symptoms, by avoiding the trigger. It is reassuring to know that few cases of eczema persist beyond childhood, and an eczema rash does not scar. Eczema is not contagious. In the UK, up to 20 per cent of all children of school age have eczema and 60–70 per cent of those children are virtually clear of the condition by the time they reach their mid-teens.

What happens

Atopic eczema is thought to be a hereditary condition. It is the commonest form of eczema and results from an allergic reaction (page 16) to something in the environment. The allergic reaction produces inflamed, irritated and sore skin. The commonest symptom is itchiness, which can be almost unbearable. Other symptoms include overall dryness, redness and inflammation. Constant scratching can cause the skin to split, and this makes it prone to infection. In infected eczema, the skin may crack and weep.

Allergic contact dermatitis is not common in babies. It develops when the body's immune system reacts against a substance in contact with the skin, and often develops over a period of time through repeated contact.

Irritant contact dermatitis is a type of eczema caused by frequent contact with everyday substances, such as detergents and chemicals that irritate the skin. It may occur as a reaction to washing powders on clothes.

Action plan

To make an accurate diagnosis it is best to have the help of an allergy specialist, a nutritionist or a paediatrician. Occasionally, cradle cap (page 163) is mistaken by parents for eczema.

There is currently no cure for eczema though research continues to shed new light on the condition. However, there are many ways to minimise discomfort and distress. The foundation is an effective skin care routine and there are many treatments available, including prescription creams and complementary therapies.

Care for your baby's skin by washing gently and avoiding scented soaps and any other preparations that may irritate the skin.

Emollients
- Emollients provide a barrier and reduce water loss from the skin, preventing dryness and reducing itching.

- They are safe to use as often as is necessary and are available in various forms including ointments, for very dry skin, and creams and lotions for mild to moderate or 'wet' eczema. Some are applied directly to the skin, while others are used as soap substitutes or can be added to the bath.
- Test a small amount on your baby's skin first (for example, on the forearm), as emollients contain substances to which some people are sensitive.
- You may need to try several types before you find one that suits your baby.

Medicines
- When eczema is under control only emollients need to be used.
- If the eczema flares up and the skin becomes inflamed, a corticosteroid cream usually reduces inflammation. It is very rare that corticosteroids are needed in young babies because other forms of treatment usually work. Topical corticosteroids (applied to the skin) come in different strengths and only the mildest is suitable for infants, as they may have side effects if used in high potency for a long time. Oral corticosteroids are rarely if ever needed under nine months of age.
- If the skin becomes infected an antiseptic cream may be needed. Antibiotics may be prescribed.
- Use of antihistamines, such as chlorpheniramine, most well known under the trade name Piriton or in a preparation known as Phenergan, to discourage itching is often effective. It is especially useful at night when itching is disturbing sleep. Your doctor will advise you about doses.

Other treatments
In the early months, your doctor may discuss wet-wrap bandaging to soothe dry, itchy skin. There are specialised creams available, but you need to seek expert advice for any treatments.

Helping your baby to be comfortable
Itchiness can be very distressing and you may be able to make your baby more comfortable and reduce her urge to scratch.
- Cotton clothing and bedding keep the skin cool and allow it to breathe.
- Using a non-biological washing powder and avoiding fabric softeners can help.

- Keep your baby's nails short and use scratch mitts if itching is very bad.
- Soap is best avoided as it may reduce skin's natural protection mechanisms (page 418).
- You may try using a pure oil in your baby's bath. A few drops of natural oil (almond, wheat germ, olive or grapeseed) may nourish her skin. You could also rub it into her skin as part of a MASSAGE.
- Touching your baby lovingly (massage may be really important) is very positive – many people shy away from touching the dry skin of eczema and this can undermine self-esteem. Touching lets your child feel loved.

Avoiding allergens

If you suspect or identify an allergen, avoid it or minimise exposure (page 15). It can be useful to keep a diary of foods or environmental agents and your baby's skin condition to try to spot any foods or substances that trigger the condition. When you wean your baby, do so slowly and watch for skin reactions.

Complementary therapies

Many people explore complementary therapies in addition to conventional treatments. It is essential to let your doctor know if you are starting another course of treatment, since interactions can occur between certain medications. Conventional treatments should not be stopped suddenly, without consulting your doctor.

- ACUPUNCTURE works to release the body's toxins.
- HOMEOPATHY views eczema as a complaint of the whole system that manifests itself through the skin. *Calendula* cream, *Aveeno* cream and bath sachets, *chickweed* cream and M-folia cream and ointment can be very helpful. There are excellent remedies available but it is best to consult a homeopath who will consider your individual case.

Emotions

The transition to parenthood is one of life's greatest emotional adventures. During pregnancy and after birth you will experience many new and intense feelings. Some will be like guides, helping you decide what feels right for you and your baby, some may be like echoes of your past and some may be troubling.

Emotions are fundamental to our nature. Thousands of emotions – inner drives involving cells, nerves, organs and fluids – occur every minute on an unconscious level. They help us adapt and survive, to move away from danger and towards safety. Those that we are aware of we can call feelings. Listening in to your feelings offers guidance on your personal journey through parenthood.

Humans are at their most emotionally sensitive as babies and your baby will express her emotions openly, and invite you to do the same. Meeting your baby as a sensitive, feeling person, while being in touch with your own feelings, will help you and your baby feel safe and free to explore, and provides a great environment for bonding in your family.

Feel, do, then think

Your baby and you experience a feeling, act on it and then think about it. This is the order of things, now clearly understood by many modern scientific disciplines including neuroscience and endocrinology. In the past, psychologists believed that the order was think, then feel, then do. The current view shows the importance of feelings in how we live from minute to minute.

BABIES' EMOTIONS

Not so very long ago, there was a popular misconception that babies could not feel pain. For decades, even surgical operations were performed without anaesthetic. Fortunately, this practice stopped when it was proven that babies are much more sensitive to pain than adults.

It is similar with babies' emotions. A misconception that they had no emotions allowed a belief that we arrive at birth as blank slates, feeling little or nothing. Today, neuroscience offers proof beyond doubt that all humans are emotionally sensitive, months before birth. It is exciting that science backs up what parents, grandparents and siblings have known for millennia. Science shows how emotions are involved in every action and experience. Fear is driven principally by the ancient 'reptilian' areas of the brain, while emotions including rage and the urge to bond and play evolved later and persist thanks to the 'mammalian' brain structures. These parts of the brain develop early in foetal life and are involved in every thought and action, however old we are.

We look at emotions in the following entries, and you may also enjoy reading about the big feelings (overleaf) that you and your baby share:

- Bonding and attachment
- Care and nurturing
- Explorative urge
- Fear and anxiety
- Playfulness
- Rage and anger
- Separation anxiety

Expressing emotions and feelings

Your baby expresses her needs as they arise and does this powerfully through the body. Adults' body language is also very strong. Your baby will show you many ways in which emotions are shown, including:

- with facial expressions
- via body language, maybe stretching arms out to you or holding them protectively across her chest
- via voice and crying
- by inviting or refusing eye contact
- via appetite and the way she suckles at your breast
- via digestion and bowel movement
- via sleep and waking pattern
- through body symptoms, such as a rash, or with a headache or pain. (Though physical and genetic factors contribute to body symptoms, emotions are a part of the larger picture.)

▓ FAMILY OF ORIGIN

In adulthood, your feelings and behaviour are influenced by your experiences through life. This includes the way you felt as a baby. The influence of your 'family of origin' is strong, and your emotional 'inner baby' still has a powerful presence. You may have felt lovingly nurtured or abused. You may have been understood or felt abandoned as a baby.

Foundations of infancy

Science shows that the experience we have as babies affects brain and body development and forms a foundation that has repercussions

throughout life. Many patterns of neural networking, brain-body interaction, cell sensitivity and hormonal rhythms form before the first birthday. These are influenced by emotions as well as by genes and physical health, and affect the way we rate ourselves and form relationships in later life. The foundation reflects nature – genetic potential – and to a greater extent nurture – the physical, emotional and social environment we experience. We each carry our own unique foundation with us, and we tend to behave towards our children in ways we ourselves were parented – replaying our 'family of origin'. Usually this is unconscious.

Your baby is an individual and you cannot control how she feels or mould her foundations according to your wishes, yet you do play a very important role because you are the centre of her world. You and other carers help to create the environment your baby experiences.

Inner baby, adult self

When your emotions are unconscious it is difficult, if not impossible, to change behaviour, but your baby will encourage you to go into your feelings and as they rise into awareness, it is easier to make choices and to avoid repeating family patterns that do not suit you or your baby today. It is possible to change automatic actions and recurrent states of mind by being aware of your feelings.

It is useful to remember that your baby does not cause your feelings, which are your personal reactions. Some of your feelings are a product of your own family of origin. They may repeat themselves until you become aware of them. Then you are in a position to accept them and to step out of old patterns. You may spend time in self reflection, keep a journal, or try spontaneous writing, drawing or painting. For most people, the best way to increase awareness and to make practical changes is with the support of another person, possibly a professional (page 162).

You may appreciate that some feelings arise from your inner baby, and others from your adult self. Parents find that distinguishing between the two makes it easier for them to be present for their babies, and to care well for themselves.

▦ BIG FEELINGS

There are many models to describe fundamental human emotions. The list here is based on brain science research and fits well with what is known about human and primate baby and adult behaviour. We are indebted to Margot Sutherland for her insights in this area.

Babies live in a world of vivid emotional colour and do not filter their feelings or think rationally about them. You may be surprised that, even though you imagine your own life is rational and controlled, your emotions drive you. Your baby gives you a precious opportunity to welcome and accept your own big feelings.

Your baby is able to move very rapidly from one state, such as fear, to another, such as playfulness. Equally, several feeling states may co-exist. Your baby may feel anger as well as fear if separated from others and may be playful and explorative and bond powerfully when with you. Your experiences are similarly dynamic and there is almost always overlap between feelings.

Your baby experiences other important feelings such as sadness and joy, jealousy and many others. We have chosen to focus on the following seven feelings for simplicity and because they cover a wide spectrum of how it feels to be human:

- Bonding and attachment
- Care and nurturing
- Explorative urge
- Fear and anxiety
- Playfulness
- Rage and anger
- Separation anxiety

It is an extremely valuable experience for babies when their carers permit and encourage them to be in their feelings. It is important for babies to feel safe, to see their feelings reflected in the people around them and to consistently discover that their needs are being understood and met. This supports their self-belief and a lifelong ability to trust their emotional feelings, and to form strong and loving relationships. Who wouldn't wish this for their baby?

▦ BIG FEELINGS IN ACTION

Emotions rise and pass away all the time. A strong feeling intensifies muscle tension, hormone release and cellular and brain activity, and when it passes, body functions return to a more relaxed state. When a feeling is intense, your baby needs practical and loving support to cope with the feeling and then to relax, as he is still physically and emotionally immature. Without regulation, body tension and surges of hormone flow may continue, your baby may feel confused and upset, and may remain distressed. Babies usually express emotional tension vocally, although it may manifest through tummy pain or another physical complaint – each baby is different. Intense emotions may also disrupt rhythms such as sleep and digestion.

The way to help your baby lovingly and effectively depends on what he needs. You may offer a feed or change his nappy or simply hold him and say something like, 'I see you are angry, you are really angry. That is okay and I am here for you.'

The picture is similar for you. If you are able to express your feelings and allow them to pass in a safe relationship you are likely to feel calmer and more focused. Being loving, open and honest, and taking your own and your baby's feelings seriously nurtures all your relationships, and may raise your confidence as you care for yourself and follow your dreams.

The following is an 'action plan' that may help you stay present for your baby and for yourself. Many of the suggestions may feel like common sense; if so, your instincts are helping you parent lovingly and effectively.

1. Touch and be close

The need for physical contact is powerful for all humans. With the security and reassurance of loving touch, your baby is able to feel and express emotions as they rise and fall, knowing you are there. You may spend lots of time skin to skin (page 517), enjoy feeding (page 88) and MASSAGE, and sleep together (page 487).

2. Nourish your baby

Your baby makes no distinction between the way he feels emotionally and the way his body feels. Having basic needs met – food, warmth, love, acceptance and touch, and hearing and smelling you – is essential as you care for him (page 120). Your baby learns that showing feelings helps get his needs met, and learns to trust you.

3. Nourish yourself
You will care for your baby most effectively when your own needs are met. Caring for yourself and giving time and loving attention to other relationships – particularly with your partner – are crucial (page 121).

4. Make quality time together
Having clear boundaries around time and space (page 433) allows you quality time to be with your baby without distractions. This may help you stay present and be calm and listen to your baby without feeling the need to do something else. If you are anxious or angry this does not offer safety. It is sometimes better for your baby to be in the safe presence of another person while you take a break or complete a pressing task.

5. Take your baby's feelings seriously
All your baby's feelings are important. Acknowledge them, tell your baby how you think he feels, using age-appropriate language and a loving tone and energy, and listen to your baby. If your baby feels heard and loved, whatever he is feeling, he is likely to communicate with increasing enthusiasm, joy and contentment.

6. Take your own feelings seriously
Your feelings remind you what you need today, and are useful guides, whether they are comfortable or uncomfortable. Some will remind you of what you felt when you were a baby. Taking your feelings seriously will help you care for yourself, distinguish between the adult-you and your inner baby, and be present for your baby. All your feelings are okay – they are part of who you are.

7. Communicate honestly
You communicate all the time, with sounds, words, touch and eye contact and by listening. When you are honest and open, your baby will feel safe. It is fun to let a conversation – which always has verbal and non-verbal elements – unfold.

8. Be present for the good times
Allow yourself the peace and time to be with your baby when you are both happy, contented, playful and peaceful. This really is a precious time and passes all too quickly.

9. Be present for the difficult times
You may sometimes find being with your baby very challenging. If you are afraid or uncomfortable as your baby expresses his feelings that is okay. You do not need to take them away – you just need to be there. It may be very difficult to stay present when your baby is in meltdown. If you are able to stay calm and distinguish between your baby's cries and your feelings of distress (your inner baby crying), you are home.

10. Play and explore
Your baby is spontaneous and follows a strong urge to explore and play. There are many opportunities for this. Smiling and laughter are important for emotional wellbeing. When things seem difficult or life feels too serious, play is a wonderful way to lighten the mood and enjoy one another.

If things aren't ideal
We all have ideals. If your pregnancy or life with your baby have not fitted your expectations, or you are concerned that the birth experience or family stress may affect your baby, it may help to remember that healing is always possible. Repair can take place at any time and you and your baby are on a journey together that will involve many ups and downs.

Practical measures may help, including appropriate healthcare for you both. For instance, cranial OSTEOPATHY or massage can ease pain after birth, and more support may improve BREASTFEEDING or create the chance for you to rest.

A powerful way to make repair and let go of anxiety is to tell your baby your story; you cannot tell a baby what he experienced, you can only imagine. For example:

'I was so excited to be pregnant with you and looked forward to the birth and holding you, and I was so upset when you had to be taken away to be looked after by the doctors.

'I imagine it was difficult for you, too. You may have felt frightened or lost. I am sorry this happened, but pleased there were people who helped you when you needed it. I am here now and I love being with you. I will do my very best to support and love you.'

Creating safety
Your baby picks up on your feelings and will frequently mirror you. Talking with honesty

conveys love rather than anxiety, and will help you and your baby feel safe. Simply letting your baby know: 'I'm feeling anxious, but it is not because of you, there is nothing you need to do ...' allows your baby to relax without taking on your anxiety. You will also be letting him know that you are not demanding anything of him, and accept and love him without conditions. This is a very powerful message for your baby: it profoundly respects him as an individual, and nurtures his self-acceptance and growth, allowing him to be delightfully self-expressed, and at ease with you. This is a key ingredient in any recipe for contentment.

Emotions
Anger

See Emotions, rage and anger.

Emotions
Blues

See Emotions, sadness and happiness.

Emotions
Bonding and attachment

See also Emotions, love.

Many parents find the deep love they feel for their babies is among life's most rewarding experiences, and bonding often happens easily with a force that is surprising, wonderful, deep and permanent. Sometimes, it takes a few days or weeks. Occasionally, there is no bonding.

Bonding has many aspects, including feeling safe and connected to another person, feeling loved and accepted, and being in love and being loved. The urge to bond and form relationships is one of your and your baby's seven big feelings. You and your baby have a genetic biological drive to bond. Many things happen spontaneously to support bonding. The delicious intimacy of lying in bed together; and looking into one another's eyes; and successful feeding are examples.

In pregnancy, mum and baby begin to build a bond through the exchange of hormones and other chemicals – including those specifically related to feeling loving, loved and bonding. You will also feel one another's movements. You may enjoy seeing your baby during an ultrasound scan. Your baby will hear and recognise your voice. Some people feel a strong spiritual connection with their unborn baby.

The mother-baby dyad

The intimate bond between mum and baby has been called a 'dyad' – a group of two that should not be separated – and this bond is really crucial for a baby. It not only ensures survival in babyhood, it also provides training for being in relationships and the skills learnt in babyhood contribute to survival and wellbeing through life. The bond between dad and baby has a different quality and may be just as powerful.

How babies and parents bond and attach

All babies need to attach to someone who will care for them. Usually, mum is the most important figure, followed a close second by dad. A baby will attach in the best way possible – it is a matter of survival.

As a baby you may have bonded securely and felt loved and safe. Alternatively, you may have been ambivalent, because you received inconsistent care or mixed messages, or you may have avoided intimacy because you felt afraid. Many babies experience a mix of these.

Your baby has a different perspective from you. This is influenced by your baby's:
* personality;
* experiences in the womb;
* experience of birth and the moments after birth; and
* how your baby feels met and cared for in the months and years that follow.

The way you bond with your baby reflects your own experience as a baby in your family of origin (page 207), as well as your circumstances and relationships today, and your experience of pregnancy, birth and beyond. You and your baby have a unique relationship and the bond will continue developing and changing throughout your lives together.

If the bond doesn't feel good

Secure bonding and attachment are ideal but in everyday life there are many things that could interfere. Examples range from grief in pregnancy, conflict in your partnership, intervention during birth, separation from your baby after birth, difficulty with feeding, lack of support, money worries, feeling stressed or finding parenting really challenging. Your own style of attachment (based on your experiences as a baby) will also be significant.

Fortunately, there are many ways to enhance bonding and to make repair when it is not secure, and repair can be made at any time. Some people repair distant or difficult relationships very late in life, but it is preferable for your baby to have a secure relationship early in life. Following the action plan on page 208 is one way of building a loving bond, including touch and breastfeeding, honest communication and play. There are further practical tips in the section on CARING FOR BABY. It is never too late to nurture a loving and lasting bond.

Emotions
Caring and nurturing

See also Caring for baby; Caring for you.

Of all mammals, human babies are reliant on others of their kind for the longest period after birth. The need to be cared for and the urge to care for others are human instinct.

For your baby, to be cared for and nurtured means:
* not being separated;
* having his needs met;
* feeling understood and comforted;
* having his big feelings acknowledged, and being supported to experience them; and
* being in a home where he feels cared for and nurtured.

Your baby will show you the benefits when his needs are met as they arise. If your baby doesn't feel cared for he may react in many different ways, perhaps with anger, by withdrawing, through anxiety, or with resilience and determination.

You also need to be cared for and you will unconsciously react if your needs aren't met – even if you have become accustomed to 'getting by' or 'going without'. There may be times when you resent your baby for taking all your caring

energy, or you resent your partner, or you feel neglected. This is where boundaries become very important, as you create time for yourself and for each member of your family (page 433).

You may feel deeply nurtured by your baby's loving affection and intimacy. This is one of the precious gifts of parenthood. Your baby cannot care for you fully, however, and it is important to use your existing and potential support network. The section CARING FOR YOU gives further tips.

Emotions
Depression

See Depression and anxiety, pre- and post-natal.

Emotions
Explorative urge

See also Emotions, playfulness.

Every human being is born with an inner biological desire to explore and this is very strongly developed in all babies. Your baby needs to explore extensively to learn about himself and his environment and the people around him, and he will actively experiment. Although he is not able to get up and walk around, his senses develop at a rate that supports exploration – with his hands, eyes, through hearing and smell, and with his mouth as he suckles, tastes and swallows. The safer babies feel, the more freely they will explore.

Your baby begins exploring in the womb. Then he will explore your breast and face and gradually extend his range. Exploring gets more eager and fun as your baby grows. There is a myth that babies need to be left alone so they can learn how to explore. This is not correct – feeling safe and supported is the best foundation for active exploration, and it is enjoyable and encouraging for your baby to explore and to share the joy of discovery with others.

Your explorative urge is also strong. Some adults need permission to really follow this feeling. Go ahead, it is fun and necessary and can be playful or tender and loving. It is basic to all mammals, who need to explore their babies first to get to know them, and then to check they are well, and to spot any problems as soon as they arise. Your sex drive is one of your in-built drives to explore, and there are many other ways to play and to experience new feelings. You will inevitably be exploring yourself and life's possibilities as a parent in your growing family.

A wonderful thing about the urge to explore is that it helps you to slow down to your baby's pace. It will heighten your sense of smell, touch and visual acuity and sensitise your ears as you get to know your baby. If the chance to do this is denied you may understandably become upset, as will your baby – so it's worth making time for it and creating quality time to be together.

Emotions
Fear and anxiety

Fear is a natural emotion that alerts us to danger. Everybody has it. Fear is one of the brain's most fundamental drives: it triggers an unconscious body-wide process that stimulates us to act in the interests of survival by running or by protecting ourselves (the 'fight or flight' reflex).

Its positive values include protecting yourself and accurately assessing your safety. It may be negative – if it is chronic, frequently repeated or very intense, for example – as it keeps your body on high alert and physical fear-sensations such as tension, restlessness and shallow breathing are not pleasant or conducive to wellbeing. These are common symptoms of stress-related anxiety, which is recognised as a widespread health concern among adults today.

Fear for baby

Fear is a very common emotion for babies, who experience so many new physical and emotional sensations in their first months. It is okay for your baby to be afraid for short periods – it's normal and is important because through experiencing fear your baby learns to cope with it. Yet he will need you as his supporter. You will often be able to keep threatening experiences to a minimum and offer safety and physical holding when your baby seems afraid. Your baby may ask

for your protection by crying and will feel better for reassurance. The advice on page 208 gives practical guidance.

If babies are often afraid, they learn to protect themselves. Some babies who are frequently afraid seem very nervous and develop a range of defensive behaviours. Possible reactions vary from 'shutting down' and being introverted, quiet and physically less sensitive, to being hyperactive, vocal and hypersensitive. Each individual baby is unique. Neuroscience now shows that excessive fear in the early years can prime a person for anxiety and fear in later life (page 311).

There are many things that might trigger fear for a baby:

In the womb
- Being unwanted can be very frightening. Hormones and other chemicals linked with maternal stress and fear are one way in which a baby may pick up such a message. Babies may react by producing their own stress hormones.
- The womb environment may be difficult, for example in the case of a dysfunctional placenta and growth restriction. This does not feel secure.

Birth
- The experience of labour may be very frightening for mum and baby.
- The environment and sense of welcome a baby meets at birth have a big effect. If a baby is left alone and separated from mum this can be terrifying.

After birth
- Being very cold or very hot is scary.
- Wanting to feed but having no food forthcoming is frightening.
- A roughly handled baby will be afraid.
- If babies do not feel comforted, both physically and emotionally, they may be afraid and angry.
- If a baby's family are generally fearful, he will be aware of this. Some babies bring loving and courageous energy into the family; others repeat an established pattern of being fearful.
- If a baby feels unable to meet the expectations of the parents, he may become anxious – particularly if there has been a previous loss, the mother or father wanted a baby of a different gender, or the parents are in conflict.

Fear for parents

You will feel afraid from time to time. Becoming a parent is a big deal and everybody feels confronted at some point. A lot depends on how secure you feel in your relationship, with your work, home and so on, but even when life is stress-free the normal transition of pregnancy, labour and birth, and the responsibility of parenting, typically involve some trepidation. It is helpful for you to have a way of acknowledging your fear, feeling safe and supported, and moving on. The alternative is for fear to persist, which may drain your energy, affect your relationships, and might lead to chronic anxiety and DEPRESSION.

During labour and birth, many women admit to being afraid of dying. The sensation of 'coming through the other side' is intense relief and euphoria.

Many people find fear difficult to accept and it may be confronting to work through personal fears if previous experiences have been overwhelming. Learning to face fear, go into it, discover its limits and its positive guiding qualities is something many people experience in adulthood, often in the context of a supportive and loving relationship. It is never too late to alter an old pattern, and letting go of the burden of fear can be liberating. Acknowledging your feelings and caring for yourself (page 121) is a positive start if you are afraid.

Emotions
Guilt

Guilt is the emotion you experience when you believe you have done something wrong or not well enough. It is an essential emotion that enables you to function as an active member of society and to love and nurture yourself and other people in an appropriate way. When you're feeling guilty you may describe it as feeling 'bad'. Guilt drains energy and is a hindrance to loving and feeling loved. It is a 'tight' feeling and has a destructive element. Yet it can be a valuable prompt to make changes where necessary.

People who feel absolutely no guilt about destructive, harmful or malicious acts are called psychopaths. Sigmund Freud described guilt as the struggle between the ego and the superego, which is set by parental imprinting. Guilt is closely related to conscience and it has been described as a struggle of doing something while hearing your parents' voices in your head, judging it as wrong.

What happens?

Guilty feelings are often useful guides. Guilt can be a powerful barometer of whether your actions, thoughts and feelings are appropriate. For instance, it may arise if you have caused harm or upset, or neglected yourself or others. It may bring about a change in your perspective or your behaviour and it can be an important ally.

Guilty feelings may sometimes signal a need to love or be loved, both essential aspects of wellbeing. The balance might have tipped. The guilt arises from your unconscious and is a call for you to take note of your personal needs and the balance in your family and your life. In this case it is not a sign that you have done something wrong, rather it is an invitation to make some changes.

Guilt can be inappropriate when it persists although you are not acting harmfully. There may be factors outside of your control, or your life or your behaviour may not meet your expectations. Persistent inappropriate guilt is draining and it may signal low self-esteem or fear, anxiety or depression. Being excessively guilty clouds your vision and happiness.

Learning on the job as a parent
You may think you will not be able to mother your baby well, and feel guilty that you are unsure or nervous. Rest assured that parenting is a steep learning curve for everyone, and confidence builds over time.

You may feel guilty if you are dishonest. If so, being truthful (which may take great courage) is the best remedy. Being truthful may begin with accepting and sharing your feelings without apologising for them – they are natural .

The influence of your past
Low confidence and anxiety are frequent companions of guilt. They often have roots early in life and may be influenced by genetic make-up and your experiences in your family

of origin (page 207). For instance, as a child you may have strived to be good or perfect, or you may have feared chastisement for being wrong, dirty or bad. You may have been teased, or seen women around you being put down. Such experiences impact on self-esteem, and for some people feeling wrong or not good enough may begin in infancy and linger through life. A feeling of being unworthy might be triggered by abuse or rape, and if abuse is still continuing (page 547) these feelings will still be strong.

Your life experiences and beliefs determine the way you value your right to feel emotions, to care for yourself, to have an opinion, to ask for support, to expect mutual respect and fairness, and so on. If you lost sight of some of these rights in infancy, this was not your fault. You had little say or ability to change things then. An infant learns about her own value in the world from her family of origin. If you find it hard to speak up or act up for yourself or for your baby now, you may feel guilty. The good news is that the effect of early experiences need not continue. If you explore your early thoughts about self-worth it will be easier to distinguish between feelings that are echoes of your past and those that relate to what's happening now. This may be a catalyst to make practical changes.

Society and religious pressures
You or your partner may feel guilty because your parents or your friends expect you to do something one way, and you prefer to do it another ('*My mum says babies should..., but I feel my baby does...*') Your religion may create expectations. The triggers will be unique for you and although it can be very difficult to let go of guilt, parenting your baby is a great opportunity to accept difference and change.

Mums and dads
Women are often more inclined to feel wrong or at fault than men. A female tendency to guilt may be based on cultural attitudes. Your religious, cultural or family background, including beliefs about the different sexes, will feature in your perception of your worthiness, successes and mistakes. Even if you have adopted a way of life that differs from your ancestral culture, experiences in

childhood may continue to influence your feelings today.

Guilt often increases in intensity when you become a parent. A 'mother's guilt' can relate to any number of factors, such as eating chocolate or smoking or drinking alcohol, over-working, not wanting sex, not having a natural birth, having a crying baby or a baby who doesn't eat happily or is not gaining weight. A 'father's guilt' may be triggered by drinking, smoking or gambling, spending too much time at work, not earning enough, not being home enough, not feeling able to care for the baby, having a baby of the 'wrong' gender, losing touch with friends, and so on.

Work and quality time
How many adults value work above parenting? Knowing your value as a parent is important, particularly if your peers or family disagree or you feel under pressure from colleagues, clients or the media. Guilt is a useful tool to help you balance your time and re-evaluate your relationship with work (whether you feel guilty for being at home too little or too much, or for not working, or for working hard). You may decide to reduce your hours or to stay with a high level of commitment, and to look at how you spend quality family time. Quality time is not always about number of hours. Its essence is in 'being present in the moment'. In other words, it is about focusing your love and attention on your baby, allowing you and your baby to love and feel loved, to play, to explore and to rest (page 437). When you are present and attentive, being with your baby is wonderful and guilt free. Being similarly focused at work can also be fulfilling.

Guilt and your big feelings
Some emotions may bring up guilty feelings – particularly resentment, anger or regret. Anger is one of your fundamental feelings (page 208) and you may find it beneath the surface of your guilt. Sometimes another basic emotion – separation anxiety – may underpin guilt, such as an uncomfortable feeling when you are apart from your baby (page 220). You may feel guilty that you have done something wrong ('*It is my fault, I am wrong, my baby is wrong*') even though your feelings are perfectly normal and appropriate. Letting go of guilt and accepting that anxiety and

anger can be guides may help you devise practical solutions. Weighing up decisions is an ongoing challenge of parenting – one that is easier when guilt is used as a signal for acceptance and a prompt for appropriate action in each unique situation.

Guilt, perfection, responsibility and your baby

You may sometimes feel overwhelmed by responsibility and feel guilty that you are not up to scratch. If you take on too much, guilt is more likely. Guilt is closely linked with your expectations. If you often feel guilty this may be because you have high expectations or a drive for perfection.

Guilt may be your best friend if it helps you to take an honest look at your expectations, identify your ideals and accept reality. This includes lovingly accepting yourself and your baby, even when times are tough (page 208). This may help you feel greater pride and confidence in what you are doing.

Some parents feel guilty about what their baby does: 'It is my fault my baby is not sleeping enough, crying too much, not gaining weight' and so on. The need to be a good parent is yours, not your baby's. It is useful to remember that your baby is a unique individual and your expectations belong to you and not to her. Your baby follows and acts on her feelings as she strives to get her needs met. She cannot feel guilt because the part of her brain that allows self-reflection and rational thought is not yet mature.

Action plan

Guilt is often appropriate and might be a useful pointer to a feeling or a situation that needs to alter. The sections CARING FOR YOU and CARING FOR BABY may help you make emotional and practical changes.

Some of the suggestions below may appeal to you.

- You may ask yourself, why do I feel guilty? The answer may or may not be immediately obvious. If it is not obvious the origin may be in your early years. When you identify a cause, maybe with the help of someone whose opinion you trust, choosing what to do will be easier.
- You may decide your guilt is unjustified, drop it and then feel much better.
- You may decide that re-organising your days to

create quality time for you and your baby may make a big difference. As you enjoy one another you will both grow more confident.

- It might become obvious that your guilt is a sign that you are neglecting your own needs or expecting too much of yourself or others. It may be useful to care for yourself better and ask for practical help from other people.
- If you have a destructive habit (anything from eating, smoking or drinking to neglecting yourself, your baby or your partner) thinking over your behaviour might help you try some changes. You may need to reach out for help. If your habit is abusive, or you are being abused, do not delay in finding support.
- If your guilt is linked to your partnership (such as a lack of intimacy, anger, being attracted to someone else) being honest with one another is a powerful step. Active listening (page 462) presents a chance for you both to talk without interruption, and to be heard. It can be a very effective way towards acceptance and change.
- If you often feel anxious or depressed, attending to your feelings is a priority.
- You may not be able to understand your guilt and/or feelings connected with it, in which case spending time with a counsellor or therapist could be very valuable.

You cannot control or reason away your emotional feelings. Guilt can be a wonderful ally and as a new parent it is healthy to question things, to stumble, to learn, to feel good and to feel bad. You can help yourself and your baby by accepting the reality of the good and the bad times. Allowing yourself time, even five minutes a day, just for you, may broaden your perspective and you may move from guilt to acceptance and positive action. Doing your best is certainly good enough and you deserve to love and to be loved.

Emotions
Love

See also Emotions, bonding and attachment; Parenting.

When you acknowledge and accept the big feelings in you and in your baby, you are likely to meet your baby's needs and help him feel good, as well as care for yourself. When your feelings are similarly accepted by someone else, you will feel good, too. Accepting your baby for who he is, rather than for what he does, is to be loving.

Love in action includes feeding, nourishing and giving protection, playing with your baby, staying up with him through the night, listening with an open heart, and ensuring your baby feels safe and comfortable. When others actively love you, they will care for you in similar ways.

▓ FALLING IN LOVE

Babies bring enormous joy into the world. Most parents would say that love for their children is like no other feeling – deep, powerful, gentle and fiercely protective. And, usually, it comes like a tidal wave soon after birth – and sometimes sooner. Loving feelings may be strongest, initially, for mums because of the hormones of pregnancy, birth and when breastfeeding, but it would be flippant to suggest that hormones are the only important thing, and many factors are involved. Dads, too, frequently fall head-over-heels in love with their babies. It is part of human nature to do so.

Falling in love is part of bonding (page 210) and this happens at different rates, and with differing intensity, for each baby and parent. It often begins in pregnancy. Love is not always instant, though, and if you do not have loving feelings immediately after birth it may be reassuring to know that this is normal. Your baby has the capacity to trigger a heart-opening and deeply loving experience, but you may not be fully ready for this yet.

One of the most crucial things is for you and your baby to be together. If you are separated after birth, you may need to wait until you are resting together, relaxed and undisturbed, to feel a loving connection. Equally, if you are stressed or upset, if the birth was exhausting, frightening or traumatic, loving feelings may be delayed. Sometimes it takes longer, and your own fears and worries can get in the way.

Being fully 'in the moment' with your baby, free of concerns or distractions, is a good way of reflecting your baby's open-hearted love. It may be difficult to be loving if you are depressed or very anxious (page 174).

Sometimes love takes time to grow. Occasionally, it remains absent. There are many ways you can enhance love and the suggestions on page 208 may be useful.

Does my baby love me?

Some parents worry whether their baby likes them, particularly when there is a lot of crying, or she asserts the desire to be independent. You don't need to do anything special to make your baby love you. You will be loved for who you are. Your baby has a biological urge to love and bond with her parents. Although your baby's demands are intense and ongoing, the rewards for you are huge. As she grows, and the physical distance between you increases, her eagerness to explore reflects the background of love and trust she felt in infancy.

▓ IN YOUR BABY'S MOCCASINS

Your baby feels pleasure for months in your womb. Part of the chemical soup in which she is immersed consists of emotive love hormones (page 307). Even if you have been stressed or afraid, love hormones flow, and your baby's brain develops naturally to help feel loving towards you. After birth, your baby will feel love when with people who love and accept her.

When babies breastfeed, it is as if they drink love juice on tap (as breast milk is full of love hormones). When lovingly held, particularly with skin-to-skin contact, softly spoken to and having eye contact with people who love him, your baby experiences pleasure and a sense of connection.

You and your baby mirror one another in a loving dance. When your baby feels delight, she will reflect love back to you. When your baby rests with you, open-hearted and accepting, you will reflect her love back to her. The alternative is for your baby to feel fear or confusion. By far the best situation for your baby is to have the opportunity to grow in a loving environment. When safely held, met well, understood and accepted, even though your baby will also have feelings of fear and anger from time to time, she will be in a loving, trusting space.

▓ THE PHYSIOLOGY OF LOVE

You may be interested to know some of the ways in which your body – and your baby's body – is set up to love and to feel another person's love.

The mammalian part of your brain (page 207) is involved in every thought and feeling and is one of the seats of loving feelings. It's automatically activated when you are in a loving situation, and responds to reflect love when others show it to you. It's ready to reflect your baby's love. The same is true for your baby, who similarly is ready to be loving and to feel and reflect your love.

Loving feelings also involve hormones and other chemicals that are part of your body's internal sea. Love hormones (page 307) flow most strongly when you feel loved, when you're in good company, with touch and pleasurable sensations. There are many other body functions linked with loving states of mind. When you're with your baby, your various body rhythms synchronise and you can pick up and mirror one another's calm contentment, just as you may mirror anxiety, tension and anger.

▓ YOUR HISTORY OF LOVE: YOUR PAST AND WHAT'S HAPPENING NOW

Your baby is on the steepest learning curve of life. The love she feels plus her experience in relationships affects her developing brain. This in turn will influence the way your baby experiences relationships, feelings and events for the rest of her life. You, as parents, are central to her early experiences of love and trust.

When you were a baby, you laid down foundations just as your baby is doing now. Your early experiences are still significant and contribute to how you love today. If your early relationships, particularly with your mother, were not comfortable, feelings such as fear, anger or sadness may be more familiar to you than loving acceptance. Love may be linked with an urge to please, with deceit or with pain and a loss of trust. If your early relationships were secure and close, love, intimacy, trust and comfort may be familiar for you.

When you have your own baby you may experience a strong and accepting love, and if this is new for you it may feel like a fresh lease of life. Alternatively the love and dependence your baby expresses may re-activate some uncomfortable feelings you had years ago. If this happens you can alter the pattern to replace emotional discomfort with pleasurable feelings, and enjoy a close bond with your baby. It is never too late to repair, or to change (page 210) if the bond doesn't feel good.

The key is to remind yourself of two levels of feeling – those connected with your early life and your relationship with your mother, father or carer, and those linked with your own baby, here and now. This simple awareness may automatically open your heart in one of the most important relationships of your life. And perhaps the greatest lesson your baby will teach you is how to love freely and accept people for who they are, and enjoy being loved and accepted in return.

Emotions
Playfulness

See also Emotions, explorative urge.

Playfulness is a fundamental feeling, a biological drive that helps us feel pleasure, make friends, feel bonded in our families and communities, explore and learn. Your baby is ready to be playful and may get a lot of pleasure from tumbling and moving in your womb. After birth, he may show his playful side frequently as he explores and gets close to you. Babies often reawaken the playful child in their parents.

Life is so much more fun for adults when children are there to explore and play. Your baby will do this frequently if he feels safe and nourished, and when he knows he is heard by you and involved in your life. You do not need to conduct elaborate games – play can be gentle, you can use your voice, your eyes, movement and music. Babies most love playing with people. When babies are older they love playing with toys, pots, pans, animals – almost anything interests them. However, having fun with other people still has the greatest potential to be deeply nourishing and enjoyable. If all the seven big feelings (page 208) are welcomed in your family, the energy is likely to be playful.

Emotions
Rage and anger

Rage and anger are strong feelings linked with human drive to survive. You need them to protect yourself. These emotions are linked with activity in the deep brain stem as well as with many 'bodymind' sensations. Anger and rage are associated with adrenaline release, which speeds up the heart and other organs and increases sensitivity to pain. Though it may be disturbing, anger is a positive emotion that drives us to express our needs and stand up for our rights. Fear often gives rise to anger.

Babies may feel and express rage when their basic needs are not being met. These include the need to feel loved, held, warm, fed and heard. A baby may not consciously identify these needs, but nevertheless feels an emotional response when they are (or are not) fulfilled. Rage may similarly be one of the emotions we have as adults when we feel our needs are being denied.

Your baby's rage may arise for a number of reasons, such as:
* pain;
* separation;
* hunger that is not satisfied;
* rough handling;
* being too hot or too cold;
* darkness;
* birth trauma; or
* being in the presence of another's anger.

Your rage may be triggered by many thoughts and events, including:
* tiredness;
* pain;
* feeling overwhelmed and having difficulty coping;
* lack of time to yourself;
* loneliness and lack of support;
* being with angry or critical people; or
* the voice of your inner baby saying you are not good enough.

It is okay and normal for your baby to be angry, and you will be supporting him well if you are there to provide love. It is also okay for you to feel angry. The action plan on page 208 may give useful guidance if you find anger upsetting or difficult. If your anger feels destructive or

painful you will probably find that being with someone who listens to and supports you will help you benefit from your anger and begin a process of change. It will be enriching for you and for your baby and family when you get the support you need.

Emotions
Sadness and happiness

See also Depression and anxiety, pre- and postnatal.

To be sad is in many ways the opposite of happiness, a term that you will understand in a way that's unique to you – a feeling of ease, joy and optimism. When you are sad, you may feel tired, upset, and not at ease.

You may be sad because something has not gone as you expected. You might have a sense of loss. You might be distressed by illness or health complications - your own or your baby's – or by conflict in a relationship. Sometimes a reason for sadness is not immediately obvious, and, as with any other emotions, the roots of your sadness may be in your early life, part of your inner baby (page 207). Babies, like adults, can and do feel sad at times. Feeling sad about being isolated, unacknowledged or hurt in infancy is an emotion that may continue into adulthood. Some people liken sadness to feeling 'worn down', or having a tendency to perceive life as negative. If you feel sad most of the time you are probably depressed.

Sadness as a friend
Sadness may not be a comfortable feeling, and is not normally seen as positive – a whole industry exists to suppress it with pills and distractions – but it can be a useful trigger for slowing down and caring for yourself. And it is entirely normal – up to 90 per cent of women admit to feeling down at some point after birth, and at times in pregnancy. The numbers are similar for men. Fortunately, only around 15 per cent of parents are diagnosed with depression (page 174); nevertheless, feeling sad has a considerable impact on life. Welcoming sadness and allowing yourself time to be in the feeling, however uncomfortable, is often more productive than ignoring it or

distracting yourself: it is as important to acknowledge your sadness as it is to embrace and celebrate joy. Accepting the *see-saw* of emotions that come with parenting may alter your perspective and usually helps to reduce the downs. It has also been said that sadness is the key to the soul. As such it can be a wonderful guide.

Feeling sad in pregnancy

Recent studies have shown that it is almost as common for women and men to feel low in the last trimester (three months) of pregnancy as it is after the birth. Antenatal depression is also becoming more widely recognised. There are all kinds of possible reasons for feeling low, and you may identify with some:

* You may find it hard to cope with your changing body, hormonal fluctuations, tiredness, apprehension about labour and the future and current challenges.
* You may feel overwhelmed, confused by mood swings, worried about money or housing, or about the health of your baby.
* You may be nervous about being a parent.
* You may feel upset about losing your independence and about changes in your relationship.
* You may become anxious in the presence of medical professionals, whether or not there are any health concerns.

Feeling blue after birth

It's normal for lows to be interspersed with incredible highs. The 'Third Day Blues' usually occur for women a few days after birth, although they may come over you for the first time, or be repeated, weeks or months later. Commonly the blues are linked with your reaction to the birth of your baby, and to hormonal changes and tiredness. Being with a tiny baby also triggers deeply buried memories and feelings, and some of your sadness may be linked to your own birth and how you felt welcomed as a baby. The blues usually pass. They are more likely to persist or develop into depression if you lack support, feel isolated, if you have been depressed in the past or if you have ongoing anxieties or concerns that are draining your energy.

Have you lost something?

After the birth, despite all the love and hope the new baby brings, it is common to sense loss. You may feel physically and emotionally 'empty' now that your baby is no longer part of you; an intense intimacy is gone. You may be upset by a loss of independence. Hormonal changes after birth can increase the feeling if you loved the feeling of being pregnant. You may mourn a loss of intimacy with your partner.

Feelings of grief and sadness pass with time but while they are strong you may be irritable or upset. Anger is a common way to show loss or sadness. Emotionally it can be confusing to have the gift of a new baby as well as feeling that you have lost an important part of yourself.

Fathers and blues

Fathers can be ecstatic and euphoric when their baby is born, and feel a slump later. In the build-up before birth, you may use a lot of energy tuning into your partner, supporting her, fitting work in and just keeping going. A feeling of anti-climax may make you feel confused or guilty. Many men feel rejected and excluded from their baby and/or partner. Strangely you may feel envious or angry about the love affair between mother and baby. Many feelings of sadness are echoes from your own experience as a baby.

Feeling blue one day or week, and bright the next, is part of the cycle of being a parent. You may mirror the way your baby goes from one feeling to another. Things don't always get easier quickly, however. A potential pitfall is that when you're down if your self-esteem falls, and you lack motivation to exercise or eat well, or see the bright side, you may enter a cycle of blues. If you feel blue more often, or are constantly feeling down, you may be depressed. Then you will need loving support to accept and address your depression (page 176).

What to do when you feel sad

There are many ways to care for yourself (page 121) and boost your mood. Yet it is not realistic to be 'happy' all the time: the reality is that you will have a range of feelings and sometimes feel low. In most cases things will get easier, or sadness will pass, either later today, tomorrow, or next week.

When sadness comes up for you, it is okay to feel it – in fact this will help it to pass. The tips on page 208 may help you accept your feelings during easy and difficult times. It may help to remember that it is difficult to reduce or let go of sadnesses on your own. While it is true that we all have many inner resources, being disconnected from others is isolating and tiring, especially as a parent of a new baby. Family and friends may be around for you, and being in touch with other mums and dads helps. If you need to extend your community, you could do this through groups: if you become friendly with just one or two people, this can make a huge difference.

You may value COMPLEMENTARY THERAPIES such as homeopathy, and feel better from regular EXERCISE or YOGA. If you continue to feel bad the advice in the entry on depression may be useful.

Emotions
Separation anxiety

Separation anxiety is universal in all human beings and in all primates. It is a biological drive that acts as a natural warning sign. As babies we need contact to be fed and kept warm, and to feel loved and safe – we need our mums and the ideal is for the 'dyad' of mum and baby not to be separated. As children and adults we need to be with other people to learn, thrive and enjoy ourselves and our lives.

Your baby may express separation anxiety when he feels alone. This feeling is particularly strong if he is afraid, angry or in pain. The feeling stirs your baby to call out for you so that you can, ideally, reassure him with your comforting presence. As an adult, you are not as dependent as you were as a baby. Nevertheless, separation anxiety is one of your fundamental emotions and will often affect the way you feel and behave.

Feelings of fear and separation anxiety are inseparable. If a baby is separated for a prolonged period, or the feeling of separation is intense, there will be an abnormally high release of stress hormones (page 310) and physical tension. Being in a persistent state of separation anxiety may make it difficult for a baby to form secure relationships or to trust that others will

be there in times of need. A reduced ability to trust and be intimate with others can persist later in life.

Minimising separation anxiety is usually straightforward. The tips on page 208 will help you offer your baby loving security. All babies and parents are different, but for very young babies and new mothers even five minutes apart is a long time.

After birth

Separation anxiety may be very strong immediately after birth when your baby has the sensation of physical separation for the first time. It's extremely important for your baby to feel safe and held and to be in contact with your body as soon as possible and contact will be most comforting and reassuring for your baby if you hold him, naked, against your skin. If there is a medical reason why you and your baby need to be separated, you can come together as soon as the medical procedures are finished. It may be possible for your partner or another caring adult to hold your baby if you require extra care. You can keep close with kangaroo care (page 518).

Many mums feel distress when they cannot see or hear their baby. This feeling is driven both by separation anxiety and by the urge to nurture and bond – together they ensure you will respond if your baby calls out for you, even if you are asleep.

When you need time on your own your baby can feel safe and have minimal separation anxiety if he is with another caring adult. When you know your baby is safe and lovingly cared for your own distress may reduce.

In your older baby

Initially your baby is not aware of being a separate person. It seems to him that the people around him are an extension of him. Around the age of nine months, he begins to sense that he is separate. He will also be able to understand that mum and dad exist even when they are out of sight. Before this time, your baby may have felt separation anxiety when you weren't close at hand. With his new understanding, he can be anxious when he thinks you are going to leave.

Separation anxiety is at the root of many

tears and screams, of 'clingy' behaviour and of attachment to comfort objects, of complaints about being left with child carers, and of crying at bedtime. Many parents wonder if something is wrong, or suggest that their baby is 'difficult' or 'naughty' or 'playing up'. Quite the opposite: it is totally natural for your baby to feel and express anxiety about separation from you. You may feel it in yourself at the same time.

Leaving your baby with another person

In some contexts, for example, when your baby is left with your partner or your mum, he may quickly feel safe and secure. In others, however, such as when being left at a new nursery or with a new childminder (see page 134), your baby may complain loudly and take weeks or even months to feel safe without you. Each case of separation is unique so there is no way of predicting how your baby will react. The important things are that:

* your baby's feelings are acknowledged;
* your baby's feelings are accepted and your baby is not chastised for the behaviour; and
* you offer safety and reassurance when you change location or leave your baby with another adult.

For parents

Parents express separation anxiety in many ways. You may become irritable or anxious, confused or forgetful, or fret about having things perfectly in place prior to a period of separation from someone you love. This often shows when you are getting ready to go on holiday or someone leaves at work.

The way separation anxiety affects you now reflects the separation anxiety you felt as a baby. If it was very painful for you then, you may find it hard to leave your baby now and become anxious at times of separation and change. Sometimes there is separation anxiety but you may not be aware of it: it may be a root cause when a mum or dad feels deeply uncomfortable without quite knowing why. It is common in dads when they have less time with mum or do not have enough time with their baby after birth. It is one of the big feelings that underpin jealousy and envy. If you notice this is what's happening, the remedy is usually simple – being honest

about what you feel, and creating some quality time to be with the person you are missing.

Emotions
Stress

See also Hormones; Post traumatic stress disorder (PTSD).

Stress arises when we feel under pressure – maybe too much is going on, or what is happening is difficult to cope with. There are many elements of life that may contribute to stress, and birth and parenting are among these. Stress is not an emotion on its own, but it is your reaction to a range of emotions and to demands on your body, time or energy.

Relieving stress

If you feel stressed it is time to take stock (page 123). There will be ways to ease the load and care for yourself. This applies whether you perceive your life as easy ('I shouldn't be stressed') or you are coping with illness or practical challenges that other people acknowledge as stressful. Taking time for yourself and being in loving company are often the most important aspects of a self-care plan that will support you in body, mind and spirit – the basics are listed on page 122.

Your family background
It can be helpful to remember that stress can be a family trait: part of your family of origin. If so, you may discover that distinguishing between the present and the past lightens your mood. Today, you have strengths, a support network and other tools for dealing with daily challenges that you didn't have as a child, or that your mother may not have had. You also have the option and the ability to say 'no' and to take time out (even though it may take some practice to do this).

Being with your baby
Your baby has a wonderfully slow pace. Looking into his eyes and letting go of the need to be active, to talk or to fix things can be deeply refreshing. As your baby entices you into his space, where he has no concerns outside of the

221

connection between you, your stress may evaporate and be replaced by calmness and smiles. You might fall asleep together and rest peacefully. Dancing or bathing together can also be extremely relaxing. When your baby is relaxed he often enters a state of meditative calm, and you may join him, breathing deep and slow, and let go. Just five minutes can help stress disappear. If you feel stressed again later, turn to your baby and re-enter this space, or alternatively focus on your breath to bring you back to a place of calm (page 105).

Time for you

It is not always easy to be calm, present and fully open and there will be times when you feel challenged. All parents need breaks. You need time for you, and it is really important to find support from other adults if you become exhausted or out of control.

Your baby is sensitive to your emotions and he is also coping with his own feelings. With your loving presence, you help him to feel safe and regain balance as strong feelings ebb and flow. If you are stressed you may not have the capacity to be there in a supportive way for him and he may feel overwhelmed and afraid. This does not mean you need to be perfect, or always present and never stressed – that isn't realistic. Rather it is an invitation to acknowledge when you are stressed, and then do what you can to let go and replenish yourself.

You could say to your baby, 'I can see that you are afraid/angry/upset. I am also finding this hard. It is not your fault and I will get the help and support I need. I am asking my friend to stay with you for a while when I take a break.' You may then think about ways to delegate some chores; maybe you can take some exercise – even a 20-minute walk can make a huge difference, and you can do this with your baby; or you may pamper yourself (a nap, a VISUALISATION, a MASSAGE, some time with your partner or some complementary treatment). Whatever helps you feel more grounded and recharges your batteries may help you to feel lighter and happier.

Using your support network

If some of your stress relates to relationships, making time to tend to these may make a huge difference. A relationship might be a trigger for

your stress; and that same relationship may be a valuable source of support, fun and pleasure. You might begin by talking over issues that are upsetting you or causing conflict. If you find yourself putting this off, or being unable to let go of blame or anger, practising 'active listening' may be very helpful (page 462).

If there are practical issues (such as finances, page 415) it may be useful to talk to your health visitor, to other parents or to a local parenting network who may give you advice that could relieve some money worries. You may want further personal advice if you feel chronically anxious (page 174).

Emotions
Support and treatment, complementary therapies

Many people use one or more complementary therapies instead of, or alongside, drug therapy to aid emotional healing. Therapies cannot cure emotional problems, however, any more than drugs can. For instance, they cannot take away the cause of grief when you lose someone close to you. But they can help as you process a recent or previous event in your life.

Aromatherapy and massage

These can be very relaxing and are particularly suitable for depression. Use the oils in appropriate doses (page 36) for MASSAGE, bathing or inhalation.

For anxiety

Neroli brings peace, *jasmine* inspires confidence and *clary sage* helps to put things in perspective (but does inspire vivid dreams so don't use it at night). *Sandalwood* sedates while *patchouli* helps bring you down to earth. After Week 24 of pregnancy you can use *lavender*, a traditional soother, and *frankincense* in low doses, which helps to overcome fear, cut links with past uncomfortable experiences and encourages calm breathing.

For depression

Bergamot can be particularly effective for depression. However, it can cause sensitivity to sunlight. If you feel very low and tired, *melissa* and *lemongrass* are uplifting. You can also use *lavender* or *chamomile* as a general soother and *neroli* to promote sleep – this is particularly good with an oil and a gentle facial massage.

Herbal remedies

Herbs can powerfully assist emotional healing, but while you are pregnant or breastfeeding it is important to consult a medical herbalist who is clear about what herbs and dosages are safe. European, Chinese, Ayurvedic and Native American herbal remedies can all have powerful effects.

* *Kava* has a relaxing effect and helps reduce anxiety, tension and restlessness without withdrawal symptoms.
* *Valerian root* has a strong sedative effect promoting relaxation and deep, restful sleep.
* *Passion flower* has mildly sedative properties, and is often combined with *chamomile*, and *valerian*.
* *Chamomile* is used as a mild sedative to help alleviate insomnia.
* *St John's wort* is a traditional remedy for anxiety and moderate depression, with a therapeutic effectiveness similar to antidepressant drugs but far fewer side effects. It is usually taken for between two and 10 weeks. It can be used with drugs of the SSRI class but not with monoamine oxidase inhibitor drugs (page 176). It can make the skin very sensitive to sunlight.
* Restorative herbs that renew vitality include *Siberian ginseng, ginkgo biloba* extracts (particularly good for headaches, emotional tenderness and anxiety) and *dong quai*, which has a calming effect.

Acupuncture, acupressure and reflexology

These treatments may be calming and re-balance underlying tension patterns in your body.

Homeopathy

Homeopathy offers a vast range of remedies that may help when you feel emotionally overwhelmed or out of balance. When a remedy is right for you it may take the intensity out of a feeling, so you feel calmer and more able to do something that will help you feel better.

Alternatively, it may help you go into a difficult feeling, and then move on without having to carry its weight. As your underlying mood or symptom picture changes, so too will the remedy that you require. In the main, receiving personal recommendation from a homeopath is most useful for emotional support. In time you (and your homeopath) may assemble a core group of remedies that work well for you and help you feel emotionally alive yet stable in the midst of life's challenges and demands.

While you are waiting to see your homeopath one of the remedies below may suit you. Initially, while symptoms are intense, you may take the remedy in 200c potency, three times a day. After two days, re-assess your choice and consult your homeopath. The following remedies are grouped in the context of shock, anxiety and depression etc., but your feelings may not be clear-cut, in which case you may wish to look in more than one section.

For shock/bad news

* *Aconite* for an emotional shock that is accompanied by panic, fear and restlessness.
* *Arnica* after a physical trauma or shock to the system.
* *Ignatia* is the first remedy to think of after hearing bad news – a bereavement or a difficult medical diagnosis. There is a sensation of feeling numb with a lump in your throat.

For anxiety

* *Aconite* for fear/anxiety so overwhelming that you are afraid you may die, you feel sudden terror and panic in certain situations such as before an amniocentesis or caesarean, or during labour.
* *Argentum Nitricum* if you have anticipatory anxiety that can result in panic attacks and makes you feel constantly rushed, impulsive, forgetful and tormented by recurring thoughts that persuade you something has gone wrong. This may be useful before you attend an appointment or you are worried about hearing bad news.
* *Arsenicum* if you worry about everything, can be quite obsessive, need to control your life, look for meaning in everything, and project the worst scenario onto ordinary events. This remedy suits feelings of raw fear and panic, particularly in the early hours of the morning, perhaps triggered by a story you have heard, or

you may have recurring thoughts about what might happen to you or your baby.

- *Gelsemium* if you fear losing control or worry about something that is about to happen (such as impending labour) to the extent that you become stiff or shaky, dizzy or apathetic or weak and uncoordinated.
- *Lycopodium* for anxiety with a sense of inadequacy, although you may be critical of others and appear haughty, and anxiety can be accompanied by digestive bloating or severe abdominal wind.
- *Phosphorous* for a sense of free-floating anxiety, when you may not be sure what the anxiety is about but it drains your energy, and reassurance from others and company helps.

For blues and depression

- *Pulsatilla* if you feel weepy, sensitive, vulnerable and exposed, your moods change rapidly and you want attention and others' advice but become overwhelmed by the variety of opinions. This is extremely helpful for the transition in the early days of parenting and often suits someone who feels worse in hot, stuffy rooms and is characteristically not thirsty.
- *Ignatia* for the days after labour, particularly if you feel shocked or out of control, maybe your ideal hopes have not been realised, you may reproach yourself and your moods will swing wildly, with lots of crying and sighing.
- *Sepia*, a hormonal balancer, after labour if you feel complete exhaustion, great despondence, indifference and detachment and little bonding with your baby – you may cry yet shun consolation and become snappy, and one thing that makes you feel better is vigorous exercise.
- *Staphysagria* after a 'high tech' labour, perhaps with stitching, or an emergency caesarean where a number of medical procedures were involved and you feel violated, humiliated, cross or resentful but you keep quiet, behave over-sensitively and go over events on your own, perhaps in the night.
- *Cimicifuga* if you feel very low yet agitated and jittery, swinging from depression and withdrawal to excitement and chattiness, and feel trapped by responsibility, and paranoid that something terrible is going to happen.
- *Aurum Metallicum* if you feel overwhelmed by sadness and grief and guilty because you could

have done better in labour and could do better as a mum. It suits people who are characteristically driven and perfectionist, successful and responsible, yet are thrown by motherhood, and is useful as you settle and grow more comfortable with your new role.

- *Natrum Mur* if you have suffered bereavement in pregnancy and the true extent of your feelings does not hit you until after the birth with deep sadness. You are extremely vulnerable and sensitive, yet may appear defensive, withdrawn and reserved and find it difficult to cry. You feel better on your own but this also makes you feel isolated and contributes to your sadness.

For anger

- *Nux Vomica* if you are driven and domineering, have a quick temper but let go easily, become angry through frustration, or from being contradicted or hindered, and usually express this verbally but may occasionally throw or smash things.
- *Lycopodium* if you feel deeply insecure, self-doubting and not good enough, although outwardly you are domineering, egotistical and sarcastic, perhaps charming away from home but prone to sudden angry shouting while at home.
- *Arsenicum* if you are anxious about your future and your health, and you become fastidious about controlling your environment and agitated when things don't go as you wish. You do not suffer fools gladly and can present a cold, rather self-righteous face.
- *Sepia* if you can become extremely irritable and fly into a rage in seconds, sometimes being very nasty or picking on someone when you are exhausted and have not got the energy to deal with things calmly.
- *Staphysagria* for suppressed anger that builds over time into deep resentment. If you are usually pleasant, compliant and unassuming but feel indignant from a well of suppressed anger that finally explodes into uncontrollable anger, this remedy may be extremely helpful.

For grief

Any mourning process can be complex, confusing and full of any combination of different emotions – shock, anger, disbelief, denial, indignation, a sense of abandonment, disconnectedness, self-reproach, loneliness – the list is unique to each individual. The remedies suggested below can in no way suppress or eradicate your grief, but they may support you and allow your grief process to unfold so that you deal with your loss in a manner that is appropriate for you. In the early stages, you take the most appropriate remedy from the list below in 200c potency three times per day for two days.

* *Aconite* in the first instance when the loss is unexpected and you are deeply shocked and afraid.
* *Ignatia* in the early days when your emotions are all over the place and often contradictory (laughing/crying, shaking/still, silent brooding/agitated). You may feel constantly on the brink of tears with lots of sighing and a lump in the throat.
* *Arsenicum* if you are acutely agitated and 'hyper', which may lead to insomnia, and you are frightened by loss of control – diarrhoea is a common symptom in this acute phase.
* *Pulsatilla* for feelings of grief with long bouts of weepiness and a need to be supported and consoled with loving company.

Thereafter, one of the following remedies may be beneficial: you may take the most appropriate remedy in 200c potency three times per day for two days, then re-assess.

* *Natrum Mur* if you feel hurt to the core yet bottle up your feelings and do not want to break down in public. You may want to withdraw and spend time alone. You may feel unable to cry, to let go, feel depressed and joyless.
* *Aurum Metallicum* for grief with a deep, black despair; a sense of hopelessness, self-blame and a feeling of having failed, leading to deep depression.
* *Staphysagria* is often needed in the established phase of grief where emotion has been suppressed or after a succession of losses that have never been dealt with and you feel strong anger and resentment towards the person who has died and towards yourself for being in some way to blame.
* *Sepia* for grief characterised by emotional apathy, withdrawal and indifference even to your closest friends, with strong mood changes, irritability and extreme fatigue, often leading to depression.

Please do consult a homeopath for longer-term prescribing.

Emotions
Support and treatment, counselling and psychotherapy

See Counselling and psychotherapy.

Elbows that click

See Knees or elbows that click.

Engorgement

See Breastfeeding, difficulties.

Epilepsy

See Fits and epilepsy, mother.

Episiotomy

See Labour and birth, mother, episiotomy and tears.

Epstein Barr virus

Epstein Barr virus (or EBV) is a member of the herpes virus family and one of the most common human viruses. Most people become infected with EBV at some time during their lives through contact with infected saliva (hence its alternative name, kissing disease), and it is likely you have developed immunity. Your baby will be susceptible to infection once antibody protection inherited from you disappears, normally by six to eight months. EBV may cause no symptoms, or a mild, brief illness.

In the unlikely event that you are infected for the first time in adulthood, you may develop infectious mononucleosis, with fever, sore throat and swollen lymph nodes ('glands'). Sometimes, the spleen may swell or the liver may be affected, and rarely the heart or nervous system is affected. There are no known associations between active EBV infection and problems during pregnancy, such as miscarriages or birth defects.

There is no specific treatment for infectious mononucleosis other than treating the symptoms. Some doctors recommend corticosteroids to reduce the swelling of the throat and tonsils.

EBV symptoms tend to disappear within one or two months but they can linger, and may cause chronic fatigue.

Exercise, mother

During pregnancy and after birth your body is primed for exercise. This is a perfect time to make exercise part of your daily life, or continue an existing habit. Exercise is one of the best ways to feel good. Hand in hand with nutrition, it is a cornerstone of health. If you already exercise regularly you need to make adjustments while you're pregnant and after the birth. If you're not in the habit, when you are pregnant your body will adapt quickly and easily. Provided you stay within your personal comfort zone and within safety guidelines, there are many options that will benefit you and your baby.

It is possible to achieve a lot in a relatively short time. Exercising for 20–30 minutes, three to four times a week, will have a huge impact and can be done simply at home or just by walking. If you follow a programme, take guidance, start gradually and increase time and intensity as you get fitter.

A balanced exercise programme combines building muscle strength (strength training) with continuous motion, such as walking or swimming (aerobic conditioning).

Tips

- For best results you need to exercise regularly, on an ongoing basis. If you stop, the benefits can quickly be reversed.
- Listen to your body, noticing any feelings of strain or discomfort. Pushing yourself beyond your comfort or pain zone can have detrimental effects.
- Rest is an important companion to exercise. You may want to increase the quality of your rest with YOGA, meditation or VISUALISATION.
- Set your own personal goals. Each person is different. Try not to compare yourself to others, nor to your own past performance. It's good to begin with easily achievable targets and

adjust your routine as the months pass. It is useful to have goals but please ensure they are realistic for your flexibility and fitness, for your stage of pregnancy and as your body makes adjustments after birth.

Aerobic exercise

Aerobic exercise is any continuous activity that raises your heart and breathing rate and yet can be sustained for long periods. If you have to stop because you are getting breathless, cut back. Around 20–30 minutes of continuous aerobic exercise, three to four times a week, is the most important part of a balanced fitness programme.

Step and low-impact aerobics

- These are safe and effective. Always work at your own pace and avoid moves that may affect your balance.
- You will need to adjust your programme as pregnancy progresses. For instance, you may ordinarily do a step routine on a 20-cm (8-in) platform: by Week 25 a 10-cm (4-in) platform may suffice and still give a good aerobic workout.
- Using a step machine is not the same as step aerobics, and is not recommended.

Walking

Anyone can walk their way to fitness. All you will need is a pair of supportive, well-fitting athletic shoes and a place to walk.

- The pace is under your control. It can be gentle, moderate or brisk if you are already fit.
- Take comfortable strides and let your arms swing naturally. You can create a faster swing by bending them at the elbow, which will make your legs move faster.
- Push off each step with the toes of your rear foot and land heel first.
- Be aware of your posture. Walk from the waist and pull your navel towards your spine: this keeps your back from arching, and helps to tone your back and abdominal muscles.
- Walk for a minimum of 30 minutes. If you walk at a mild pace, you will need to walk for longer to achieve the same training benefits resulting from a short walk at a quicker pace. If you do decide to increase your pace, remember, it must be at a pace you could sustain for longer if you wanted to.

- If you find your pelvic joints hurt when you walk, choose an alternative form of exercise that puts less strain on your joints, such as swimming.

Swimming

- Swimming is great for cardio-vascular fitness and soothing too. The feel of water on the skin triggers the release of natural chemicals that help you feel relaxed and contented and reduces aches and pains.
- If you can, go swimming regularly, and gradually increase the duration or the number of lengths you do. Aim to maintain a steady rhythm, and slow down or take breaks if you become breathless. You will get an excellent aerobic workout.
- The water takes your weight and you'll feel light. This may be particularly welcome in the last weeks of pregnancy.
- Because your bones are not bearing your weight (as they do while you're walking, for instance) swimming does not increase your bone density and so needs to be part of a wider fitness programme.
- Don't swim if your waters have broken.

Cycling

- In early to mid-pregnancy, cycling is a good form of aerobic exercise. If using a conventional bicycle, the main risk comes from falling off. This does not apply to exercise bikes in the gym.
- In late pregnancy, the discomfort of sitting on the saddle may rule out cycling, and your large uterus could alter your technique and make your legs turn out at the hip, putting uncomfortable pressure on your joints, particularly at the knees.
- In the gym, upright rather than recumbent bikes will be more comfortable.
- Spinning classes are not appropriate for pregnancy.

Jogging, running and high-impact sports

- Jogging and running are only advisable if you were already practising regularly before your pregnancy. Running in late pregnancy is not advisable.
- It's important to reduce your speed and the length of your runs and remember your joints are more vulnerable: speed walking is a good alternative.
- High-impact sports such as tennis and squash

are not recommended in pregnancy. You need to avoid rapid twists, jumps and high impact.

Strength conditioning and weights

Strength conditioning is the fastest and most effective way to tone and shape your body, and build up stamina and strength in preparation for pregnancy and labour. But if you haven't already been doing it – don't start in pregnancy. If you already use weights, you'll need to modify your programme and it's important to take advice. In the last six to eight weeks of pregnancy, you may wish to replace your normal programme with a gentle regime.

The goal of weight training is to maintain joint stability and improve posture, but not to make great advances. It is impossible to make big strength gains because pregnancy hormones soften your joints. It's important to go easy: you may damage your joints if you exceed your limits.

If going to the gym is not an option, you can buy a set of dumbbells in 1kg, 2kg and 3kg weights to use at home for 20 minutes three to four times a week. Start with the lightest and build up as you get stronger.

▓ IN PREGNANCY

Many sports centres and health clubs run exercise sessions for pregnant women including 'aqua' exercise, which is held in a swimming pool. At a designated class you will receive professional instruction and advice, and motivation and support from other mums. Your local club or centre will have details.

Keys to safe exercise in pregnancy

The following advice can help you keep fit without putting your own health or your baby's at risk:

- Ask your doctor or midwife to confirm that what you're doing is safe during each trimester (three month period).
- Exercise regularly and keep within your personal limits.
- Don't aim to increase your fitness beyond your pre-pregnancy level as your fitness will tend to reduce as pregnancy progresses: only 10 per cent of women maintain their pre-pregnancy fitness level.

- If you feel hot, dizzy, faint, sick or out of breath, or experience any bleeding or pain, stop immediately.
- You must be able to talk during a workout. Lower the intensity if you are too breathless to talk, and take regular breaks. Never exercise to the point of exhaustion.
- Avoid twists, jumps, high impact and rapid shifts in direction.
- Avoid exercises that take any joint to its maximum point of resistance. Take care not to over stretch.
- Wear light clothing to avoid overheating and drink water as you exercise.

First trimester (Weeks 0–13)

- Most exercises are safe providing you don't feel nauseous or tired.
- Avoid the step machine, which may overstretch ligaments attached to the uterus.
- Begin pelvic floor exercises (page 438). This will help prevent prolapse in the postnatal period.
- If you suffer from sickness, dizziness, palpitations and fainting you may need to stop or reduce the amount of exercise you do until it wears off (normally Weeks 12–15).

Second trimester (Weeks 14–25)

- If you have varicose veins, avoid using ankle weights.
- If you are lifting heavy weights, be sure not to push yourself; you may need to reduce the repetitions or the weights you are using.
- After about Week 20 you may feel more comfortable to limit your exercise programme to swimming and walking, combined with a gentle strength-training programme.

Third trimester (Weeks 26–40)

- After Week 25 you may start to feel uncomfortable performing exercises lying on your back. The weight of your growing uterus on blood vessels can affect blood flow. If you feel dizzy or faint do the exercises in an inclined or sitting position or while lying on your side.
- This is now a perfect time for aqua workouts (exercising in a pool), low-impact exercise and step classes.
- Walking and swimming are great.
- If your pelvic or hip joints are painful (page 43) take care to avoid over-stretching them (for instance, you could do back stroke in the pool

instead of breast stroke to avoid opening your legs wide).
- If you enjoy continuing with weight training, reduce the duration and the weight.

+ Red flag

If you have pain, bleeding or contractions, see your doctor as soon as possible. If you experience severe breathlessness, palpitations or faintness before or during exercise stop immediately.

■ POSTNATAL EXERCISE

After the birth, it is important to continue a regular exercise programme. You will feel energised and, over the months, find it much easier to regain your pre-pregnancy body weight and shape. Your body needs time to heal and adjust, though, so please take it easy.

What happens

After birth, some pregnancy hormones stay in your system, particularly if you are breastfeeding, so your joints remain flexible but may be unstable. You also need time to heal from a vaginal birth (with or without intervention) or a caesarean.

As your baby grew in pregnancy, your body adapted to the increasing load and became more efficient. Your heart and lungs have adapted to pump an increased amount of blood and circulate more oxygen than before. So when you begin a new exercise programme after birth, your body will respond well.

+ Red flag

Stop exercising at once if you experience pain or an increase in postnatal bleeding, or you become breathless or faint, or have palpitations. It is safest to set goals that are a little short of what you believe you can do: after birth you need time to build up strength and stamina.

Action plan

Listen to your body and begin at a pace that suits you. Each woman is different. Appropriate exercise is energising, but too much is tiring and can hinder recovery and reduce the energy you have for your baby. There is no rush and there are many ways to exercise with your baby.

Within days of birth

* You can begin gentle exercises in bed within days of birth. As soon as you have sensation in your vaginal muscles (this may be within a day or two), try pelvic tilts. Do pelvic floor exercises (page 438) as often as you remember. You can do them anywhere.
* After a couple of days, even following caesarean, you can start to do some gentle walking. Being active within your comfort zone will help your recovery, stimulate your circulation and reduce fluid retention and stiffness. It will also encourage your digestive system to return to normal.

In the first month

* Within two weeks or as soon as you feel up to it, you can return to light exercise.
* Walking is the perfect way to begin getting back into shape after childbirth. Build up slowly. There may be a walking club for mums in your area.
* Gentle yoga is energising and relaxing.
* PILATES is strengthening.
* If your back or pelvic joints are painful (page 43) ask your midwife for advice. Remember that strengthening your muscles protects your joints and your spine and can help to relieve discomfort.

After six weeks

* Allow at least six and preferably 12 weeks before you return to demanding exercise.
* If you want to return to strength training, wait until week six at the earliest and start with low weights.
* Gradually increase the distance you walk while carrying your baby – ideally in a sling or papoose. This helps your bones and your baby's bones lay down more calcium and become stronger. It also increases your cardiovascular workout.
* A balanced combination of aerobic conditioning

and strength training is the most effective way to reduce excess fat and build a strong, fit body.
* It is fine to continue with yoga and pilates.

After caesarean

* Gentle postnatal yoga stretches and pelvic floor exercises (page 438) are fine to do within three to four days.
* You could start a graduated programme of walking in the first week, and swim or use an exercise cycle within one to three weeks. Begin with five to 10 minutes of exercise, and gradually increase to 20–30 minutes over weeks.
* If you begin gently and take care you'll have no problems using free weights at the gym.
* Abdominal exercises must be delayed for six to 10 weeks.
* It's best to delay a return to intensive aerobic exercises for 10 weeks.

Motivation

If you cannot muster the enthusiasm or find the time, rest assured that many women feel the same. Making exercise part of every day may not be as hard as you think. There are many ways to exercise with your baby, including stretching at home and walking together. You won't need a babysitter or a crèche, you can walk with a sling or big-wheeled stroller. The motion is usually very restful.

When you are ready to exercise without your baby, there may be people in your family or community who can care for her for up to an hour. This could create two or three opportunities for exercise each week – perhaps swimming or cycling or going to the gym.

Gentle progress

* Try not to set goals that are too ambitious – keep your aims moderate.
* It will take time to regain your pre-pregnancy shape. Try not to judge your progress by your weight – now is certainly not the time to cut down on calories. If you are building up your muscles the scales may actually show a gain simply because muscle weighs more than fat – but your body shape will improve. It is best to judge your wellbeing by the way you look and feel, and to exercise as part of a wider programme of caring for yourself (page 121).
* If you are breastfeeding, you may lose weight

gradually, or continue to carry a couple of extra pounds of energy so your body can produce enough milk.

■ PROBLEMATIC AND COMPULSIVE EXERCISE (ANOREXIA ATHLETICA)

Exercise beyond the level needed for good health is a disorder called anorexia athletica. It is often linked with an obsession about weight and diet. Compulsive exercise can be a way of avoiding facing up to emotional problems or challenging relationships. It may be used to relieve stress or guilt, especially if you have been bingeing. In pregnancy, exercising excessively and addictively may be a problem if you become overheated, dehydrated or exhausted or if the exercise carries a risk to your baby, for example from excessive running or high-impact activities. With a good diet the risks to a baby are minimal but there is a higher risk of intrauterine growth restriction (IUGR) and premature birth. After the birth, excessive exercise may reduce breast milk flow. If you exercise inappropriately the support suggested on page 201 may be useful.

Expressing milk

See Breastfeeding, advice.

Extra digits

Straight after the birth, the counting of fingers and toes is all part of the ritual of welcome. Accessory digits (extra fingers and toes) are usually simple to spot. If they are present it is reassuring to know that this is a common situation and causes no problems.

Extra digits are one of the more frequently occurring congenital abnormalities. Usually they appear next to the little finger or smallest toe. The extra digit may be attached by a narrow band of tissue and be very small. It may have a nail and contain an artery, vein and nerve but probably no bony tissue.

The best treatment is for a plastic surgeon to cut off the accessory digit at the base. This is usually done at the age of three to six months, under an anaesthetic. Once removed

there is no problem with either walking or using the hand.

A much rarer type of accessory digit occurs beside the thumb or at the site of the big toe. These can sometimes be associated with other defects, including heart abnormalities, and need to be investigated. The extra digits are often complete duplications of the thumb or big toe and treatment will be advised by a paediatric plastic surgeon.

Occasionally, an infant is born with an extra little toe on one or both feet, a relatively common condition called polydactyly. Though alarming to parents, this condition simply requires surgical removal of the additional toe to avoid problems with wearing shoes and walking, as well as for cosmetic reasons. The procedure is usually done before walking begins. Once the toe is removed, your child's foot will develop normally, and he will run, jump and play just like every other child his age.

Eye crossing and squinting, baby

Eye crossing or misalignment is common in the first three months because your baby's eyes do not work in synchrony until after 12 weeks. If her eyes cross after she is four months old, or beyond the sixth month she seems to have a squint (strabismus) where one eye points in a different direction to the other, you need to visit an ophthalmologist who can assess her visual development.

A squint may result from long- or short-sightedness. This leads to poor focusing and the brain does not merge the images received by each eye. As a result each eye adopts its own position, and if they are not aligned with each other the central black spot (iris) appears off centre. Treatment with glasses to correct the impairment allows the eyes to realign so they look straight and move together. If the squint is not treated then binocular vision, which is required in order to judge depth and distance, will not develop. Glasses for young children are safe and come in a range of fun colours.

Some squints result from a weakness in one of the eye muscles. The muscle may be strengthened by exercises, wearing glasses, and finally by an operation to either lengthen or shorten it.

Operations are usually done for cosmetic reasons and often a loss of depth-perception can occur despite early attempts to correct vision.

PUPILS OF DIFFERENT SIZES

Occasionally, differing pupil size, also called anisocoria, is inherited and there is no underlying disorder. If other members of your family members have this condition, the differing size is likely to be genetic and will have no effect on your baby's eyesight. Some believe this occurs in up to 20 per cent of individuals, and appears more commonly in those with blue eyes.

Rarely, different-size pupils might indicate a problem in the eye, optic nerve or in the brain, and your doctor may recommend referral to a specialist.

RETINOBLASTOMA

Retinoblastoma is a rare type of eye cancer that is typically limited to children below the age of five and is rarely a cause of squinting. Between 40 and 50 children develop this type of tumour each year in the UK. Although this can be very distressing and frightening for the child and their parents, over 90 per cent of children are cured with the right treatment.

Retinoblastoma is often picked up early when parents notice that one eye does not show the red reflection to flash photography. This can be seen in the photograph. The pupil may look white, like a cat's eye that is reflecting light, and your baby may not be seeing well. Alternatively, the eye may be red and inflamed. If you are concerned, ask for your baby to be checked. The earlier treatment is given, the better the outcome.

Retinoblastoma can occur in two forms:

An inherited (genetic) form

Here there are often tumours in both eyes (bilateral) or sometimes only in one eye. This accounts for around 40 per cent of cases. People with the defective gene, known as the Rb gene, have an increased risk of developing other types of tumour later in life. Not all children of an affected parent will inherit this gene. However, all children with a family history will usually be checked after birth and every few months for five years, so that treatment can be started early if a tumour does develop.

Non-inherited form

Here there is a tumour in only one eye (unilateral). The cause remains unknown.

Treatment and support

The discovery of a cancer and the course of treatment will affect the whole family and you will all benefit from support. Your child and any brothers and sisters may have a range of powerful emotions and need emotional care.

Following treatment, an eye specialist will frequently examine your child's eye under anaesthetic to check that the cancer has not come back. Follow-up is usually in a clinic for childhood cancers (a paediatric oncology clinic) and your child will be given genetic counselling when she is old enough to understand it, if the retinoblastoma is genetic.

The aim of treatment is firstly to get rid of the tumour and secondly to try to keep the sight in the eye. A small number of children lose some of their sight.

For small tumours, treatment is given to the eye itself (local therapy). More than one treatment session may be needed (usually at monthly intervals). Methods include freezing (cryotherapy), laser therapy, the use of a plaque (a small disc containing a radioactive substance stitched over the tumour on the outside of the eye, for two to four days), or thermotherapy (using laser-directed heat), often in combination with chemotherapy or radiotherapy.

Larger tumours can be treated in a number of ways, including chemotherapy, radiotherapy or, if the tumour is very large and vision has been lost, surgery to remove the eye (enucleation) and fit a false eye.

Eye infection and swelling, baby

If your baby has swollen, puffy or red eyes, or there is pus in the eyes, he may have an infection. Your doctor will be able to diagnose the problem. The most important measure is for you to keep your baby's eyes clean. Homeopathic and/or medical treatment may be appropriate. Common causes of eye problems are:

- Blocked tear ducts – typically causing weepy eyes.
- Conjunctivitis – typically causing sticky eyes, swollen eye lids, and sometimes pus in the eyes.
- Stye – typically causing a red spot on the edge of the eyelid that enlarges and then bursts.

At birth, you may see a blood-red spot in one or both of your baby's eyes. This is not a sign of infection but a result of pressure during birth that has caused blood vessels on the white of the eye to break (conjunctival haemorrhage). The blood will be reabsorbed and disappear within a few weeks.

■ BLOCKED TEAR DUCTS

About 5 per cent of babies are born with a blockage to the tear duct, which stops tears draining away down the back of the nose. This is usually noticeable within two months of birth when one or both eyes water continuously ('weepy eye') and when your baby cries, you may see that the nostril on the affected side remains dry. From time to time, your baby may also have 'sticky eyes' caused by a mild infection resulting from the blockage (below).

Action plan

The best thing to do is to keep your baby's eyes clean and care for them well.

- Clean the eyes using cotton wool soaked in fresh, boiled and cooled water. Use a separate piece of cotton wool for each eye. Gently wipe the cotton wool up the bony part of his nose, over the inner corner of his eye, then out over the eyelids. This also massages the tear duct and may open the blockage.
- If you are BREASTFEEDING, squeeze a couple of drops of milk into the affected eye.
- In general, antibiotics are not needed, but occasionally, if the eyelids become unusually red and swollen, antibiotic treatment may help.
- Your baby's tear ducts are likely to be normal within 18 months, without treatment. There is a small chance (5 per cent) that discharge may continue for longer and the ducts will need to be cleared by a specialist. This is done as a day case, under anaesthetic.

■ CONJUNCTIVITIS (STICKY EYE)

The conjunctiva is a transparent membrane than lines the inside of the eyelid and covers the front of the eye. Conjunctivitis occurs when the conjunctiva becomes inflamed. This may be the result of a bacterial or viral infection or may happen if your baby gets a chemical (such as a perfume spray) in his eye. An infection usually affects both eyes. If just one eye is affected, check to see whether your baby has something lodged in his eye or has any sign of injury. Conjunctivitis may be a symptom of ALLERGY, although this is rare in babies below one year of age.

Conjunctivitis infection most commonly occurs following a blockage of the tear ducts. Usually, aided by blinking, tears flow across the front of the eye and drain into the tear duct, passing down the back of the nose and throat. Anything that blocks the passage of tears can lead to infection. Newborn babies often have partially closed ducts and have a tendency to recurrent sticky eyes for a few months.

Uncommonly, conjunctivitis may be a symptom of GONORRHOEA infection, especially if sticky eye appears within 24 hours of birth. This needs prompt treatment because it may cause permanent eye damage. If your newborn has conjunctivitis your doctor will also consider other infections, such as CHLAMYDIA, particularly if he also has a cough. Both infections need careful specialist treatment with antibiotics and eye ointments.

Bacterial conjunctivitis

Yellow sticky pus in the eyes (hence 'sticky eyes') is the classic symptom of bacterial conjunctivitis, which is common and highly contagious. It usually rapidly settles after treatment with antibiotic drops and ointment. The drops wash out quickly and so need to be given every few hours during the day. The ointment works well at night, forming a film over the eye that helps prevent the eyelids sticking together in the mornings. If your baby wakes up with crusty eyelids, wipe his eyes with cotton wool soaked in warm, previously boiled and cooled water. While your baby (or any other member of the family) is infected do not share towels.

Viral conjunctivitis

Conjunctivitis caused by viral infection often makes the affected eye feel gritty and there may be a slight discharge. Viral conjunctivitis will not respond to antibiotics and can take two or three weeks to settle without treatment. It is important to clean your baby's eyes carefully, and he may respond to homeopathic remedies (see below), which speed the healing. If his eyes are very sore, lubricant drops may give some relief. Conjunctivitis may recur when another virus is present and your baby may have other symptoms such as a sore throat. If the infection is MEASLES, RUBELLA or HERPES, your baby will need specialist treatment and will be prescribed antiviral drops.

Homeopathic treatment

You may give the most appropriate remedy (30c potency) three times a day for three days and then re-assess. In addition, you may bathe your baby's eyes with *Euphrasia Tincture*, which must always be diluted: eight drops to 250ml (½ pint) of boiled, cooled water. This may be repeated three times per day. *Euphrasia Tincture* should never be used undiluted.

- *Arg Nit* is a specific remedy for conjunctivitis in newborns, where the eyes are red, the lids swollen and there is a creamy or yellow discharge.
- *Pulsatilla* if the lids stick together with a bland, yellowish discharge (often the left eye is worse)

and your baby is clingy or whiney and feels better in the open air.
- *Apis* for puffy eyelids and if your baby is irritable and fidgety, rubs his eyes and seems sensitive to light.

STYES

A stye (also known as a hordeolum), is a bacterial infection of a gland or hair follicle on the edge of the eyelid. A stye starts as a red spot and slowly enlarges over three to four days, slowly filling with pus. It then bursts and will subsequently heal over five to seven days. If your baby rubs his eyes a lot, another stye may occur in his other eye.

The infection may be fought off naturally by his body, but antibiotic ointment can help. Rarely, infection spreads and causes cellulitis of the eyelid, which requires oral antibiotic treatment. If the same gland gets infected over and over (a chalazion) your baby will be referred to an ophthalmologist who may recommend very minor surgery to drain the gland, after which the infection will not recur.

Homeopathy
The most commonly used remedies for styes are *Pulsatilla* and *Staphysagria*. You may start with *Pulsatilla* (30c potency) three times a day for two days and continue for a further two days if there is improvement. If there is no improvement after two days then you may give *Staphysagria* (30c) for two days and re-assess. If there is no improvement please seek alternative medical advice.

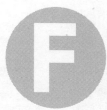

Fainting

See Blood pressure, low and fainting.

Family

See Parenting.

Father

For the majority of men, being a father is one of the most wonderful experiences in life. Throughout this book the advice for enjoying parenthood and caring for yourself and your baby amid the challenges of everyday life relates as much to dads as to mums. This entry is more specifically for you.

Despite dads having a much greater involvement in family life today than was the case in the past, many men still question their role. Do I protect my partner and our children? Is it okay for me to cry? Can I still enjoy football and nights out when I'm a dad? Does my child need me when my wife is there to feed and hold him?

The answer to all of these is 'Yes'. You bring a unique male energy to your family and to your baby. Your baby will look to you for love and comfort and will enjoy the difference between you and his mum. He will benefit from having you both around to care for and play with him. In the early months, an important role for you is to care for your partner so that she can care for, feed and nurture your baby. To do this well it is essential to care for yourself. Focusing on the

three of you – without neglecting yourself – is the best recipe to ensure you all feel calm, happy and healthy. You may enjoy dipping into the section CARING FOR YOU.

You may or may not want to base your way of parenting on the example set by your father. This may depend on the relationship you had with your father and on changing attitudes towards fatherhood by society as a whole. Now you have an opportunity to establish your own role model for your son or daughter. Daughters need your male energy as much as sons. You can bond and play with them and nourish them in a way that feels good for you both, and enjoy a close and loving relationship. The tips on page 120 give an overview. Laying strong foundations now will set up a good relationship for life.

▨ BIRTHING WITH YOUR BABY

See also Labour and birth, baby; Labour and birth, mother.

Being present for the birth takes many different forms. Some dads are fully involved and choose to welcome their baby's head and assist at the final moment of birth, then cut the cord; others prefer to be beside their partner's head; others choose not to be in the room at the moment of birth. These days most fathers have a choice about their level of involvement – but even with planning, things do not always go as expected. You may become either more or less involved than you had anticipated. On the day you will respond to the mood and needs of your partner and baby, and the encouragement or requests of the midwives.

It's important that you talk with your partner prior to labour so that you understand her wishes and she knows how you feel. If you wish to be hands-on, useful preparation includes rehearsing positions, breathing together, trying MASSAGE and maybe practising VISUALISATIONS. You may be in charge of the music, preparing the birthing space, and on the day she may appreciate having you there to liaise with the birth team. Your partner will benefit from your love, encouragement and patience. You'll be able to give her the best possible support if you are relaxed and keep up your own energy levels.

If you do not wish to be present for the birth and the decision feels right for you both, it is important to talk about when you do want to join your partner, either in early labour but not later, or within minutes of the birth, or after she and your baby have had a longer period of undisturbed time together. You may change your mind on the day. There may be ways you can be there without watching the actual birth. You and your partner may want to ask another person to be present, either in addition or instead of you.

Tips

* Talk things through in advance. You may want to create a birth plan together.
* Most dads feel the benefit of talking to other fathers (and expectant fathers) as well, and attending one or more antenatal meetings or birth classes.
* Ensure you are well nourished so your energy levels stay topped up. Labour can go on for hours.
* It is both okay and necessary to rest. You may want to leave the room from time to time, for a nap or to freshen up.
* Don't take it personally if your partner doesn't want you there or doesn't like what you're doing. She is likely to enter a state of consciousness you have never witnessed before and her focus is on the contractions and her baby.
* Try not to engage your partner with difficult questions, as this could draw her out of the birthing space and slow her progress.
* You may want to read about labour and birth and talk to midwives – this reduces your anxiety on the day and may be useful if interventions or special care are needed.

* You may find it difficult to see your partner in pain and distress. It is useful to chat about this before the birth.
* Arrange to have practical support at home after the birth so you can spend time with your baby and your partner.
* If there are problems or birth doesn't go as planned, it is important to acknowledge that you may be shocked, frustrated or upset. Many dads in this situation focus on being strong for their partner and baby. Some cannot keep it up and become stressed. It usually helps to talk to a good friend or to one of the medical team.

Meeting your baby

If you are in the birthing room you have the opportunity to meet and greet your baby as soon as he is born. Many men describe this as the most incredible experience of a lifetime. If your baby and your partner are well and do not need medical support, the time immediately after birth is for them to enjoy skin-to-skin contact (page 517) and the intimacy of feeding. This is the best possible start for your baby and is an important part of bonding.

When your partner is ready, or while she is having medical care, it will be time for you to hold your baby for the first time. If you hold your baby naked against your bare skin, this is likely to deepen your connection and will help to flood your body with joyful love-hormones (page 307). This early contact, whether it comes minutes or hours after the birth, is extremely precious.

▓ BONDING WITH YOUR BABY

See also Emotions, bonding and attachment.

Bonding is not the preserve of mums. Many dads wonder in advance whether they will be able to bond with their baby, and find that any concerns are unfounded. The key is to spend time with your baby. The more time you spend together, the closer the bond between you is likely to be. Your baby will feel secure if you offer a calm, loving and accepting space and you are able to focus on him and slow down to tune into his needs.

Bonding is a two-way process in which your baby also attaches to you, and he will always play an important part in your relationship. Remember that your baby is genetically programmed to bond and wants to feel close to you. There are many practical things you can do to build and deepen the connection. These include skin-to-skin contact, eye contact, talking, watching and listening and they are discussed on pages 208–9).

If you do not feel you are bonding with your baby, the remedy may be as simple as spending more time together. It is useful to work through any problems in your partnership (page 461) so that you are relaxed at home and the environment around your baby is peaceful and playful. For some dads, bonding gets a lot easier when anxieties are shared with a good friend or a counsellor. It can be reassuring to know that not all fathers bond the instant their baby is conceived or born, and also that when a bond is formed, it tends to last for life.

There is no 'perfect' situation. What matters most is the quality of time you spend together – if your baby feels you connecting with him, his psychological health is bound to be enhanced and the relationship between you will flourish. Think of the first few months as an introduction. If you met an adult you would get to know them through spending time with them. The same applies to your new baby. In the first months the pace is slow. Getting to know one another may be the easiest thing you have ever done. On the other hand, if you are ambivalent about being a father it could take time to settle into your new role.

The sex of your new baby may be important to you. Some men find it easier to bond with a boy. Others feel a stronger bond with a girl. In some families there is a cultural preference, or pressure from one or both sets of grandparents. You might choose to ask at the ultrasound scan during pregnancy about your baby's sex. The sex can usually be identified from around Week 20. If you know whether your baby is a boy or girl and you feel disappointed, you have time to get used to the idea and accept your baby for the individual person he or she is. Talking with friends or family about the issue could be very helpful if you feel ambivalent or upset.

The way you bond with your baby is also influenced by the way you bonded with your own father and mother. Your earliest relationships and the lessons you unconsciously learnt about loving, trusting and communicating affect the way you behave now. You may prefer not to recreate your own family experience, if it was an unsatisfactory one. On the other hand, if your family life was idyllic you may be keen to repeat it. Either way, bear in mind that your experience with your child will be unique.

As you build a relationship with your new baby you will discover that he is an individual. Your baby will let you know what he needs and likes. The most important thing for him is to feel heard, accepted and loved for who he is. Feeling you love and delight in him will help your baby delight in himself, feel settled, and encourage a progressively deeper bond.

▓ CARING FOR YOU

Although cultural expectations of men and of fathers are changing, a stereotypical image of men being strong, resilient and supportive has not disappeared. Many men tend to be driven, albeit unconsciously, by these qualities. They are incredibly valuable but can be draining if you do not also care for yourself. It is not rocket science to know that if you are well cared for, you will be stronger and more supportive for yourself and your family.

Popular hero figures glorify masculinity as a combination of superhuman powers, strength and high achievement and rarely focus on the need for rest, good food, good friends and time with a new baby and time out for you – or the need to play and to be loved and nurtured.

When you care for yourself well, you are likely to enjoy:

* Enhanced energy and health.
* Growing confidence as a parent.
* More enjoyment with your baby.
* Better communication and intimacy with your partner.
* Greater satisfaction at home and at work.
* Good times with your friends.

What do you need?

Many adults – men and women alike – are unsure what they need in order to feel well and happy. This uncertainty often has roots in babyhood. All children need adults to help them understand and trust their feelings and their needs. Children who do not have quality time with mum and dad in a close and secure relationship may cut off from their emotional feelings, or believe their needs are not important.

You may have been raised in a family of regimented feeding and sleeping times, or in a family where children should be 'seen and not heard', or in a family where stressful work commitments reduced the time your parents had with you. You may not have been encouraged to acknowledge or express your feelings and ask for your needs to be met.

Alternatively you may be clear about what you need, including time with your baby and family, exercise, friends to confide in, time to relax, a chance to express your talents and skills through work or play. These are among the basics (page 122). Knowing your needs may help as you deftly balance your life and prioritise in the months after birth when your lifestyle may change significantly.

Priorities

Your priorities are likely to shift from week to week, and you will need to juggle your needs with the needs of your baby and family. Some men give family commitments low priority and put most energy into work – often there is a feeling of pressure from financial and emotional demands and a desire to be single and carefree. Others put work in second place and rate family time as high priority. Being 'hands on' as a father and family man is not wasted time: it is very precious and nurtures skills that will serve you well in your future career as well as in your personal relationships.

If you tend to give your needs a low priority, you may expect your partner and your child to feel the same as you do. You can change within a loving relationship where you are encouraged to listen to and care for yourself, and it is okay to voice your needs – this may be the best way to get support and to notice what your baby and partner need. Your family and your new baby offer you the wonderful opportunity of slowing down, spending time together, and feeling the rewards of your relationships growing. You may begin to recognise more of your needs and fulfil them within the new context of family life. You, your baby and your family will benefit from your own wellbeing.

■ EMOTIONS AND FEELINGS

Becoming a father is an intensely emotional time of life. It is a wonderful opportunity to enjoy the richness of strong feelings: delightful, rocky, turbulent, calm and frightening. Some men love the emotional ride, while others find the intensity overwhelming. Your emotions affect your wellbeing, your energy and your relationships. If it was the norm in your family of origin to suppress emotions, including joy, anger, love and fear, it may be difficult to be comfortable with the emotional journey you are on now.

Your big feelings

We look at emotions in depth on pages 206–25. They are common to everyone – men, women, babies and children – and you may enjoy reading about the big feelings that we all share: bonding, care and nurturing, explorative urge, fear and anxiety, playfulness, rage and anger, separation anxiety. You may recognise some of these 'big feelings' in the range of views below, some positive and some negative:

Positive feelings
* I am so in love, this feeling is incredible, the best of my life.
* I feel so strongly linked with my baby.
* I am so clear now about my purpose and I love providing for my family, it feels so right.
* I love the feeling of playing with my baby, it's so easy; we have so much fun together.
* I feel even more deeply bonded with my partner now, this is really special.

Negative feelings
* I'm worried about my baby's health – what if there's something wrong or something bad happens during birth?
* There's no time for me any more – my baby and my wife only have eyes for each other.
* I can't stop worrying that my colleague will get that promotion I wanted – he's not distracted by a baby.
* I get so angry when I come home from work and my baby is crying and my wife is grumpy.
* I'm jealous I can't be as intimate with my baby as my wife is.
* I'm nervous around my baby, it seems I can't do anything right.

* It upsets me that I hardly have any time with my baby.
* Will we ever have sex again? I don't know how long I can hold out for.

It is okay to have whatever feelings arise, and it's helpful to accept and welcome them. Your feelings are your guides and even the uncomfortable ones invite you to acknowledge and possibly change some aspect of your life.

There will be many practical things you can do to alter an uncomfortable situation. For example:

* Create time to be with your partner.
* Negotiate a night out with your mates.
* Massage and play with your baby.
* Sleep with your baby and partner.
* Ask for extra help around the house.

These and other suggestions are discussed in more detail elsewhere in this guide. Please remember that these early days do not last long and it is great for you, your baby and partner to spend time together. You are all on a journey and you are likely to feel better if you talk and keep intimacy alive (page 471).

Feeling left out – separation anxiety

The 'mother cat with her kitten' instinct often surfaces in a new mother. If your partner is like this, it may be hard for you to take an active part in baby care – she may not give you time with your baby, or she may criticise you for doing things in the wrong way.

Men also play roles. The 'upset little boy' sometimes emerges, and a man expects to be mothered by his partner and feels neglected. These feelings often arise from childhood experiences.

The first months are for 'trying on' the roles of parents and juggling all your needs. Your partner's hormones focus her on your baby. Try not to take this personally. Nature has ensured that she concentrates on nourishing and protecting your baby. This is a time when some men begin new relationships. If you feel left out, it may be useful to think about alternative ways you can be involved at home. It may take weeks to feel at ease around your partner and your new baby.

When you're upset

When you feel upset or confronted you may carry this energy into your relationship – perhaps being snappy with your partner – and then feel more upset and angry. She may behave in a similar way when she is upset. There is advice on resolving differences on page 462) that may help you accept your feelings, step back from the 'blame game' and feel heard. Reducing your emotional stress will improve your energy, and you'll be pleased of this after the birth when you may be short of sleep. Try to keep love and acceptance – of yourself as well as your baby and partner – to the fore.

■ SLEEP

Fatherhood inevitably means your sleep pattern will alter, probably for a few months, perhaps for years. This may begin before the birth, if your partner finds it difficult to get comfortable in bed or wakes frequently at night.

There are tips for getting good quality sleep on pages 495–6. One of the tricks is to focus on quality rather than the number of hours. You can still be well rested, even without getting six to eight hours' sleep at a stretch. Remember that night time can be a wonderful opportunity for intimacy. If your baby is in your bed you will both benefit from skin-to-skin touch. It's also important to sleep well. It will be okay for you to spend a night in a different room if you need to be fresh and alert the following day.

If tiredness becomes a problem it may be useful to attend to what happens in the day – work demands, exercise, nutrition and rest – as well as your sleeping habits at night. There are tips for improving energy on pages 515–6.

Fear

See Emotions, fear and anxiety.

Febrile convulsions

See Fits, baby.

Feeding

See Bottle-feeding; Breastfeeding, advice; Weaning.

Feelings

See Emotions.

Fever, baby

At some point your baby will almost certainly develop a high temperature. This is a natural mechanism that helps her body fight infections. The average baby has around seven to eight viral illnesses a year, which invariably result in fever. Fever is also called febrile illness. When the temperature rises rapidly, some babies may be susceptible to febrile seizures (page 241).

Taking your baby's temperature

The average childhood body temperature varies from 36.5 to 37.5°C. A fever is an abnormally high body temperature that is at least 0.5°C above normal on two recordings taken at least two hours apart. Your baby's 'normal' body temperature is individual to her. To find out what this is, simply take your baby's temperature when she is well, using the same method as you would if she was unwell with a fever.

It is important to read your child's temperature before giving any fever-reducing medicines. A satisfactory temperature reading can usually be obtained by placing a digital display thermometer in the armpit, directly against the skin, and holding the arm gently against the chest for the time recommended by the thermometer manufacturer or instructions that come with the thermometer. Digital thermometers usually give a reading within a few seconds. The armpit, also called the axillary, reading will be 0.5–0.6°C lower than it would be if the temperature was measured with a thermometer in the mouth (oral). For accurate guidelines, see the table overleaf.

Accompanying symptoms, such as your baby seeming unwell or too warm, having sweaty

+ Red flag

Call your doctor or the emergency services immediately if one or more of the following occur:
- Any fever below eight weeks of age or, when older, a temperature more than 0.5°C (0.9°F) above normal.
- A FIT (seizures) or convulsion.
- Uncontrolled crying or restlessness.
- A sudden rash or bruising.
- Difficulty breathing (page 102).
- Drowsiness or irritability.
- Fever related to heat/humidity exposure (heat stroke).
- A rash that does not fade when a glass is pressed against it. Your baby may also have a stiff neck. This could indicate infection with the bacteria Meningococcus, which causes MENINGITIS.
- Ear pain (or ear rubbing).
- Your baby becomes limp and floppy. A very sick baby may not show a fever, but may get cold instead (page 315).
- Persistent DIARRHOEA and VOMITING.
- Your baby looks or acts sick and refuses feeds.
- Your baby's temperature does not fall in response to the usual treatments (see below). Your baby may get one illness closely followed by another, giving the impression that the fever is long lasting but it is best to be safe.

The key is to establish the source and site of the infection causing the fever. This is often a viral infection of the ears, nose or throat, the digestive system or the urinary tract. Viruses usually disappear without treatment and cannot be treated with antibiotics.

skin or being generally out of sorts, are also important. If your baby has a fever, her hands and feet may feel icy cold, and look a bit blue. If you are worried, follow your instinct. Feeling your baby's forehead is not an accurate measure of temperature – use a thermometer to be sure.

239

Your paediatrician may refer to the following figures:

	Normal	*Fever*
Mouth	37°C (98.6°F)	37.5°C (99.5°F)
Armpit	36.4°C (97.6°F)	37°C (98.6°F)
Rectum	37.6°C (99.6°F)	38°C (100.4°F)

Forehead strip readings are accurate enough to confirm the presence of a fever, and to use as you decide whether to give your baby paracetamol (page 429), but not accurate enough to determine that fever with any precision. They are more accurate than just feeling the forehead with the back of your hand. The temperature detected by both these methods, however, will be affected by high room temperatures, which do not affect electronic digital thermometers.

When reporting a fever to your doctor, it is best to just report the reading on the thermometer, saying how you took it, instead of trying to add or subtract a degree yourself to see if the temperature is significant or not. The temperature reading is just one of the factors that your doctor will consider when deciding how best to treat your child.

Stopping further temperature rise

The goal is to stop the temperature rising any higher, and this will make your baby more comfortable and reduce the small risk that a rapid rise in temperature will lead to a febrile seizure (fit or convulsion). Use the 'take temperature, treat temperature, take temperature' approach.
- Give loving care.
- Keep your baby's room cool but avoid cold draughts.
- Keep your baby lightly dressed in cotton for comfort or take all her clothes off.
- Do not bring your baby into your bed where your body heat may boost her temperature.
- Use infant paracetamol in the correct dosage (page 429) to treat the fever and reduce pain. It cannot mask more serious symptoms.
- Give favourite nutritious foods and drinks. She may enjoy juice or ice pops.
- Sponge your baby with lukewarm (never hot) water. But make sure the water is not too cold

because if it is this will reduce blood flow to the skin and that may make your baby's temperature increase. The ideal water temperature is the same as your skin. It often takes 20–30 minutes of this to reduce the fever significantly. If your baby starts to shiver, stop sponging – the shivering will raise her temperature again.
- Try to keep your child calm because exertion may raise the temperature.
- Do not put a baby with febrile convulsions/seizures in a bath or use alcohol on her skin.
- Aspirin-containing preparations must never be used in childhood. Aspirin intake during a viral infection has been associated with an increased risk of Reye's syndrome, a rare condition that causes brain and liver damage and sometimes death.

Fevers generally get better within three to four days. If your baby continues to have a high temperature or any rash does not settle, visit your doctor to exclude other illnesses including bacterial infections requiring antibiotics.

Because your child may be infectious, it is best to keep her away from other children for 24 hours after the fever has cleared.

Homeopathy
Homeopathic remedies may be an effective method of reducing temperatures. As you get to know which remedies work best for your baby, it becomes much easier to prescribe. If your baby's temperature is very high you must seek urgent medical attention (above). You may give the most appropriate remedy (30c potency) every hour for the first three hours and then re-assess. If your baby seems to improve, continue with the same remedy every two hours for a further six hours and re-assess. If after one hour there is no change, look at giving a different remedy and consult your homeopath.
- *Belladonna* for sudden onset of symptoms – often around 3pm: a 'Belladonna look' with flushed face, red lips, dilated pupils, glassy eyes, skin hot to touch on the body, feet are usually cold, a strong racing pulse. Your baby may feel worse from bright light, and from any jarring movement.

- *Aconite* for a sudden onset of symptoms, usually around midnight (sometimes after the baby has become chilled), with a dry heat, great thirst, contracted pupils, anxiety and restlessness.
- *Chamomilla* if your baby has a burning heat, usually with sweating, particularly around the face and head and perhaps alternating with chills, or one part of the body is hot while another is cool, one cheek may be red and the other pale, she is irritable and demanding and often wants to be carried.
- *Arsenicum* for symptoms that are worse between midnight and 2am, a high fever with sweating, thirst, laboured breathing and perhaps vomiting or diarrhoea.
- *Ferrum Phos* for fevers where there are few other symptoms, without sudden onset or intensity, nor irritability or restlessness, but with fever worse in the late afternoon and at night, relieved with cold compresses and lying down.
- *Bryonia* for a fever that has a gradual onset with heat, sweating, irritability and thirst, symptoms are worse for movement, and your baby wants to be left alone and quiet.
- *Gelsemium* for a slower onset of symptoms. Your baby may look heavy-lidded, drowsy and weak with no thirst although the mouth and lips may look dry.
- *Pulsatilla* for a fever with chilliness and changeable symptoms. Your baby may feel weepy, clingy, whiny, wanting to be held and carried. She may feel better in the fresh air and is characteristically not thirsty.

▓ FEBRILE SEIZURES (FITS OR CONVULSIONS)

A febrile seizure, or fit, is a convulsion brought on by a fever. It appears to be related to a rapid rise in temperature, rather than the height of the temperature itself. It usually has no serious or long-term effects but witnessing your child having a fit can be terrifying. These types of fit occur in around 4 per cent of children between the ages of six months and six years and tend to run in families. The advice below applies to babies and small children.

What happens

During a febrile seizure your baby will lose consciousness, the eyes may roll back into the head and there is usually stiffening followed by rhythmic jerking of the arms and legs. This lasts no more than 10 minutes and stops without treatment. Your baby will probably be sleepy after the seizure but get back to normal – often within 60 minutes – except for feeling ill from the fever and the illness causing it. If the fit continues for longer than 10 minutes, your baby needs help to stop the seizure because a prolonged fit may lead to damage. Call for an ambulance.

After the fit, your baby may continue to shake or shiver – this is called a rigor, and is a response to the high temperature. The rigors will stop as the temperature comes down. Many children thought to have had a febrile convulsion have, in fact, had a severe rigor. These carry no risk of epilepsy or any other complication.

Action plan

If your child has a febrile seizure, attend to the convulsion, which will be short lasting. Then your priority is to help reduce the temperature as you would for a fever. As soon as you can, or if someone is with you, call your doctor or the emergency services.

Although you may be frightened, it is most helpful to stay calm. Taking a dose of homeopathic *Aconite* (200c potency) yourself can be very calming. Once you're calm it's easier to do the best for your baby and to observe the fit so you can describe it to a doctor. In particular, note whether it affects the whole body or just certain parts. The fit may seem to last longer than it actually does. Your doctor will ask you how long the fit lasted. Refer to a clock or watch so you can give an accurate account, rather than estimating.

- While your baby is jerking, lie her on the floor on her side and check that her throat is not obstructed: your baby may be dribbling or vomiting and so should not be upright.
- Do not put anything in the mouth or restrain your baby.
- Soothe your baby with your voice and a gentle touch and watch closely.

- When the fit has passed, unless already undressed, remove your baby's clothes as a first step to cooling her. Do not cuddle your baby, as this will prevent heat loss.
- Sponge your baby with water that is cool/lukewarm (but not cold). It should be roughly the same as your body temperature. If you have flannels or cloths to hand, soak them and lay them over your baby's body for a short time. Do not leave them there because they will soon begin to trap heat.
- Turn off any radiators or move your baby to a cooler room or use a fan and await the arrival of your doctor or the ambulance crew.
- Stay with your baby and reassure her that everything is all right and you are there, but do not cuddle your baby. Your baby may take around five minutes to regain consciousness and register your presence and then go back to sleep.
- If you have not given infant paracetamol in the last four hours, give a dose as soon as your baby is able to take it. Paracetamol is also available as a suppository and this may be suitable if your baby is vomiting. Suppositories can be bought over the counter at larger chemists and pharmacists, where a pharmacist can discuss the dosage with you (page 429).

If your baby is prone to febrile convulsions, consult with your homeopath who can prepare a group of remedies that might be required.

Medical care

Not all doctors recommend admission following a febrile convulsion. Your doctor will advise you. If your baby is in hospital:

- She may be kept in isolation if there has been vomiting or diarrhoea. Her temperature will be taken regularly and she will be kept calm and regularly given infant paracetamol.
- Your doctor may check to exclude bacterial infection or meningitis-related illness. A urine test will check for urinary infection.
- If the doctors are happy that your baby has fully recovered and have observed her for six hours, she will be allowed to go home. Her temperature, depending on the initial cause, may remain high for three to four days. Further fever-related fits are unlikely.
- If your baby is still having fits when help

comes, medical staff will give oxygen and may give anticonvulsant medication. After a prolonged fit, your baby will be monitored, with full medical follow-up that may include tests for infection.

What are the implications?

- If your baby has had no previous signs of neurological problems and the seizure is related to a fever, there is no increased risk of developmental problems.
- If your baby has had a rigor there is no risk of complications.
- Once your baby has had a febrile seizure, the risk of having another is around 35 per cent. Next time your baby's temperature rises, take early steps to reduce it.
- A febrile convulsion cannot cause epilepsy. If your child is predisposed to epilepsy, however, the first febrile convulsion may be a trigger.

Fibroids

A fibroid is a thickening of the muscle fibres in the uterine wall. Fibroids can vary from pea-size to grapefruit-size, or bigger, and may occur singly or in groups. They are benign (non-cancerous) and usually reduce after pregnancy. Their cause is unknown. They are more common in women of African origin and may run in families. Most women with small fibroids are able to have a normal labour and birth. Although the most common symptom is pain, many women have fibroids without symptoms.

What happens

Fibroids can form on the outer surface of the wall of the uterus, in the wall itself or impinge into the internal cavity of the uterus – the last are more likely to be troublesome. During pregnancy the muscle fibres of your uterus and the fibroid enlarge and symptoms are more common.

- If the fibroids are near the fallopian tubes, they rarely cause difficulty conceiving and an ectopic pregnancy is slightly more likely.
- A fibroid in the internal cavity of your uterus may prevent conception because it acts like a foreign object.

- An early MISCARRIAGE is slightly more likely. Larger fibroids very uncommonly cause a late miscarriage. Fibroids may be associated with bleeding in early pregnancy, a sign of a threatened miscarriage. Usually the bleeding stops and the pregnancy is unaffected.
- Large fibroids may swell by retaining fluid. This is called 'degeneration' and may cause pain, usually after Week 12. The fibroid stops swelling by Week 20 and after pregnancy it may shrink and even disappear.
- Very rarely, extremely large fibroids may lead to PREMATURE BIRTH.
- Fibroids low down in your uterus may prevent your baby's head from engaging. Your baby may breech, or his head may fail to engage for birth – either event means it is safest to deliver by CAESAREAN SECTION.
- Large fibroids may cause bleeding after birth because they can prevent the wall of the uterus from retracting to seal the blood vessels supplying the placenta. You may require an oxytocin hormone injection to speed up placenta delivery and minimise bleeding (page 391).

Action plan

If you have abdominal or uterine pain, with or without bleeding (page 1), it is important to contact your doctor or midwife immediately. An examination and ultrasound can detect whether this is due to fibroids. Treatment of fibroids during pregnancy depends on an accurate diagnosis of the number and the site of the swellings.

- Fibroids causing pain and discomfort are best treated by rest. You may have to cut down on work and intense physical activity. If pain is severe, analgesic medication may be needed.
- Homeopathic remedies may help reduce pain and swelling and need to be prescribed on a case-by-case basis.
- After the birth, fibroids tend to shrink and soon may become even smaller than before conception. Unfortunately, new fibroids tend to form and recur until the menopause, even after surgery.
- Most small fibroids can be safely left. Surgery is not done during pregnancy because of the risk of bleeding. A number of new techniques have been developed to treat fibroids after pregnancy

or to assist conception. If you have had an operation to remove fibroids and the cavity of your uterus was not opened during surgery, a normal labour is feasible in a subsequent pregnancy. If the cavity of your uterus was opened it may be safer to have a caesarean section because of the small risk of the uterine wall rupturing during labour.

First aid

See Accidents and first aid, baby.

Fits and epilepsy, mother

See also Blood pressure, high and pre-eclampsia.

Fits (seizures or convulsions) are rare. If you have epilepsy, it is important to receive specialist care while you are pregnant and preferable to have counselling before conceiving. Specialist medical advice is constantly being updated and over 90 per cent of epileptic women who become pregnant have completely normal pregnancies. In pregnancy, a possible cause of fits is eclampsia, resulting from very high blood pressure (page 68).

Risks to your baby

There is little risk of passing epilepsy to your baby (page 245), although the risk to you in pregnancy will depend on your type of epilepsy and its severity. Some anti-epileptic drugs may increase the risk of nervous system abnormalities. Your specialist doctor will be able to advise you with an accurate diagnosis and a change of medication.

If you are susceptible to fits you need to take anticonvulsant medication. Some medications have been linked with an increased risk of CONGENITAL ABNORMALITY in babies (2–5 per cent higher than normal). It is preferable to use single medications rather than a combination.

If you have pre-eclampsia with high blood pressure that is kept under control, the risk of eclamptic fitting is very low. Eclamptic fits are more prolonged than epileptic fits and carry a higher risk to mother and baby.

Although your baby is usually protected,

243

severe trauma from an intense seizure may very rarely cause placental abruption (page 444) or foetal asphyxia (page 249). There is also a small risk you may injure yourself.

Action plan

It is important to advise your doctor of any seizures and remain in contact with a neurological specialist. Avoid potential triggers for your seizures where possible.

If you have a fit

* Whoever is with you needs to call for medical help immediately.
* You need to be protected from injuring yourself, without being tightly restrained. It is best for you to be laid on your side, and tight clothing loosened. The person with you needs to check you can breathe freely. A medical team can administer drugs to control your convulsion.
* If your fit is eclamptic, you will be given medications to control fits and blood pressure. You may need artificial ventilation and intensive care. If pregnancy is sufficiently advanced, the team will deliver your baby by emergency CAESAREAN SECTION.

Medical care

* Your specialist will assess your medication and may advise adjusting the dose, changing medication or withdrawing medication altogether if you have not had convulsions for at least two years.
* If you wish to stop treatment, you must discuss this fully with your doctor, as having a convulsion may pose a greater risk to you and your baby than any possible effects of the medications.
* In early pregnancy, natural fluid changes and vomiting may reduce the levels of the drug in your blood. It is best to measure the levels monthly so you are given the most effective doses.
* Some anti-epileptic drugs, particularly phenytoin, primidone and phenobarbital, reduce the levels of vitamin K reaching your baby. You may be given vitamin K in the last eight weeks to boost the levels.
* During pregnancy, ultrasound scans are helpful

to check your baby's heart and brain and rate of growth.

Lifestyle and diet

* Taking care of yourself is very important to avoid potential triggers for seizures: a good diet will help to avoid fluid and mineral imbalance, adequate rest can prevent sleep deprivation and loving support may help you avoid emotional stress. See page 121.
* Some doctors recommend combining medication with attention to diet. Your specific mineral needs will be indicated by your type of epilepsy and advice from a nutritionist may help. Some epileptics have a reduced number of fits if they eat more B6, vitamin D, zinc, magnesium or calcium.
* For some people, alcohol as well as evening primrose oil trigger attacks, so avoid these.
* Increasing your intake of folic acid and other vitamins and minerals prior to conception and in pregnancy might also decrease the risk of foetal nervous system abnormalities including spina bifida, associated with the use of anti-convulsant medications in pregnancy.

Care during labour

During labour it is important to have access to anti-convulsants. Your doctor will advise on the optimal drug, if one is needed, to avoid depressing your baby's breathing reflex after birth.

Care after birth

Caring for yourself remains important. The treatment you and your baby receive depends on the medication you had during pregnancy. The higher the level, the more intense observation and treatment need to be.

* You will be advised to allow your baby to have a vitamin K injection (page 63), to prevent abnormal blood clotting and bleeding.
* Your baby will be watched for bleeding and signs of withdrawal (page 192) from any drug you have been taking.
* If you are BREASTFEEDING and taking anti-epileptic medications, your baby is unlikely to be affected. If she continually appears drowsy, inform your doctor.
* It will help to use medical support: your health

visitor, neurology nurse or occupational therapist may have good advice to fit your lifestyle.

* If you are prone to seizures, it is safer to feed and change your baby on the floor. If you are alone, give your baby a wash with a sponge rather than a full bath. Always use a safety harness in a pram or pushchair and precautions against everyday hazards – a fire guard and stair gate, for example – will keep your baby safe if you have a seizure and while you are recovering.

Fits, baby

A baby's developing brain is an incredibly complex collection of cells, connections and chemical reactions. When something causes this system to malfunction the resulting change in brain activity may cause a fit, or convulsion, which is also known as a seizure. A tendency towards repeated fits (seizures) is called epilepsy.

Most fits are less serious than they appear, and a baby becomes calm within 10 minutes. If there is no improvement within 10 minutes you must call for immediate medical assistance.

What happens

In a baby, a fit or fit-like activity is not the same as seen in children and adults where there is usually loss of consciousness and shaking of the limbs. In a baby a fit may cause only excessive lip smacking or staring, with a slight shaking of the limbs, often down one side or other, and sometimes a colour change to bright red or pale white. There may be no change in the baby's level of wakefulness, and feeding may be unaffected.

When fit-like activity does not affect a baby's level of consciousness it is called a partial seizure. When consciousness is lost, the fit is said to be generalised. Babies who have had a genuine fit tend to fall asleep or appear sleepy for two to three hours after the fit. They then usually wake up and appear quite normal, unless the fit was due to an infection in the brain (MENINGITIS), when the level of consciousness may remain altered.

A prolonged fit lasting over 30 minutes can cause further damage to the cells of the brain, usually by causing low oxygen levels in the blood supply to the brain. The brain may then swell but internal bleeding does not usually occur as a result of the fit.

▮ APPARENT AND ACTUAL FITS

Many babies who are thought to be fitting are often not fitting at all, but the activity causes a lot of anxiety for parents and grandparents alike.

* One cause may be reflux of feed and stomach acid (regurgitating), which can be distressing for the baby and retching may appear like a mild convulsion.
* It is also quite common for a baby's limbs to jerk in a way that mimics fits because the immature nervous system is still developing (see 'Jitteriness and myoclonic jerks', below).
* A convulsion connected with a high temperature (FEVER) may be a genuine febrile convulsion but could also be a rigor (page 241), which is not a fit.

Jitteriness and myoclonic jerks

The commonest abnormal movement seen in babies is jitteriness. This looks like shivering, stops when you touch the shaking limb gently, and is not associated with any other unusual activity, such as strange eye movements, sleepiness or poor feeding. Jitteriness or shuddering is quite normal and can persist to the age four to six months. These movements may be caused by an immature and active developing nervous system.

Myoclonus

This is similar to the jitteriness described above, but is a larger, more rhythmic movement, which occurs only during sleep and mimics a seizure. The condition can be alarming to parents and professionals, but does no harm. Sometimes only one limb may move rhythmically, again only during sleep, and can be associated with grunting and shaking of the cot. To exclude the possibility of these harmless but alarming movements being fits video brainwave monitoring can show no abnormal electrical activity during these events. This is called 'benign sleep myoclonus'. Myoclonic jerks are sometimes described as benign, meaning that they are not part of a more significant problem in the brain.

'Funny turns'

Babies and young children often have strange episodes of blankness, blinking, shaking, head turning and nodding, and a range of other movements that might surprise their parents. To differentiate this wide range of movements from a fit the child's level of consciousness will remain normal, whereas in a fit the level of alertness will be reduced, and he may appear sleepy. Most of these are harmless and are merely habits and others are made for enjoyment. Most stop as a baby grows older.

In a small number of babies in the first six months after birth there may be an underlying problem causing a 'funny turn'. It is often discomfort like acid reflux, tummy pain, ear ache or head ache. Rarely are they signs of fits. A change in heart rhythm, causing temporary reduction in blood flow to the brain because of low blood pressure, is usually associated with a colour change to blue or white (pallid attacks). It may happen if the heart rate (normally 120 beats per minute) exceeds 250 beats per minute, called supraventricular tachycardia. Treatment needs to address the heart rhythm disturbance.

▓ EPILEPSY

Epilepsy is the name given to the condition of recurrent seizure activity, unrelated to fever. There are several different types, named according to the type of seizure involved. *Grand mal* epilepsy is what most people think of when the term is mentioned. *Grand mal* seizures are the most dramatic, involving stiffening and jerking of the entire body, breath holding and turning blue (cyanosis), and loss of bowel and bladder control (incontinence). *Petit mal* epilepsy or absence attacks generally affects school-age children and involves brief periods of 'blanking out', staring without seeing, which can be so brief that they are misinterpreted as normal pauses in speech, or attention deficit disorder. Body tone is not lost and the child does not slump over or shake, but the eyelids may flicker. There may be 100 of these little attacks a day, severely disrupting a child's ability to learn and function in school.

Infantile spasms

Infantile spasm is a specific type of seizure seen in an epilepsy syndrome of infancy and early childhood known as West's syndrome. The onset is predominantly in the first year, typically between three and six months. The typical pattern of infantile spasms is a sudden bending forward and stiffening of the body, arms, and legs; although there can also be arching of the torso. Spasms tend to begin soon after arousal from sleep. Individual spasms typically last for one to five seconds and occur in clusters, ranging from two to 100 spasms at a time. A baby may have dozens of clusters and several hundred spasms per day. Infantile spasms usually stop by age five, but are often replaced by other seizure types. West's syndrome is characterised by infantile spasms, abnormal, chaotic brain wave patterns EEG, and learning disability with often severe developmental delay. Other nervous system disorders, such as CEREBRAL PALSY, may be seen in 30–50 per cent of children with infantile spasms.

There are many other types of recurrent seizures, or epilepsy, many with their own specific name. If your child has been newly diagnosed or has had suspected seizures you will need a specialist opinion to diagnose the condition and determine the cause. Often a specific cause cannot be found.

Children known to have convulsions frequently are often provided with medicines called anti-convulsants, to help stop prolonged fits. If your child is epileptic it is essential that everyone who cares for him knows about the condition and what to do in the event of a seizure. The outlook today for most forms of epilepsy is very good with modern drug therapy.

▓ FEBRILE CONVULSIONS (FEVER FITS)

Convulsions with associated fever (page 241) are said to affect about 4 per cent of children between the age of six months and six years, and may run in families. Each fit is relatively short, lasting less than 10 minutes. They are generalised (there is loss of consciousness) and the child will have a fever either before or after the event. Complete recovery is expected and the cause may be an infection requiring a medical examination; urinary infections are often the cause.

Sometimes the first fit or convulsion in a child who goes on to develop epilepsy is triggered by a fever. However, epilepsy is no more common in children who have had febrile convulsions than in children who have never had a febrile convulsion.

▩ FITS FROM BIRTH TO ONE MONTH

The neonatal period is the first 28 days after birth for a baby born at term, or one month after the due date in a premature baby. Neonatal seizures occur among roughly one in 1,000 babies. They can be difficult even for neonatal nurses and doctors to spot. Most neonatal seizures occur within a few days of birth, most by the tenth day. Of babies who have neonatal seizures roughly half show no long-term effects and do not have seizures in later life. Of the other 50 per cent, some do have long-term learning or developmental difficulties. Some babies have a family tendency to neonatal fits, others may fit because there is a problem in the brain or nervous system and it is important to investigate a possible cause.

If no cause is found, a family history of neonatal seizures may suggest a good outcome. A condition that usually has a family history, occurs within 48–72 hours of birth, but stops by age two to six months, with normal long-term development, is called benign familial neonatal seizure. A similar condition where fits start around the fifth day, and can be quite severe, but settle down by the tenth day, with normal long-term development, is called a benign idiopathic neonatal seizure.

When there is a fit before the first VACCINATIONS the immunisation programme may be delayed until the paediatrician agrees that they can begin.

Possible causes of fits at birth:

- Brain injury from severe FOETAL DISTRESS AND ASPHYXIA called neonatal hypoxic ischemic encephalopathy (page 301). It results from insufficient oxygen supply in pregnancy or during the birth process and if the HIE is mild the baby makes a complete recovery. For one in 1,000 babies, HIE may be severe and lead to serious brain damage or death.
- Bleeding in the brain (intracranial haemorrhage) is uncommon and mainly affects premature babies where the blood vessels are fragile and bleed easily. It may occur after a birth injury but this is very rare now. The blood is usually absorbed but it may occasionally need to be removed surgically.
- Infection (including meningitis). The infection may very rarely have been contracted during pregnancy (such as LISTERIA, TOXOPLASMOSIS or CYTOMEGALOVIRUS). After birth the most likely organism is Group B Strep (page 269) and premature babies are more susceptible. A tiny number of babies are infected with genital HERPES during delivery and it may be severe.
- HYPOGLYCAEMIA or low blood glucose levels may cause fitting. The brain depends on glucose for energy. Low glucose levels occur after delivery in some premature or small IUGR babies and may occur among babies of diabetic mothers. The risk of low blood sugars is greatest in the first 48 hours and can be avoided if the baby is receiving regular feeds.
- Drug withdrawal (page 192).
- Less commonly, a rare chemical disorder or abnormality of brain development can result in fits.
- Injury to the head or being shaken can also cause fits.

▩ FITS FROM ONE MONTH ONWARDS

Fits may occur in as many as 1 per cent of children between the age of one month and 14 years.

Between one and six months

The period from one to six months is an unusual time to develop a seizure, and if your baby has not had fits in the first month then a fit between one and six months usually signifies illness. Idiopathic epilepsy (two or more seizures with no apparent cause) does not begin until the end of this time period and febrile convulsions are very rare under six months of age. Some fits are due to developmental abnormalities of the brain, which would have been determined at conception.

Below six months the likely cause is an infection of the nervous system, such as a bacterial meningitis or a viral encephalitis. Reactions to vaccinations may be another cause of a seizure, but even though there may be a fever at this time, the fit is not considered to be a febrile convulsion. The cause is usually due to a direct infection of the brain or the lining membranes.

Many children who experience a first-time seizure in this time period may never experience a second seizure. However, a seizure at this time may be the start of a more serious medical condition and extensive tests to rule out causes may be needed.

Yet another cause of fits, breath holding is usually seen in babies over three to six months of age. For more on breath holding, see page 101.

Six months and over

Over six months of age fits may be due to one of a number of causes:

- A reaction to high temperature, with febrile convulsions (page 246).
- Breath holding, which may begin from three or six months of age, is another possible cause of fits. For more on breath holding, see page 101.
- Infantile spasms (West's syndrome, salaam attacks) occur between four and eight months and consist of clusters of spasms upon awakening (see page 246).
- *Petit mal* epilepsy involves blanking off or staring in frequent short episodes, perhaps as many as 100 times a day (see page 246).
- A small number of fits after six months relate to causes that can give earlier fitting and have had a long-term effect, such as foetal distress, infection, bleeds, developmental anomalies and hypoglycaemia.
- Injury to the head or being shaken can also cause fits. Non-accidental head injury now accounts for about 15 per cent of all new cases of epilepsy. This cause of epilepsy is largely avoidable.
- Benign rolandic epilepsy occurs in children aged four to 10 years at night. Juvenile myoclonic epilepsy (JME) occurs in the teenage years, usually on waking.
- Infection and meningitis account for about 15 per cent of older children with epilepsy.

■ SUPPORT AND TREATMENT

Watching a child of any age have a fit is terrifying. You may feel certain that your child is going to die, and this often leads to confusion and panic. Despite this natural reaction, it is important that you do all you can to remain calm and to help your child breathe. He is likely to be very frightened and will need reassuring, either straight away or when he has come round from a brief spell of unconsciousness.

✚ Red flag

What you can do

A – Keep the **Airway** open.
B – Make sure your child is **Breathing**.
C – **Call** for help – this is a frightening experience.
D – **Do not** panic.
E – **Even now** remember that complete recovery will take place.

- Do not pick up your child because if he thrashes around, you may drop him. If he begins to have a fit while you are holding him, lie him down on the floor, on his side, as soon as you can. Being upright increases the chance of vomiting and fainting.
- If your baby is unconscious deal with the **A B C** (airways, breathing, circulation: page 3) immediately.
- If your baby is hot, cool him by removing clothing, opening a window, or gently fanning. Do not put him in a cool bath – this may bring on a renewed fit and he may breathe in the water.
- Give a medicine designed to reduce fever, such as infant paracetamol suspension if he is able to swallow. Do this even if there is no apparent fever because often a fever follows a convulsion.
- If recovery is complete, with return to normal behaviour, normal pupil size, and your baby is fully conscious within 30 minutes then arrange for the child to see your GP within 24 hours.
- If recovery is not complete within 30 minutes, or the fit continues beyond 10 minutes, call an ambulance or GP. For a continuing fit your baby needs oxygen and anti-convulsant medication and follow-up may include a brain scan.

Homeopathy
If your baby is prone to fits, please consult your homeopath who can provide you with advice or remedies for future use.

After a fit

Following a seizure your main concern may be whether your baby will be completely normal. If he was normal before the fit, then the chances of any problem as a result of the seizure are low.

* If the cause of the fit (for example, low blood sugar) is corrected then the risk of damage and the risk of further fits are considerably reduced.
* If the fit was caused by a febrile convulsion, then the risk of any damage at all, even subtle damage, is extremely low, and you can be reassured that there will be no long-lasting effects.
* If the fit was very prolonged and difficult to stop, taking 30–60 minutes to bring under control, then the risk of a longer-lasting problem begins to rise. If the cause is a viral illness there is a risk that this has damaged the brain, and will lead on to longer-term problems.
* For the large proportion of babies who have a fit, at any time, there is no change to the baby. It may, however, take some time, anything up to five years of close monitoring and assessment, to ensure that there have been no subtle signs of damage.

The chance of future fits

It is difficult to give a definitive prognosis after a single seizure, and you will need to talk to your child's doctor about the underlying cause and any test results. Some general rules do apply.

Children who have a single, short, generalised seizure along with normal neurological development have a 40 per cent chance of having a second seizure. The prediction can be more accurate after an EEG (electroencephalogram, to record brainwave patterns): a normal EEG gives a recurrence risk of only 25 per cent, whereas an abnormal EEG gives a 50–70 per cent risk of recurrence.

Children with developmental problems, abnormalities of the brain structure, or neurological abnormalities have a higher risk of recurrence of fits.

Flat feet

Babies' feet normally appear flat because children are born with a pad of fat in the arch area. Also, foot and leg muscles aren't developed enough to support the arches when children first begin to stand. The arch doesn't usually become apparent until around two and a half years old.

Flatulence

See Bloating and flatulence.

Flu, baby

See Influenza (flu), baby.

Flu, mother

See Influenza (flu), mother.

Foetal alcohol syndrome (FAS)

See Drugs, alcohol.

Foetal distress and asphyxia

The term 'foetal distress' is used to mean that a baby in the womb is showing signs of stress from potentially threatening conditions, whatever the cause (for example, infection, a knot in the cord, etc.) Among other things, foetal distress may be a sign that there is poor blood flow or circulation. The term for poor blood flow is ischaemia. When blood flow is restricted, oxygen delivery to all organs, and most seriously to the brain, is reduced. The term for low oxygen is 'hypoxia'. The term 'asphyxia' describes the process that results in the hypoxia: and a baby shows evidence of this with 'foetal distress'. These terms may at first appear confusing but the distinctions between their meanings are important for healthcare professionals attending to a baby with foetal distress.

In the majority of cases where there are signs of foetal distress, the birth team intervenes and the baby is born safely with no long-term difficulties. Less commonly, the problem is severe and presents a significant risk for the baby. Prolonged lack of oxygen may lead to changes in the physiology of the cells in a baby's body, which may be damaged or die. If distress is spotted early, measures can be taken to reduce the risks. This is why modern obstetric care is geared to checking babies regularly in pregnancy and during labour. Monitoring will be more intensive if yours is a 'high-risk' pregnancy.

Susceptibility
During pregnancy, the majority of babies are able to build up sufficient reserves of glycogen (the form in which glucose is stored in the body), mostly laid down in the final 10 weeks. A baby draws on these stores for energy if oxygen levels fall. Babies who are born early (page 453) or have INTRAUTERINE GROWTH RESTRICTION (IUGR), and the few who have a developmental disorder or infection, may have low glycogen reserves and are more susceptible to asphyxia if the oxygen concentration drops. On the other side of the spectrum, a very small number of babies who develop asphyxia at birth do not show signs of foetal distress in pregnancy or during labour. This happens even with the most developed obstetric care and in apparently normal healthy pregnancies.

While labour is the most common time for asphyxia to occur, some babies are susceptible during pregnancy. This is rare, and is more likely in high-risk pregnancies (page 302). When antenatal monitoring indicates this, early birth is advised. Very rarely, asphyxia in the womb may be a cause of stillbirth (page 501).

What happens

Side effects will be mild provided oxygen is restored within a reasonable time period. More serious damage is rare and occurs if lack of oxygen continues and a baby's energy reserves have been used up. When this happens, the tissues use other chemicals to produce energy. This results in the production of an acid, called lactic acid. Normally this is carried away by the bloodstream, but if blood flow is poor, levels of lactic acid build up. High levels of lactic acid cause a state called 'acidosis', and this presents a problem as the acid may poison the cells, which become damaged, or die. The changes may affect all the body organs, including the heart, lungs, kidneys and liver, but the brain is the most

sensitive. Damage may be temporary, for instance when the affected organ (such as the kidney) recovers completely. Sometimes damage is permanent, for instance if brain cells are affected and do not recover.

Foetal distress and asphyxia in labour
The most common time for oxygen flow to be interrupted is during the contractions of labour, but this is intermittent and the flow returns between contractions. In labour, the main indicator of wellbeing is your baby's heart rate (page 335). Variations from the normal rhythm may suggest foetal distress, and this may occur in labour for a number of reasons.

- If blood flow to the placenta falls excessively, this may affect the delivery of oxygen to your baby. The flow may fall if the uterine muscle contracts excessively, sometimes following the use of oxytocin or prostaglandin to boost contractions or to induce labour. The flow may fall if you lie flat in bed and your uterus presses on the blood vessels supplying the placenta.
- Epidural anaesthetic may cause reduced blood flow, particularly if you lie flat on your back.
- Oxygen flow may be reduced if the umbilical cord becomes compressed because the amount of amniotic fluid is reduced or the cord has become tight around your baby's neck.
- Placental abruption (page 444) can reduce blood flow.
- If your baby has reduced energy reserves she is more susceptible to distress (see above).

Asphyxia after birth (neonatal asphyxia)
If a baby has been deprived of oxygen during labour, she may be born asphyxiated and have difficulty breathing after birth. This is called neonatal asphyxia. When mild, it is easily corrected by administering oxygen at birth. In a minority of cases neonatal asphyxia is severe. When breathing cannot be established, a baby is stillborn after labour. This tragic event occurs in one in 2,000 deliveries in the UK.

Signs of foetal distress

Heartbeat monitoring (cardiotocograph or CTG)
This is an integral aspect of modern obstetric care in preventing and diagnosing foetal distress. Although heartbeat monitoring is not

100 per cent reliable, it is a good indicator and an abnormal variation prompts the medical team to monitor and observe the baby and the mother's progress more intensely.

- Sometimes the foetal heart pattern will alter but there is no asphyxia: this is called a false positive (the pattern looks abnormal but there is no distress).
- In intense asphyxia, an abnormal heartbeat is usually detected and continuous heart monitoring may be needed to confirm the diagnosis. In some hospitals when the foetal heart pattern indicates asphyxia, a sample of blood is taken from the baby's scalp (below).
- Heartbeat monitoring is explored in detail on page 335.

Meconium staining of amniotic fluid

Another sign of possible distress is greenish meconium staining of the AMNIOTIC FLUID, evident when the waters break, which indicates that the baby has passed his first bowel motion in the womb.

- The bowel movement can be normal – it happens in 30 per cent of labours without apparent foetal distress. It is more likely in babies after 40 weeks and is rare before 36 weeks.
- It does not indicate foetal distress unless the baby's heart rate is abnormal or the meconium is very thick and there is a reduced volume of amniotic fluid.
- The greatest risk associated with passing meconium is that it may be breathed in by the baby (page 253).
- Some units have a grading system dependant on the thickness of the meconium, but this is not universal.

Blood oxygen levels

If foetal distress is indicated by the baby's heart rate during the first stage of labour, a doctor may take a blood sample from the baby's scalp. This is known as foetal blood sampling. A speculum is used to visualise the cervix and prick the baby's scalp. Blood is then collected and the oxygen and carbon dioxide content assessed within 10 minutes. The results help the doctor to decide whether it is safe for the baby to continue with the labour. There is a risk of scalp infection to the baby and transmission of HIV and HEPATITIS virus from the mother.

Possible effects

The effect of low oxygen depends on the:
- *Severity of reduced oxygen.* Fortunately it is very rare for oxygen flow to stop completely but healthy babies are hardy and they can recover completely after 10 or more minutes without oxygen by drawing on glycogen energy reserves.
- *Strength and maturity of your baby.* A full-term mature baby who has been well nourished in pregnancy can withstand reduced blood flow for longer than a baby with low energy reserves.

Asphyxia and brain injury (HIE)

If there has been insufficient oxygen to the brain and other vital organs, a baby may show signs of brain injury with hypoxic ischaemic encephalopathy or HIE (page 301). This is uncommon and in its severe form affects one to two in 500 babies.

Asphyxia and cerebral palsy

Rarely, asphyxia during labour may be the underlying cause of CEREBRAL PALSY. Cerebral palsy is uncommon and there are many causes. In fewer than one in 500 babies with cerebral palsy, the cause can be attributed exclusively to asphyxia and sub-optimal care in labour.

▇ ACTION IN PREGNANCY AND LABOUR

If your baby shows one or more signs of foetal distress, the healthcare team will be keen to monitor the situation and intervene if doing so is likely to improve your baby's safety. Routine monitoring is part of a baby's general care.

In pregnancy

One of the aims of antenatal care is to identify any factors that may make pregnancy 'high-risk'. Routine checks also look for signs that a baby may be receiving reduced oxygen before labour begins, or may be susceptible to foetal distress during labour. This is the main method of preventing damage from oxygen reduction, although not all high-risk pregnancies are detected before labour.

If your baby is at a very high risk of asphyxia (the process that leads to a reduction in oxygen in your baby's circulation) an elective CAESAREAN SECTION may be suggested. You will need to give birth in a hospital with a SPECIAL CARE BABY UNIT

(SCBU), particularly if giving birth before term (page 453). If the risk is not high but is still significant an INDUCTION of labour (see LABOUR AND BIRTH, MOTHER) will be considered. Early birth usually means that factors which could lead to asphyxia are avoided.

In labour

Close monitoring during labour (page 335), particularly in high-risk pregnancies, empowers midwives and obstetricians to intervene at the most appropriate time. Despite the availability of monitoring, however, not all cases of asphyxia are detected.

Expediting birth

Because there is a risk of damage to the brain if oxygen deprivation is prolonged, particularly if your baby is premature or has low glycogen reserves, the obstetrician may be keen to hasten the birth. The action chosen will depend upon the level of foetal distress, the stage of labour and your preferences.

- If significant foetal distress is apparent in the first stage, the birth team will address the obvious causative factors (helping you get upright if possible, reducing an oxytocin infusion, adjusting fluid replacement and your position during epidural anaesthesia). If this is not successful a caesarean section will be advised, particularly if your baby is at high risk.
- If there is concern during the second stage when you are pushing, the birth team may recommend using an upright position to improve your power, or an assisted delivery with forceps or ventouse or a caesarean section.
- Delay in the birth caused by SHOULDER DYSTOCIA will be actively treated by the birth team.
- If the foetal heart pattern at any time indicates a significant risk of neonatal asphyxia that could lead to HIE and brain injury, the baby needs to be born within 10 minutes. When there is concern a paediatrician will be called to be present at the delivery and check the baby at birth.

▓ ACTION AFTER BIRTH

At birth, the midwife or doctor will check your baby immediately. If there is asphyxia, she may have difficulty establishing breathing, her heart rate may be slow and her muscle tone floppy:

she will be given assistance, and may be transferred to a special cot with all the equipment required, called the Resuscitaire. Most babies who receive help to begin breathing are fine within a few minutes.

Your baby's state is measured according to the Apgar system (page 337). If the score is below seven (out of 10) at one minute then a baby may require resuscitation with oxygen, and this is usually a simple and effective procedure. A score below three at one minute, and especially if still below three at five minutes and not improving, usually indicates severe asphyxia and the possible need for more intense resuscitation.

- The first step is to remove liquid blocking the airway. This is done gently, using a plastic suction catheter in the mouth or nose. Contact with the cooler air in the room on a baby's skin normally stimulates breathing.
- If the onset of breathing is delayed gentle stimulation, perhaps through drying the baby with a towel, will probably initiate breathing, and extra oxygen may be blown on the baby's face.
- If after one minute a baby is not breathing regularly then artificial ventilation is started, initially using a face mask, but a plastic tube may be inserted into the baby's airway (intubation). In mild asphyxia the initial gasp of air or oxygen is enough for breathing to begin.
- For a tiny number of babies more treatment is needed and will be given by a paediatrician or midwife. The lungs may be ventilated after intubation. Usually this is sufficient to restart breathing and the tube can be safely removed after five or 10 minutes.
- If the asphyxia is severe it may indicate HIE (page 301). Ventilation will be continued and intensive resuscitation with medication may be needed. This may include cardiac massage and intravenous fluids and adrenaline to correct fluid balance, heart rate and acidosis. Following severe asphyxia a baby needs to be cared for in an SCBU.

Umbilical cord oxygen and acidosis measurement

After the umbilical cord has been clamped and cut, a blood sample is taken from the vein and the artery on the placental side. The baby will not be aware of this. The oxygen and acidosis levels are measured to indicate the severity of asphyxia at birth.

Meconium aspiration

Meconium aspiration into the lungs can only occur if there is reduced amniotic fluid volume (oligohydramnios). The usual causes are postmaturity and intrauterine growth restriction (IUGR). When this is combined with the baby passing copious amounts of meconium into the amniotic fluid, severe asphyxia may make the baby gasp in the uterus, and inhale meconium before birth.

- If there has been intense meconium staining, the midwife, obstetrician or paediatrician present at birth will apply suction to the back of the baby's mouth to remove meconium from the throat and larynx. Once this has been carried out the baby is likely to respond well and may begin to breathe easily.
- In about one in 500 births, the lungs contain thick meconium and oxygen cannot enter easily. These babies require the insertion of a tube into the trachea for suction and assistance with breathing. They are transferred to a special care unit for oxygen monitoring, ventilation and antibiotics to prevent a chest infection. The meconium clears in a few days but the baby may be very ill during this time. This is more common in pregnancies going beyond 42 weeks, and among boy babies.

After birth, if there has been foetal distress, recovery for your baby and for you may take time, as you welcome one another and integrate your feelings about what happened. Fortunately, foetal distress is usually mild with no long-term problems. Your need for practical and emotional support will be greatest if there are concerning effects for your baby.

Food allergy

See Allergy and intolerance, foods.

Food and eating, mother

See also Eating difficulties, mother; Weight, mother.

'You are what you eat' remains as true today as it was a thousand years ago. The term 'nutrition' includes what you eat, drink, smoke and inhale – all the elements that your body absorbs, uses, stores and excretes.

Questions about food are extremely common in pregnancy, when many women wonder if it's okay to eat a certain food, or the ideal diet for the growth and health of their baby. When you eat well before conception and during pregnancy this gives you and your child optimal nutrition. It is also important to focus on good nutrition after birth. This applies to dads as well.

The balance of your nutrition affects you from moment to moment and from month to month. It influences your hormones, your feelings and energy, your skin and hair and, of course, your weight. In pregnancy your baby consumes what you consume. It is the basis for long-term health.

The way you choose to eat depends on what's happening in your life and how you feel. It also reflects habits in your family, at work and in your community.

Food and eating, mother
Action for healthy eating

See also Food and eating, mother, safe eating.

The entries on the following pages explore different aspects of nutrition. You can scroll through and read any that interest you. With a strong foundation, it's okay to be flexible and enjoy treats without counting calories (page 256) or feeling guilty. There are many different components that combine to meet your needs. Getting an overall balance helps you to absorb the goodness from each component: the better the balance, the better you'll feel. Here are some tips for healthy eating during and after pregnancy:

Colour counts
Make as many meals and snacks as possible from whole (unprocessed foods). As a general guide, opt for a rainbow of colours on your plate. Bright green, red, yellow and orange fruit and veg are rich in vitamins, minerals and antioxidants. The browns of rice, grains, nuts, wholegrains and meat, and the pinks and light colours of oily fish add protein, essential fats and useful bulk. Try to achieve a balance of fish, meat and veg and avoid a diet high in meat and dairy.

Fresh foods

Fresh foods have more goodness than processed foods, and are free of additives including added sugar and salt. Eat organic whenever you can, avoiding toxic pesticides and artificial growth-promoting hormones. To get full nutritional benefit, it is best to eat plenty of raw or steamed vegetables and avoid frying and cooking with saturated fats. Roughly 30 per cent of your vegetable intake could be raw (such as salads, snacks and crudités).

Enjoyable eating

There are three important ingredients that make eating fun: taste, abundance and company. You can eat in abundance when the tasty food you choose isn't calorie laden (page 256). When you're in good company, the combination of tasty food and love helps your feel-good hormones flow – great for you and for your baby. After birth, your baby can join the dinner table, while BREASTFEEDING, or maybe while resting on your chest (page 518) or lap, or sleeping nearby.

Simple cooking

Fresh foods and easy recipes abound – try books, the internet, friends and family tips.

While you're pregnant, you could get into the habit of cooking double (or triple) quantities and freezing meals for a later date, and practise time-saving techniques.

Relaxing

If you always sit down to eat and take care to finish one mouthful before taking another, eating is more relaxed, food tends to be more enjoyable and you're more likely to eat what your body needs. It takes 20 minutes to know if you feel full. If you rest before getting busy again, you help your body make the most of the nutrients and you're less likely to suffer digestive discomfort.

Be sugar and salt aware

It is so easy to reach for a sugar fix and ride the roller coaster of sugar highs and lows (page 261). Sugar is a potent source of weight gain and low energy and anxiety, and is best kept to a minimum. Salt, too, can cause problems when added to excess. Limit how much salt you add to cooking or at the dinner table, or better still add salt-free condiments, herbs and spices instead.

Balance

For nutritional balance, include something from all the food groups (see table, below).

Guidelines for nutritional balance

Recommended % of daily intake	Food groups	Food type	Approximate number of servings each day
5%	Fats - unsaturated	Oils, nuts, seeds	Cook with olive oil – other seed or plant oils are good, too, e.g. hemp, sesame etc. Use oil in a salad dressing. Add a handful of nuts/seeds a day
10%	Proteins	Meat, fish, eggs, pulses, nuts and seeds	Each week 3 servings of fish; up to two servings of meat or poultry; 2-4 eggs
Up to 25%	Complex carbohydrates and protein	Vegetables, and pulses (e.g. peas and beans)	Four to six servings per day; veg at lunch and dinner, 70% cooked, 30% raw; 2–3 meals with pulses a week
Up to 15%	Complex carbohydrates (slow burners)	Fruit	Around two or three pieces a day – with skins if edible
Up to 45%	Complex carbohydrates (slow burners), roughage	Wheat (bread, pasta), rice, oats, corn, barley and grains	Four to six servings

Gradual changes

Make one change at a time. Change tends to last longest if it is gradual. It's okay to slip up when you are learning new habits.

Bounty and your budget

Most people in the UK live within a few miles of local farm producers who offer vegetables, milk, fruit, eggs, cheeses, fishes and meats that are full of flavour, free of additives and may undercut supermarket prices: arrive at a market towards closing time for bargains. Other options include clubbing together with friends or family to buy in bulk – organic produce may be more easily affordable in bulk.

Emotions and feelings

If you feel uncomfortable around food or as you try to change some habits, take a look at your feelings. Your eating experience is intimately bound up with your emotions, and changing one influences the other. Pregnancy and a new baby provide a great opportunity to begin a process of change.

Seek help if you need it

If you begin pregnancy with an EATING DIFFICULTY, or a difficulty surfaces after conception, it is important to seek support and care for yourself (page 162). If you have a difficulty such as anorexia and bulimia there is professional help available to you.

Nurture your body

Your body responds to what you eat and you'll feel a difference if you eat well In addition, taking a 30-minute walk or swim three times a week or cycling helps to balance your appetite, improve your digestion and use up fat stores. YOGA also supports your digestive system. These are all part of a wider programme of caring for yourself (page 121).

Food and eating, mother
Cravings and pica

In pregnancy, you may find you go off some foods you enjoyed before and develop new and even unusual tastes. Although some cravings might be due to hormonal, smell and taste changes, many cravings could point to a need to replace some elements that are lacking in your diet. Vitamin and mineral supplements may reduce the craving. In some cases, your body may call out for some foods because they quell nausea.

Usually a craving does not cause long-term health risks, although if cravings are for high-calorie or high-sugar foods you'll need to be aware of the effect this could have on you, particularly weight gain. You may need to make an effort to keep 'empty calorie' indulgences (sugary foods that lead to weght gain without any nutritional benefit) to a minimum.

When the craving is for a non-food, such as mud, coal, paper, starch or ice (and stranger things...) and you consume it, there may be risk. This more unusual craving for something with no obvious nutritional value is known as pica. Women who practise pica are often ashamed of the compulsion and hesitate to admit it. The cause is not clear but pica may be linked to a lack of certain minerals.

What happens

The most common cravings are for sweets and dairy products, sour fruits and spicy or salty foods and junk foods, which have a high salt and sugar content.

- Cravings for salty foods such as pickles or crisps may indicate a need for more minerals including sodium.
- You may crave sugar because it is a quick energy source and helps you to feel good. Recurrent cravings for sugar might reflect a diet containing too many fast-burning carbohydrates (page 261), too little EXERCISE, or a deficiency of magnesium.
- Another cause of sugar cravings may be anxiety, which is associated with adrenaline release and this stimulates the appetite for sugar.
- Smoking and caffeine can also increase sugar and food cravings.

Action plan

Cravings are not a problem if you can fulfil them without causing an imbalance in your diet or putting on excess weight. Eating a balanced, nutritious diet and drinking adequate water (six to eight glasses a day), and taking vitamin and mineral supplements, may help. At times, you may need to think of alternatives, such as an orange instead of orangeade, or nuts instead of chocolate. The initial energy hit may not be as rapid but your body will feel satisfied for longer.

Cravings usually fade as pregnancy progresses, although some women continue to want something specific for the entire nine months. Pica usually disappears.

A craving for sugar and chocolate may intensify after the birth if you feel anxious, overwhelmed or depressed, or if you are not eating regularly and nutritiously. If a craving becomes a problem, the Action Plan for eating difficulties and disorders may help you step out of your habit (page 201).

Food and eating, mother
Dieting

There is an enjoyable alternative to dieting that involves plenty of delicious food and no guilt. It is about changing the way you eat to benefit you, your baby and family. Pregnancy is a great time to introduce changes that can stay with you and your family for decades.

A diet that involves denying yourself vital nutrients is not appropriate during pregnancy – and indeed doesn't pay off at any time. A dieting cycle typically alternates between eating too much, eating less and losing weight, and then eating more and gaining again. The overall trend with recurrent dieting is to put on weight progressively. This is known as 'yo-yo' dieting. For some women, pregnancy seems a good excuse to eat too much, followed by cutting back after birth, a cycle that mimics the fluctuations of dieting.

Calories
The term 'calorie' describes the energy-producing property of food. Everyone needs calories but in excess they contribute to weight gain.

In pregnancy and while breastfeeding, women are advised to consume an extra 300 calories a day, bringing the recommended total daily intake to roughly 2,400. You can get the extra 300 calories easily and nutritiously, for instance with a single avocado (packed with vitamin E), or a bowl of porridge oats (beneficial fibre), or an extra handful of nuts or seeds (brimming with healthy fats). Depending on your personal

metabolic rate, you may sometimes need to consume a little more – particularly while you are breastfeeding when a total daily intake of 2,500–2,550 calories may suit some women without leading to excessive weight gain.

Please remember that in pregnancy eating for two does not mean eating twice as much. Do not use your pregnancy as an excuse to overeat. If you already consume food in excess, pregnancy may be the time to reduce to the recommended amount. This is not dieting – it is optimal eating.

Try focusing on whole foods that are slow burning (page 261) and avoid saturated fats. This is a simple way to reduce calories and to stabilise your energy throughout the day. Snacks are fine – if you keep them nutritious. If you add a small amount of protein to each snack the energy effect lasts longer. For drinks, stick to water or teas: fruit juices and colas can be a potent cause of weight gain. Remember that sugary foods are empty calories that put on weight but do not add the vital nutrients your body needs.

Why dieting doesn't work

Eating less than your body needs sends it into 'famine' mode and you actually reduce the calories you burn by slowing down the rate you use energy, and storing as much of the remainder as you can. When you diet, you may feel colder and more lethargic than usual, and tire easily.

When you diet the first thing you lose is muscle and the first thing you put back on is fat, in preparation for the next 'famine'. When you return to your normal intake you will put on weight rapidly. Being on a diet also involves a heightened awareness of emotions such as guilt and being 'not good enough' and these will drain your energy.

Eating well and avoiding dieting is important in pregnancy. It may be helpful to remember that while you are pregnant your body is highly efficient at using the nutrients you consume for your health and for your baby's growth.

Avoiding the diet trap

Replacing dieting with a new way of eating may be much easier than you think. You may want to begin with the tips under healthy eating advice (page 253) and use other entries in this section. Here are a few pointers:

Eat well

A good place to start is to choose foods that are good for you, and that you love. Creating ways to enjoy them may be fun to do with a friend, or with the help of a nutritional therapist. With a nutritional balance you can let go of calorie counting and this could change your whole approach to eating.

Exercise

Let exercise and eating well go hand in hand. Exercising helps your body draw on unused fat and sugar stores, reduces cravings, and helps you feel good.

Re-assess your body image

One of the underlying themes of dieting is often low body image. Although reaching your target weight may mean a change in your outer appearance, it may not change your basic image of yourself, which comes from the way you feel inside. You may find it easier to introduce new eating patterns when you also tend your self-image (page 72).

Maintaining control

Dieting is also about control, particularly when a food regime is strict. It may help to lighten up – maybe ask a friend to try new food habits with you. You may also need to avoid eating when you're not hungry. Take it one step at a time and don't worry when you slip up: it's okay to re-assess and begin again.

Taking a long-term view

If you are overweight (page 566) at the beginning of pregnancy it is preferable to take the long-term view of reaching your target weight nine months after the birth. Eating well in pregnancy will prevent excess gain, so you'll have less far to go after the birth.

Food and eating, mother
Drinking

Your body always needs fluid and the most powerful drink at your disposal is water. Many people do not drink enough and this has a negative effect on their energy and wellbeing. There are, of course, individual variations from person to person, but a guide for optimal intake is to have between 1.5 and 2 litres (2.5 and 3 pints) or 6–8 glasses daily. It is best to drink earlier in the day to avoid disturbing your sleep at night. If you breastfeed, you'll need to drink more than usual. Drink as much as you feel you need to satisfy your thirst. The majority of women crave a drink (usually a big glass of water) when they sit down to breastfeed.

What happens

Your body needs fluid to maintain all its cells and tissues, maintain blood levels, and aid digestion – in short, to survive.

In the womb, babies need fluid for their growth. Your body needs extra fluid to cope with the huge increase in your blood volume (this doubles by Week 28) and to sustain amniotic fluid around your baby. It is also needed to maintain flexibility and in your muscles and joints. By the end of pregnancy, your body may be supporting 7 litres (12 pints) more water than before pregnancy. When you breastfeed you need extra fluid to produce milk.

If you don't drink as much water as you need, you may feel the effects as fatigue, headaches or dizziness, or feel hungry more often than usual. Your susceptibility to urinary tract infections (page 170) may also rise. It is unlikely that your baby will be deprived – except in severe dehydration, your body and the placenta work together to ensure your baby stays well nourished.

If you drink more water than you need the most likely consequence is frequent urination and you may also deplete your body of minerals passed in the urine.

Drinking for health

Drink water – it's by far the best fluid for you and your baby.

Which water?

The cheapest form of purified water is filtered tap water. If you prefer bottled water, choose those sold in glass bottles – there is a risk that synthetic or foreign oestrogens (xenostrogens) may be absorbed from plastic containers and these can affect your baby. Water that is labelled 'sparkling water' does not necessarily come from a pure or natural spring source, and may simply be tap water with carbon dioxide added to it – better to drink still water. Fizzy drinks and sparkling water (which contain phosphates) can interfere with calcium and mineral absorption.

Fruit juices
The food industry has promoted bottled and carton fruit juice as healthy but these juices have a very high sugar content (some of it added), contribute to sugar highs and lows (page 261) and could be a potent factor in excess weight gain. It is best to avoid them. You may enjoy experimenting with a range of fruits, and perhaps add vegetables like carrots. Remember that it's still cautious to keep your fruit intake (and the sugar it contains) within reasonable limits. Two pieces of fruit or a glass of freshly squeezed orange juice using two or three oranges is enough for one day.

Colas, diet and fizzy drinks
Colas are full of sugar. Diet drinks contain sweeteners that can confuse your body – the sensation of having something sweet is not followed by a rise in your blood sugar and you will feel hungry or thirsty within a short time. If you follow your urges your calorie intake will be too high. Many colas and diet drinks also contain caffeine. Cut them out!

Tea and coffee
Indian tea and all coffees (except decaffeinated) contain stimulants including caffeine that cause a rise in blood sugar and give a short-lived energy rush (page 261). Drinking too much depletes your energy resources. Caffeine is also addictive, and you can pass the addiction on to your baby in the womb. It can also interfere with your body's absorption of nutrients, especially iron and zinc. As a diuretic, caffeine can increase the excretion of nutrients in your urine. Best to keep caffeine to a minimum. It may take a few weeks for your body to withdraw from caffeine and get used to the subtle effects of fruit and herb teas (below).

Herbal teas and drinks
Water is the first and best drink. You can jazz it up with a slice of lime or have it hot with lemon for a revitalising drink that's also good for digestion. There are many other alternatives using herbs and fruits:

- *For wellbeing*: redbush or rooibos tea is a refreshing drink and a source of antioxidants – vitamins and minerals essential for normal cell development.
- *For birth preparation*: raspberry tea strengthens the uterus and may assist contractions, so try drinking a few cups each day from Week 34 of your pregnancy. Red clover and lady's mantle have similar properties and all three encourage hormonal balance.
- *For breastfeeding*: fennel tea aids digestion, reduces water retention and bloating and encourages milk production after birth.
- *For digestive comfort*: peppermint tea aids digestion and relieves heartburn, wind and nausea, so it's an ideal drink after food. Some women cannot tolerate peppermint, however. Herbs with similar effects include lemon balm and spearmint.
- *To boost immunity*: marigold is a useful tonic for boosting your immune system, as is echinacea. As a preventive measure, drink echinacea 15 days on, 15 days off.
- *For nausea relief*: ginger tea is one of the most effective ways to prevent and alleviate nausea (page 552).
- *To improve relaxation and sleep*: chamomile tea helps relaxation and can diminish morning sickness.
- *To reduce stress*: if you're feeling emotionally turbulent, an infusion of lime flower, lemon balm, and chamomile may have a calming effect.

Food and eating, mother
Emotions

Eating and emotional feelings are closely bound. Through life we all develop associations between particular feelings and certain foods, and how we feel when we eat in company. These associations are largely unconscious, although most people can identify with comfort eating.

The link between feelings and food is psychological and also physiological. The mutual relationship between your brain and stomach, known as your 'brain-gut axis', involves a complex and constant exchange of chemical, hormonal and nervous signals. So, your feelings affect your appetite, your digestion and even blood sugar levels, just as what you eat affects the way you feel emotionally. Gradually altering eating habits may help you feel more emotionally stable and content, while attending to emotions may help you step out of unhelpful food habits.

Pregnancy is an emotional time and your attention is naturally directed inward, and to the needs of your family. The potential benefit of this is that you may grow more skilful at recognising your emotions and sitting with them, even those that are uncomfortable, and use food less often as a method of distraction or comfort. If your emotions around food are intense or you notice you are 'using' food, focusing your emotions (page 206) may help you avoid poor eating habits. If you feel addicted to food or are depriving or punishing yourself, extra support may be important (page 201).

Love

Sharing food and nurturing another person can be an expression of love, and eating may be like the feeling of being loved. This is how it is for a baby who is lovingly fed. The early experiences of eating and being fed are always linked with emotional feelings and you have an opportunity to offer your baby love together with food.

The love you have for yourself will affect the way you nourish yourself. Low self-esteem (page 72) can lie beneath destructive eating habits or resistance to healthy eating. How you are loved by people around you is also central, and if they provide delicious food you will feel really good.

Rhythms and control

Your baby shows you natural rhythms of hunger and thirst. We are all born with inherent rhythms, but we can lose touch with them. We may have been fed when we were not hungry, or denied food when we were. Early experiences shape each person's unique ability to remain in tune with body signs of hunger and fullness. This has been proven in relation to bottle-feeding, which can deliver more calories than a baby needs and may predispose a baby to being overweight or obese in later life. Over-feeding may continue in childhood with pressure to 'eat

everything on the plate', even if the portion size is not suitable for the individual child's needs (which alter from day to day). The teenage years are very important.

You may use food as a way of being in charge, and food and eating may be used as a way of rating behaviour in your family: a baby is good (eats everything) or bad (doesn't eat everything), and parents are good/loved (when baby accepts food) or bad/unloved (when food is rejected).

Children left to their own devices signal when they are hungry and tend to eat what their body needs and when they need it. It may be difficult for you to believe this if your background is one of rigid meal times and if food has been a controlling factor in your life. Babies who are breastfed on demand are not overfed, and tend to complain less.

Comfort and habit

We all know about comfort food, used to mask or suppress uncomfortable feelings including sadness, anger, anxiety and pain. Usually, comfort food is highly sugary or salty. The immediate physical effect of eating – a rise in blood sugar and a flush of feel-good hormones – is to feel better and temporarily forget the uncomfortable feelings. Food can temporarily soothe a crying baby who is giving vent to his feelings but is not hungry.

It is okay to enjoy comfort food from time to time. But if you are in the habit of doing this every day you may wish to look at other ways of expressing your feelings. The habit may have originated in your childhood and can be surprisingly easy to alter now.

Stress

Stress alters your appetite, and demands on time and energy make it harder to eat well. There may be a cycle where you eat on the hop and have mainly processed foods and caffeine, because of lack of time, but these foods actually increase your stress from sugar rushes, reduce your energy reserves and disturb your hormonal balance. Eating when you are stressed – indeed stress on its own – can also contribute to digestion problems. You may find the suggestions on page 222 helpful to reduce the pressure.

Food and eating, mother
Safe eating: what to eat and avoid

You can be sure of a good balance of nutrients if you eat a varied mixture of nourishing foods.

Foods to focus on

- Fresh vegetables, including their skins.
- Raw, steamed or stir-fried vegetables, and salads.
- Fresh, whole fruits (two to three daily – avoid more). Avoid fruit juices and dried fruits with excess sugar.
- Wholemeal bread and pasta, brown rice and whole grains (oats, barley, millet, corn).
- Beans and pulses.
- Tofu and soya.
- Fish (deep-sea white fish, sardines, salmon and mackerel – but some fish are best avoided, see 'Foods to avoid', below).
- Meat – at most 90g (3.5oz) a day. Choose poultry and prime cuts of lean, red meat – organic where possible – and grill or roast so that some fat drains away.
- Eggs (well cooked, not fried – see 'Foods to avoid', below).
- Water and fruit and herb teas – six to eight glasses a day.
- Live organic unsweetened yoghurt, in moderation.
- Nuts (except peanuts if you have a personal or family history of peanut allergy, page 21) and seeds in their natural state (without salt).
- Cold pressed oils – olive for cooking, sunflower, walnut, sesame.
- Seaweeds (wakame and nori arame).

Foods to reduce

These foods are best reduced and you may choose to avoid them. This is not because of a risk of infection or a potential impact on your baby's development, but because they do not contribute to your nutrition or to healthy growth for your baby, and may be a factor in excess weight gain and unstable patterns of energy release. It is better to satisfy your appetite and your need for beneficial calories, vitamins and minerals with nutritious foods.

- Biscuits, cakes, white bread, white pasta and white rice.
- Chocolates, sweets and crisps.
- Added sugar, ready made fruit juices and smoothies (keep to minimum because sugar content is still high, and avoid concentrates).
- Added salt.
- Saturated animal fats (sausages, burgers, bacon and fatty meats including salamis and sausages).
- Excess full-fat dairy produce, such as cheese (semi-skimmed or skimmed milk contains less fat, and calcium can be obtained from many other foods, see page 263).
- Fast foods and food fried in animal fats.
- Tea and coffee.
- Foods containing additives ('E numbers'), especially preservatives and colourings.

Foods to avoid

- Liver and cod liver oil (an excess of vitamin A can cause birth defects).
- Raw meat, meat pâtés and ready-to-eat poultry (risk of LISTERIA).
- Raw and smoked fish, including sushi (risk of listeria).
- Fish with potentially high mercury content such as marlin, shark and swordfish. (No more than two portions of oily fish – or two tins of tuna – per week. There is no risk with white fish.)
- Raw egg products – including handmade mayonnaise and mousse made with raw eggs – it is important to cook eggs well (risk of listeria).
- Unpasteurised soft or blue cheeses such as Camembert, Brie, Stilton (risk of listeria).
- Colas and concentrated fruit juices (sugar high).
- Recreational (or 'street') drugs, smoking and smoky atmospheres.
- Alcohol (see page 190).
- Peanuts need to be avoided if you have a family history of allergy (page 21).

Watch out for...

Wheat
Wheat is a staple and although it offers benefits of fibre many people have wheat intolerance without being aware of it. The symptoms vary

and can include bloating, bowel pain, weight gain, fluid retention, low energy, low moods and even DEPRESSION. Food manufacturers add a lot of salt and sugar to many wheat products.

It is safe to cut out wheat-based foods such as bread, pasta, biscuits and cakes (all of which also contain sugar). There are other good sources of fibre such as brown rice and vegetable skins. You may miss the bread and pasta but there are alternatives such as oat cakes, rice cakes, rice, rice noodles and other grains such as polenta and quinoa. After a week you may notice a boost in your energy. There may be a reduction in weight gain (more noticeable when you are not pregnant). As you bring wheat back into your diet you may notice a reaction and you can then decide to keep it to a minimum.

Sugar

Sugar is the main cause of excess weight gain. It is hidden in many processed or refined foods and in colas and fruit juices. Anything with 'ose' in the list of ingredients – such as fructose, lactose, sucrose – means added sugar. See below for more information.

Food and eating, mother
Sugar

Eating sugary and processed food gives a short-lived energy high followed by a slump – plus an adrenaline-fuelled anxiety rush. It is the commonest cause of excess weight gain. It can disrupt your hormone balance, add to emotional swings and depression and increase your cravings. Artificial sugars are worse: they intensify sugar cravings and weight gain and they may alter your mood.

Highs and lows

When energy is released from food it raises your blood sugar levels and this affects the way you feel, your energy and mood and the way your body functions, including your digestion, circulation and hormone production. In pregnancy, your baby's blood sugar levels and hormonal fluctuations are affected by what you eat.

Many women are on a roller coaster of blood sugar highs and lows. When your blood sugar levels are high (hyperglycaemia), you're likely to feel energetic and positive. When they are low (hypoglycaemia), they may bring on feelings including lethargy, tiredness, anxiety and stress, you may be tense and irritable, have difficulty concentrating, be dizzy or thirsty, have a headache and crave sweet food.

Fast burners

A large part of your diet will be made up of carbohydrates, which are your chief source of energy. Some foods release this energy quickly. These are 'fast burners' that provide a quick energy release – but the sugar is quickly burned up and a slump in energy follows. If you eat only fast burners your blood sugar levels rise and then fall dramatically in 90 minutes. Fast burners are 'empty calories' – they provide little goodness and increase weight gain.

As a guideline, refined sugar is a very fast burner. When food is refined, carbohydrates are simplified and other supportive ingredients such as fibre reduced – so eating white bread is less sustaining than eating brown bread. Refined wheat in cakes, biscuits and pastries is an example of a simple carbohydrate that your body breaks down quickly. Sugary sweets, chocolate, honey, colas, fruit juices and sweetened yoghurts are all fast burners, too.

Slow burners

Some foods give a sustained energy release because your body takes longer to break them down. Complex carbohydrates (such as beans and pulses, brown rice, brown bread and brown pasta, and fruit and vegetables with skins on) are 'slow burners', and when you include fibre (roughage) and protein in a meal, this helps sustain the energy release. Eating 'slow burners' protects against the roller coaster of sugar peaks and troughs and can help to stabilise your appetite, your weight, your moods and hormones.

Glycaemic index

The scientifically based glycaemic index scores foods according to the rate of energy release, showing which are slow burning and which are fast burning. A high score is a fast burner and a low score is a slow burner. Foods only appear on the index if they contain carbohydrate.

Sweeteners

Sweeteners are chemicals that taste sweet but it is not true sugar sweetness. The chemicals cause your body to release hormones and enzymes as if you had eaten sugar. During the 90-minute roller-coaster cycle you will feel the full symptoms of intense hypoglycaemia and the need to consume food and calories. You may put on weight. The chemicals may have other potential long-term health risks. It is best to avoid them.

Avoiding the sugar trap

The best scenario is to eat every three to four hours, with slow burners as the foundation of your meal or snack. To slow the energy release even more, add a small amount of protein to a carbohydrate snack, such as an apple or a few uncooked nuts.

You may want to buy or download a list showing the glycaemic index of foods and pin it up for reference, along with a table of basic food groups. Ensure your diet is rich in variety and interest and fits your appetite during and after pregnancy, and if you are still reaching for sugar, it may be worth assessing your exercise levels and your feelings (page 226).

Food and eating, mother
Timing meals and snacks

It is not only the content of your meals that is important for healthy eating. Other factors such as when you eat and how much you eat in any meal are important considerations, too.

Timing

It is best to eat small amounts every three to four hours. This is a guideline, since the exact time it takes your own body to break down and use energy depends on the food you have eaten and on your own metabolic rate. Your meal times are not the same as your baby's, who has a smaller stomach and a different digestive system and so may need to eat every two to three hours.

Snacking

Eating every three to four hours means you will need to eat snacks – oat cakes, nuts or fruit, for example – as well as main meals. If you are bored, you may be inclined to 'graze' so ensure sweet and fatty snacks are not in your cupboards. If you have fruit or other carbohydrate food, add a small amount of protein such as a handful of natural nuts. This will prolong the effect of the snack by an hour or more.

A snack before you sleep – such as a few oat cakes with cheese or hummus, a glass of milk, an oat-based cereal or a sandwich – can help you sleep soundly and reduce feelings of nausea the next morning.

Portion sizes

Portion sizes are important when eating main meals. Eating small- to moderate-size portions will help you feel energised. It takes your brain 20 minutes to register fullness, so it's preferable to keep quantities small. If you are still hungry half an hour after eating a main meal, you can take a second helping. It may take you a month or two to adjust if you change to smaller amounts. This may go against your conditioning of what a full meal looks like – big is not better. Eating large portions doesn't mean you will be able to go without food for longer. Your body stores the energy (calories) you do not use. Smaller portions and snacks spread your calorie intake over 24 hours and reduce the sugar 'roller coaster'.

Breakfasting

It is optimal to begin the day with a nutritious meal. If you are not a breakfast person, try a nutritious snack. This is particularly important when you are pregnant or breastfeeding, because a cup of tea or a glass of juice alone begins the pattern for a day's sugar highs and lows.

Habits, old and new

It is worthwhile looking at your eating habits. You may carry some from your family of origin, such as enjoying a biscuit to ease boredom or pain, or feeling guilty if you do not finish everything on your plate. Your transition to parenthood is a good time to review habits and to talk about points of difference with your partner, as you will both strongly influence your baby's relationship with food and eating. Your baby's early experiences with food are important and shape his behaviour around food as an adult.

Food and eating, mother
Vitamins, minerals, EFAs and supplements

During pregnancy your need for numerous vitamins and minerals increases. A balanced, varied diet with nutritious meals at regular intervals could supply the vitamins and minerals you and your baby require during pregnancy and beyond. But you may have days when you skip meals or eat meals with low nutritional value. Even with a balanced organic diet, there may be deficiencies, depending on the soil in which a food is grown, and the method of cooking. Taking a supplement ensures you get the nutrients you and your baby need.

Where parents are well nourished there is a lower rate of miscarriage, birth abnormalities and low birth weight. After birth, supplementation helps replace any elements your body has lost and keeps you nourished when the demands on your energy are high and your sleep is broken.

Antioxidants

Antioxidants 'mop up' damaging by-products of natural body functions known as free radicals, also produced by other sources including cigarette smoke, traffic pollution, UV-rays and heated fats.

The chief antioxidants are the 'ACE' vitamins and the minerals zinc and selenium. Vitamins A and C are abundant in brightly coloured fresh fruit and vegetables (such as raspberries, kiwis, yellow peppers, parsnips and melon). Good sources of vitamin E include cold pressed seed oils, olive oil, wheat germ and avocados.

Vitamin A is sourced from animal meats as retinol, and from vegetables as beta carotene, which your body converts into vitamin A, provided your zinc sources are sufficient. All red,

yellow and orange and dark green vegetables are good sources of beta carotene. The conversion only occurs when your body needs the vitamin so there is no risk of getting too much vitamin A from vegetable sources. Animal sourced vitamin A, if not used by your body, is stored in your liver. Excess retinol in pregnancy can lead to foetal abnormalities, so avoid high-dose vitamin A supplements, animal-sourced vitamin A, cod liver oil and liver.

Nuts (such as brazils) and seeds (such as pumpkin) are good sources of zinc and selenium. Antioxidants have many other benefits, too. Vitamin C, for instance, boosts immunity, while vitamin A improves skin health.

Calcium

Calcium is the only mineral whose requirement doubles during pregnancy as it is essential for the development of foetal bones. If calcium is in short supply, it will be leached from your bones and may even lead to pregnancy-associated OSTEOPOROSIS. Drinking an extra pint of skimmed or semi-skimmed milk per day supplies additional calcium. Make sure the milk is organic. Milk is not essential and if you prefer to keep your dairy intake low, or you have a dairy intolerance, you can get all the necessary calcium from nuts, seeds, fish and green veg.

EFAs (omega oils)

Essential fatty acids are vital to health. The term 'essential' does not refer to their importance but to their source: they must be obtained from food sources as the body cannot make them from other nutrients. EFAs are also referred to as omega oils. The most important EFAs for the development of the foetal brain and nervous system are omega-3 and 6. In pregnancy your baby draws on your reserves so it is important to increase your consumption. Tiredness may be a sign that you are not getting enough, and if your baby is using all your omega-3 reserves, the effect on your brain may lead to depression.

The best sources are nuts, seeds and cold pressed oils (especially hemp oil and flax seed oil), wholegrains and dark green leafy vegetables. Oily fish including mackerel, herring, salmon, trout, sardines and pilchards are particularly rich in omega-3 oils. The FSA recommends a limit of two portions from this selection per week. It's best to include various sources in your diet, and easy to do with, for instance, a handful of powdered seeds and an oil salad dressing. Some people have physical difficulty making use of omega-3 oils from plants and so oily fish is the best source.

Folic Acid

Folic acid is important for cell formation and function in your baby and you, and reduces the risk of heart disease. Taken in early pregnancy (and ideally before conception) it reduces the incidence of neural tube defects, such as SPINA BIFIDA.

Natural sources include wheatgerm, sprouts, asparagus, sesame seeds, broccoli, cashews, cauliflower, avocado and walnuts, and fortified cereals and bread. All pregnant women are advised to take supplements. If you have epilepsy, it's important to take specialist advice as some epilepsy medication can reduce the absorption of folic acid.

Regardless of diet, all women are advised to take folic acid supplements daily during this time and it is typically included in multivitamin and mineral supplements for pregnancy. The recommended supplemental dose of 0.4 mg (400 mcg) per day is particularly important before conception and during the first 12 weeks of pregnancy. If you have previously had a child with a neural tube defect you may be advised to take a higher dose of 800 mcg folic acid per day.

Iron

Iron helps your red blood cells transport oxygen and enables your muscle cells to function normally. Women can absorb up to six times their normal amount in pregnancy. If your natural iron stores are low you may feel tired and become anaemic (page 26). Natural sources include egg yolk, molasses, wheatgerm, almonds, parsley, pumpkin seeds, cashews and prunes and all dark green vegetables.

Vitamin K

Vitamin K is essential for blood clotting and is important after birth to help your uterus heal, and to stem postnatal bleeding. It is produced by naturally occurring gut bacteria, and is found in cauliflower and green leafy vegetables. Babies cannot produce their own vitamin K and supplements are recommended at and shortly after birth (page 63).

Zinc

Zinc is vital for cell growth and chemical balance, for you and for your baby. It also offers some protection against toxic metals, such as lead, promotes healing and skin health, and helps to prevent depression. Low rates may inhibit optimal foetal growth. In the latter stages of pregnancy, your baby draws heavily on your zinc stores, so eating more ensures you do not become depleted. Natural sources include wholegrains, oysters, fish, apricots, eggs, pumpkin seeds, rye, oats, almonds and pecans.

Choosing supplements

Choose your supplements carefully – not all are equally effective, and absorption can be improved if you take a combination. For example, minerals such as zinc, iron or calcium need to be part of a wider vitamin and mineral programme to be absorbed effectively. Some iron supplements are difficult to absorb and can cause digestive problems, especially CONSTIPATION. You may find iron EAP or a tonic works better for you. Finally, check the labels: the effect of supplements reflects their qualities and it's worth avoiding pills containing ingredients such as sugar, talc, lactose and preservatives.

Supplements formulated for pregnancy ensure you will avoid taking a potentially dangerous excess of one or more nutrients. If you are in any doubt about a suitable mix of supplements, talk to your GP or midwife, or consult a qualified nutritional therapist. Please beware of the temptation to treat supplements as a substitute for good food: they work best and are most efficiently absorbed when taken in conjunction with a healthy diet.

It is ideal to begin taking pregnancy supplements before conception and continue after birth. It may take a few weeks or months for you to notice the impact of a fuller nutritional programme on your energy and moods.

It is best to include supplements of omega-3 and 6 essential fatty acids. These are available in capsules derived from fish oils formulated

Your personal requirements	Recommended supplements
Minimum supplementation for pregnancy and after birth	Multivitamin and mineral designed for pregnancy: 1 daily, with breakfast.
Moderate supplementation for pregnancy and after birth	Multivitamin and mineral designed for pregnancy: 1 daily, with breakfast. * Essential fatty acid: 1 at breakfast, 1 at dinner.
Maximum supplementation for pregnancy and after birth This is necessary if your iron level is low or you have anaemia	Multivitamin and mineral designed for pregnancy: 1 daily, with breakfast. * Essential fatty acid: 1 at breakfast, 1 at dinner. * Vitamin C (500 mg) plus Iron EAP**: 1 daily, one hour before food (lunch or dinner).
If you feel down or depressed	Multivitamin and mineral designed for pregnancy: 1 daily, with breakfast. * Essential fatty acid: 1 at breakfast, 1 at dinner. Zinc citrate (15 mg): 1 at breakfast, 1 at dinner.
To reduce sugar highs and lows	Multivitamin and mineral designed for pregnancy: 1 daily, with breakfast. * Essential fatty acid: 1 at breakfast, 1 at dinner. Chromium (100 mg): 1 daily, at dinner.

* Avoid essential fatty acids and vitamin C supplements if you are taking aspirin or heparin or if you have epilepsy.
** Take iron 1 hour before food to increase absorption and avoid black tea.

specifically for pregnancy and breastfeeding. If you are vegetarian, hemp oil is a possible alternative. Avoid taking cod liver oil, though, which is too high in vitamin A and can harm a foetus.

Forceps and ventouse

See Labour and birth, mother, forceps and ventouse.

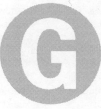

Gastroenteritis

See Diarrhoea, baby.

Genes and genetics

See also Congenital abnormalities.

Genes are what determine how every person functions and their traits, such as blood type, body build and personality. Genes are made of deoxyribonucleic acid (DNA), the chemical code that is the basis for life. All the genes are contained in chromosomes, which are, in effect, long strips of genes all linked together. Each healthy cell in the body normally has 46 chromosomes – in 23 pairs. The first 22 pairs of chromosomes are said to be autosomal (matching pairs) and are common to males and females. The 23rd pair is the sex chromosomes. Males have one X and one Y chromosome, while females have two X chromosomes. Mothers always contribute an X chromosome. Fathers contribute an X or a Y chromosome and hence determine the sex of the baby.

■ DISORDERS IN GENES AND CHROMOSOMES

Genes are found in pairs, one of the pair is on one chromosome and the other is on its matching chromosome. One member of each gene pair is inherited from the mother, and the other is inherited from the father. Some genes are dominant over others and, depending on the

combination of the gene pair, different characteristics will be expressed. The dominant gene will be expressed more forcefully and an obvious example is eye colour. The other gene is recessive.

If a chromosome carries a faulty gene that can potentially cause illness it can have an effect if it is dominant, but not if it is recessive – unless paired with another recessive gene. Even if a recessive gene does not cause illness in an individual, it may be passed on and have an effect in a future generation. In girls, the general rules about dominant and recessive genes apply to their two X chromosomes. But boys only have one X chromosome and so if this contains a faulty gene it will usually cause illness. This is called X-linked inheritance.

On rare occasions, a fault can occur in the pairing of chromosomes, resulting in an abnormal number of chromosomes. One example is DOWN'S SYNDROME, which is caused by having 47 chromosomes. Although rare, this is the most common chromosomal disorder tested for in antenatal screening (page 31). Most chromosomal disorders cannot be passed on. In rare cases, an extra chromosome may become attached to another chromosome and can sometimes be inherited from a parent.

■ GENETIC TESTING

Examining genes and the chromosomes to which they are related, or the enzymes that they influence, has become an increasingly accurate way of detecting developmental disorders. Genetic testing is offered to selected parents who wish to know the likelihood of their baby inheriting a genetic disorder when there is a family history. It is also increasingly used in standard antenatal screening for everyone.

The main purpose of genetic testing is to establish a diagnosis and enable the parents and the medical team to make informed decisions. The ethical and religious debates surrounding genetic testing are intense. There are different guidelines for testing in different countries and in different hospitals within a country. Some parents choose not to be tested.

Genetic counselling

Genetic counselling provides emotional and practical support before, during and after pregnancy and if there is bereavement. Clinical geneticists are specialists with up-to-date information.. They advise parents and other professionals about tests and the likely outcome for mother and baby. In many hospitals, the midwives, obstetricians and paediatricians perform this role. For guidance on what happens when an abnormality occurs, see page 148. Advice on personal and emotional support is given on page 46.

Diagnostic testing

Diagnostic testing is used to identify an abnormality or a condition in a parent or a baby. The information is helpful in determining the course of a disease and treatment. The tests include identifying chromosomes or doing biochemical tests for individual genes. Some of these tests are offered in pregnancy.

Prenatal studies before implantation
Pre-implantation studies are used following in-vitro fertilisation to diagnose a genetic disease or condition in an embryo before it is implanted into the mother's uterus. This enables unaffected embryos to be implanted. There are rules governing pre-implantation diagnoses which are constantly under review.

Carrier testing
Carrier testing determines whether an adult carries an altered gene for a particular disease. Follow-up tests during pregnancy can determine whether the baby has inherited the condition. Tests may be based on a family history but they are increasingly offered to all pregnant women. Many conditions are detectable including CYSTIC FIBROSIS, sickle cell anaemia (page 476) and disorders of blood clotting (haemophilia).

Prenatal diagnosis
Prenatal diagnosis is used to detect a genetic disorder in a developing foetus and includes maternal blood screening (page 30), ultrasound (page 33), AMNIOCENTESIS AND CVS (chorionic villous sampling).

Some of the diagnostic tests such as ultrasound scans or blood tests may be offered to all pregnant women. Tests such as amniocentesis or CVS (explained in detail on page 21), are selectively used if parents have a family history of a condition, a previously affected baby, or a scan or blood test indicates the baby is at risk of a condition. There is a risk of miscarriage after the test. The cells obtained in the test are examined to check the baby's chromosomes or look at the gene being investigated. There are more than 200 gene defects that can be detected.

Newborn screening
Newborn screening for certain genetic diseases is standard across the UK. The tests are usually on blood taken in the heel prick test (page 338) performed by the end of the first week in an otherwise healthy baby. The blood is tested for a range of conditions, including biochemical disorders such as hypothyroidism (page 513), PHENYLKETONURIA and cystic fibrosis as well as sickle cell disease and thalassaemia (page 476) that may cause ANAEMIA. Early diagnosis may allow early treatment to begin, leading to a better outcome and fewer complications for the child and family.

Genitalia, ambiguous

See also Congenital abnormalities.

When a child's genitals do not appear clearly male or female, this is extremely distressing for the parents. Fortunately, it is very rare, affecting only around one in 25,000 babies per year in the UK. Most commonly, a female has severe virilising (overproduction of male hormones) and appears to have a small penis, or a male has an abnormally small penis that resembles a clitoris. Very few affected babies have genitals that are so ambiguous that a gender determination cannot be made at birth.

True hermaphroditism, where a baby has both male and female internal genitals and the external genitals may be indistinct, is extremely rare. The ideal care is a team approach, including parents, neonatologists, geneticists, endocrinologists, surgeons, counsellors and ethicists.

What happens

In many cases the cause cannot be identified and the genetic disorder appears to occur by chance, but there are some known causes. Congenital adrenal hyperplasia (CAH), present in about one in 15,000 babies, is the most common cause of females to become masculinised. The condition is related to a gene that affects the overproduction of male hormones from the adrenal glands and a deficiency of cortisone that leads to salt deficiency in the body's tissues. A paediatric endocrinologist may suggest medication to suppress the production of male hormones and replacement cortisone. In families with the disease, the diagnosis may be established by antenatal testing and cortisone steroid treatment for the mother may begin before the birth.

Action plan

The discovery is usually unexpected. You will be offered counselling and put in touch with support groups. In most cases, gender can be determined relatively soon and a chromosome analysis will be carried out on a sample of your baby's blood.

Treatment depends on the type of the disorder, but usually includes corrective surgery, hormone replacement and close follow-up. Some children born with ambiguous genitalia may have normal internal reproductive organs that do not interfere with fertility. At puberty, treatment with oestrogen and progesterone may be used for girls with absent or non-functioning

ovaries to bring on pubertal changes of breast development, body proportions and body hair. In some girls the vaginal opening may need to be enlarged.

There is controversy concerning issues of gender because gender assignment by doctors and family may not correlate with gender preference by the patient in adulthood. The most important organ for gender assignment is the brain, which may undergo hormonal imprinting in the uterus.

German measles (Rubella)

See Rubella.

Gingivitis

See Teeth and gums, mother.

Glue ear

See Ear infection and pain, baby.

Gonorrhoea

Gonorrhoea is a sexually transmitted bacterium that tends to infect the cervix and sometimes the urethra, rectum or, less commonly, throat. In men it infects the penis, urethra and prostate. Around half of the women infected don't experience symptoms. Others have a vaginal discharge and may have vaginal pain and redness and perhaps pain when passing urine. Men have symptoms such as abnormal discharge from the penis or burning sensation when urinating.

Gonorrhoea is now relatively rare and is usually easily treated. It is, however, highly contagious through sexual contact. If you have unprotected sex with someone who is infected you have a 90 per cent chance of catching it. It can be spread through oral, vaginal and anal sex. When gonorrhoea is present there may be an accompanying infection of CHLAMYDIA and TRICHOMONIASIS.

What happens

Gonorrhoea usually responds to treatment, which can be given in pregnancy to reduce the following potential complications. Resistant strains of the bacteria are very rare.

- If the infection is not treated, it may cause pelvic inflammatory disease, which may cause blockage of the fallopian tubes and increase the likelihood of ECTOPIC PREGNANCY and infertility.
- Although rare, gonorrhoea may lead to severe pelvic inflammation after delivery.
- If the bacteria are present in the cervix and vagina during birth, it may affect your baby's eyes, leading to severe conjunctivitis with redness, swelling and discharge. This needs to be treated to prevent long-term scarring and vision problems.
- In a baby infected in the womb, gonorrhoea may rarely cause septicaemia (blood poisoning) and need intensive antibiotic treatment.

Action plan

You may not be offered routine testing for gonorrhoea. If you have another sexually transmitted disease or suspect you may have been exposed to gonorrhoea it is worth being tested to reduce the risks to your baby. The test involves a vaginal or urethral swab. If you test positive there is a high chance you may also have chlamydia, so it is good to be checked for the range of sexually transmitted diseases (page 476).

The standard treatment for gonorrhoea in pregnancy is penicillin by injection. If you are allergic to penicillin or the bacterial strain proves resistant, there are alternative safe antibiotics. You will need a vaginal swab after the treatment to ensure that the bacteria have been eliminated. Your partner also needs to be treated.

After you have given birth, if you are infected your baby's eye may be swabbed. If your baby is infected (*ophthalmia neonatorum*, literally newborn eye infection) the eyelids are likely to swell and produce pus. This can be treated with penicillin eye drops and intravenous penicillin for five to seven days to prevent infection elsewhere in her body. Long term, the outlook is fine, providing the cornea or other eye structures have not been damaged during the infection.

Group B streptococcus (Group B strep or GBS)

One in four pregnant women carries the Group B streptococcus (GBS) bacterium in her body, usually in the bowel, vagina, bladder or throat. Adults who carry the bacterium are usually not harmed by it and it does not usually require treatment. In labour, however, an infected woman may pass GBS to her baby during vaginal delivery. A small number of babies become infected, leading to a risk of critical illness. If you test positive for GBS, your medical team will advise extra precautions during and after birth. These measures are very effective in reducing the GBS risk to your baby.

What happens

Infection in pregnancy

Few GBS carriers are aware of being infected. Occasionally, GBS may cause a vaginal discharge or a urinary tract infection. It may also cause a postnatal pelvic infection. In women with HIV that is untreated, GBS can cause a dangerous infection that spreads around the body.

Infection in a baby

Only 1 per cent of babies born to infected mothers are themselves infected, accounting for around one in 1,000 babies. They acquire GBS during birth: this usually occurs after the membranes rupture and vaginal bacteria enter the amniotic fluid and are inhaled or swallowed by the baby (page 391). The risk increases with the length of time after the membranes rupture, particularly after 12 hours. Bacteria may invade through the skin of the baby after birth.

The risk is greatest in premature babies, particularly where the membranes ruptured many hours before birth. It is less common in full-term babies, and rare after one month of age. There are two forms of GBS disease in infants early onset and late-onset.

Early-onset GBS disease is the more common and more serious form. Typically, an infected baby will show signs within hours of birth. These include grunting, poor feeding, lethargy or irritability, abnormally high or low temperature, and rapid heart rate or breathing rate. Early-onset GBS disease can lead to infection of the lungs with pneumonia (page 446), infection throughout the bloodstream causing septicaemia, a potentially life-threatening condition, or MENINGITIS, an infection of the membranes (meninges) and fluid surrounding the brain and spinal cord.

Late-onset GBS disease develops one to 12 weeks after birth. About half of all babies with late-onset disease acquire the infection from their mothers. The source of the other cases is unknown. The warning signs may include fever, poor feeding and/or vomiting, change of consciousness, a shrill cry or whimpering, dislike of being handled, a tense or bulging fontanelle, jerking movements or floppiness, altered breathing patterns, and pale or blotchy skin.

Despite antibiotics, both late- and early-onset GBS infection can be fatal. A minority of infected babies die and of those who survive, some have permanent neurological damage, including seizures and hearing loss, particularly following meningitis. The impact of late-onset GBS is typically less severe.

Action plan

Routine testing is not current in all UK hospitals, and is not 100 per cent accurate as it may produce a false negative, which would suggest an absence of infection when it is in fact present. For this reason, any mother who has had a previously infected infant will be treated, whatever the test result. Your baby is more likely to be exposed to GBS if you have the organism and one or more additional risk factors, which include the following:

• A cultured vaginal swab, which tests positive for GBS at any time during pregnancy.
• A urinary tract infection caused by GBS.
• A previous baby with GBS disease.
• A fever (37.8°C/100°F or higher) during labour.
• Ruptured membranes 12 hours or more before delivery.
• Labour before Week 37.

Treatment

Antibiotics are not recommended in pregnancy because they do not reduce the risk of GBS in your baby. If you have a urinary infection caused by GBS, this is treated in pregnancy to prevent damage to your kidneys.

In labour, if you have GBS in your vagina only, but no other risk factors, you may not be offered routine antibiotics. If you have more than one risk factor, antibiotics such as penicillin or ampicillin are recommended when labour begins or when the membranes rupture. If you're allergic to penicillin, you may receive clindamycin or a similar alternative. Doctors and midwives generally try to give two doses of antibiotics by intravenous drip four hours apart before birth. If you have a long labour, you may receive additional doses. If you do receive antibiotics during labour, each dose takes 30 minutes to run in and then the drip is capped off till the next dose is needed. GBS does not affect your ability to breastfeed safely.

Medication is not necessary if you have a caesarean section. Having a positive GBS swab is not on its own a reason to have a caesarean, because the antibiotic schedule is easy to administer and very effective in labour.

After birth

The GBS bacterium can be passed through touch, so it is very important that all adults make sure their hands are clean before handling your newborn baby.

If you have tested positive in pregnancy, your baby will be checked by a paediatrician. He will not require treatment unless there are clear indications of infection. If you have not been able to receive antibiotics for at least four hours prior to delivery and the membranes have been ruptured for a significant time, your baby may be offered antibiotics until the doctors are certain he is not infected. Opinions vary and many paediatricians do not recommend routine antibiotic treatment in these circumstances.

If after the birth your baby shows signs consistent with early- or late-onset GBS infection or meningitis, call your doctor immediately. Early intensive treatment could prevent potentially serious consequences.

Growth and development, baby

See also Autistic Spectrum Disorders (ASD) and developmental concerns.

Your baby is genetically inclined to grow and develop but the precise path is not predetermined. There is a mix of nature and nurture. How your baby is met, held and listened to by other people, what is in his environment, what he eats and drinks and his emotional experiences, and unique style and personality, will all affect the way he adapts and passes through each stage of development. As parents, you are in a powerful position. This may feel daunting but at the same time there is much to reassure you because nature sets the stage for you and your baby. You don't need a scientist's insight or a medical degree – what your baby needs most from you is for you to tune in, follow his lead, be there for him, and trust your instincts.

Your baby will be unique, but there are some key points:

- Skin-to-skin contact is excellent for growth (see page 517).
- Carrying your baby encourages bone strength and allows him to explore from a safe place, with a good view of the world. With a strong spine, the rest follows naturally.
- Do not leave your baby for long periods in a car seat or other seat that causes his back to slouch. For optimal development he needs to lie on his back and spend time on his stomach.
- Tummy time is incredibly important. There is no other way for your baby to develop optimal strength in his spine, shoulders, neck and upper arms. Give your baby time on his tummy each day – you can do this by lying him across your lap, and on the floor.
- From Weeks 4–6, you can begin using developmental MASSAGE techniques to build your baby's natural flexibility and strength.
- Your baby will lead the way, showing you when he is keen to try sitting, rolling, crawling and standing. These milestones are covered in the following pages.

Sequence of physical development

All babies learn basic motor skills in a similar sequence, but the age at which your baby masters each skill depends on genetics and environment. There is wide variation between babies, just as there is with the rate of growth. Some babies are ahead of the average in one area but not another. For example, one baby may never crawl yet may walk at 12 months. Another may be crawling by six months and not walk until 16 months. Babies usually learn in spurts and can master a skill in days: wobbly attempts

to sit on Monday are replaced by confident sitting on Friday, for example.

Is my baby on track?

Many parents are tempted to compare their baby to others, or are drawn into this in conversations at the local baby group, supermarket or health centre. ('Is she sitting yet? When did yours roll over? How many hours does he sleep at night?') Although curiosity and a degree of anxiety are natural, try not to take the timing of your baby's developmental stepping stones too seriously. Early achievement is not an indication of greater intelligence or co-ordination, nor of better parenting. Some babies walk early; others have a different emphasis, such as talking. There is no need to worry about delays unless your baby is months behind, in which case your GP or health visitor will help you determine the cause of any problems.

The following entries give a brief overview of developmental areas. Your health visitor or doctor can give more precise guidance in the light of your baby's unique circumstances.

BODY

Babies are rarely still. In the womb, they roll and turn, hiccup, stretch their arms and legs and move their tongue, lips and eyes. They push and press on the walls around them and bring their hands to their mouth as they explore. After birth, they continue to move, even in their sleep.

Most early movement is involuntary or is spurred by a reflex to move towards a source of love and protection, or away from danger. And every movement informs future development. The slightest twitch strengthens muscles and helps them process information. Inside a baby's head, the brain fires, linking cells, and a baby learns, unconsciously, to connect sensory experiences with conscious bodily awareness, and to co-ordinate and then consciously control movements. This learning begins in the womb and continues apace after birth. As each day passes, your baby develops and adapts to the environment, and there is a general rule: use it or lose it (page 274). The bodily structure and function that develop in your baby's earliest months provide a foundation for childhood and beyond.

Physical growth and progressive control

At birth, all your baby's muscle fibres are in place, but muscles take time to thicken, strengthen and move when instructed by the brain. In the same way, the skeletal structure is present but takes time to change from cartilage to bone, a process that continues into early adulthood.

Your baby is curled up in the womb and uncurls the spine from head and neck downwards after birth. This may occur very gradually. Your baby opens his legs and arms from shoulders and hips to fingers and toes. Gentle massage is a lovely way to help this natural process of unfurling from the foetal position.

Muscular control progresses from the top of the body downwards, beginning with the neck, then the upper body and shoulders, then the arms, lower trunk (enabling sitting) and then the legs. Finer (motor) control develops outwards from the centre of the body: your baby can control his arms through swiping before being able to control his hands; his fists before his fingers.

As babies become stronger and more mobile, they follow this natural course of development. You can learn a lot from your baby: how to sit with a straight spine, how to roll over and get up, how to stand with your head held high, and how to relax completely.

Stepping stones in mobility and control

Stepping stones are guidelines – they cannot be spaced precisely as each baby is unique. The sequence, though, is significant as each stage builds on the one before. Some stages may be skipped completely.

In the womb: Babies explore, using their hands, mouth, legs and body. Their movements are reflexive and help build strength and flexibility.

At birth: There is little voluntary control over bodily movements, yet your baby has strong reflexes to suck, to locate your breast, to seek and maintain eye contact, to touch you.

One to four weeks: Early swiping movements are gradually refined and at around three or four weeks babies may reach for things that they see or hear within reach. Babies will enthusiastically exercise their legs and feet by kicking. If actions produce a result, like a bell ringing on a toy, your baby will try it again and again; repetition is part of learning. He may kick in excitement, as a way of saying hello, and when he cries: kicking is an important part of body language.

Six to eight weeks: Babies begin to hold their head up without support. They can lift their head while lying face down on their belly and may confidently push up on their arms.

Three months: By this time, babies can grab an object within reach and learn that they own and can control their hands. Your baby's legs get stronger and he may enjoy being supported in a standing position on your lap and bouncing.

Four months: When supported, babies can sit without their head flopping forwards. In this position your baby may bring his hands together and hold something, and can judge shape and size and prepare the position of his hand to hold an object securely. He may now start to shake things (especially noisy objects), explore them with his mouth, and hold a different object in each hand.

Five months: Babies at this age begin to roll from front to back, and often enjoy touching their toes, and then bringing their feet to their mouth.

Six months: Your baby by now may begin rolling from back to front and may sit with support.

Seven months: Your baby may now sit without support – with a beautifully straight back. Head movements are more pronounced and confident, and affect balance less and less.

Nine months: If your baby is going to crawl, he has probably started by now. This is the foundation for walking. Hand use becomes more refined, with stroking as well as patting, and using a pincer grasp to pick up raisins and beads. This helps with all kinds of experiments, and your baby may now reach many more tempting objects.

Ten to 12 months: By holding onto another's hands, or furniture, your baby may pull up to standing position, and may be eager to walk. Babies begin walking on average anywhere between 10 and 18 months.

Flexibility and strength

When a baby is born he is free, for the first time in months, to uncurl from the foetal position. The process of straightening the spine is gradual. Babies are flexible, with ligaments and joints that are soft and malleable, and this provides a foundation for their growing strength.

It is a rule of nature that form follows function. As your baby grows you play an important role in helping him build strength and balanced posture. Strong beginnings are likely to bring benefits not just in infancy but also years later in adulthood.

- Carrying your baby in a sling or papoose helps him develop strength as it encourages his bones to lay down calcium and become increasingly strong. Ensure that the way you carry your baby suits his head and neck control, dependent on his age.
- Ensuring babies can lie flat on their back gives the best support for the spine. Avoid leaving your baby in a car seat except when driving.
- With gentle MASSAGE you can help your baby strengthen the spine and develop strength in the neck, upper arms and legs.

Tummy time

Giving your baby time on his belly while awake is very important – this will help him develop strength in his spine, as well as his shoulders and upper arms, and the confidence to lift his head. You can begin to do this within days of birth, starting by lying your baby across your legs while you sit, and gradually helping him to straighten his spine and open out his chest.

Bum shuffling

Some babies get around happily by 'bum shuffling'. From a sitting position, they use one or two arms to lift and move from A to B. This can be as fast or faster than crawling. A minority of babies favour bum shuffling over crawling, and some never crawl yet walk without a problem. This is normal and you need not worry: but do ensure your baby gets plenty of playing time on his belly.

Baby walkers and bouncers

Baby walkers and bouncers may seem like a novelty for your baby before he is independently mobile, and the look of delight as your baby moves may be magical. It might also be convenient for you, if you need a 'break' from hands-on entertainment. These items can be fun, but they do not support optimal development. If you wish to use them, limit your baby's time to 15 minutes a day.

■ BRAIN

The increasing sophistication of brain-monitoring tools in the last few decades and the new insights gained in neuroscience as a result have shed a great deal of light on child brain development. A few key points may add to your understanding of the sequence of development and help you support your baby.

Critical period

- Your baby's brain develops at its most intense rate between conception and the first birthday. This is a critical period when nerve cells form and millions of neural network patterns develop. Many persist for life.
- Your baby's brain is genetically primed to help him focus on the people around him, to form bonds and to communicate, and to mimic his parents and other people in his world. Your baby learns from what you do rather than from what you say.
- Your baby's brain is programmed to assist bodily control, and at the same time responds to physical experiments and movement. Babies need practice to fulfil their genetic potential, and each step forward in muscular and joint control is linked with brain development and improved coordination. For instance, if one eye is covered for the first year, the brain misses the opportunity to develop links, and vision in this eye can never be optimal.

Emotional brain

The parts of the brain that are involved in emotional sensitivity are highly developed and fully 'on line' even before birth (page 206). The emotions that arise for any individual baby most often and most strongly determine the perceptions that particular child forms about

273

himself and the world, and the lessons he learns about relationships. In other words, self-image forms very early in life. In the earliest months many of your baby's feelings may arise in relationship with you.

All babies are able to recognise familiar things – sounds, feelings, smells – even before birth, but they do not rationalise. The frontal cortex in the brain matures sufficiently several months after birth to allow a certain degree of prediction and thought. Even after this a baby's emotional feelings remain in the driving seat; in fact, the form and function of the brain ensure that emotions are influential in every thought, feeling and action, throughout life.

Use it or lose it
Your baby's brain has more cells than there are stars in the sky. The early months are critically important because during this time some brain cells connect through being used repeatedly, and others are pruned back through not being used at all. Your baby has the potential to learn just about anything, but he needs experiences to do this. The saying is, 'use it or lose it'.

At birth, babies can hear the subtle distinctions between every language in the world. But by 10 months they have lost the ability to hear tones they have not been exposed to. This process of development ensures your own baby recognises his mother tongue and learns to communicate with his family. This specialisation goes on all the time as your baby adapts to his world.

Plasticity – capacity for change
With growth comes the need for adapting, and within the brain existing connections can be changed, and new connections form when there are new experiences. This is known as 'plasticity'. Even if your baby has had a rocky start, it is useful to know that brain development is an ongoing process: it is never too late to make repair.

Into adulthood
The critical early period of brain development is part of a foundation that informs your baby's view of the world, the way he relates to other people, the way he perceives and values himself,

and his unique fears and passions. This foundation will be built on through life, and will still have an influence when your baby is an adult.

Your own foundation from infancy is with you today, although it is mostly unconscious. Healing early traumas is possible, although this may take considerable time and perhaps intense therapy. Offering your baby strong foundations sets him on a positive journey through life.

◼ GROWTH CHARTS

Growth charts provide a useful tool for you and for the health professionals overseeing your baby's development. Using these in conjunction with measurements of weight, height and head circumference, your baby's growth can be plotted. Any abnormal growth patterns can be easily spotted this way. In the UK, health checks are spaced at increasingly wide intervals, and you will keep the charts in your child's 'parent-held' record book. In the first weeks you may be keen to chart your baby's growth frequently and reassure yourself that all is going well. As your baby gets older, or with your second or third child, providing he appears to be healthy and well, you may be less concerned about measurements.

Standards for growth charts

In April 2006, the new World Health Organization (WHO) Child Growth Standards stated that children born anywhere in the world and given the optimum start in life have the potential to develop within the same range of height and weight. Naturally there are individual differences among children, but across large regional and global populations, the average growth is remarkably similar. Differences in children's rates of growth up to the age of five years are influenced most strongly by nutrition, feeding practices, environment and healthcare, rather than by genetics or ethnicity.

The new standards are based on breastfed children being the norm, allowing for varied eating habits as the months pass. In the past, growth charts were based on bottle-fed babies. This shift is very significant as it most closely reflects the natural rate of growth, and offers a realistic guide to parents who breastfeed their children – which is universally recommended as the best feeding option for babies.

Using the charts

There are separate charts for boys and girls, because their average birth weight and rate of growth differ. On both charts, however, the principle is the same. Your health visitor will weigh and measure your baby and help you to record his growth curve.

The lines already marked on every growth chart are called centiles. The central line is the 50th centile, so called because 50 per cent of children fall below this line and 50 per cent above. The top and bottom centiles represent the extremes of height and weight. Small deviations from the fiftieth centile are not a cause for concern. Every baby fluctuates from his average with natural growth spurts and as a result of minor illnesses.

Downward sloping lines

If your baby's measurements join to form a downward sloping curve, this suggests he may not be growing optimally – the term used is failure to thrive (page 559). In over 80 per cent of babies, a downward trend is temporary, yet it is best to consult your health visitor or your doctor to check your baby's wellbeing. Your health visitor will advise you. Rarely, a physical illness needs treatment.

Upward sloping lines

Lines that slope upwards and cross the centiles usually indicate catch-up growth. This is common among pre-term or low-birth-weight babies, and if your baby is recovering after a short period of weight loss. More rarely, it may happen after treating an illness. If a baby's weight for height or length is 50 per cent more then expected this may be because of overfeeding: early weight gain is now recognised as the first indicator for obesity in early childhood.

Prematurity

If a baby is born prematurely, the weight will be first plotted at the week of birth rather than at '0'. For instance, if your baby is born at 36 weeks, birth is plotted at Week 36. The chart is usually marked in this way until the end of the twelfth month after birth.

Post mature babies

Babies born at 42 to 43 weeks are usually plotted from 40 weeks, as a correction for two weeks makes no difference.

Breastfed or bottle-fed: growth rates

Healthy breastfed babies tend to grow more rapidly than formula-fed infants in the first two to three months after birth, and then less rapidly from three to 12 months. Current growth charts reflect this differentiation and your healthcare worker should have the appropriate charts to hand, depending on whether your baby is bottle-fed or exclusively breastfed, accounting for your baby's age and whether he is eating solids.

Unfortunately, not all healthcare workers are aware of the difference in growth rates between bottle-fed and breastfed babies partly because, prior to 2006, WHO growth charts were based on bottle-fed babies (opposite) who on average weigh more than breastfed babies aged six to 12 months. Occasionally, a healthcare worker may wrongly assume that an exclusively breastfed baby is not gaining weight adequately, basing measurements on an outdated chart, and advise supplemental feeding or, in some cases, recommend a mother stop breastfeeding.

If your healthcare worker raises concern about your breastfed baby's weight gain, but your baby is well and is gaining weight according to the charts reflecting exclusive breastfeeding, there is no cause for concern. If you and your healthcare advisor consult the appropriate charts and your baby's measurements have fallen across two or more percentiles, only then is it appropriate to investigate and alter feeding methods (see page 559).

▦ HEARING

See also Hearing difficulties, baby.

Babies have a finely tuned and fully developed sense of hearing by the time they are born. They have been hearing sounds around them, including the sounds of their mother's heartbeat and voice, since at least Week 15 of pregnancy. They are genetically geared to tune into voices above all else, and they learn about language and tone very early in life. At the end of pregnancy they will already tune into your mother tongue and will associate some sounds with the way they feel. If you are relaxed each time you listen to your favourite music or become excited and energetic when you dance or sing, your baby will feel it too. If you are tense and afraid when someone shouts at you, your baby will feel the effects of your adrenaline. Such responses can become habitual in pregnancy, and shape aspects of a baby's behaviour after birth.

Babies are primed to hear melodic and high-pitched speech, which most adults and children use automatically. This has been called 'motherese'. As your baby watches you speak he connects your facial expressions and body movements with your intonations and the combination helps your baby to learn about the way you feel, and what your words mean. These early lessons inform your baby's understanding about communication in relationships. And it is not all about hearing. Your baby will expect to be part of your conversation. Babies work at a slower pace than adults, and you will often need to allow your baby time to register what he hears, and answer in his own time, in his own way – whether with a look, body movements or his voice.

Although babies are powerfully driven to learn through hearing they also have the ability to shut down (like adults who 'selectively' listen) and may appear not to hear. This may happen when your baby is relaxing, slipping into a meditative state, or has had enough stimulation, is bored, or has shifted his attention to something else.

Stepping stones
In the womb: Babies can hear from at least Week 15, and recognise their mother's voice from Week 32.

At birth: Hearing is fully developed. Providing there are no hearing difficulties, your baby recognises your voice, his mother tongue and familiar music. Babies are inclined to tune into voices above everything else and will be startled by a loud noise, like a door slamming. Babies at birth can locate sounds produced in front of them.

Eight weeks: Hearing has developed sufficiently for a baby to turn to locate the source of noise made to the side.

Five to six months: Your baby can now locate sounds made behind him.

Six months plus: There is a greater focus on language, connecting the shape your mouth makes with the words your baby hears.

▓ SMELL
A baby's sense of smell is far more acute than an adult's. This sense is really important as scents help him to identify where he is and to feel secure with familiar people and objects. It is so strong at birth that your baby is able, if laid on your abdomen, to locate and wriggle up to your nipple. In pregnancy, the watery environment will smell (and taste) different according to what you eat and drink and the hormones in your circulation, and from the moment of birth your baby will know your smell. He may react adversely if you use a new soap or perfume – and in time you will learn which smells upset your baby. You may suggest other people reduce the quantities of their perfume or aftershave!

The nose offers a more direct pathway to the brain than the other sense organs (except for the skin) and smells are thought to be central to emotional reactions and to memory formation. When babies sense a comforting smell (usually mum and dad are favourites) they are likely to settle quickly. Your baby may enjoy sleeping with an item of your clothing in his pram or cot when he is not with you. Later your baby may have a favourite 'security' blanket.

Stepping stones
In the womb: Babies smell the amniotic fluid. At around the sixth month of pregnancy the sense of smell is more acute than at any other time of life.

At birth: The sense of smell is acute. Your baby distinguishes his mother's smell above all others – this is one of the reasons why skin-to-skin contact with mum, and breastfeeding, is usually so pleasant for a baby. Babies quickly become familiar with other people with whom they are often in contact.

Eight weeks: The sense of smell is a key element in survival. It tells your baby whether you have entered the room and lets him know when a stranger is around. Your baby has already formed memories that may be triggered by scents in tens of years.

Five to six months: Exploring objects with his mouth and tongue boosts your baby's learning as the sense of smell and taste are combined with feel, texture and temperature.

SMILING

Babies can smile from birth. There are also suggestions that babies smile in the womb: they have been observed during highly detailed ultrasound scanning. A true broad grin, however, usually begins from around week 4 or 6, and marks a new stage in loving and playful communication between babies and their parents. Your baby will love to see his own smile reflected in your face.

TASTE

The nerve endings around the mouth are some of the most sensitive in the body. In your baby's brain the pathways relating to the tongue, mouth and lips are among the first to develop. The mouth is the first tool for exploration as he sucks his hands in the womb. As he tastes different flavours in the amniotic fluid, some may be accompanied by a physical response. For example, when you eat chocolate, your blood sugar rises and you feel temporarily energised: your baby shares in your reactions. Taste associations continue beyond birth.

At birth, a baby's suckling power is incredibly strong. Over the next few months the tongue gradually separates from the floor of the mouth, growing from the tip and lengthening considerably. The growth allows increasing control over vocal sounds and enables him to use the mouth to explore flavours and textures.

Although there's a general tendency to enjoy sweet flavours (breast milk is sweet), your baby can grow to like bitter or sour flavours. But it's not true that all babies can grow to like all flavours – there is a genetic disposition to like or dislike foods, and your baby's temperament will play a part in his acceptance of food when beginning to eat solids. As with all aspects of development, taste preferences reflect personality, physiology and experiences before and after birth.

Stepping stones

In the womb: A baby's sense of taste is powerful and closely connected to the sense of smell. The 'flavour' of your amniotic fluid changes

according to what you eat and how you feel, and by Week 16 your baby is already able to distinguish sweet and sour.

At birth: Your baby is likely to love the taste of your skin and especially your nipples and your breast milk. The flavour of your milk reflects what you consume and how you feel.

Eight weeks: Your baby's tongue is growing, and lots of muscle exercise from sucking, yawning and grimacing allows him to produce an increasing range of sounds.

Five to six months: With good hand control your baby will bring just about anything to the mouth for a taste. By six months a 'sweet tooth' can be established – perhaps in response to drinking juice from a bottle, which is not advisable for any baby (page 564).

VISION

See also Eye crossing and squinting, baby; Sight problems and blindness, baby.

Babies can see well at birth provided they are looking at something roughly 20cm (8in) away. So while your baby rests in your arms and feeds at your breast, he can see your face in perfect focus. A baby can detect muted colours and will home in on areas of contrast, such as your eyes, eyebrows and lips. Within a day, your baby can recognise you.

Your baby will invite and maintain eye contact (and can repel it) and can 'read' your emotional messages from the expressions on your face. This is due to genetic inheritance. Your baby will also mirror you and any others around. If you stick your tongue out, your baby may try too. As your baby watches you smile, he will practise grinning, too. When you mirror your baby, he will feel good – babies need this mirroring to learn about, and feel good about, themselves.

Babies' eyes soon strengthen, and as eyes and brain develop together they are able to focus at a greater distance, and track moving objects more accurately.

The best 'exercise' for your newborn baby's eyes is to look at exactly what is in front of him – your face. As your baby's vision improves, the world in focus will expand and he will enjoy exploring all the new sights. Babies are particularly attracted to faces, as we are in adulthood, too, and anything that moves or has bold and contrasting patterns. Being with you in nature is perfect for your baby. When you expose your baby to everyday sights and interesting things to focus on you are helping the formation of nerve connections in his brain that are essential for normal vision and visual memories.

By about eight months, babies see almost as well as an adult, providing they have plenty of practice in using their eyes, and there is no developmental delay. If a squint (page 230) persists beyond this time, it is important to get it checked.

Stepping stones
In the womb: Babies open their eyes at around Week 25.

At birth: Your baby focuses perfectly on your face (at a distance of about 20–25cm or 8–10in) when you hold him in your arms, at your breast. Your baby is programmed to explore and recognise your face, and to focus mainly on your eyes. A baby's visual capacity is lower than an adult's.

Eight weeks: Your baby recognises your face, even in a photo or if you wear a hat. Babies can see details so clearly that no two faces look the same to them: even in a line of people from an unfamiliar race (or a line of chimpanzees), faces that may seem indistinguishable to you are distinct to a baby.

Ten weeks: Your baby's two eyes begin to work together, and he is better able to follow the movement of his hands.

Five to six months: A baby of this age can predict the movement of objects. He can judge texture, size and shape from what he sees.

Six months: A baby of this age can scan the entire room while sitting up proudly. He can detect distance and tries to point to objects that are out of reach, instead of apparently swiping at them. Visual capacity, especially depth perception, and visual experience are growing quickly. Peripheral vision is still relatively poorly developed, so keep approaching your baby from the front and continue to place toys in front of him.

Nine months plus: Your baby can now no longer distinguish between similar faces of an unfamiliar race as he has adapted to distinguish most keenly between faces of familiar race(s). Vision continues to mature, and focal range and muscular control continue to develop.

Guilt

See Emotions, guilt.

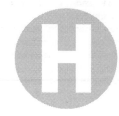

Haemoglobinopathy screening

See Blood screening, baby.

Haemorrhoids

See Piles (haemorrhoids) and anal fissure.

Hair pulling

See Behaviour, baby, difficult.

Hair, during and after pregnancy

During pregnancy the condition of your hair may change, probably exaggerating your normal state (greasy or dry). Your hair may darken, and its growth may slow down, but baldness is not a result of pregnancy. After birth or perhaps when you stop breastfeeding your hair may thin and more than usual may fall out when you brush or wash it. This is because growth slows during pregnancy; when the follicles resume growth, new hair develops from the roots and old hair comes out. Provided that you are adequately nourished with vitamins, minerals and iron, your hair will return to normal within a few months. If you wish to colour your hair, see page 469 for safety tips.

Homeopathy for hair loss

If you have continuing hair loss after childbirth, it is advisable to seek good, ongoing constitutional treatment. In the short term, the following remedies may assist. You may try the most indicated remedy in 6c potency, morning and evening for two weeks, and re-assess. If there is little improvement, please consult your homeopath.

- *Sepia* if hair loss is accompanied by recurrent headaches and heightened sensitivity at the roots of the hair; you may feel generally exhausted, over-sensitive, irritable and easily offended, although you feel better for exercising.
- *Lycopodium* when hair feels brittle and dry or there is premature greying of hair after childbirth; you may find yourself feeling generally anxious, forgetful, moody and irritable on waking.
- *Natrum Mur* if you are anaemic or where you suffer hair loss after a bereavement; your scalp may feel dry and flaky; you may find yourself wanting time on your own and feel better in fresh air.

Hand pain and carpal tunnel syndrome

See also Pain, mother.

During pregnancy, body fluid increases significantly and this can commonly cause slightly puffy fingers. If your fingers feel numb, your tissues may be retaining fluid and your finger joints may ache. This happens to roughly

5 per cent of women. When fluid is retained in the carpal tunnel, which is made up of bone and ligaments in the wrist, this puts pressure on the median nerve, often leading to numbness, pins and needles and pain in the thumb, index and middle fingers. Sometimes pain radiates up the arm. When there is general swelling, all the fingers may hurt. Symptoms are often worse in late pregnancy and, because fluid collects throughout the day, at night.

Action plan

- If your sleep is disturbed, your doctor may suggest wearing a wrist splint to relieve pressure on the nerve. Try sleeping with your hands raised on a pillow.
- You could try massaging your wrists, concentrating on the front of the joint near the hand.
- You can gently stretch your ligament to encourage fluid to dissipate: kneel with the palms of your hands on the floor and your fingers pointing towards your knees (wrists facing away from you) and keep your elbows straight. Slowly move your knees back until you can feel a stretch in the wrists. Repeat three to four times a day, including last thing at night.
- The advice for SWELLING contains tips for reducing fluid retention.
- When the syndrome is bad, you may be offered mild painkillers in the form of non-steroidal anti-inflammatory drugs (NSAIDs). These are usually only necessary in late pregnancy. (See page 408.)
- This condition normally resolves after delivery but very occasionally simple surgery is needed to release the ligament on the front of the carpal tunnel.

Homeopathy

One of the remedies below may be taken in 30c potency, three times per day for one week; then re-assess the situation.
- *Ruta* for sore, aching pain when the affected area feels stiff and bruised, worse on first moving and better with warmth and by rubbing the area.
- *Calc Carb* if you have tingling and numbness in your fingers, swelling in your wrist and pain from elbow to wrist, usually on the right side, worse from grasping an object.

- *Rhus Tox* if you have a tearing pain, stiffness and your hand and wrist, feel hot and better from continual gentle motion, worse in the morning and in damp weather.
- *Causticum* when the finger tips, first finger and thumb are most affected with a raw, tearing pain with tingling, numbness and stiffness that is better from warmth and wet, damp weather.

Hand, foot and mouth disease

Hand, foot and mouth disease (HFMD) is a common illness in children, characterised by fever, sores in the mouth, and a rash with blisters. It is caused by the virus coxsackie A16. HFMD is often confused with foot-and-mouth disease of cattle. Although the names are similar, the two diseases are not related and are caused by different viruses.

The risk of infection is higher for pregnant women who do not have antibodies from earlier exposures and who have close contact with young children. If you are infected in pregnancy, the evidence suggests there is no risk to your baby. The only small risk to your baby arises if you are infected shortly before birth. Usually the impact is not serious. Most infected newborns have a mild and self-limiting illness, but, in rare cases, they may develop an overwhelming infection within two weeks of birth.

What happens

The onset of HFMD tends to begin between three and seven days following infection with the baby feeling sick or off colour, often with a sore throat, a poor appetite and mild fever. One or two days after the fever begins, painful sores develop in the mouth, usually on the tongue and gums and inside the cheeks. They begin as small red spots that blister and often become ulcers. Over one or two days, a skin rash may develop with flat or raised red spots, some with blisters. The rash does not itch, and it is usually located on the palms of the hands and soles of the feet. It may also appear on the buttocks. A person with HFMD may have only the rash or the mouth ulcers.

Action plan

The virus causing HFMD is common and prolific, and the chances are that you are already immune. You can take preventive measures by following good hygiene practices, particularly if you are in close contact with babies and children.

A blood sample can be tested for the most common of the coxsackie viruses including A16. There is no effective treatment other than general care to make your baby comfortable until the illness passes. The disease is usually a short, self-limiting illness, even in babies, thus testing is not usually necessary.

Hayfever

See Allergy and intolerance.

Head and head shapes

Nature prepares your baby for the pressures of birth by ensuring the skull bones can easily slide over one another. As a consequence, the head may mould into an alarming shape. The moulding will smooth out within a few days, but two areas known as fontanelles remain soft for longer. They are a part of the skull structure, enabling it to expand as the brain enlarges. The average head circumference of a newborn is about 32cm (13in).

Each fontanelle consists of a sheet of tough fibrous material that bridges the gap between the growing bones. This area is no more sensitive than any other area of the skull and is immensely strong. When your baby is quiet you may be able to see or feel his pulse here. The posterior (back) fontanelle marks where the skull bones at the back of the head join. It cannot usually be felt beyond the fourth month, although being unable to feel the posterior fontanelle before this is not abnormal, nor is it uncommon. Very rarely, the posterior fontanelle may be closed, when the bones have fused too early, usually before the third month. This is usually linked with an unusually shaped or small head. The larger fontanelle at the front of the head (the anterior – 'front' – fontanelle) remains obvious until it

closes at around 18 months. Early or late closure of the anterior fontanelle is not usually a cause for concern.

The fontanelles do rise and fall with normal breathing, and this is of no concern. If they appear sunken, accompanied by a dry mouth and perhaps sunken eyes, this may be a sign of dehydration (page 182). If they appear to bulge it may indicate MENINGITIS or hydrocephalus, when there is swelling within the brain (see below). If your baby's fontanelles appear shrunken or swollen, visit your doctor.

■ FLATTENED HEAD (PLAGIOCEPHALY)

If your baby's head appears flattened on one side behind the ear, this is most likely due to his sleeping position as he habitually turns his head to one side. He may have a bald patch on the favoured side. You could alter your baby's head position from night to night to cure this. Otherwise, it will right itself when your baby begins to sit. Typically, flattening improves at around four to eight months, and is usually gone by 2–2½ years of age. Recently a range of helmets has been offered (at a cost), with the claim that they speed up what is a naturally occurring healing process, but their usefulness is highly questionable. The flattening is likely to disappear naturally, and you can help your baby by ensuring he has lots of playtime on his tummy and is carried in a sling by you or other adults. Some professionals suggest that flattening may arise when babies are left lying on their backs, or sitting in a car seat or rocker chair for excessive amounts of time. This is referred to as 'positional plagiocephaly'.

Rarely, a flattened head may be a sign of WRY NECK, where there is tightness or tearing in one of the strap muscles. This can be treated with physiotherapy or OSTEOPATHY.

■ HYDROCEPHALUS

The term hydrocephalus comes from two Greek words meaning 'water in the head'. It affects one in 6,000 babies in the UK. The 'water' is cerebrospinal fluid (CSF) that does not drain away as usual. Because it is constantly produced but cannot get out, CSF accumulates, causing raised pressure, the brain tissue stretches and is squashed, and the head gets larger. The effects of hydrocephalus include pressure on the eyes that may lead to a squint or impaired vision, and symptoms related to raised intracranial pressure, such as VOMITING, drowsiness, FITS and failure to thrive (page 559). Later in childhood, there may be effects on concentration, memory or co-ordination.

PREMATURE BIRTH is the most common cause of hydrocephalus because there is a higher risk of BLEEDING into the brain, which may block the absorption system. Before birth, a CONGENITAL ABNORMALITY such as SPINA BIFIDA or infection with TOXOPLASMOSIS may be a cause. Meningitis after birth may also cause inflammation that blocks the CSF pathways. Cysts and tumours are extremely unusual causes.

Action plan

Hydrocephalus may be diagnosed in pregnancy by ultrasound scan. After birth, every baby has a head measurement to check for an unusually large head. Early diagnosis allows treatment to begin soon, and improve the outcome.

- Hydrocephalus is usually treated with an operation that allows the CSF to drain, via a shunt, into the bloodstream. Occasionally a shunt may be put in place using amniocentesis during pregnancy and will be replaced with a permanent shunt after birth. More recent techniques for making an opening in the skull instead of using a shunt are suitable for some types of hydrocephalus.
- Most children with hydrocephalus are educated in mainstream education – sometimes with extra help if they have learning difficulties. If the treatment is working effectively, the prospects are good. The system of shunting has been used since the 1960s and many adults have grown up with shunts without complications.

▓ LARGE HEAD (MEGANCEPHALY)

A larger-than-normal head (megancephaly) is usually noticed at the six-week check. It is rarely a cause for concern, and often runs in families, so it is useful to check a parent's head circumference. It can prompt further investigation, however, due to confusion with hydrocephalus.

▓ SMALL HEAD (MICROCEPHALY)

About 40 per cent of babies whose heads are small for age and gender have no abnormalities related to development. However, in some 60 per cent of cases the head size relates to an abnormally small brain and there are associated learning difficulties, perhaps also a high-pitched cry, poor feeding, fits, or stiffness of the limb muscles (page 126).

A small brain is usually caused by early failure of brain growth in pregnancy due to chromosomal abnormalities, infection, recreational DRUGS or excess alcohol intake. After the birth, microcephaly may occur as a result of severe FOETAL DISTRESS AND ASPHYXIA with brain injury, infection, or an underactive thyroid gland. Close follow-up is usual, but the extent of the problem is usually not evident for seven to nine years.

Microcephaly may be associated with fusion of the skull bones earlier than the usual fifth or sixth month after birth. Early fusion can restrict space for the brain to grow and may make the head look small or oddly shaped, depending on which skull bones fuse. Sometimes surgery may be needed to prevent damage to the developing brain.

Head banging

See Behaviour, baby, difficult.

Head pain, mother

Headaches are common during and after pregnancy. The most likely cause is tension due to changes in muscles and ligaments. There are also less common but potentially serious causes, so it is important to call your doctor if you have a sudden or intense headache.

What happens

Everyday causes

- Tension headaches are due to changes in muscles and ligaments and usually involve the brow, often worse on one side, sometimes radiating to one eye. Tension headaches are

+ Red flag

Serious causes

- An intense headache may indicate high blood pressure and severe pre-eclampsia (page 68), particularly if it is associated with visual changes, swelling in your legs and upper abdominal discomfort. In rare instances, pre-eclampsia can lead to eclampsia itself, involving seizures (fits) and is extremely dangerous. Prompt treatment can prevent this.
- Very rare but acute problems involving bleeding or blood clots in the brain can cause headache. Severe pain that comes on suddenly and is associated with vomiting or muscle weakness warrants a full neurological examination.

more common in women with backache. They often stem from poor posture.

- Conditions unrelated to pregnancy may cause the problem. Tooth pain and sinusitis are examples that can be treated.
- Pain or imbalance in your back (page 43) may cause head pain.
- Tiredness and anxiety are common causes.
- Not eating well, such as consuming insufficient nutrients, and/or an excess of caffeine or sugar, can contribute. Each woman reacts in her own way to food components.
- Persistent headache may be related to ALLERGY and is often linked to smoking.

Migraine

- Migraine may occur for the first time in pregnancy but is more likely if you have had it before. It may be associated with other symptoms including visual disturbances and VOMITING. This may also signal pre-eclampsia (page 68) so it is important to have your BLOOD PRESSURE checked.
- Migraines are often reduced by avoiding triggers such as stress, hypoglycaemia (page 261) and allergenic substances (page 15).

After birth

- Headaches in the early weeks and months are often due to tiredness or stress, and to the way you hold your baby. They may reflect dehydration too if you are not drinking enough fluids.
- A spinal or epidural anaesthetic might lead to an alteration in the cerebrospinal fluid pressure, giving a 'low pressure headache' that usually disappears within five days. It is most effectively treated by resting flat in bed (page 385).

Action plan

If a headache is new or severe, a full examination is needed to exclude pre-eclampsia and rare causes. For a moderate headache, you may find relief by caring for yourself, resting, and maintaining good posture. Much of the advice on reducing back pain (page 44) also helps to relieve headaches.

Pregnancy and the few weeks following the birth are excellent times to focus on releasing tension in your muscles and improving your strength and posture. You may also need to tend to anxieties. Feeling emotionally at peace is a great step towards reducing headaches.

It may be possible to alter an underlying tension pattern through:

- rest and having help with caring for your baby,
- adopting good posture (page 451) when lifting your baby and baby equipment,
- YOGA or OSTEOPATHY, and
- a balanced diet, avoiding sugar highs and lows and consuming plenty of water.

If your headache is related to another medical condition, treating that cause will often relieve the headache.

Homeopathy

Prescribing homeopathic remedies for headaches can be tricky, as the symptoms have to closely match the right remedy. It's best, then, to seek advice. Try to describe the symptoms specifically. For example, describe the type of headache (splitting, throbbing, and so on), where it is situated and what – if anything – makes it worse or better.

For acute headaches, one of the following may suit you. The recommended dosage is 30c

283

potency, three times a day for two days; then re-assess. This is by no means a comprehensive list and you may want to consult your homeopath for advice.

- *Bryonia* for a bursting, crushing, severe headache that often settles above one eye or travels down to the neck. It is worse for any movement, particularly stooping. There's a desire to apply firm pressure to the pain and to keep as still as possible. This is a very useful remedy for a sinus headache or a headache brought on by mild dehydration.
- *Gelsemium* for a congestion-type headache that gives the sensation of having a tight band around the head or over the eyes. Pain tends to move from the back of the head forwards, you feel heavy-lidded, often dizzy and exhausted and may have flu-type symptoms with muscle pains in your neck and shoulders.
- *Sepia* for headaches with shooting pains that often settle over one eye (usually left), that can come on because you skip meals. You feel heavy-headed, exhausted and worn out. It may be accompanied by nausea and dizziness or backache, and improves for fresh air or some form of exercise.
- *Nat Mur* when your head is being hammered with pain settling on the top of your head or over your eyes. It is worse from coughing, moving your eyes or direct sunlight, and better when you are alone, quiet and in the fresh air.
- *Nux Vomica* for headaches that follow over-indulgence of food or drink or a period of stress and loss of sleep, that give a dull pressure headache, often with nausea, and make you extremely irritable and sensitive to noise and light.

Healing

Healing means, literally, 'to make whole'. For thousands of years healing has been acknowledged as a powerful gift. It is becoming more popular across the globe and may be used for relaxation, as part of an adjunct to medical care for relieving symptoms or treating problems, and to restore emotional balance and lift vitality.

Each healer has a unique set of skills and sensitivities that allows them to pick up information about another person, and deduce where healing may be needed. Most healers sense energy flow within the body, and may also tune into energetic fields around the body (which include magnetism, cell vibration and auras). Others tune into bodily rhythms (including breathing, circulation and heartbeat), and some connect at a deep spiritual level.

Healers have an ability to channel energy. They focus on restoring balance. Healers may use guided VISUALISATION, deep breathing, MASSAGE or go into a meditative space and practise without touching or talking. This may be very useful if you have experienced physical or emotional trauma in the past.

During healing, as your energy changes, your body reacts with warmth, altered metabolism and reduced tension. As the impact goes through you, there may be a change in your circulation, hormonal balance and cell vibration. You may experience new sensations, including intense emotions, memories, smells, colours and pulsing vitality. After healing, most people feel relaxed, as if body, mind and spirit are in harmony. Many people say that the impact may take hours, days or weeks, as the deep inner-body shift and a change in energy become apparent.

Some healers offer house healing. You may be interested in this if you are moving into a new house, or if there are areas of your house that feel uncomfortable.

Health checks after birth, mother and baby

See also Caring for baby; Labour and birth, mother, your 'bodymind' after birth; Vaccinations.

■ IN HOSPITAL

If you are in hospital, midwives may be on hand to talk to and advise you, help you and your baby get used to breastfeeding, and give you assistance if you need it. They may guide you as you bathe your baby for the first time. You may be visited by a physiotherapist who will talk to you about caring for your pelvic floor and regaining pelvic floor tone and control. Before you are discharged, a paediatrician or a specially trained midwife will give your baby a standard postnatal check (see below).

When you are discharged depends on hospital policy, the birth, your baby's health and your personal feelings. How much support you have at home will influence your decision. If special care is required by you or your baby, the nature of care and the date of discharge will depend on your individual situation.

Baby checks

All babies born in the UK are routinely offered a full examination within 72 hours of birth (page 337). The findings will be documented in your baby's notes, or in your postnatal care plan. Soon after, your health visitor will give you a personal 'child health record'.

It is normal for baby clinics to give mums information about the routine VACCINATION programme in the first two to eight weeks. Your baby is also offered a developmental and physical check, usually by your GP, but sometimes from a health visitor, to assess early development, such as social smiling, and visual following and fixing. Your baby may have been given an electronic neonatal hearing screening test (page 288), although this can be carried out successfully up to three months of age.

▓ AT HOME

In the UK, all families have access to a general practice where a health visitor oversees routine care for babies, with the support of one or more GPs (doctors trained in general practice with a focus on family care).

A midwife will visit you and your baby for 14 days after birth (often excluding weekends), and if you or your baby require extra help or have any concerns you may be visited more frequently. She will check your baby's wellbeing and ensure her umbilical cord is healing well (page 529). She will help you both with feeding and check your postnatal recovery. Most mums appreciate the company and find it helpful to ask questions about feeding, sleeping and other aspects of care.

Some time in the first 14 days you may have a visit from your GP. Your health visitor will come round as well. She is trained to support families and may offer advice and a listening ear for years to come. Although she makes just one statutory visit (at 11 or 14 days) she'll leave a phone number so you can contact her if you have any concerns. The health visitor will arrange a heel prick blood spot test on your baby (page 338) six to eight days after the birth. This is a tiny prick in the heel and a squeeze to collect blood which will be tested for thyroid activity (page 512), phenylketonuria (page 439) and a group of disorders known as haemoglobinopathies (page 72). The blood may be tested for other diseases, depending on where you live. It is important that feeding has been established by the time the test is done, so do tell your health visitor if feeding is a problem.

Your midwives and health visitors are there to:

* give you information to help you make informed decisions;
* give you advice, including tips on staying well, caring for your baby, and minimising risks of SIDS (page 503);
* listen to your concerns;
* encourage and support you;
* check your baby's wellbeing;
* assess the healing of your baby's cord stump;
* weigh your baby;
* check your physical and emotional wellbeing;
* assess your postnatal healing, including any tears or vaginal stitches and the contraction of your uterus; and
* support you to breastfeed.

Your emotional health is one of the strongest influences on both your and your baby's physical health, and it is important therefore to tell your midwife, health visitor or doctor if you are concerned about your mood or EMOTIONS. Many women enjoy being able to talk to a friendly – and often familiar – midwife about their labour and their feelings as they adapt to parenting. This is an important part of your recovery.

Many health visitors focus care on first-time mums and vulnerable families. If you are not visited by your health visitor frequently, you may still get in contact, usually through your surgery.

Concerned?

If you have concerns about your health or about your baby's wellbeing it is best to contact your health visitor or GP. In an emergency your hospital will provide backup.

Parents' concerns about their babies' health in the first six weeks are usually related to relatively straightforward issues, typically whether feeding, sleeping and CRYING patterns are normal. Common problems arising in the early weeks that are usually easy to address include rashes, particularly nappy rash (page 418), and THRUSH, CONSTIPATION (especially in bottle-fed babies), reflux (page 554) and COLIC. Issues such as FEVER, DIARRHOEA and VOMITING will need your doctor's help and advice, and sometimes specialist advice, too.

■ AT THE HEALTH CENTRE

You will be invited for regular checks until your child is five years old. In most areas, routine checks are recommended at standard vaccination times (page 538): months two, three and four, and then at nine months, 18 months and 21 months. Some health visitors carry out pre-school weight checks, due to the rise in childhood obesity.

Your health visitor will weigh and measure your baby and chart her growth, do tests to check her development (such as vision and hearing), and talk to you about nutrition and vaccinations, and anything else you wish to discuss. In most general practices, a doctor is available for consultation at each regular check-up.

The six-week check

You will be offered an examination either in your GP's surgery or in the hospital six weeks after the birth. The doctor will ask you how everything has progressed for you and your baby. You may also discuss contraception (page 154). You will be offered an examination that may include a vaginal check. If you have had a CAESAREAN SECTION your scar will be checked. Many doctors offer a cervical smear at this visit but it is better (because of accuracy of result) to wait until your menstrual cycle recommences.

After one year

You will be visited by your health visitor a year after your baby's birth for a general check-up. This is mainly to listen to any concerns you may have, and to assess how you're doing. Part of the assessment includes asking a list of questions (the Edinburgh Depression Scale) intended to assess your state of mind and your risk of postnatal DEPRESSION. It really is worth answering honestly. Many mums feel guilty or somehow at fault if some of the answers are not positive (such as 'I am not happy, most of the time', or 'I feel anxious a lot'). But if you are finding parenthood difficult, being honest with your health visitor may be a good first step towards feeling supported and enjoying parenthood more. At present there is no similar questionnaire, nor a routine visit, aimed at fathers.

Non-routine tests and special care

Health checks for your baby begin with the first antenatal scan. If this or later scans detect an issue that needs attention after birth, or you or your partner have family or genetic conditions that may be significant, further tests may be recommended. Please turn to the relevant entries for more information. If your baby requires special care, health checks are likely to be more frequent and specialised according to her needs. There is further information from page 497.

Hearing difficulties, baby

If your baby appears to have difficulty hearing, or hears nothing at all, it might be comforting to know there are three types of hearing loss, and deafness may be temporary. For most babies, the problem is a conductive hearing loss, caused by wax blockage or glue ear (page 198), that improves with treatment. If your baby's hearing loss is permanent you can then consider the best course of action and get support. The sooner you do this, the greater her chance of developing language and communication skills at a similar rate as hearing children. About one in 1,000 babies born in the UK each year is deaf.

Signs of hearing difficulties

- In the first days and weeks a baby with hearing difficulties will not startle, blink or open her eyes in response to a sudden sound.
- At one month she won't stay still to listen if you make a sudden, continuous sound.
- At three months an affected baby doesn't calm down as your voice quietens.
- At six months she will not turn towards the sound of your voice when you are across the room or when you make a quiet noise to one side of her head.
- At nine months normal babbling will not have begun, nor will the baby look towards the source of a sound that is made by something she cannot see.
- At 12 months there will be no response when her name is called.
- As time goes on, you may notice your toddler is late learning to speak, shouts and is inattentive, especially at story time. She may not respond to music, may give inappropriate answers to questions and have difficulty distinguishing between similar-sounding words, particularly when the words begin with f, sh or s. She may turn her head to favour one ear when listening.

What happens

Conductive hearing loss
This reflects a problem with the middle ear and includes temporary hearing loss caused by ear infections such as glue ear, colds and ALLERGIES. It is usually mild but can delay understanding and language development if the underlying cause is not treated.

Sensory hearing loss
This is also called central hearing loss. It occurs when there is malfunction of the inner ear or damage to the auditory nerve or the auditory centres of the brain. This problem can be genetic, or may be caused by an infection contracted by the mother while the baby is in the womb, such as RUBELLA or LISTERIA, or after the birth, such as MENINGITIS. When the nerve is damaged, hearing loss may be permanent. Premature babies and those who have severe asphyxia (page 249) at birth may also suffer deafness.

Action plan

All newborns are now screened with tests that detect problems early on (page 288). If your baby has hearing difficulties one of the following approaches may be recommended:

- If deafness is caused by glue ear arising from an infection, the problem may resolve without treatment (it often does). Otherwise a simple operation to fit a grommet can correct your child's hearing (page 198).
- If your baby's hearing difficulties may be helped by a hearing aid, you will need to visit a specialist. Hearing aids work by amplifying sounds and can be used from as early as six weeks.
- If your child is given a hearing aid and this does not help, a cochlear implant into the ear may be considered. This is an electronic device that turns sounds into tiny electrical pulses, and, without needing to use the middle or inner ear structures that do not work properly, sends the signals directly to the hearing centres in the brain. Cochlear implants improve hearing but cannot yet restore hearing to normal. A cochlear implant needs to be fitted with a surgical operation.

If your child is deaf

As soon as you know that your child is deaf you can begin to communicate without using sounds. If you have no experience of deafness this will be a challenge but your role is integral to your baby's learning and development. It is best to seek support and find out as much as you can, as soon as possible. You may need emotional support, advice and training as you learn to communicate by signing, which can enrich communication from a very early age, and as your baby learns to lip-read.

What happens once your child's hearing difficulty has been diagnosed depends on the degree of hearing loss. You will be given extensive support from the medical team and your local education service will probably arrange for you to be in contact with a visiting teacher of the deaf. You may find national support groups for the deaf have valuable information and can put you in touch with other parents of deaf children.

Many parents emphasise that communication without sound can never begin too early – babies have an inexhaustible capacity for expression and understanding, and facial expression, eye contact and touch are all part of communication.

Hearing screening and tests, baby

All newborn babies are offered a hearing test as part of the Newborn Hearing Screening Programme (NHSP). Your baby will be tested either before you are discharged from hospital, or afterwards during a visit from your health visitor. At the time of writing (2007), the standards are for all babies to be fully screened by the age of three months.

The benefit of this early screening to detect full or partial hearing loss is that any child who cannot hear well can be lovingly supported. Without others' awareness of its hearing difficulties, many babies can feel disorientated, ignored and frustrated, and parents and carers may worry about the child's intelligence or ability to engage in conversation. This can hinder bonding and the baby may find it difficult to trust and fully engage with the world around her. Awareness of a hearing difficulty early on allows an appropriate intervention plan to begin (page 287) to help your baby enjoy conversations and build relationships, and develop self-esteem.

Screening (Oto-acoustic emission / OAE and AABR screening)

The most commonly used screening test is the Oto-acoustic emission (OAE) screen. This involves placing a small soft-tipped ear-piece in the outer part of your baby's ear and playing quiet clicking sounds. The cochlear in the ear produces sounds in response to the clicks and these are recorded and analysed by the computerised screening system. It usually takes a few minutes and can be done at the bedside when your baby is asleep. However, it is not always possible to get a clear response, particularly in the first 24 hours after birth. In this case, you may be offered the AABR screen.

The automated auditory brainstem response (AABR) screen involves placing small sensors on your baby's head and neck and then presenting quiet clicking sounds through tiny soft headphones. A computer analyses the responses to sounds beyond the cochlear.

Heart defects, baby

Around eight in 1,000 babies have a heart that has not formed correctly. For many the defect is not serious. Symptoms may not show until weeks or months after birth, and sometimes a defect may not become apparent until adulthood. Some of the heart abnormalities may cause breathing and circulation problems, which may begin early after birth. Increasingly, an abnormality may be detected in the womb by means of an ultrasound scan.

It is good to know that with increasingly sophisticated surgical skills many conditions can now be treated – either by complete correction, or by reconstruction of the heart, and ultimately with a heart transplant in the rare case where other treatment is unavailable. In some cases, the defect presents few problems or relatively simple surgery is required and the outlook is very good. For other babies a series of operations may be necessary. In up to 1 per cent of babies with a significant heart problem little can be done and the focus is on supporting the baby and parents.

If you receive the news that your baby has a heart problem, your initial response will soon be followed by the need to make practical plans (page 45). The specialists caring for your baby will be able to give you details of your baby's condition, the options for treatment and the long-term outlook.

Causes and symptoms

In a normal heart there are four chambers – the two ventricles and two atria. The left side of the heart receives blood that has passed through the lungs and been oxygenated. The left ventricle sends the blood to the aorta, the main artery to the body, from where it is passed to all the organs. Blood then returns to the right side of the heart through veins, and is pumped from the right ventricle into the pulmonary arteries and on to the lungs where it is oxygenated, and back into the left side and around the body once more. Most defects of the heart reduce normal blood flow between the heart, lungs and body, or cause the blood to flow in an abnormal pattern.

After the birth, a heart defect may cause one or more symptoms. These include:

* breathlessness or rapid, shallow breathing;
* blue appearance;
* a heart murmur (some murmurs may not be a sign of an abnormal heart);
* poor feeding;
* listlessness;
* slow growth and failure to gain weight; or
* susceptibility to respiratory infections, such as pneumonia (page 446).

Causes of heart abnormalities

A baby born with an abnormal heart is said to have a congenital heart defect. In most cases the cause is not known. Rarely, a viral infection in pregnancy, such as rubella, may interfere with heart development. Some chromosomal abnormalities such as DOWN'S SYNDROME can involve the heart. If a mother consumes an excess of alcohol, or recreational drugs such as crack cocaine, this may increase the risk of having a baby with a heart defect.

Action plan

Diagnosing a heart defect

A defect may be suspected during pregnancy through the appearance on the ultrasound. If an antenatal heart defect is suspected you may be referred to a specialist in foetal cardiology. Alternatively, after birth your baby will be referred to a paediatrician who specialises in cardiology. Your baby may be given a chest X-ray and an electrocardiogram (ECG), which monitors electrical activity of the heart, and an ultrasound Doppler echo test that shows the anatomy of the heart and the direction of blood flow, and can indirectly measure the pressures in the heart.

Treatment

Abnormalities that interfere with healthy heart function are numerous. If your baby is diagnosed with a heart condition, specialist care will depend on her exact condition.

The course of action and outlook for recovery and resumption of normal health depend on the type and extent of the abnormality and whether or not surgery is needed. You and your family need to be supported as you absorb the news, live with the difficulty and await the results of tests and operations, and look towards the future. Your medical team will be your first line of help and there are support groups.

With almost all cardiac defects there is a risk of a heart infection during any form of surgical treatment, including some dental work. To reduce this risk, it is important for your baby to take antibiotics after surgical procedures.

■ CYANOTIC HEART DEFECTS (BLUE BABY)

This is an incomplete or incorrect formation of the heart that stops blood from being oxygenated sufficiently before being passed around the body. These conditions account for about 25 per cent of congenital heart disease. The blood contains less oxygen than normal, causing blue discoloration of the skin (cyanosis). The term 'blue babies' is often applied to infants with cyanosis. They require expert surgical and medical care. The outlook depends on the severity of the defect.

Tetralogy of Fallot involves a ventricular septal defect and a narrowing (stenosis) of the pulmonary valve and an abnormal aorta. If the condition is severe, an operation shortly after birth, called a shunt procedure, is required to improve blood flow to the lungs. Most children with Tetralogy of Fallot have their corrective surgery pre-school. Transposition of the great arteries is when the aorta is connected to the right side so most of the blood bypasses the lungs and the pulmonary artery is connected to the left ventricle, so most of the blood returning from the lungs goes back to the lungs again. Babies with this condition are very ill. The long-term outlook depends on the severity of the defects.

Tricuspid atresia is a lack of a tricuspid valve, which means no blood can flow from the right atrium to the lungs for oxygenation unless there is also an abnormal opening in the internal heart walls (a septal defect) to allow the baby to survive. Surgical shunting procedure is needed to increase blood flow to the lungs.

Pulmonary atresia is a lack of the pulmonary artery so blood can't flow to the lungs from the heart. The only source of lung blood flow is the patent ductus arteriosus (overleaf). A surgeon can create a shunt between the aorta and the pulmonary artery to help increase blood flow to the lungs.

▦ HYPOPLASTIC LEFT HEART SYNDROME

This syndrome accounts for fewer than 10 per cent of congenital heart defects. The left side of the heart is underdeveloped and to keep blood oxygenated the heart relies on the patent ductus arteriosus. A baby may seem normal at birth, but when the ductus naturally closes at between days two and four, and at the latest within the first seven days, she will become ashen, have rapid and difficult breathing, often associated with grunting, and also have difficulty feeding. This heart defect is often fatal, either in the first few days, or over the course of the treatments. Modern surgical techniques have improved the outlook, but treatment is complicated and involves two or three serious heart operations in the first few years after birth.

▦ PATENT DUCTUS ARTERIOSUS (PDA)

This is an improper closing of a natural passageway in the heart that allows a baby to draw oxygen from blood flowing through the placenta during pregnancy and bypass the lungs. This passageway normally closes after birth (page 408). PDA accounts for 10 per cent of congenital heart diseases and is more common in premature babies. When the passageway remains open, some blood that should flow to the body returns to the lungs and the rest of the body does not receive enough oxygen. The persistent ductus may close by itself (60 per cent) or require the drug indometacin or surgery.

▦ STENOSIS

This is an obstruction of blood flow in the heart or the veins or arteries connected to it. Pulmonary stenosis involves the valve on the right side of the heart and this may cause cyanosis (blueness) because less blood reaches the lungs. Aortic stenosis is narrowing of the aortic valve leaving the left ventricle – it usually causes no symptoms and remains undetected until adulthood. The aorta itself may be narrowed (coarctation) and less blood flows to the lower part of the body. Symptoms can develop early or not until adulthood. Surgery may be needed if stenosis or coarctation is severe.

▦ VENTRICULAR SEPTAL DEFECT ('HOLE IN THE HEART')

This accounts for 50 per cent of congenital heart disease cases. It is an opening or hole between the chambers of the heart, allowing blood to flow between the heart's right and left chambers, which are normally separated by a muscular wall. Oxygenated blood from the lungs mixes with deoxygenated blood.

Atrial septal defect is an opening between the atria, the two upper chambers, and may cause few symptoms. Ventricular septal defect is an opening between the ventricles, the lower chambers. If small, it doesn't strain the heart but there is a loud murmur. If large, the heart has to over-work to pump extra blood and may enlarge. When this is combined with pulmonary high blood pressure and an abnormal aorta (in Eisenmenger's complex), the condition is very serious and may be fatal if untreated. Atrioventricular canal defect is a particularly large hole in the centre of the heart involving the atria and the ventricles. As a result of its size, it often inhibits normal growth and makes a baby look blue. Many babies with septal defects require surgery.

Heart disease, mother

Heart disease is uncommon in pregnancy. If you are aware of a previous problem, it is best to consult your cardiologist about the effect of the increased load on your heart in pregnancy. A heart problem may be discovered for the first time in pregnancy.

Action plan

You will be advised to eat well and take supplements to prevent anaemia so the load on your heart is minimised. It has to deal with the largest volume in the 12 hours after birth when the placental pool of blood is squeezed into your circulation before the fluid is excreted by your kidneys.

Your doctor may advise rest and frequent visits to review your symptoms and alter drug treatment. If a very irregular heartbeat is adversely affecting the function of your heart, you may be given beta-blocking drugs to regulate the heart rate.

At delivery, you will be asked not to bear down in order to keep the load on your heart to a minimum. Your contractions may provide enough downward force but there is an increased chance your baby will require assistance with forceps or ventouse (page 373). You can have an epidural, but given with care to prevent you being given too little or an excess of fluid, which would increase the volume in circulation and raise the load after birth.

Birth of the placenta will be carefully controlled to ensure you do not lose excess blood because a sudden drop in blood volume may cause shock and compromise your cardiac function. Ergot type drugs are not used to assist this stage as it can raise blood pressure and increase the strain on your heart. Oxytocin alone can be used.

Women with cardiac problems are usually offered antibiotics to cover labour and birth to prevent an infection developing in one of the heart valves.

In the days following birth, your heart will be monitored as the fluid in your circulation returns to normal.

Your baby's heart may be checked with ultrasound by a specialist ultrasonographer performing foetal echocardiography around Weeks 16–20. This check is particularly important if you were born with a heart problem as the condition may run in families. This check helps ensure that the baby's heart is developing normally and it also monitors growth and development. (See also HEART DEFECTS, BABY.)

Heart rhythms and murmurs, baby

See also Heart defects, baby.

Babies often have minor abnormalities of heart rhythm. The most common is a fast heart rate called supra ventricular tachycardia (SVT). This rarely causes serious problems, but can be picked up before birth, and it may lead to emergency delivery as the fast rate is interpreted as foetal distress. A slow heart rate may be caused by drugs given to either baby or mother, such as beta-blockers to control anxiety and blood pressure. Another cause of a slow heart rate in an otherwise normal baby is when the electrical impulse that

governs the heart rate is blocked and unable to make the heart rate change – this is called congenital heart block, and may occur in some babies whose mothers have lupus antibodies. Babies with fast or slow heart rates may require medication after birth, and sometimes a pacemaker is inserted to control the rate.

Heart murmurs are commonly heard in just under 10 per cent of newborn babies. Most arise from the sound of blood flow through the heart and the blood vessels, and are completely innocent. If the murmur is found with other signs of possible heart problems, then further investigations are needed.

Heart rhythms and murmurs, mother

See also Heart disease, mother.

Pregnancy hormones widen your blood vessels, increasing blood volume, and also affect the way your heart responds to this increased fluid load. Initially, your heart copes by increasing the amount of blood pumped out with every heartbeat, but if this is not sufficient your heart rate (and pulse) may also rise. You will probably not notice the different beat unless you are exercising.

■ MURMURS

A murmur may be detected during a routine examination. The most common cause in pregnancy is the sound that the increased blood flow makes as it passes through the valves in your heart. This effect occurs in many women with a normal heart. Occasionally the increased flow during pregnancy brings to light an abnormality of one of the heart valves and the murmur is due to the blood flowing through the abnormal valve.

■ PALPITATIONS

You may experience palpitations, which are fast or irregular heartbeats. They are very common during pregnancy as your heart has to work up to 25 per cent harder to keep the blood circulating around your body. Palpitations usually cease after birth. They are rarely linked with an underlying heart condition.

- Palpitations are more common with TWINS or if you have ANAEMIA or iron and vitamin deficiency.
- If you are very anxious, your heart may beat faster.
- Heart rate may increase if you get hungry or your blood sugar falls: this triggers a release of adrenaline to raise blood sugar, which also increases heart rate.
- If your blood pressure falls when you sit still or stand suddenly ('postural hypotension'), your heart may compensate by beating faster.
- During and after labour you may be aware of palpitations if you become dehydrated. The effect is intensified if you lose blood excessively during the birth. Your midwife will help to keep bleeding to a minimum and provide you with fluids to prevent dehydration.
- An abnormal electrical circuit that transfers the tiny electrical signal for every heart contraction at each beat may lead to palpitations and an irregular beat. This is called an arrhythmia and may require medical treatment. Your doctor will need to arrange for tests to find out the underlying cause.
- Coronary artery disease is very rare.

Action plan

If you are well nourished, including vitamins and minerals, and look after yourself with a balance of exercise and rest, this will encourage good circulation. Be aware that what you eat can affect your blood sugar levels (page 261), with a knock-on effect of adrenaline on your heart. Maintaining stable blood sugar is important. With attention to your posture it is easier to avoid a dip in blood pressure when you stand.

Medical care

If you have frequent palpitations, it is best to see your doctor and request a heart examination. This consists of listening to your heart to detect a murmur, and possibly an electrocardiogram (ECG) to check the regularity of your heartbeat. Although heart disease is rare, your doctor may want to investigate further.

- Your blood may be tested to see if anaemia may be a cause.
- If a murmur is detected, an ultrasound scan will allow your heart valves to be examined. If you

do have an abnormal valve you will be offered antibiotics to prevent infection during the birth.
- If the beat is irregular and symptoms are intense, you may have to wear an ECG monitor for 24 hours to help diagnose the problem.
- If a problem is detected, you may be advised to have further tests to monitor your heart after the birth.

Homeopathy

For palpitations you may use the remedy below that matches your symptom picture in 30c potency three times a day for two days and then re-assess.

- *Aconite* if palpitations occur suddenly, usually after a shock, and are worse at night.
- *Arg Nit* when there is anticipatory anxiety or a sense of being out of control or you're worried about your health.
- *Natrum Mur* when there's a feeling of heat – of being 'hot and bothered' – constriction in the chest and your heartbeat feels as if it is shaking your whole body.

Heartburn and indigestion

See also Bloating and flatulence.

Hormones produced during pregnancy soften muscles and ligaments throughout the body to allow space for your developing baby and to make labour and childbirth easier. However, an unwelcome side effect is that those hormones can also relax the muscles in the valve between the oesophagus and the stomach. This, combined with the pressure that your expanding uterus places on your stomach, may allow stomach acid to flow back up into the oesophagus. This irritates the sensitive lining of the oesophagus, causing indigestion and heartburn.

What happens

Heartburn and indigestion may make you feel:
- Discomfort in the upper abdomen above your belly button.
- A burning feeling extending up into your chest when food and gastric acid reflux back into the oesophagus.

- Bloated.
- A colicky pain when your intestine contracts as your food is digested.
- Excess wind/flatulence, nausea or VOMITING.

Heartburn often becomes more severe in late pregnancy and when you lie down at night. It may also be related to a change in the food you eat and is more likely if you are overweight and have a LARGE BABY or TWINS.

Very occasionally, pregnancy may reveal a hiatus HERNIA, where there is a weakness in the valve between the stomach and the oesophagus, and heartburn is more intense.

Stomach or duodenal ulcers are very uncommon during pregnancy and tend to improve as the pregnancy continues.

Action plan

Food and eating
- It is best to eat a healthy, balanced diet with small meals every three to four hours. Don't rush, and always sit straight to prevent acid reflux.
- Before bedtime, eat a light, slow-burning snack (page 261) such as a rice cake, oat biscuit or raw carrot.
- Avoid alcohol, strong coffee, fizzy drinks, highly refined food, smoking and large, fatty or heavy meals.
- Heartburn may be eased by milk or yoghurt, but for some women these foods cause the stomach to react by producing more acid 30 to 90 minutes later. Light acids such as a fruit tea can reduce acid production. Some people get severe heartburn after eating acidic fruits such as oranges. If you try different foods you should find out what works for you.
- Cut down on the amount you drink with your meal to reduce the volume in your stomach, and maintain your daily fluid intake by having drinks between meals.
- Mint tea is a traditional herbal remedy for heartburn, but choose mild mint rather than peppermint, which may exacerbate indigestion (and avoid minty sweets).
- Iron supplements may cause heartburn. You may find you tolerate an elemental iron preparation taken one hour before a meal.

Lifestyle
- Posture has a significant effect: avoid slouching and remind yourself to sit upright. It is best to avoid sitting on a couch when you watch television or read. A good alternative for you may be to sit on the carpet or a cushion with your back against the couch, or to ensure you have a chair that gives your back necessary support. Regular YOGA or PILATES may help you assume an upright posture with little effort and there are further postural tips on page 451.
- Adjust your sleeping position, perhaps by supporting your upper body with pillows or raising the head of your bed safely.
- Make sure your clothes are not too tight, to reduce pressure on your abdomen.

Medical care
- If your indigestion is severe, it is worthwhile visiting your doctor or midwife for practical tips on reducing discomfort. Heartburn usually settles completely after pregnancy, unless there is an underlying cause such as hiatus hernia.
- There are a variety of over-the-counter antacids available on the market. Most preparations are safe in pregnancy but avoid any with a high sodium or aluminium content. Your pharmacist can advise.
- H2 blockers and proton pump inhibitors reduce gastric acid production. They are usually very effective but you must check with your doctor or pharmacist that they are safe in pregnancy. It is best to avoid them during the first half of pregnancy.

Homeopathy
You may match your symptoms closely to one of the remedy pictures below and take one tablet in 30c potency three times a day for three days and then re-assess.
- *Nux Vomica* if you have an unpleasant, sour, acidic taste in your mouth, feel stressed, uncomfortable around two hours after eating, have a headache, constipation, or nausea, feel the food heavily in your stomach and you feel irritable and chilly.
- *Lycopodium* for an acidic feeling with bloating and lots of rumbling in the abdominal area, burning from the stomach up to the throat, and belching with an acidic taste and indigestion that's worse from eating cabbage,

beans, onions and cold food and drinks and comes with anxiety.

- *Arsenicum* for burning heartburn often accompanied by nausea when you are chilly, restless, and agitated, you feel worse at night, better from sips of warm drinks and being propped up, and you crave company.
- *Pulsatilla* for heartburn and indigestion after a meal of rich or fatty food giving a dry mouth without thirst, weepiness and reduced symptoms after a good cry, company and fresh air. Do not take *Pulsatilla* until Week 13 of pregnancy.
- *Carbo Veg* for heartburn with bloating and shortness of breath, when there is a sensitivity to rich and fatty foods and although you may feel hungry, you feel full after eating very little.

Aromatherapy

Use lemon or ginger oil in the bath, in massage or as a compress. From Week 24 try lemongrass in low dosage and chamomile.

Hepatitis

Hepatitis is infection of the liver that may be caused by a number of different viruses (hepatitis A, B, C, D and E). It is extremely rare for women to be infected in pregnancy. Hepatitis infection in children is uncommon except in areas where the viruses are endemic, for example in the water, or when a child has been exposed to the infection at birth.

Not all people who contract hepatitis have symptoms, and this is particularly true among children. When symptoms appear they typically include pain in the abdomen, dark urine, fever, jaundice with yellowing skin and whites of the eyes, enlarged liver, malaise and tiredness, nausea and vomiting. Less common symptoms include joint pain, diarrhoea or light coloured stools and itchy skin.

Most cases of acute hepatitis lead to recovery within a few weeks. In some cases, however, more commonly when the sufferer is malnourished or has contracted HIV infection, hepatitis can lead to severe illness. Pregnancy does not appear to increase the risk of chronic illness, nor does infection in pregnancy increase the risk of complications for mum or baby.

Infection with hepatitis

- Hepatitis A and E are present in the stools of infected individuals and also spread through water and food that has been contaminated by faecal material and through close personal contact. Hepatitis A can survive for over 12 weeks in water and cases have also been reported of infection from swimming in contaminated water.
- The main transmission of hepatitis B is from mother to child in pregnancy, or through blood and body fluids (injections or sexual transmission).
- Hepatitis C is mainly transmitted by injection or by sexual contact.
- Hepatitis D is only present with hepatitis B.

HEPATITIS A

Hepatitis A is the most common form of hepatitis in children, usually as a mild infection with few symptoms. It is not significant in pregnancy but babies are susceptible in the first nine months. Sometimes an infected child has DIARRHOEA (gastroenteritis). In many developing countries where sanitation is poor, nearly all children have evidence of previous hepatitis A infection.

Rarely, hepatitis A may cause severe illness. Occasionally it relapses months after apparent recovery, but there is no chronic form.

Vaccination for adults is available and effective, and is advisable if you are travelling to an area where the infection is endemic, where you also need to take care about drinking unpurified water and water-based products (such as ice and soft drinks) as well as uncooked food, especially meat and fish. Vaccination is not recommended in pregnancy. Attention to hygiene, particularly if you are changing nappies, is also an important preventive measure. Research is still being conducted on the best method of vaccination for young children.

HEPATITIS B

Hepatitis B is potentially more serious than hepatitis A. Although most people make a full recovery, in 10–15 per cent of cases chronic infection may lead to cirrhosis and, in a small number of cases, liver cancer. This risk does not appear to rise with pregnancy. The risk of developing chronic infection is greatest with a childhood infection. Hepatitis B cannot be passed through breast milk, but the virus may pass through blood if a mother's nipples are cracked and bleeding. There is no risk of transmission through kissing or cuddling.

A blood test can indicate whether you are infected and very highly contagious, have been infected or vaccinated and are no longer susceptible, or have a chronic infection and are a carrier. Risk of transmission to a baby is higher if the mother is a carrier.

Infection in pregnancy

In pregnancy, if blood tests show that you are infectious, it is best to consult a liver specialist regarding your own health. It is advisable for your whole family to be checked and vaccinated if necessary. Your baby can be protected against infection with active and passive immunisation – this has a success rate of 85–95 per cent. Hepatitis B vaccines are composed of inactivated components of virus and do not pose a risk of infection.

* Passive immunisation consists of injecting hepatitis B antibodies (immunoglobulin) within 12 hours of birth. This gives your baby sufficient protection against infection until he develops his own antibodies.
* Active vaccination begins 12 hours after birth and stimulates your baby's immune system to develop its own antibodies. This takes some time so a repeat vaccination is given at one to two months and again at six months. Between 12 and 15 months your baby's blood will be tested to ensure the vaccination has been affective.
* Your baby may react to the vaccination with soreness at the injection site. A few children develop a fever. Severe allergic reactions are rare. Homeopathic remedies can offer support alongside vaccination, and need to be personally prescribed.
* In the very unlikely event that your baby does develop hepatitis B, he is likely to make a full recovery with specialist treatment. However, there is a risk that the infection may become chronic and follow-up may be recommended.

▨ HEPATITIS C

Hepatitis C infection is becoming an increasing health issue, with infection rates of up to 6 per cent world-wide. Infection is most prevalent

among intravenous drug users or people who received infected blood during a transfusion (although from 2007, all blood products are screened for hepatitis C). It can be spread through sexual contact but this is rare. Acute hepatitis C causes no symptoms or only mild fatigue for most people. For 25 per cent of people, though, it causes jaundice (yellowing of the skin) and it is estimated that 25 per cent of all infected people develop liver cirrhosis, with a smaller number developing liver cancer – whether or not they have symptoms of the initial hepatitis infection. The risk of this happening does not appear to increase with pregnancy.

The hepatitis C virus has 80 subtypes. Because of this there is not yet a hepatitis C vaccine. Antibodies to the virus subtypes do not necessarily indicate immunity – they indicate a current or previous infection with hepatitis C.

The risk of passing hepatitis C to your baby is 5 per cent, if your baby is exposed to your blood. This rises to 35 per cent if you are also HIV positive. As with hepatitis B, you cannot pass the infection to your baby through breast milk, but could do if your nipples are cracked or bleeding. You cannot spread the virus by kissing, hugging, sneezing, coughing, sharing eating utensils or drinking glasses, or casual contact, nor is it spread by food or water.

Infection in pregnancy

If you test positive for hepatitis C you may need therapy, although the drugs cannot be used in pregnancy. The usual medication is a combination of interferon and ribavirin, which is effective in 40 to 80 per cent of cases.

If you have developed hepatitis C antibodies, these will be transferred to your baby and will remain in his blood for six weeks to 15 months. Babies can be screened at 15–18 months. If your baby is not infected, no antibodies will be present. Infection in babies is extremely rare. Around one in 25 babies of infected mothers contracts hepatitis C during birth. Most infected babies have no symptoms and do not appear to suffer long-term effects. In the unlikely event that your baby is infected, you will need to see a specialist for advice. There are antiviral treatments that can be used during childhood if necessary.

■ HEPATITIS D

Hepatitis D cannot exist without hepatitis B. There is no treatment or vaccination for hepatitis D, so the best way to prevent it is to avoid infection with hepatitis B. A combination of hepatitis B and D seems to reduce the chance of infection reaching the chronic stage.

■ HEPATITIS E

There is no vaccine against hepatitis E. If you have been infected, the illness usually passes, is mild and does not appear to develop into a chronic form. Prevention relies on stringent hygiene and avoidance of potentially contaminated food and water.

Herbal medicine

Throughout human history and all over the world, people have used local plants to treat ailments and enhance their wellbeing. Herbal medicine is as old as medicine itself. There are many different forms of herbal medicine, and as world-wide communication expands, more varieties of medicinal herbs are becoming available through local suppliers or via the internet.

Some herbal treatments are available in tablet form, while others are taken as tinctures, teas, syrups, lotions or extracts. Although most substances used are from plants, Chinese herbal medicine (opposite) sometimes uses minerals or animal products.

The most straightforward way to harness the power of herbs is to use them in cooking and make them a part of your diet. You will find some advice on nutritious food and herbs in the EATING section, and there are tips for what to eat if you are unwell throughout the A–Z.

By using plants in their complete form, a complex fusion of chemicals can be introduced into the body in a gentle way. Plants have a natural balance and energy and, when prescribing, the constitutions of the plant and the person are equally considered and their 'temperaments' matched. It is relatively simple to make your own infusions (brewing leaves in hot water) or decoctions (boiling, for example, roots and bark) if you have guidance.

However, herbs can be very powerful and although many have great value in pregnancy, not all are safe for use when you are carrying a baby or breastfeeding (below). If you decide to use herbal medicines it is best to visit a registered practitioner.

■ USING HERBS SAFELY

Herbalists stress the importance of using the whole plant, as certain compounds present in the plant may be needed to counteract any toxic constituents. Side effects from herbs are rare and most likely when large doses are consumed. Nevertheless, 'natural' does not necessarily mean 'safe' and particular care should be taken during pregnancy. You should always seek the guidance and expert knowledge of a medical herbalist for conditions that would also warrant an orthodox medical opinion.

- As a general maxim, avoid herbal medicines during the first trimester (three months) unless you have been advised to continue treatment. Teas for nausea, constipation and lethargy are safe.
- Highly concentrated extracts should be avoided throughout pregnancy because the danger of side effects is considerably higher than in preparations that contain the whole plant. Use infusions or decoctions, not tinctures.
- When in doubt, or if worrying symptoms persist, seek the help of an appropriately qualified herbalist or your GP's opinion.
- From conception to the cessation of breastfeeding ensure you only use herbs that are safe. It is always best to avoid herbs known to have a stimulating, or irritating, effect on the body.

Self-medication with herbal medications from the following list is not advised:
- aloes (although external application of the gel is unlikely to cause problems),
- barberry,
- blue cohosh,
- cascara sagrada,
- castor oil,
- celery seed,
- golden seal,
- juniper,
- parsley*,
- pennyroyal,
- pokeroot,

* rue,
* sage*,
* senna,
* southernwood,
* tansy,
* thuja,
* wormwood

* okay to use in cooking

Chinese herbal medicine

Chinese herbs are administered in a combined formula containing anything from three to 15 different herbs. Each one acts to strengthen and enhance each other's properties. Herbs can be used in teas, or as concentrated powders that can be dissolved in water or put into capsules. Although herbs have been used for centuries in China, they have not been subjected to the same degree of scientific testing and surveillance as conventional pharmaceuticals, and many can have powerful effects. It is always best to obtain herbs directly from a registered Chinese herbalist following a consultation.

Hernia, baby

A hernia occurs when a section of intestine protrudes through a weakness in the muscles of the abdominal wall – a soft bulge can be seen beneath the skin. The most common hernias are around the belly button (umbilical) or in the groin (inguinal). Umbilical hernias occur in around 10 per cent of babies, with a higher incidence in Afro-Caribbean children. Inguinal hernias occur in fewer than 3 per cent of babies. Premature babies are at a higher risk of developing a hernia, as are babies with CYSTIC FIBROSIS, or if there are problems with the testicles when descent is delayed or if there is a family history of hernia.

Abdominal hernias are often reducible, which means they can be gently pushed back into the abdominal cavity. When a hernia is not reducible, the loop of intestine may become caught in the weakened area of abdominal muscle. This may lead to the blood supply to the intestine being reduced and obstruction of the intestine itself. If the blood supply to the intestine is completely cut off, in a strangulated hernia,

this is a surgical emergency. Surgery corrects the defect and saves the bowel.

Much more rarely, there may be a defect in the abdominal wall, allowing the abdominal contents to protrude into the diaphragm (congenital diaphragmatic hernia, see below). Also rare, an exomphalos occurs when a defect allows the abdominal contents to protrude in a sac near the belly button (overleaf).

What happens

Hernias are usually apparent in a newborn, particularly when she is crying or straining, although they may not be noticeable until several weeks or months after birth. If you push gently on the bulge when your baby is calm and lying down, it will usually get smaller or go back into the abdomen. If you cannot push it back, contact your doctor straight away for urgent medical examination. Your doctor will diagnose the hernia and abdominal X-rays or ultrasound examinations may be used to visualise the intestine. If the intestine is obstructed, emergency surgery may be needed.

▮ DIAPHRAGMATIC HERNIA

A diaphragmatic hernia is a rare congenital abnormality, affecting one in 3,000 babies. It results from the improper formation of diaphragm muscle so the abdominal organs, such as the stomach, small intestine, spleen, part of the liver and the kidney, appear in the chest cavity. The lung tissue on the affected side has usually not developed fully, a condition called hypoplastic lung. Breathing difficulties usually develop shortly after birth because the diaphragm cannot move effectively and the lungs are unable to expand.

The cause is unknown and there is no prevention. It is usually an isolated abnormality, but can be associated with some heart or chromosomal conditions.

Antenatal ultrasound may establish the diagnosis by Week 20 and a few specialist centres attempt in-utero surgery (operation carried out while the baby is in the womb). At birth, a baby needs immediate intensive care and ventilation to aid breathing, and a surgical operation to reposition the abdominal organs and repair the diaphragm. Multiple operations may be needed. The decision about whether to agree to surgery is extremely difficult for parents because babies who survive with a hypoplastic lung may have severe breathing problems and need long-term oxygen therapy. Life for them and their families can be very difficult.

▨ EPIGASTRIC HERNIA

This protrudes through a narrow hole in the ligament connecting the two rectus muscles that run down the front of the abdomen above the umbilicus. It is usually small and may occur between the umbilicus and the sternum (breastbone) in the chest. Sometimes fat or parts of the bowel get caught in the hernia and cause pain that mimics colic. An epigastric hernia is wide necked and will only very rarely cause the bowel to be trapped. It is only necessary to operate when the bowel is trapped and cannot easily be pushed back into the abdomen. An epigastric hernia is usually operated on after the age of three, but if it causes pain early on treatment may go ahead.

▨ EXOMPHALOS AND GASTROSCHISIS

Exomphalos (omphalocoele) is a defect in the wall of the abdomen allowing some of the internal organs to protrude from the body in the vicinity of the umbilical cord, beneath a protective membrane. The opening occurs in one in 5,000 babies. Many babies born with an exomphalos also have other serious genetic, chromosomal or organ abnormalities. It is often visible on a pregnancy scan and amniocentesis may be offered to diagnose chromosomal anomalies.

Since some or all of the abdominal organs are outside the body, infection is a concern after birth. There is also a risk that an organ may become pinched or twisted and lose its blood supply and become damaged. If the protrusion is small and there is no other abnormality, the outcome is usually excellent after an operation following birth. If it is very large, a series of operations may be needed.

Gastroschisis is similar to exomphalos but is part of a more generalised condition associated with being small for age. Excessive heat loss from the exposed bowel may make a baby very

cold after birth. There is also a high risk the exposed bowel may become twisted, and if starved of oxygen and blood flow, it could die. Early treatment is therefore critical.

Action plan

Surgical treatment is required for exomphalos and gastroschisis. The outlook depends on the extent of the protrusion and whether your baby has any associated conditions. Fortunately, there is rarely severe damage to the intestine. The relatively normal intestine can usually be returned to the abdomen and the defect closed in one or two surgical operations shortly after birth. Your baby will be in intensive care for several weeks before the intestines work well enough to allow feeding and she can come home. After this, it is most likely that your baby will feed normally and grow without problems. With very few exceptions, and these would be babies with severely damaged bowels and other problems such as heart defects, the condition is successfully treated, even if a series of operations is required.

▨ FEMORAL HERNIA

Very rarely, the bowel pushes its way down the femoral canal, which is a channel running from the groin area in the abdomen to the thigh. Because this canal is small, a femoral hernia is likely to cause bowel obstruction, which needs surgical repair. The swelling appears in the inner part of the groin adjacent to the labia in girls or the testicles in boys.

▨ INGUINAL HERNIA

As a boy develops during pregnancy, his testicles descend from the abdomen through the inguinal canal into the scrotum. If the inguinal canal does not close off completely after birth, a loop of intestine can cause a hernia. Girls also have an inguinal canal and can develop hernias here. The swelling is more common in the right groin, although it can occur on either side. In a boy, similar symptoms may arise from hydrocoele fluid around the testicles, which is harmless, or from twisting of the testicles (page 510), which needs emergency treatment.

An inguinal hernia needs to be surgically repaired as soon as possible to prevent obstruction to the intestine. Surgery is carried out under a general or local anaesthetic. After the operation, most babies feel fine within a day or two and the incision is checked a few weeks later.

UMBILICAL HERNIA

There is a small opening in the abdominal muscles through which the umbilical cord passes. This gradually closes after birth. Sometimes the muscles do not grow together and a hernia results. In most cases, an umbilical hernia is small and heals without the need for surgery. Surgery may be recommended if the hernia becomes bigger or is still present after the age of three years. Tape applied across the navel will not repair a hernia.

Hernia, mother

Normally, the muscles and ligaments of the abdominal wall protect the contents of the abdomen. A hernia occurs when there is a weakness in the wall of the abdomen (as described in HERNIA, BABY) and the pressure of walking, coughing or moving causes the abdominal organs, usually the bowel, to protrude into the defect, causing a bulge beneath the skin. If you have a hernia during pregnancy, it is unlikely to cause problems. Rarely, a hernia becomes strangulated and causes pain, temperature rise and bowel obstruction, and does need urgent treatment. Fortunately, strangulation is not common in pregnancy, perhaps because the growing uterus pushes the intestine up and away from the most common hernia sites. You may be more likely to get a hernia if you have had abdominal surgery, are overweight or have a family history of the condition.

Hernias in the groin (inguinal)
These are the most common and are called inguinal hernias. They occur above the crease with the thigh. A femoral hernia is in the groin to the outer side of the labia, but it is rarer. Varicose veins in the groin may appear similar to a hernia.

Hernias in the abdomen (umbilical/epigastric)
Hernias may occur in the belly button (umbilical hernia) or above it (epigastric hernia). Umbilical hernias are more common in African women.

Divarication of the rectus muscles
This occurs when the two strap muscles that run in the midline from the ribs to the pubic area move apart. The abdomen, mainly below the belly button, looks stretched and the uterus may protrude through the defect.

Diaphragmatic hernia
This may occur in the area of muscle where the oesophagus meets the stomach and weakens the valve that stops food from refluxing. This hernia is much smaller than diaphragmatic hernias in babies and is not visible. It may lead to painful reflux, HEARTBURN AND INDIGESTION.

Action plan

* If you are aware of an umbilical, inguinal or femoral hernia before pregnancy, it is best to have it repaired before conception. Recurrence is uncommon.
* If you suspect a hernia during pregnancy, your doctor will ask you to cough as he feels for a bulge. If a new hernia appears, it is best to wait until after the birth for surgery. An abdominal support belt may help to reduce pressure.
* Only in the rare event that a hernia becomes strangulated will you need an operation that can be performed with very little risk to you or your baby.
* Divarication of the rectus muscles is usually not treated by surgery: a support belt is useful. After the birth, abdominal exercises encourage the muscles to move closer together.
* If you have a hernia, it is possible to have an active birth. Pushing will not damage the tissues or cause strangulation. The skin on your abdomen will not burst.
* If you have a diaphragmatic hernia, you can reduce pressure by not gaining excessive weight and sitting and sleeping upright. Attention to diet and eating small meals frequently may decrease discomfort from indigestion and heartburn, which can also be relieved with antacids.

Herpes

Herpes simplex virus (HSV) invades the nerves and then gives rise to skin blisters and ulcers that heal. There are two herpes simplex viruses: HSV-1 and HSV-2. Either one can infect the mouth or genitals but, most commonly, HSV-1 occurs above the waist as oral herpes (cold sores or fever blisters), and HSV-2 below the waist as genital herpes. In general, 80 per cent of herpes infections are oral, due to type 1, and the remainder type 2, mainly genital.

The first attack is the most painful. This stimulates the production of antibodies and any further attacks, coming on when the dormant virus in the nerves reactivates, are likely to be less intense. Roughly 10 per cent of women in the UK are affected, although attacks are less likely in pregnancy.

If you have had herpes in the past but do not have an active attack when you are pregnant there is no risk to your baby. In the unlikely event that you have your first attack in pregnancy, particularly if it is active when you are due to give birth, you will need close medical care to avoid passing the infection to your baby. With a depressed immune system (for example, through HIV infection or in organ transplant patients) the herpes virus can be fatal.

What happens

Genital herpes occurs two to 20 days after contact with an infected person, giving rise to white blisters in clusters, although a single spot may appear alone. The blisters burst and form painful open sores that may make it painful to urinate, and there is often a profuse vaginal discharge. Sometimes bacteria infect the sores and cause painful swelling in the lymph nodes ('glands') in the groin.

Infection and pregnancy

During pregnancy, existing antibodies (resulting from a past infection) cross the placenta and provide protection for your baby. If you have an attack it may be painful for you but, providing there is no genital infection at birth, your baby will be unaffected.

If you have an active genital herpes infection when you go into labour, it is safest to give birth by CAESAREAN SECTION, as your baby is at risk of contracting the infection from your vagina. The likelihood of active infection in labour is tiny, however, and this is a very rare reason for a caesarean delivery.

If you have a long-standing herpes infection, your baby's immunity will be strong, and the chance of passing the virus to your baby, even if the disease is present in your vagina during delivery, is extremely small.

In the very unlikely event that you become infected for the first time in pregnancy, your baby may become infected and this can lead to neonatal herpes. The risk is lowest if you are infected in the first trimester (three month period), and highest if you acquire the infection for the first time late in the last trimester, when there is less time for you to make sufficient antibodies to give your baby protection.

Action plan

It is important to have an accurate diagnosis because herpes symptoms may be confused with cystitis (page 170) or SYPHILIS. Your doctor can take a sample from the sores before they have healed. This will go for laboratory analysis.

Diet and lifestyle

* If you have sores, take care of the affected area, keeping it dry and clean to help healing. Avoid physical contact with the area until all sores are healed.
* It is safe to breastfeed provided you wash your hands.
* Do not kiss your baby when you have active sores around the mouth, and avoid sexual intercourse when either you or your partner has active sores around the genitals.
* With genital sores, wear cotton underwear and avoid tight clothes, as moisture and heat delay healing.
* A nutritious diet with appropriate vitamins and mineral and antioxidant supplements (page 263) may increase your immunity and reduce the chance of recurrence. Lysine may be an effective agent. It is present in many foods, including fish, chicken, beef, lamb, milk, cheese, beans, brewer's yeast, mung bean sprouts and most fruits and vegetables.

Medical care

* For a first infection in the last trimester, particularly between Weeks 36 and 40, many

obstetricians recommend a caesarean delivery but some feel a vaginal delivery is acceptable if no lesions are present.

- If you have an acute vaginal attack when you go into labour, a caesarean section may be recommended. It is best done within four hours of spontaneous rupture of the membranes because the virus can travel into the uterus and infect your baby.
- If you have had vaginal ulcers, your medical team may want to keep a close eye on your baby for the first 14 days in case sores develop.
- Antiviral drugs can be used to treat you and your baby after birth, if you were infected when you gave birth. The antiviral drugs reduce the severity of the attack. They do not reduce the recurrence rate.
- The use of antiviral drugs in pregnancy for recurrent herpes to prevent an acute attack is not recommended.

Homeopathy

Constitutional homeopathic treatment under the care of a qualified homeopath is by far the best way to deal with herpes. However, in an acute attack one of the following remedies may be useful in 6c potency, three times a day, for oral or genital herpes. Re-assess if there is no change after two days.

- *Natrum Mur* for lesions that are often circular, hot, puffy and pearl coloured, with dry surrounding skin, and may appear when you feel vulnerable or after an emotional time.
- *Rhus Tox* for blisters that burn and itch, are red and swollen and then become crusty and you feel restless.
- *Hepar Sulph* for itching, inflamed sores that often converge, give stinging pain and can bleed and weep, and you can feel extremely edgy and irritable.
- *Graphites* for burning, crusty eruptions that can ooze a honey-coloured sticky fluid and with very dry skin in the surrounding area.
- *Calendula* tincture is very useful as an adjunctive treatment. Dilute 10 drops in 250ml (½ pint) water and bathe the affected area two to three times a day.

▇ INFECTION IN A BABY (NEONATAL HERPES)

Around one in 44,000 babies is born with neonatal herpes. This may cause a severe illness involving the brain, eyes, skin and lungs if the herpes is not treated early. For those few babies each year who are infected in this way, the risk of death or severe damage is about 80 per cent, with most survivors having nervous system damage.

Herpes is most commonly transmitted as a baby passes through the birth canal and inhales or swallows the viral particles from sores in the vagina. A tiny number of babies are born with herpes acquired in the womb. After birth, all babies are at risk of acquiring herpes, which can be passed on by being kissed by someone with oral herpes.

HIE (hypoxic ischemic encephalopathy)

Neonatal hypoxic ischemic encephalopathy (HIE) is rare, but is a cause of brain injury in newborn babies. HIE is graded according to severity: from Grade I, the mildest and not usually associated with any long-term brain damage, to Grade III with the greatest risk of long-term brain damage. All three grades (I, II and III) result from insufficient oxygen and reduced blood flow to the brain and other essential organs during birth, or at some time late in pregnancy. When HIE is mild there is usually total recovery. More severe HIE has serious consequences for around one in 1,000 babies.

Neonatal HIE can be diagnosed only when there is evidence of severe foetal distress and asphyxia (page 251). Another indicator is an Apgar score (page 337) below three at 10 minutes after birth, along with altered newborn behaviour that is consistent with brain injury, such as excessive sleepiness, poor feeding and excess crying or convulsions. All of these events are very stressful for any parent and support after the birth is essential.

What happens

Grade I HIE (eight to 10 in 1,000 births) involves temporary nervous system irritability with crying and whimpering, constant jerky muscular movements, normal muscle tone, tremulousness and high-pitched cry, worried look with dilated pupils and little blinking and a weak suck, despite seeming hungry. A baby with

Grade I HIE is usually better within 48 hours and will have no long-term associated problems.

Grade II HIE (four to eight in 1,000 births) suppresses the nervous system and makes a baby more sleepy than expected, and more irritable when awake. The baby will be mildly floppy. Half of the babies with Grade II HIE have seizures (FITS), a weak startle (Moro) reflex, a very weak or absent suck, and constricted pupils. The condition stabilises and begins to improve within three to five days. At follow-up 80 per cent are normal.

Grade III HIE (two to four in 1,000 births) suppresses the nervous system, making the baby floppy and unable to suck. The baby may be unconscious and will not startle (will not show the Moro reflex), intermittently stretch his limbs and have unresponsive pupils. Of the babies who have a Grade III in the first 24 hours or move between a Grade II and III within 48 hours of birth, 50 per cent do not survive. The other 50 per cent have severe brain damage, developmental disability, poor brain growth (microcephaly) and spastic cerebral palsy with all four limbs involved (quadriplegia).

The risk of neonatal HIE rises when there is severe foetal distress and prolonged low oxygen levels leading to asphyxia (page 251).

Action plan

If your baby has signs of HIE the medical team will act accordingly, giving intensive resuscitation and ongoing treatment and medication.

A definitive diagnosis of HIE is made based on the history and physical and neurological examinations. Ultrasound and CT scan reveal brain haemorrhage and swelling. MRI is valuable in severe HIE to identify pre-existing developmental defects of the brain. The interpretation of MRI in babies requires considerable expertise. Considering all the clinical factors is important.

In its mild form, HIE presents no long-term problems but if it progresses or is already severe at birth, vital organs may dysfunction and intensive treatment may be needed. The long-term outlook will be assessed by taking a number of factors into account, including how your baby responds, the acid levels in the cord blood at birth, and results from CT and MRI brain scans. Your baby will be cared for in the Special Care Baby Unit (SCBU, page 497) where you will have the support of the specialist nurses and doctors.

High blood pressure (pre-eclampsia)

See Blood pressure, high and pre-eclampsia.

High-risk pregnancy

Pregnancy is not usually a high-risk condition, and most pregnancies have a healthy, happy outcome. Around 8 per cent are identified as high-risk. This does not mean that a problem will develop, but there is a higher chance, so antenatal monitoring is more intensive, as is attention during labour and provision of facilities for care after birth. High-risk pregnancies account for 70–80 per cent of complications. There are also pregnancies where risks have not been identified that result in complications.

If you are told there is a cause for concern, you may become anxious and might need support (page 46). Your medical team will give you the facts. Their highest priority is the health and safety of you and your baby. Often, extra care is a standard precaution and the outcome is fine.

What happens

The risk may be present because of a mother's physiology or a baby's development; it may be caused by genetics or may stem from environment and lifestyle. Usually a complication is out of the mother's control. Some conditions that may prompt close monitoring are listed here. There are details of each condition within this health guide.

Mother
* Age. Girls below 15 are more likely to develop high BLOOD PRESSURE with pre-eclampsia and deliver underweight babies – premature or with INTRAUTERINE GROWTH RESTRICTION (IUGR). After 35 years of age, there is an increased risk of high blood pressure, DIABETES or FIBROIDS and having a baby with a chromosomal abnormality

such as DOWN'S SYNDROME.
- Weight. Being underweight increases the likelihood of IUGR. Being overweight raises the chance of diabetes, high blood pressure and having a LARGE BABY.
- Medical conditions. Diabetes, chronic high blood pressure, kidney disease, HEART DISEASE, epilepsy, sickle cell anaemia, THYROID problems and blood-clotting problems may increase pregnancy risks.
- Physiology. An abnormally shaped uterus may increase risks; so may an incompetent CERVIX and fibroids.
- Family history. If you or your partner has any hereditary disorders there may be a risk.

Previous pregnancies
- Loss. If you have had three consecutive miscarriages there is a chance of another. If you have previously lost a baby through stillbirth or neonatal death and the cause has been found, your team can advise whether it indicates a risk in this pregnancy.
- Premature birth. The cause of most PREMATURE BIRTHS is unknown but the more pre-term deliveries a woman has had, the greater the subsequent risk.
- IUGR. If you previously had a growth-restricted baby it may happen again, depending on the cause.
- Large babies. If you have previously had one or more large babies it may happen again (and could indicate diabetes).
- More than five pregnancies. This increases the likelihood of weak contractions and rapid labour, and of bleeding after birth.
- Rhesus incompatability. This is rare now that anti-Rh D immunoglobulin is routinely given to rhesus negative mothers.
- Hypertension and pre-eclampsia. These are only likely to recur if you have underlying high blood pressure.
- Genetic disorders or birth defects. These may or may not recur – your obstetrician or geneticist can predict the risk.
- Placental abruption. With antenatal bleeding this may recur.

Events in pregnancy
- Exposure to chemicals or radiation.
- Infection that may present a risk of infection in the womb or complicate delivery.

- A medical condition related to pregnancy (such as CHOLESTASIS).
- DRUG consumption, including smoking.
- Excessive alcohol intake.
- BLEEDING caused by placenta praevia or placental abruption.
- AMNIOTIC FLUID excess or reduction.
- Premature rupture of the membranes (page 391) and premature labour.

Baby
- Restricted growth (IUGR). Predisposes to problems such as FOETAL DISTRESS AND ASPHYXIA.
- Excessive growth (being large). May add to complications during vaginal delivery.
- TWINS or more babies. Are more likely to be born prematurely or receive inadequate nutrition in the womb.
- Postmaturity. When a baby remains in the womb beyond Week 42 placental reserves may fall.
- CONGENITAL ABNORMALITY. This may require special care.
- Breech position. May require extra attention in labour.

In labour
- Care in labour is intended to prevent foetal distress and asphyxia and birth injuries.
- Babies with high-risk pregnancies are more susceptible to distress, particularly if they are fragile from prematurity or IUGR.
- Premature and very large babies are more likely to be injured during birth, as are babies who are not positioned optimally (page 341) or who are subjected to a prolonged labour.

Action plan
Before conception
- If you are aware of any health problem or condition that may place you in a high-risk category, it is best to consult your doctor prior to conception.
- Many conditions can be treated before pregnancy to reduce risk, and if you need to take medications you can check the safety issues and take alternatives if necessary.
- If you take other drugs, drink alcohol or smoke you may need support to give up (page 189).
- Being optimally nourished (page 260) improves your and your baby's health.

* You may need to consult a genetic counsellor (page 267) if you have had a baby with a developmental problem, or have a family history of a condition. You may choose to consult before pregnancy even if you believe you are in good health.

In pregnancy
It is best to remain as healthy as possible by caring for yourself (page 121). If your pregnancy holds risks, your medical team can recommend steps to improve safety. Some conditions simply require extra observation, some can be managed easily and some need specialist attention. You will be able to discuss tests and options for care. If a problem is suspected additional tests are often required for diagnosis (see ANTENATAL TESTS).

If your baby is considered to be at high risk in the second half of pregnancy you will be checked frequently. The following tests may be suggested to help you and your doctor to decide on when and how your baby is born.
* You will need more frequent antenatal visits so your midwife can examine and record your baby's growth and the amniotic fluid volume and treat any medical disorder.
* You will be asked to observe your baby's movement. Normal movements (page 379) indicate health. Movements may reduce when your baby sleeps, but if you are concerned that there are fewer than 10 movements a day, ask to be examined and checked.
* You may be offered regular ultrasound scans with Doppler blood flows with a frequency depending on the degree of risk associated with your pregnancy. In combination with foetal heart tracing this gives an indication of when it is safest for your baby to be born.
* Foetal heart tracing (CTG non-stress test) is useful between scans and is done with a foetal heart monitor on your abdomen. As the predictive accuracy of health improves on scans, foetal heart tracing is used less frequently. If the pattern is normal, you can be reassured your baby will be fine for 24 hours; if there is an abnormality the test will be repeated and acted on if it is confirmed.

Your birth team will assess the results of the tests on an ongoing basis. If they consider the risk to your baby is high, an elective caesarean section (page 108) may be suggested and it is essential to give birth in a hospital with a special care baby unit. In rare instances, being premature is less hazardous than remaining in the uterus. In a lower-risk situation an induction of labour will be considered when your baby is sufficiently mature. When the risk is not so significant, you can wait for labour to begin spontaneously and go ahead with a vaginal delivery.

In labour and birth
* A high-risk baby will be closely monitored during labour and birth to detect and prevent foetal distress and asphyxia.
* In the highest-risk situation you will be advised to have a caesarean section.
* When the risk is lower you will be advised to be upright to maximise the blood flow to the placenta and choose a mobile epidural and adequate fluid replacement if you require these. Precise recommendations depend on the nature of your unique situation. For instance, if your baby is large, you will need careful help in the second stage to reduce the chance of your baby's descent being obstructed (page 397).
* In the event of bleeding, premature birth or foetal distress, your doctor may request the help of a paediatrician to care for your baby and provide resuscitation if needed.
* After birth high-risk babies are monitored to prevent HYPOGLYCAEMIA (low blood sugar) and HYPOTHERMIA and to maintain breathing and oxygen flow. Early feeding helps prevent hypoglycaemia and aids weight gain.
* Premature babies or babies with specific problems have special requirements that are routinely checked.
* Often labour progresses normally and the baby is fine. It is always best to be prepared to improve the outlook for mothers and babies.

Hips, congenital dislocation

As part of the routine newborn baby examination, the midwife or doctor will bend and flex each of your baby's hips in the Barlow and Ortolini's test. If there is a click, it is probably due to the natural sliding of the ligaments (hence its commonly used name, 'clicky hip'). The test is repeated at six weeks. In roughly one in 300 babies a click indicates congenital dislocation of the hip (CDH) so every click is followed up with further investigation. You may also hear this referred to as developmental dysplasia of the hip (DDH).

CDH affects girls more often than boys and is more likely to occur in the left hip. In about 25 per cent of cases both hips dislocate. It can be caused by the way the legs are positioned in the womb. It is more common in breech babies (page 342) and may run in families. It is more likely to occur in TWINS and may be associated with other congenital conditions such as SPINA BIFIDA or DOWN'S SYNDROME. There is no way to prevent the condition or to detect it in pregnancy.

What happens

With CDH the hip joint forms incorrectly so the head of the thighbone can be dislocated from the joint located in the pelvic bone. Usually the socket in the pelvis is shallow, allowing the femur to slip out. The most common symptom is the 'click'. CDH may also lead to unusual skin folds on the upper legs and some babies have trouble spreading their legs for a nappy change. The condition does not give any pain, yet if it is not treated the joint may continue to develop poorly and there is an increased chance of arthritis and pain in adulthood. CDH does not delay walking, but could lead to a waddling gait.

Action plan

All babies with clicky hip, breech position or a family history of CDH are offered an ultrasound within six weeks of birth. The ultrasonographer can see how the head of the femur and the pelvis socket are formed. A baby found at the newborn examination to have CDH will be referred immediately to a specialist orthopaedic surgeon – early treatment increases the likelihood of normal hip development.
* If there is a click but the hip joint appears to be functioning normally, it used to be advised that the joint may be painlessly splinted by using two nappies instead of one for a few weeks. However, current advice is that this is unnecessary, and so is no longer routinely recommended.
* If there is an obvious dislocation of the hip

socket on doing the hip test, or the ultrasound scan shows the joint is shallow, an orthopaedic brace, sometimes called a Pavlik's harness, may be used for a few months. The harness has Velcro straps to hold the legs in a frog-leg position to put the hip ball into the socket. It is painless. The brace can be removed in seconds for nappy changes and does not interfere with feeding, bathing or sleeping. It needs to be worn until the hips are felt to be stable in the socket and then, usually by six months, the harness can be removed. A baby may need time to grow accustomed to being without the harness.
* If treatment is needed after six months, a plaster cast may be used. For a small number of babies, surgery is performed to enlarge the socket. This is usually carried out before the baby starts walking.

Hitting

See Behaviour, baby, difficult.

Home birth

See Labour and birth, mother, at home or hospital.

Homeopathy

Homeopathy has been in use for over 200 years. A gentle and powerful system of medicine, it is rooted in a deep knowledge of physiology and emotions and the integration of mind and body. Homeopathic remedies trigger your 'bodymind' to give a healing or balancing response. It is founded on the principle that 'like cures like' and uses minute doses of substances that, if taken in higher doses, would cause the same symptoms in a healthy person. The word homeopathy is derived from two Greek words: *omnio* meaning 'same' and *pathos* meaning 'suffering'.

The remedies are specially diluted and succussed (mixed according to homeopathic principles) to promote a curative response. A remedy may have a rapid effect to relieve acute symptoms, or work over a period of time to shift a chronic complaint (constitutional treatment).

Remedies are prescribed to meet the unique needs of each individual at any given time.

People react differently to the same illness. For example, five people may have a cold, but each expresses their symptoms differently. Effective homeopathic prescribing requires matching an individual's 'symptom picture' to the corresponding symptom picture of a remedy. As your symptom picture changes so, too, will the remedy that suits you.

Homeopathy in pregnancy

During pregnancy it's usual to respond quickly to homeopathic remedies because nature provides tremendous vital energy when new life is nurtured. The same applies to babies and children. Homeopathic remedies aim to encourage balance, increased vitality and support on many levels.

Homeopathy can be used alone or in combination with other methods of treatment, such as conventional ('allopathic') medicine, YOGA or EXERCISE, MASSAGE, AROMATHERAPY, ACUPUNCTURE or CRANIAL OSTEOPATHY.

Finding the right remedies for you and your baby

By far the best way to become accustomed to using homeopathy is to visit a qualified homeopath who can advise you on the remedy and potency (see below) that suits your current symptoms. In time and with advice from your homeopath, you will learn which remedies work for you in which situations, and you may become reasonably adept at basic homeopathic first aid. For optimal home-prescribing, a comprehensive book presenting a variety of symptom pictures for first aid and acute complaints will be useful, alongside a kit of basic remedies.

Prescribing for babies involves perception and awareness because babies cannot verbalise how they feel. Babies have powerful body language and often present very clear and uncomplicated symptom pictures. The pictures presented throughout this A–Z are designed to help you use your baby's body language to gauge her needs. The most important symptoms are those that differ from your baby's usual state of being, such as if your baby is usually very alert and active and becomes floppy, or is typically thirsty and refuses to drink anything.

Potency

Homeopathic remedies are prepared according to a variety of scales, most commonly the decimal (x) and the centesimal (c) scales. The figure of potency denotes how many times a substance has been diluted and succussed, and the letter indicates which scale has been used.

Lower potencies, such as 6x and 6c, are usually most suitable for treating localised symptoms over a short period. Medium potencies, such as 30c, are often used as a first-line treatment for an acute case. These potencies are the usual ones for first aid and home-prescribing. They are widely available in chemists or health food shops.

Higher-potency remedies, such as 200c, have a powerful action and are typically used when a situation is intense, such as in labour. Higher-potency remedies are only available from specialist homeopathic pharmacies or homeopaths who can supply labour kits with a selection of appropriate remedies.

How to take remedies and what to avoid

Remedies usually come as small sugary tablets or pilules, occasionally as powders or liquids. Creams, ointments, lotions and tinctures are also available for external use. Tablets should be taken in a clean mouth and no other substance should be put in the mouth for at least 15 minutes either side of taking the remedy (not even toothpaste). The effects can be reduced by coffee, peppermint, menthol, eucalyptus and camphor, which are best cut out of the diet completely while treatment continues.

When administering remedies to your baby, the simplest option is to use soft tablets (lactose based) that dissolve almost instantly on her tongue, and have little or no taste. Alternatively, you could crush the harder pilules (sucrose based) and put the powder in her mouth or diluted in a little boiled, cooled water on a sterilised teaspoon.

Remedy responses

- Homeopaths believe in the 'less is more' approach. Frequently evaluating and re-evaluating the symptoms is the best way to administer remedies appropriately.

- The ideal response to a well-chosen remedy is a steady improvement in all symptoms, and when this happens the remedy can be stopped.
- If symptoms return, then a remedy may need to be repeated.
- If there is no change at all after two doses, then re-assess the situation and seek advice.
- If symptoms change then the remedy may need to change.
- Always seek professional advice if you are unsure or if the symptoms do not improve.

Safety

+ Red flag

In cases where there is an underlying acute or serious medical condition that requires urgent medical diagnosis or treatment it is crucial to seek medical care, and not to use homeopathic remedies (see list on page 147). The use of homeopathic remedies can not be regarded as a replacement for professional medical treatment and advice, and as with any medicine, homeopathy is most safely used with the advice of a qualified practitioner.

Throughout this A–Z guide where self-prescribing may be appropriate, symptom pictures are given that may help you decide whether any of the remedies listed may suit you or your baby. Typically, self-prescribing is only appropriate for first-aid and mild acute situations. For treatment of long-standing problems, for certain major acute illnesses (such as measles, MENINGITIS, etc.) or where a remedy picture does not match your symptoms, it is always advisable to seek professional advice. If you are in any doubt, consult your homeopath, midwife or doctor.

Hormones

Your hormones affect your entire being and your energy all the time. In pregnancy, you will notice the impact of your hormones on your body and emotions particularly strongly. Although the focus is traditionally on women, hormones are universal to all humans, men as well as women,

and are in action from the moment of conception.

Hormones are involved in every physical function and emotional feeling. The mind and body are not separate. In the 'bodymind' (page 73), hormones are produced in one part and are transferred to affect the activity of another part. For instance, love or stress hormones can be produced in the brain and also in the bowel. There is now a much deeper understanding of the way hormones are bound up with the way people feel, and it is certain that babies have powerful emotions (page 206). Our emotional feelings affect our hormone flow. Our bodies, and physiological changes such as pregnancy, labour and birth, all trigger intense hormone flows that impact on the way we feel emotionally.

The flow of certain hormones – including the 'love hormones' – increases naturally during pregnancy, birth and breastfeeding. Others connected with fear, anxiety and stress may also increase in response to life events, and when you are in labour. You may find it interesting that there are ways to enhance feelings of love and happiness, and reduce stress, by influencing hormone flow. The entries that follow provide a brief guide to a range of hormones that are particularly relevant for you and for you baby.

■ BONDING AND LOVE HORMONES

See also Emotions, bonding and attachment; Emotions, love.

Although it would be simplistic to suggest that love is purely a reflection of chemical activity, research in the late 20th century has shown how closely hormones are connected with loving feelings. What's really significant is how important these hormones are for babies, for mums in pregnancy, during childbirth and afterwards, and for dads, too. These hormones trigger feelings of love, pleasure and bliss, and they play a fundamental part in our drive to form attachments with one another – crucial for bonding. They flow in increasing quantities through pregnancy and assist the physiological process of natural birth and breastfeeding. In pregnancy, at birth and when breastfeeding, you and your baby get the benefit of these love chemicals more than at any other time of life.

The flow of these powerful hormones is influenced by what is happening in your 'bodymind'. For instance, fear, pain or chemical interventions can reduce the flow; while security, warmth and kindness enhance it. Not everything about your life is in your control, and everyone faces challenges; but there is a lot you can do to set the scene for love and pleasure for you and for your baby.

What happens

Everybody has 'love hormones', a term coined by French obstetrician Michel Odent. In fact, love hormones are common to most of the animal kingdom, contributing to the basic feeling of being alive and knowing pleasure. In humans, love hormones are produced by many different parts of the body, including the brain, gut, reproductive organs and heart. In pregnancy, they are also produced by the placenta. Your baby produces his own love hormones and responds to the hormones that flow from you.

Love hormones influence your emotions and thoughts, your organs, muscles, tissues, senses, vitality and behaviour, and may give you the sensation of loving and being loved, prompt a blissful, tingly feeling, and relax you. They also help to reduce the sensation of pain, relieve stress and improve the quality of sleep.

These hormones are really important for your baby – not just because they help him feel pleasure, but also because they help him feel loved and connected to you. Without this sensation, a baby can feel very insecure and the important foundations of self-esteem and trust are poorly supported (page 206).

Oxytocin and prolactin

The main love hormones are oxytocin and prolactin. Their effect may be heightened when endorphins (opposite) also flow, and by oestrogen and progesterone.

Oxytocin is mainly produced by the pituitary gland in your brain. It helps the uterus contract during labour, and flows strongly during breastfeeding. In a natural labour, levels rise continually until peaking with the force of birth. With this peak, mum and baby feel loving and a powerful urge to touch one another and be together. This magical connection is repeated during breastfeeding, and each time mum and baby rest together. The flow of oxytocin at birth also affects the way mum and dad bond with one

another. When dad is present, touching and making eye contact with mum and after birth with his baby, bonding deepens.

Prolactin, also known as the 'mothering hormone', also mainly comes from the pituitary. Its flow increases in pregnancy and in labour, and most significantly during breastfeeding, when it stimulates milk production and maternal feelings – including love, tenderness and protectiveness.

Action plan

The flow of love hormones increases in everyday life when you are having fun, experience joy, when you are loved and in good health. During birth, the flow is supported if you feel secure and loved; if you are warm; when birth progresses naturally without intervention and when your environment is comfortable and familiar.

The flow is inhibited if you:
- are stressed;
- are threatened or in pain;
- feel isolated; or
- have sad or upsetting thoughts.

During birth, your natural oxytocin production may fall if:
- you feel afraid, exposed or cold;
- lights or noise are intrusive and distracting;
- pain is overwhelming;
- you are asked to focus on a rational problem; and
- certain chemical interventions are used.

If you feel down (page 218) or if labour becomes difficult, it may be reassuring to know that there are some simple, practical things that may help you feel a little better. When your love hormones flow, they influence your stress system (page 310) and help you feel less anxious. Even after a traumatic birth or if you and your baby have been separated for medical reasons, there are many ways to create the right conditions for love and bonding.

Your love hormones can be boosted by:
- Being with people you love – this is part of good health and happiness.
- Feeling safe and comfortable.
- Loving touch, from holding someone's hand to a full body massage. It's wonderful for your baby and for you when he rests naked against

your skin. This contact is really important for every baby in the first hour after birth (page 332).

- Eye contact, with a loved one, with a trusted health worker, with your baby. Your baby feels love when he makes eye contact with you.
- Positive VISUALISATION and meditation.
- Being at a comfortable temperature – this is something you need to help your baby with, too.
- Eating delicious food – typically linked with pleasure and love.
- Pleasant smells such as your baby, breast milk, aromatherapy oils, fresh coffee, warm bread and so on. For your baby, the most delicious smell is you.
- Breastfeeding – this delivers love hormones on tap to your baby and increases the flow in your body too.
- Being close together and having eye contact during bottle-feeding – this is a good bonding opportunity for dad and you may hold your baby skin-to-skin during a feed to enhance the effect.
- During sex.

The effects of synthetic oxytocin and epidural

If you are given synthetic oxytocin in labour to boost the strength of your contractions, it will assist contractions but it does not trigger loving feelings. For some women, it may inhibit natural oxytocin production. But because love is about more than chemicals, you may still feel powerfully loving and connected with your baby. After your baby is born, skin-to-skin touch and breastfeeding will enhance your love-hormone production. If you are given an epidural, this may also reduce natural production of love hormones. Don't worry: they can still flow powerfully after birth when you are with your baby.

Priming your baby for love

Your baby's body, like yours, is very sensitive to love hormones. In early life, while his body is adapting to new experiences and learning, receptors to love hormones will be stimulated in the brain and elsewhere. Your baby's 'bodymind' quickly forms associations and sensations of love.

Babies whose love-hormone receptors are frequently stimulated tend to be more positive and loving, and this continues into later life, as their cells are literally more open to love. Babies who receive less loving stimulation and higher levels of stress are more likely to feel stressed and anxious, and tend to be less optimistic.

Whatever happens in your baby's life, it may be reassuring to know that you – and other caring adults – are in a position to offer your baby a loving and secure environment, and give gifts of pleasure, love and optimism.

▓ FEEL GOOD HORMONES/ENDORPHINS

Endorphins have been called 'feel good hormones'. They are closely linked with other hormones that contribute to feelings of pleasure, bliss and comfort, such as the 'love hormone' oxytocin. Endorphins are released by your brain and other areas of your body when you exercise and they act on your brain like opiates, helping you feel pleasure (the so-called 'runner's high'). Endorphins are also pain relievers (the word endorphin means 'endogenous morphine'). In labour, your body releases endorphins as part of a cocktail of chemical substances, helping to reduce pain and helping you feel positive in pain-free intervals. All these substances are more likely to flow in abundance when a woman feels confident, supported in a way that's right for her, and in an environment that is comforting. The release of endorphins and other feel good hormones after birth is part of a broader 'recipe' that helps mum feel euphoric.

When endorphin release rises you may feel the effect for hours. Exercise in the middle of the day, for instance, may keep you feeling good through the evening, and sex is thought to be linked with high levels of endorphin activity in the areas of the brain involved in pleasure perception.

Choosing activities that help raise levels of mood-enhancing chemicals like endorphins (such as exercise, meditation, laughter or playing) may help lift your spirits when you feel down. Even a gentle walk can make a huge difference. Loving touch also stimulates endorphins and other feel good substances, and this is significant for you and for your baby.

■ STRESS HORMONES AND FEAR

See also Emotions, fear and anxiety.

Your adrenal glands are your guardians and supporters. They are the main producers of the hormones that protect you from danger and help you to respond to life and face its challenges. They are part of your 'fight or flight' reflex and respond almost instantaneously to signals sent by your brain when you are anxious or threatened. The hormone production of your adrenal glands also reflects what you eat: when your blood sugar is low, adrenaline production rises.

When adrenal hormones rise, your 'bodymind' shifts into a state of high alert: you are ready to act and you may feel anxious. Depending on the balance of stress hormones (adrenaline, noradrenaline and cortisol) you may feel energised and run, or you may freeze and be unable to think. Levels return to 'baseline' when your 'bodymind' senses equilibrium.

This rise and fall is as natural for your baby as it is for you, as your baby responds to the environment in the womb and after birth. After birth, your baby's brain and developing hormonal and nervous system take their cues from your facial expressions and tone of voice to gauge whether a situation or a person is safe or frightening. Your baby learns from you and will frequently mirror you. Your baby's experiences in the first year impact the way the brain–body stress system develops, and this foundation has a strong influence on how anxious, fearful or confident he will be in later life.

Labour

During labour, a slightly raised flow of adrenal hormones helps you keep going and move from one contraction to the next over a number of hours. In the second stage, when your baby is ready to emerge from your vagina, a surge of adrenaline enhances the power of birth. If adrenaline flows very strongly before the second stage, however (a likely reason is that you are afraid or in pain), it may inhibit the production of birthing hormones. You can boost the beneficial hormones and reduce stress with loving and supportive company, a safe environment and pain relief. Your baby may also have intense stress hormone release but the way he experiences the sensation is not the same as yours.

Keeping stress to a minimum for you and your baby

When there is a balanced stress-response system involving your adrenal glands and your brain, you are likely to feel energetic and deal with demanding situations effectively. You can support your adrenal glands through eating well and aiming for balance between home and work, rest and activity, and exercising well. These are all part of caring for yourself (page 121). You may also use meditation and relaxation techniques, possibly in conjunction with professional emotional support, to alter a stress response pattern that may have originated from earlier in your life.

Your baby's stress-response system is highly developed by the time he is born but continues to develop, in response to experiences, after birth. As the system matures, you can help your baby learn to calm down when he feels afraid and also to experience feeling safe. Your baby will watch your face and mirror you and if you are there for him to feel secure, emotionally and physically, your baby's stress response system will mature from this foundation. If your baby feels a lot of separation anxiety (page 220), pain or fear, and does not feel secure, this stress response system may become highly sensitised, so that high levels of stress hormones are easily triggered and your baby may be frequently anxious. Your baby's experience of any situation, and the levels of anxiety he feels, will not be the same as yours, and you cannot control his feelings: the best you can do is offer him an environment of love and safety. When you need to be apart from your baby he is likely to feel safest, and avoid intense separation distress, if he is with another loving adult.

Excess stress hormones

When you are feeling very stressed, anxious or afraid, your adrenal glands work hard. They may go into overdrive. Another trigger for being in overdrive is a diet high in sugar, caffeine and cigarettes. When this happens you may feel chronically anxious and depressed, lose interest in life, feel tired and have lowered immunity. Other signs include insomnia or cravings for sugar, coffee or cigarettes, and weight gain. A high flow of adrenal hormones can also interfere with your bowels (possibly causing DIARRHOEA or CONSTIPATION) and contribute to high pain sensitivity. Babies who are exposed to excessive levels of cortisol and other stress hormones, in the womb and after birth, or feel intensely afraid for long periods in early life, are more susceptible to physical and emotional anxiety symptoms later in life.

Anxiety cycles

If you are often anxious, your health may be affected. There is a cycle but it may not be clear what came first and acted as the trigger – a cause of stress or your underlying anxiety. The higher your levels of adrenal hormones, the more anxious you feel and the more frequently you reach for an artificial aid such as coffee. On the other hand, a difficult time in your life may provoke the hormone release from your adrenal glands. If you are in a cycle that may have begun in childhood you need courage, willpower and support to break it. Lifestyles changes, diet and emotional work preferably with a counsellor (page 162) can all be very helpful. Your 'bodymind' will respond and it is possible and worthwhile to break the cycle, even if it has been present for many years.

Human Immunodeficiency Virus (HIV), Acquired Immunodeficiency Syndrome (AIDS), baby

Among children, most cases of AIDS result from transmission of the HIV virus from mother to child during pregnancy, birth or through breastfeeding. Fortunately, advances in medical care mean fewer than 2 per cent of mothers transmit the virus to their babies when they are aware of their infection and take preventive measures (page 313).

Babies whose mothers have had good antenatal care and have regularly taken antiviral drugs during pregnancy, yet do get the HIV virus, tend to be born with a lower viral load (less HIV virus is present in their bodies) and have a better chance of long-term survival with a significantly reduced risk of developing AIDS. If your baby is diagnosed with HIV, he may be treated with a combination of antiretroviral (ARV) drugs. This slows the progress of the disease.

Symptoms of infection in a baby

A baby born with HIV infection most likely will appear healthy. But sometimes, within two to three months after birth, an infected baby may begin to appear sick, with poor weight gain, repeated fungal mouth infections (thrush), enlarged lymph nodes ('glands'), enlarged liver or spleen, neurological problems, and multiple bacterial infections, including pneumonia.

Babies who are born with HIV have weakened immune systems and are more vulnerable to developing 'opportunistic infections' and more severe bouts of other common childhood infections including MENINGITIS. Early diagnosis and treatment can help reduce susceptibility to infection.

Action plan

Diagnosis of HIV in a baby

During pregnancy your antibodies are passed to your baby, so an early blood sample will therefore test positive. This doesn't mean your baby is infected as he will keep your antibodies for months. If your baby is infected with HIV, he will make his own antibodies, thus testing positive after 18 months.

Earlier diagnosis of HIV infection can now be made using tests that show the presence of the virus itself rather than the HIV antibodies. This is 'virological testing' and can be carried out from six weeks of age (and occasionally earlier if necessary). The great benefit of this is that life-saving highly active antiretroviral therapy (HAART, see below) treatment can start early.

Drug treatment

ARV medication is effective in slowing the replication of the virus and preventing or reducing some effects of the disease, allowing people living with HIV to remain free of symptoms longer. Because these drugs work in different ways they are used in combination cocktails under the direction of a specialist HIV team. This regimen is known as HAART treatment (highly active antiretroviral therapy). The HAART drugs interfere with the ability of HIV to reproduce in the white cells. Doctors may also prescribe antibiotics to prevent opportunistic infections.

Can babies pass on infection?

There have been only a handful of reported cases where HIV infection was passed from a child to another person. All of these involved direct blood contact within a household. The typical baby secretions (such as urine, dribbled saliva, vomit, faeces) do not seem to transmit the virus, so routine care of babies with HIV is considered safe.

Despite widespread concerns, there are no reported cases of infection of the HIV virus within a nursery or baby-care setting. Infection with HIV requires direct contact with HIV-containing body fluids. Staff in day care and nursery provision should be advised to routinely use gloves when any child has a cut, scrape or is bleeding, and for mopping up vomit.

Vaccinations for an HIV-positive baby

It is very important that your baby receives VACCINATIONS, including yearly vaccination against influenza, starting at seven months of age, and the pneumococcal vaccine at age two. But he must avoid any live virus vaccines such as chickenpox vaccine. Your baby can still receive the primary vaccines at two, three and four months, as they no longer contain live polio virus. He will need the care of a paediatrician experienced in the treatment of AIDS because new technologies are constantly evolving.

Family life

Life for a family with an HIV-positive child can be very stressful. Many families find it difficult to continue the regular drug schedules, and many HIV-positive children find themselves fostered or adopted, as their parents simply cannot cope.

Human Immunodeficiency Virus (HIV), Acquired Immunodeficiency Syndrome (AIDS), mother

Human immunodeficiency virus (HIV) is responsible for acquired immune deficiency syndrome (AIDS). Becoming pregnant does not appear to endanger the health of an HIV-infected woman, but does carry implications for her baby. Yet treatment can dramatically improve a baby's outlook as well as a woman's health during and after pregnancy. Screening for HIV is routine in the UK although not everyone agrees to have the test. In many hospitals there are specifically trained HIV midwives and counsellors.

What happens

HIV is most commonly transmitted through sexual contact and through the use of contaminated needles, often with drug use. A person who is 'HIV positive' does not necessarily have AIDS, but can transmit the virus to others. Antibodies may not show up in a screening test until three months after infection. It can take 10 or more years for an HIV-positive person to develop AIDS. A person with AIDS has a deficiency of the immune system and is more susceptible to infections and certain cancers that can be fatal.

HIV and pregnancy

If you are HIV positive and become pregnant, it is sensible to take medication during pregnancy and birth and to care for yourself as well as possible. If your partner is HIV positive and you test negative, and you refrain from unprotected sex and then test negative again after three months, you are clear of HIV. Refraining from unprotected sex with your partner is the only sure way to continue protection and be certain that you and your baby will not be infected.

Transmitting HIV to your baby

The likelihood that you will transmit HIV to your baby in pregnancy ('perinatal transmission') is directly related to the number of virus particles in your body (known as viral load). If you have developed AIDS, you will have a greater number of viral particles in your circulation and transmission is more likely than if you are HIV positive without AIDS. Treatment in pregnancy can reduce the viral load, thus helping to prevent transmission.

Without treatment, transmission of HIV from mother to baby occurs in up to 27 per cent of cases. The risk of transmission can be cut to less than 2 per cent if you have medication during the last six months of pregnancy, possibly give birth by CAESAREAN SECTION, bottle-feed and introduce drug therapy for your baby.

HIV testing

You will be offered an HIV blood test in early pregnancy by your midwife as part of routine serum screening. A minority of women refuse to have the test. If the test is positive the result is checked on a repeat blood sample. Women who are HIV positive are offered a blood test. This will measure CD4 cells (also known as T cells, a type of immune system cell), and viral load, the number of virus particles present in the blood. Taken together these two figures indicate the severity of the HIV infection and the risk of AIDS developing. As HIV degenerates towards full-blown AIDS, the immune system begins to collapse. The number of CD4 cells declines and the number of virus particles increases.

HIV infection risk for your baby

A high CD4 count indicates that your immune system is functioning well and if the viral load is low your baby is unlikely to become infected. You are at low risk of AIDS developing during pregnancy. A low CD4 count and a high viral load indicate your baby has a higher chance of becoming infected and your risk of AIDS is increased.

Action plan

It is best to care for yourself with a nutritious diet, vitamin and mineral supplements, and regular exercise and rest. Try to avoid people you know to be infected with contagious illnesses. It is best to avoid smoking and taking recreational DRUGS.

The drugs that can prevent HIV being passed from a mother to her baby are called antiretroviral (ARV) drugs. Your HIV specialist will help you decide which ARV drugs to take and when to start and stop. The factors to consider are your health, reducing the risk of HIV being passed to your baby, and the side effects of the drugs on you and potential harm to your baby. There may be a difference between which drugs you would ideally take and which ones are available. Treatment usually begins after 12 weeks to reduce the risk of harm to your developing baby.

ARVs are also taken by HIV positive women who are not pregnant, to reduce the viral load and to prevent them from becoming ill. The drug zidovudine (also known as AZT) has been shown to be particularly useful for preventing HIV being passed from mother to child. It is advisable to take it. If combination therapy with other drugs is available it will probably be recommended because drug combinations are usually even more effective at lowering a woman's viral load.

Drug therapy is continually evolving and it is best to discuss all your options with your HIV specialist. They are usually effective in preventing HIV transmission to your baby.

Birth

If you are HIV positive your specialist's recommendations will reflect your viral load and your wishes. Most mother-child transmission takes place during birth or breastfeeding. Vaginal delivery is an option if your viral load is low, you are taking ARV medication, and if labour is progressing well. You will be given medication via a drip throughout labour and birth. It is important to minimise the risk that your baby will be exposed to your blood, so it is advisable to avoid monitoring with a scalp electrode and the use of FORCEPS or VENTOUSE (see LABOUR AND BIRTH, MOTHER) to assist your baby's birth.

Caesarean delivery is recommended if your viral load is unknown or is high or if you have not taken appropriate ARV medication during pregnancy. To be most effective in preventing transmission, a caesarean is best done before your waters break. It is routine to administer AZT intravenously, beginning three hours before the operation.

Treatment after birth

You will need to discuss your treatment requirements with your HIV specialist. If your viral load is low and CD4 count is high treatment can stop. If you need to continue treatment you will be offered extra support from your health visitors or HIV nurses.

Living with HIV

If you are diagnosed with HIV you will need to adapt to the changes in your body, as you would with any chronic illness, and the effects that drug therapy have on you and your family. If your baby is infected, coping with his physical symptoms may be extremely upsetting.

Perhaps the most difficult aspect is uncertainty. In the past, HIV-positive people often faced death in the near future. Today, with daily medication, the prognosis is better. Although some drugs have unpleasant side effects, there is a chance that you could feel quite well and the effect on your life could be minimal for years.

Living a normal life, enjoying your family, keeping a job and having the courage to fall in love with your children may not be easy. Help from your family and friends, your medical team and HIV support groups could help enormously. Other challenges include feeling stigmatised and worrying about your children being isolated because of your condition, and more so if they are infected. Your whole family, including your partner, will benefit from support.

Hydrops foetalis

Hydrops foetalis (or simply 'hydrops') is a severe, life-threatening problem. Hydrops develops when too much fluid leaves the bloodstream and goes into the tissues, causing oedema (swelling due to excess fluid) in a baby. It may become evident during antenatal screening, or not until after birth, and may be linked to a viral infection such as PARVOVIRUS. A baby with hydrops may respond to treatment, which is sometimes possible during pregnancy. The outcome varies depending on the cause and there may be other complications. Roughly one in 5,000 babies is affected by hydrops.

There are two main types of hydrops:

■ IMMUNE HYDROPS

This accounts for 10–15 per cent of hydropic babies. It is caused by Rhesus incompatibility (page 67), where a Rhesus negative mother's immune system regards the baby's Rhesus positive blood as foreign, and attacks the red blood cells. As a result, the baby develops ANAEMIA. It may occur when a Rhesus negative mother has not received anti-D in a previous pregnancy or responded to antenatal treatment. The hydrops will develop as the baby's organs are unable to compensate for the anaemia. The heart begins to fail and large amounts of fluid build up in the baby's tissues and organs. This is the most serious form of hydrops, causing death in 75 per cent of cases. The remaining 25 per cent of babies usually have no long-term

consequences and after blood transfusion, either before or after birth, no longer have the immune response that caused the hydrops.

■ NON-IMMUNE HYDROPS

This is more common, accounting for 85–90 per cent of affected babies. It includes all other diseases or complications that may result in a build-up of fluid. Roughly 100 babies are born with non-immune hydrops each year in the UK. Up to 75 per cent of parents who discover their babies are affected choose to terminate the pregnancy. The condition carries a high risk (75 per cent) of major structural or chromosomal conditions but in up to 25 per cent of cases a baby may survive without significant problems. The potential for healthy survival is greatest when the cause is viral.

What happens

During pregnancy, an ultrasound scan may reveal large amounts of amniotic fluid and a thickened placenta, and the baby may have an enlarged liver, spleen or heart, and fluid build-up in the abdomen. Hydrops does not always cause the same symptoms in all babies, and for accurate diagnosis, foetal blood sampling (done by placing a needle through the mother's uterus and into a blood vessel of the foetus or the umbilical cord) or amniocentesis (page 21) may be used.

After birth, symptoms may include pale colouring due to anaemia, severe swelling, especially in the abdomen, enlarged liver and spleen and difficulty breathing, due to fluid collecting around the lungs in the chest cavity.

Action plan

The specific treatment will be carefully considered, depending on your baby's unique situation. You may be offered intrauterine surgery, such as laser treatment to the blood vessels on the placenta, if the hydrops is a result of anaemia resulting from twin-twin transfusion (page 528). Your preferences are important and you may want to talk to a genetic counsellor or another specialist as you assess the situation.

After birth, a baby with hydrops may need assistance with breathing. Excess fluid can sometimes be removed from spaces around the lungs and abdomen using a needle, and there are medications that help the kidneys to remove excess fluid from circulation.

Survival depends on the skill and experience of the specialists caring for your baby, and the extent and cause of the hydrops. Any baby surviving hydrops will need long-term follow-up, at least until school entry.

Hypoglycaemia in the newborn

Hypoglycaemia occurs when the amount of glucose (sugar) in the blood is lower than normal. A mild reduction is common among newborns and usually is not serious. It does, however, carry a risk. If hypoglycaemia is prolonged and severe it can cause brain damage. Your baby's brain requires sugar to function. Fortunately, hypoglycaemia is easily preventable with close blood glucose monitoring of babies who are at risk.

Symptoms include sweating, jitteriness and jerky movements, rapid breathing, rapid heart rate, pallor or even apnoea (absence of breathing). Approximately one in 500 newborn babies develop symptoms of hypoglycaemia. Some others have low levels but no symptoms.

What happens

Glucose is a vital brain energy fuel and an important energy source for the body. There is no other food source that can be used for the energy requirements of the brain. During pregnancy, your baby receives glucose from your bloodstream via the placenta. Some is stored as glycogen in your baby's liver, heart and muscles. These stores are important for supplying the brain with glucose during labour, and after your baby is born, before feeding is established. Stores are mainly laid down in late pregnancy. This means that hypoglycaemia tends to be most profound or difficult to treat when associated with prematurity or severe INTRAUTERINE GROWTH RESTRICTION (IUGR, page 322).

Symptoms of hypoglycaemia generally come about as the body attempts to raise the blood glucose level. It does this by releasing adrenaline, the hormone that stimulates the body to release its glucose stores.

Babies who are more likely to develop hypoglycaemia include:
- Babies whose mothers have DIABETES: the mother's blood glucose is high and the baby produces high levels of insulin to break down this glucose. The insulin levels remain high after birth and contribute to the rapid fall in blood sugar once the source of glucose is removed.
- Small or growth-restricted (IUGR) babies, who may have too little stored glucose.
- PREMATURE babies, especially those with low birth weight, who often have limited glycogen stores or immature liver function, without sufficient stores of glycogen.

Action plan

If your baby appears hypoglycaemic, blood monitoring on a heel prick sample can be used to assess glucose levels. If levels are low, it's important for your baby to have a rapid-acting source of glucose. Breast milk is an excellent source, and formula milk also contains glucose. Some babies need glucose given intravenously (by injection). Your baby's blood glucose levels will be closely monitored after treatment to see if the hypoglycaemia occurs again.

For most babies, the risks of hypoglycaemia pass after 48 hours, when regular feeding has been established. Blood glucose measuring can stop once the medical team is happy that levels are normal.

On extremely rare occasions, the baby's pancreas may produce too much insulin even where there has not been diabetes in the mother. If the excessive insulin production continues there may be recurrent episodes of severe and dangerous hypoglycaemia for weeks after birth. A blood test measures insulin levels and the baby will need treatment by a specialist paediatric endocrinologist (hormone specialist) to stabilise the blood sugar levels. In this rare situation treatment may be needed for months.

Hypothermia, baby

Your newborn baby cannot efficiently regulate her temperature, and there is a risk of excessive cooling or overheating. The main factors that may make your baby too cold are being exposed to cold draughts in a cold room or outside and being allowed to cool excessively when her skin is wet. She needs your help to maintain a reasonable temperature and if she does become very cold, she will need to be carefully warmed.

What happens

If your baby becomes too cold, her temperature will fall below 35°C (95°F). A very cold baby will become apathetic and not feed, cry feebly and have depressed reflexes, a slow heart rate and reduced urine production. Deceptively, she may have ruddy cheeks and extremities, but will feel cold to the touch.

Babies do not have a shivering mechanism, which in older children would be activated to make sure major organs stay at normal temperature, and they cannot restrict blood flow to the skin, which would otherwise slow down cooling. They have little fat to insulate them, and the hormones to generate heat are rapidly used up in babies. Babies with low birth weight are more susceptible to a reduction in temperature because there is a larger surface area of skin, less fat, and low blood sugar levels. It is easier for them to lose heat than to produce it.

Severe hypothermia: cold injury

Cold injury refers to the rare event of severe hypothermia with a core body temperature of 32°C (89.6°F) or less. Risk factors include birth into a cold room or cold water, air conditioning blasting cold air on to a wet naked baby or exposure to a cold atmosphere when inadequately dressed. Severe cooling may make the body tissues become damaged and swell, giving a woody feel to the limbs. Hypothermia may make a baby have difficulty maintaining blood sugar levels, have breathing difficulties and bleed excessively from reduced blood clotting. The death rate of cold injury is high because of severe HYPOGLYCAEMIA (low blood sugar), low blood oxygen levels and bleeding into the lungs and brain. The risks are linked with rapid re-warming.

Action plan

Prevention

At birth, your baby will be at the optimal temperature if you hold her naked, against your skin. Being skin to skin helps to regulate her temperature, and your own core temperature is capable of rising or falling to meet your baby's needs (page 517). Alternatively, she will be kept warm in a warm dry towel or in a warm cot.

- Premature babies below 1.8kg (4lb) are usually nursed in an incubator and the skin temperature kept at 36.5°C (97.7°F). Sometimes, a plastic heat shield is used to lessen heat loss. Woolly bonnets are ideal for preventing heat loss through the head. Kangaroo care (page 518) offers an alternative way to keep a baby warm and tends to keep a baby's temperature more stable than it might be in an incubator.
- If your baby becomes moderately cold, a cuddle, a hat and a feed will usually be sufficient to warm her. If you are worried that she is excessively cold, you need to get medical help for her.

Treatment

If your baby becomes too cold, you need to contact the emergency services urgently.

- She will need re-warming in an incubator. Her temperature will be raised at around 1.5–2°C (2.7–3.6°F) per hour.
- She will be monitored for hypoglycaemia and treated if necessary with intravenous warmed dextrose water to prevent low sugar levels.
- The doctors will check whether an infection has caused the low temperature and give antibiotics as a precaution. They will also check the baby's blood clotting system.
- She will be given oxygen while she is being re-warmed.

When her temperature is back to normal she will be kept under observation to ensure that it remains normal at room temperature. It is best to continue to monitor her temperature for a few days after she recovers.

Incontinence, vaginal laxity and prolapse

Carrying a baby through pregnancy and, more significantly, giving birth vaginally, puts pressure on your pelvic floor area and the muscles and ligaments around your vagina. Your body is designed to cope, and will be better equipped if you are committed to performing pelvic floor exercises (page 438) that strengthen your pelvic floor and the valves of your bladder and anus. For some women, extensive stretching, increased laxity or ligament damage during birth leads to problems. Usually these are short term and there are effective methods of treatment. After a few months, the vagina recovers, the tissues regain their tone and symptoms are less frequent. Not all women recover fully, however, and occasionally a problem continues.

What happens

In pregnancy, pelvic muscles and ligaments stretch under the effect of hormones. These effects are reversed after the birth. The pelvic organs and structures are most vulnerable during birth.

- If the ligaments that attach to the side wall of the pelvis to support the vagina are torn, the vaginal walls may become lax and descend (prolapse).
- The muscles of the pelvic floor may tear, and these may include the bladder and anal sphincters. If these are disrupted incontinence may follow.

- Bruising or injury of the pudendal nerves along the side walls of your pelvis as your baby's head descends may affect their function, reducing pelvic muscle tone and adding to prolapse or incontinence.
- Damage to the tissues or nerves may cause pain in your vagina, lower back or lower pelvis, or on passing a stool.
- A first birth may carry the highest risk of pelvic floor damage but there may be a cumulative risk of damage with subsequent births. Factors that may contribute include prolonged second stage of labour, use of forceps or ventouse, being overweight, or coming from a family where there is a history of prolapse.
- Giving birth by elective CAESAREAN SECTION does reduce the likelihood of prolapse. Caesarean birth does not reduce the laxity of muscles resulting from weight bearing and hormonal changes in pregnancy.
- Routine use of EPISIOTOMY (see LABOUR AND BIRTH, MOTHER) does not prevent prolapse.

Stress incontinence of urine

This is a urinary 'storage' problem: the strength of the bladder sphincter (valve) reduces, and is not able to prevent urine flow against increased pressure from the abdomen. Small leakages of urine are common in pregnancy, usually brought on by a cough, sneeze or laugh, or a sudden movement such as running or jumping, particularly in late pregnancy. Occasionally, a heavy vaginal discharge or rupture of the membranes with the passage of amniotic fluid may be mistaken for incontinence.

Up to 20 per cent of women experience stress incontinence for a short time after birth but many find that with regular pelvic floor exercises (page 438), incontinence does not persist for more than a few weeks. Roughly 10 per cent experience occasional incontinence nine months after birth. It is more likely to affect women who have given birth vaginally.

Urinary urgency incontinence and irritable bladder

If your bladder is irritated by infection (page 170), inflammation or bruising, it may be more liable to contract. This means small volumes of urine may give a feeling of fullness and urgency, and there may be leakage when you need to pass urine and it flows before you are ready. This is also known as irritable bladder.

Urinary retention and overflow incontinence

Pressure during birth may lead to swelling of the tissues of the urethra in the bladder outlet and cause retention of urine so the bladder fills excessively and then overflows. Sometimes urine retention is due to a narrow urethra, a condition easily treated with a small operation to dilate (widen) it.

Anal incontinence

If your anal sphincter muscle has been disrupted you may involuntarily pass gas or faeces. Occasionally it can cause difficulty emptying the bowel completely. This is more likely to occur if FORCEPS or VENTOUSE (see LABOUR AND BIRTH, MOTHER) were used to assist birth. It affects roughly 4 per cent of mothers. Women who already have one pelvic floor disorder, such as prolapse or urinary incontinence, are more likely to suffer from anal incontinence as well.

Vaginal prolapse

Vaginal prolapse occurs when the vaginal walls drop below their normal limits because the supporting ligaments and muscles have been stretched by the birth. It may be associated with urinary incontinence.

- Prolapse occurs in about 10 per cent of women. It is usually mild. Prolapse symptoms sometimes do not become apparent until years after childbirth.
- Prolapse may sometimes give a sensation of a wide vagina and reduced sensitivity during intercourse.

- If it feels as if something is 'coming down' in the front or back of your vagina there may be prolapse. The front is affected if the bladder descends (a cystocoele). When the back is affected and the rectum descends, it is called a rectocoele.
- If there is a cystocoele, you may pass urine more frequently. Occasionally there may be difficulty emptying the bladder, and urinary tract infection is more likely.

If you have prolapse you may have an increase in urinary or anal incontinence in the next pregnancy but it usually settles after the birth. The next birth is likely to be straightforward because the vaginal tissues stretch easily and an episiotomy will probably not be needed.

Action plan

If you have symptoms of prolapse or urinary or anal incontinence, visit your doctor. At your six-week postnatal visit, the tone of your pelvic floor muscles and ligaments will be checked in detail if you are concerned. Few women find it easy to admit to faecal incontinence, but treatment can be very effective.

- Pelvic floor exercises in pregnancy (page 438) help strengthen your muscles and are good preparation for the pressure of birth. After birth, begin the exercises as soon as possible and build up gradually. Try contracting and releasing your pelvic floor 30 times every time you feed your baby.
- When you urinate, tighten your muscles mid-flow so the flow stops briefly, and then release and let it recommence. Do not do this every time – twice a day is fine. It may take a few weeks before your pelvic floor responds. You may hold your urine for a progressively longer time, up to five minutes, to strengthen the muscles.
- Sex is a great way to strengthen all the muscles in the vagina.
- There are no certain ways to prevent prolapse but using upright postures in birth (page 350) may reduce the time spent bearing down and the need for assistance.
- If your baby needs help to be born, ventouse is preferable to forceps. Provided it is applied only when your cervix is fully dilated, it is less disruptive on your tissues than forceps.

- Being well nourished and eating optimal amounts of vitamins, minerals and antioxidants improves the tone of your connective tissues. Eating well also allows your body to recover more easily after pregnancy and birth.

Medical care

- An ultrasound scan can identify pelvic floor damage and tears to the anal sphincter. MRI, X-ray and bladder-pressure studies can be done if the symptoms persist.
- If the ligaments are very stretched or if the pudendal nerves in your pelvis are bruised, you may find it difficult to contract your pelvic floor selectively. A physiotherapist may recommend exercises and the use of cones. They are very easy to use and within four to six weeks you are likely to notice an improvement.
- Biofeedback can assist with exercises and cones. Electrodes are placed on your abdomen and along the anal area. A monitor shows which muscles are contracting and which are at rest and you can use this to identify the correct muscles for performing pelvic floor exercises. Of the people who use biofeedback, about 75 per cent report improved symptoms.
- Electrical stimulation therapy uses low-voltage electric current to stimulate and contract the correct group of muscles. This may be done at home. The current is delivered using a battery-operated probe in the anus or vagina. Treatment sessions usually last 20 minutes and may be performed every day for months. Stimulation is effective if the pelvic nerves are functioning normally.
- It is rare, but if you have severe prolapse after the birth, your doctor may insert a ring to hold your vagina in place. The ring can be removed when your vaginal ligament tone improves.
- A surgical operation may be required to treat severe prolapse, particularly if it is associated with incontinence and/or anal sphincter damage. It is preferable to postpone the operation until your childbearing is completed. When an operation is carried out and pregnancy follows, birth is usually by caesarean section to avoid damaging the repair.
- If you have a urinary infection, treatment should improve your symptoms.
- If you have urinary retention, inserting a catheter tube to drain the urine until the

swelling reduces will help. The bladder usually recovers spontaneously within 24–48 hours.

Homeopathy

For urinary stress incontinence

The following homeopathic remedies may help stress incontinence, taken in 30c potency three times per day for five days and then re-assess:

- *Pulsatilla* if leakage occurs particularly at night or while lying down and you are not thirsty but feel weepy and your moods are changeable.
- *Sepia* if leakage is accompanied by a bearing down sensation, is worse from walking, laughing or sneezing and you are irritable and feel chilly.
- *Causticum* if involuntary urination is worse during the first part of the night and from coughing, sneezing or laughing.

For urinary urgency incontinence and irritable bladder

Once you have been checked for infection and been diagnosed with irritable bladder one of these two remedies in 30c potency, taken morning and evening for five days, may reduce the intensity of your symptoms; after this time, re-assess:

- *Equisetum* for a constant desire to urinate, often urgently, a sensation of fullness in the bladder that is not relieved by urinating, general tenderness and aching in the bladder area, and a cutting or pricking pain in the urethra while you pass large quantities of light-coloured urine, worse at the end or after urination.
- *Staphysagria* following use of a catheter and/or you have frequent urges to urinate with a sensation of pressure but difficulty urinating, burning during urination (drop by drop) with continued urging and pain afterwards.

After trauma to the bladder during birth, or for urinary retention

The following remedies may be useful (30c potency) every hour for four hours, then re-assess.

- *Staphysagria* is the No.1 remedy, particularly if a lot of intervention was used (forceps), it is very painful to urinate but you only pass drop by drop with much urging and you feel quite battered.

* *Aconite* if labour was emotionally shocking and delivery was very fast, you have a frequent urge to pass urine with pressing pains accompanied by anxiety and fear.
* *Opium* if retention follows shock and the sphincter of the bladder is in spasm. You may be feeling confused and slightly spaced-out.

Indigestion

See Heartburn and indigestion.

Induction of labour

See Labour and birth, mother, induction and augmentation.

Inflammatory bowel disease (IBD), mother

Inflammatory bowel disease (IBD) is the general name for a collection of conditions including Crohn's disease (affecting the small intestine) and ulcerative colitis (affecting the colon). It is uncommon and it rarely occurs for the first time during pregnancy. It is characterised by profuse diarrhoea and symptoms similar to IRRITABLE BOWEL SYNDROME (IBS), but there may also be mucus and blood in the stools and abdominal swelling, and you may feel very unwell. Women who already have the condition usually find symptoms improve in pregnancy.

Action plan

* To make a definitive diagnosis of IBD, a bowel X-ray and/or colonoscopy examination (inserting a finger-size camera into the colon via the anus) is needed. These will be delayed until after birth so a diagnosis during pregnancy is usually based on symptoms. If IBD has previously been diagnosed, your doctor will take your pregnancy and baby into account when prescribing medication.
* If symptoms are severe, it may be necessary to take anti-inflammatory drugs or steroid hormones, usually by enema. This needs to be done on the recommendations of a gastroenterologist (a doctor who specialises in treating bowel problems). Corticosteroid enemas are regarded as safe in low doses in pregnancy.
* Your obstetrician needs to monitor your baby's growth because it may be reduced (page 322) if your condition is severe and leads to mineral and vitamin deficiencies.
* Your nutrition will need to be monitored and blood tests will check for ANAEMIA. You may need extra vitamins, minerals and iron.
* If you choose HOMEOPATHY, visit your homeopath for a remedy to fit your precise symptom picture.

Influenza (flu), baby

See also Coughs and colds, baby.

If your child suddenly develops a high fever (above 39°C/102.2°F) accompanied by a dry cough and runny nose, he may have influenza – the flu. The fever and most other symptoms last about five days, though a cough may linger for several weeks or even longer. Other viruses, such as bronchiolitis (page 107), can cause a similar illness.

Action plan

When your child has the flu, make sure he gets lots of rest and drinks plenty of fluids. He will get sufficient fluid from your breasts, if you are breastfeeding, although his appetite for richer milk may be low. If you are bottle-feeding, he may feel better for some extra drinks of water (which must be pre-boiled and cooled). If your baby is weaned, he may not have much appetite while he is unwell.

* Call your doctor if your baby's temperature rises above 38°C (100.4°F) between birth and three months old; 39°C (102.2°F) or greater between the ages of three and six months; or if it reaches 40°C (104°F) when your baby is older than six months.
* Call your doctor if your baby has trouble breathing, appears to have ear or face pain, or looks very ill (some children develop complications from flu such as pneumonia, or ear or sinus infection).
* Take your child to the doctor if his cough lingers

for more than a week or is getting worse.
* Seek advice if he has persistent chest pain and fever, or is wheezing and coughing up discoloured mucus, as these might be signs of pneumonia or lower respiratory infection.

Antibiotics are not effective in treating flu, but may be offered if a bacterial infection such as a chest or ear infection develops.

Homeopathic remedies are outlined under INFLUENZA (FLU), MOTHER and can be given to your baby.

Vaccination against flu
Some children with chronic health problems are at increased risk of serious complications from flu. These include children with ASTHMA, HEART DISEASE, sickle cell disease, DIABETES, HIV and those undergoing cancer treatment, as well as children living in households with someone who has any of these conditions. The Department of Health advisors on immunisations recommend a flu vaccine each autumn after the age of six months for such children. It is administered through local health services such as your GP.

The NHS recommends VACCINATION of healthy children between the ages of six and 23 months. This age group is at increased risk of complications and hospitalisation due to flu. For more on immunisation recommendations and choices, see page 536.

Influenza (flu), mother

See also Coughs and colds, mother.

An estimated 10 to 20 per cent of UK residents get the flu each year. If you get flu you are likely to recover easily. There is some evidence to suggest that flu infection in pregnancy may increase the risk of complications (such as lung infection and pneumonia) for the mother and could in theory carry a risk for the baby. For this reason some health professionals are calling for free vaccination in pregnancy.

What happens

Influenza viruses are spread in the air when an infected person coughs, sneezes, or speaks. Flu can also be spread when a person touches a

surface that has viruses on it (such as a door handle) and then touches his or her nose or mouth.

Symptoms tend to start suddenly and may include fever, chills, headache, aching muscles and feeling generally unwell, together with a cough or sore throat. You may feel unwell for more than a week, and sometimes flu seems to 'drag on'. You can distinguish a flu infection from a common cold, as the latter is likely to start gradually with a sore throat and stuffy or runny nose and tends to be less severe. Flu viruses change from year to year, making each winter's flu different from the last.

Action plan

The best thing to do is to rest as much as you can and treat your symptoms as you would for a cough or cold (page 160). Paracetamol products may help to reduce a fever and pain, but need to be taken in safe doses (see page 408).

If you get flu after the birth, it is safe to continue breastfeeding your baby. Ensure you drink plenty of water.

Antibiotics are not effective against the flu virus, but your doctor may suggest antibiotic treatment if you develop a secondary bacterial infection, such as a chest infection.

Homeopathy
Generally flu runs its course in stages. The important factor when using homeopathy is to match the symptoms carefully at each stage and prescribe a remedy accordingly. This can often shorten the duration and intensity of a bout of flu. You may give the most appropriate remedy in 30c potency two hourly for the first six hours and re-assess. In the early stages, usually the most appropriate remedies are:
* *Aconite* when there is a sudden onset of a fever, usually at night, possibly with bouts of heat alternating with shivering, anxiety, agitation and restlessness, and a thirst for cold water.
* *Belladonna* when symptoms come on quickly and the fever is suddenly very high, usually coming on mid afternoon, with a flushed face, dilated pupils, rapid pulse and intense heat radiating from the body and head, although hands and feet tend to be cold, there is no thirst and you feel worse for any motion, light or jarring.

321

For the established stage of flu, the following remedies may be useful. You may take the most appropriate remedy (30c potency) four times per day for two to three days and re-assess.

- *Gelsemium* for gradual onset flu where there is an overall weakness and heaviness of limbs, droopy eyelids and aching, chills (especially up and down the spine) alternating with heat, plus exhaustion and sleepiness. There is no thirst and usually a coated yellow tongue.
- *Eupatorium Perf* for established flu symptoms that include deep aching in the bones and muscles, where even the skin feels sore, there is weakness with nausea and dizziness, a high fever with accompanying chills and a harsh cough that hurts the chest.
- *Bryonia* for gradual onset flu where everything feels dry – dry cough, dry lips, dry skin, symptoms are worse for any movement, general aching, including the eyes, you are thirsty for large quantities of liquid, but prefer to be left alone.
- *Mercurius* for flu with swollen glands and a very sore throat, often with offensive breath, increased saliva, thick mucus, anxiety and restlessness and symptoms are exacerbated at night.

Preventing flu

The nasal flu mist vaccine (LAIV) is not approved for use by pregnant women. There are studies researching the potential benefits and risks of having a flu vaccine in pregnancy. Some studies suggest a possible risk of developmental defects in the baby if the mother has bad flu in the first trimester of pregnancy. There may be a raised risk of developing leukaemia in later life among people exposed to the virus as babies in the womb. There are also suggestions that women in late pregnancy are more susceptible to the virus. You may want to consult your doctor if you are considering the vaccine.

Natural preventive measures include eating well and avoiding close contact with anyone you know to have flu. If you are in contact, avoid touching your eyes, nose or mouth before you have a chance to wash, and take care to ensure you wash your hands well and regularly.

Injury

See Accidents and first aid, baby.

Insomnia

See Sleep, mother.

Intimacy

See Sex, being intimate.

In-toeing and tibial torsion

Your baby's feet may turn in. In-toeing is commonly caused by a twist in the shin bones (tibial torsion), which will correct itself over time, as walking helps the bones straighten along the line of stress bearing.

In-toeing may also be caused by a twist in the thigh bone or femur ('femoral torsion'). The feet bones remain straight, but the softer ligaments mould more easily and cause the feet to curve inwards. This is usually nothing to worry about – if your baby's feet straighten when you gently hold them in a forward-facing position, they will straighten over time. If they feel stiff or you are concerned, visit your doctor or health visitor.

Occasionally gentle physiotherapy and foot stretching exercises help to loosen them and assist the natural process of straightening. Some one in 3,000 babies are seen by a specialist orthopaedic surgeon who may arrange for special boots or apply plaster casts to the feet to speed the straightening process.

Intrauterine growth restriction (IUGR)

There are two types of low birth weight: being born PREMATURE (early) and intrauterine growth restriction (IUGR). If the exact date of conception is known, IUGR indicates the baby has a weight that would be attained by fewer than 5 per cent of normal babies at that stage of pregnancy. Other terms for IUGR include small for gestational age (period of development in the womb), 'small for dates' and foetal growth restriction. Premature babies may also have IUGR. Many babies with IUGR have a low birth weight of less than 2.5kg (5lb 8oz) after Week 37. Some babies who weigh over 3kg (6lb 8oz) are genetically meant to be bigger – possibly over 4kg (8lb 12oz) – but do, in fact, have IUGR.

During antenatal checks, if your midwife or doctor thinks your baby is small, he or she may refer you for an ultrasound scan. Measurements are considered together with your baby's gestational age and sex and your ethnic origin, weight and height. Some 70 per cent of babies who have IUGR are small and constitutionally healthy; around 28 per cent need intensive monitoring and only 1–2 per cent are severely affected.

Some babies who are suspected of having IUGR are born normal in size and perfectly healthy. Some are genetically small and very healthy. At the same time, some babies with true IUGR remain undetected. This includes babies who are below their potential birth weight. For instance, a baby who is genetically programmed to weigh 4kg (8lb 12oz) at birth and weighs 3kg (6lb 8oz) may not be considered small but will have IUGR.

A baby will usually thrive if IUGR is mild and birth goes ahead without complications and feeding begins soon. But babies with severe IUGR are more susceptible to FOETAL DISTRESS because their energy reserves may be low. With increasingly sophisticated care, it is possible to time birth to minimise this risk. Where IUGR is severe, a baby may require more medical support after birth until feeding has been established and weight gain begins. If a baby is premature and has IUGR, there is a higher chance that special care will be needed.

What happens

The normal pattern of growth during pregnancy can be divided into two main phases. In the first 20 weeks there is rapid division of cells as the building blocks for body and brain are laid down. In the second 20 weeks the rate of cell division slows but the cells enlarge, and after Week 28 fat

and muscle accumulate. Your baby gains over 90 per cent of her weight during the last 20 weeks of pregnancy.

Growth inhibition during the first 20 weeks produces a smaller than usual baby who is said to have symmetrical IUGR – so called, because the growth of the head and body are affected equally. If there are factors inhibiting growth after Week 20, a baby compensates by releasing noradrenaline and selectively diverting blood to the heart, brain and the head, where growth continues. Meanwhile growth of the other organs slows down. This is a phenomenon called the 'brain-sparing effect'. It leads to asymmetrical IUGR where the head is relatively larger than the abdomen. These babies have fewer fat stores and a smaller liver, with lower glycogen stores (so there are lower energy reserves during labour). Ultrasound measurements of the abdomen and head can distinguish between symmetrical and asymmetrical IUGR. Sometimes babies with IUGR have a combination of symmetric and asymmetric growth restriction.

What may cause IUGR

Modern testing can detect IUGR and can often determine the cause, so that complications may be reduced or avoided. However, not all IUGR babies are spotted in pregnancy. Some may only be detected when they are weighed at birth. Medical care increases the chances of a baby reaching her full growth potential.

Maternal health
Your baby's environment for growth in the womb partly depends on your health. Usually a baby is efficient at obtaining all the necessary nutrients, and minor illnesses, including morning sickness, do not have an adverse effect. More intense health problems may have an impact by reducing the efficiency of the placenta and IUGR is more likely.

* If you have already had a baby with significant IUGR, there is a higher risk of recurrence. IUGR may run in families.
* The importance of nutrition in foetal development is undisputed. The current consensus is that low maternal weight before pregnancy, and a gain of less than 10kg (22lb) during pregnancy, is a risk factor. Many studies point to malnutrition or vitamin and mineral

deficiency before conception or in early pregnancy as most significant.

- DRUGS may significantly affect development, and there is a correlation with the type of drug and the amounts consumed. Smoking is probably the most significant cause of IUGR world-wide, perhaps causing as many as 40 per cent of small babies – but alcohol, cocaine, amphetamines and heroin are powerful drugs that affect growth.
- An underlying medical condition may reduce placental efficiency. The most significant are: high BLOOD PRESSURE and severe pre-eclampsia, particularly if the elevated blood pressure was present before conception; blood-clotting disorders (thrombophila) with excess clotting; sickle cell and thalassaemia forms of ANAEMIA, and severe medical disorders requiring intensive medication.

Abnormality of the placenta and blood flow

IUGR may occur when there is a reduction in the function of the placenta, reducing blood flow, oxygen and nutrients to the baby. This may be for one of several reasons:

- If placental cells do not embed deeply enough when they implant and do not invade the arteries in the uterus, this may lead to a reduction in blood volume flowing to the placenta. This is most commonly beyond a mother's control but is more likely to happen if she has poor nutrition or a medical disorder such as high blood pressure.
- IUGR occurs in 15–25 per cent of TWIN pregnancies and is particularly likely with identical twins where one baby receives less blood from the placenta (page 525).
- Placental function may become less efficient if there is significant BLEEDING during pregnancy that leads to placental abruption. This is uncommon but significant.
- Occasionally, the umbilical cord contains a single artery in place of two (page 530): this may result in reduced cord blood flow.

Abnormality in the baby

Some developmental abnormalities reduce growth and lead to symmetrical IUGR, with the head and the body retaining the usual proportions.

- About 5 per cent of IUGR babies have CONGENITAL ABNORMALITIES such as DOWN'S

SYNDROME or heart defects (page 288) or skeletal defects.

- Approximately 10 per cent have restricted growth because of maternal infections in pregnancy, such as RUBELLA, CHICKENPOX or CYTOMEGALOVIRUS. Some infections, such as SYPHILIS and TOXOPLASMOSIS, can be treated during pregnancy.

Action plan

Once IUGR has been confirmed in your baby, your care team will help you plan for the remainder of your pregnancy and for the months that follow. When measurements confirm IUGR, the course of action depends on the extent of growth restriction. Only a minority of IUGR babies are ill. In the majority of cases screening tests confirm the baby is growing well. The lower the weight, the higher the degree of risk. Often, extra vigilance is needed to assess and treat coexisting issues such as infection, twins or high blood pressure.

Detecting and diagnosing IUGR

IUGR can be best diagnosed with ultrasound scans where the date of conception is known. The rate of detection increases progressively beyond Week 20. External estimations detect about 70 per cent of IUGR babies. An external examination may miss an IUGR baby, particularly if a mother is overweight, or mistakenly suspect IUGR, particularly if the date of conception is wrong (and your midwife expects your uterus to be larger when its size is normal for the true dates).

- *Scan 1* (Weeks 12–14) can accurately assess the date of conception. Markers of some congenital abnormalities, such as Down's syndrome, can also be seen.
- *Scan 2* (Weeks 18–22) checks growth. After Week 20, a Doppler ultrasound scan can measure the rate of blood flow in the uterine artery: this may reveal a likelihood of IUGR developing. In most hospitals this is the last routine scan.
- *Scan 3* (Weeks 30–36) can check foetal growth and assess placental function, and can help to distinguish between asymmetrical and symmetrical IUGR and babies who are constitutionally small but healthy. A routine third-trimester scan often detects unsuspected IUGR.

• *Scan 4* (or more) is carried out as necessary to monitor a baby with suspected IUGR. Measurements observe movements and analyse growth of the head and abdomen, the amniotic fluid volume and blood flow in the umbilical and cerebral arteries to check the baby's wellbeing.

Antenatal care

If your baby has IUGR you are likely to be examined more frequently. If she is small but growth is steady and there is no evidence of ill-health, then no extra care is needed, although your baby will continue to be monitored as a high-risk pregnancy. In a minority of severe IUGR cases detected early, an amniocentesis may be offered to check for congenital abnormalities. If the cause of slow growth is treatable (such as high blood pressure or poor nutrition) you may be able to decrease the risk.

Extra care during labour and birth

The majority of babies with mild IUGR have a natural labour and birth. Birth teams are more inclined to recommend a CAESAREAN SECTION at an early stage if there are signs of distress because growth restriction may mean there are lower stores of glycogen to provide energy in labour.

• In labour, it is important to monitor foetal heart rate continuously or frequently in accordance with procedures for a high-risk pregnancy.
• Babies with moderate IUGR may require INDUCTION of labour, particularly if the amniotic fluid volume is reduced (page 375).
• Babies with severe IUGR are more likely to develop foetal distress and asphyxia with low Apgar scores (page 337).
• Severe IUGR may necessitate a caesarean section prior to labour.

After birth

If birth goes without complications and your baby begins feeding soon to boost her blood sugar levels, she is likely to thrive. Your team will be alert for problems related to a low birth weight (below). A paediatrician will assess the IUGR to exclude any underlying problem and provide extra care if necessary.

Potential difficulties after the birth include:

• *Hypothermia.* Low fat reserves and a low capacity for producing heat increase the risk of low body temperature. It is important to keep your baby warm, preferably with skin-to-skin contact, and stay in a warm room.
• *Hypoglycaemia.* A smaller baby may have low sugar stores. If these are not boosted sufficiently after birth, there is a risk of reduced glucose and oxygen to the brain. This can usually be avoided with early feeding, and occasionally with medical support.
• *Polycythaemia.* If an increased number of red blood cells formed because of a reduced concentration of oxygen before the birth, this may lead to JAUNDICE.
• *Prematurity.* If your baby is born early and has IUGR, she may have additional problems if some body systems are immature – usually the lungs and breathing are affected. Assistance and treatment in a SPECIAL CARE BABY UNIT (SCBU) may be the best option.

Growth and development

With good feeding, catch-up growth with weight gain can be rapid (within days), particularly if your baby is born in good condition with asymmetric IUGR. If your baby is genetically small, she will remain small. If the IUGR is severe and if there is an underlying cause, she may remain small. The only way of assessing growth is by monitoring it for a few years after birth.

Except where IUGR is linked with a congenital abnormality or is very severe and began in early pregnancy, small babies tend to develop perfectly normally when given loving attention and good nutrition. Touch, loving contact and frequent feeding in the days and weeks after birth can have a very positive effect on development. Many of the care issues relating to premature babies (page 454) apply to IUGR babies.

The long-term effect depends on how long and how severely nutrition was reduced during crucial stages of brain development. In humans, there is an intense brain growth spurt beginning in mid-pregnancy and continuing until the age of two years. If asymmetric IUGR occurs in the second half of pregnancy, with the 'brain-sparing' effect, there may be no long-term effects on mental development. If there was an underlying cause such as an infection or chromosomal problem or severely reduced placental blood flow, it may affect future development. Conditions that begin early in pregnancy are likely to exert a greater effect. Yet even with severe IUGR most children develop normally.

Behaviour and relationships

A small number of babies whose growth has been severely restricted, where birth weight is below 2.5kg (5lb), may behave differently from babies with normal growth. There will always be big differences from baby to baby, yet with severe growth restriction there is a general pattern of passivity and becoming inconsolably upset. These babies can seem more emotionally volatile, perhaps as a consequence of feeling that some basic needs were not met in pregnancy and/or after birth (page 120). Some show a reduced ability to concentrate during the first year.

Some people comment that IUGR babies 'speak a different language' and some parents and carers find this challenging. It may sometimes feel hard to engage attention and have a normal interaction. Accepting your baby for who she is, whatever feelings she is expressing, rather than seeing her as a 'difficult' baby, might make it easier for you. Vulnerable babies have a higher risk of emotional difficulties if they are not understood and you may need to summon extra patience and effort to enjoy quality time together so you can learn your baby's language and develop a close relationship. The rewards will be considerable for you both and as your baby grows the challenge becomes easier. It is important, for your whole family, to get as much practical and emotional support as possible.

Irritable bowel syndrome (IBS), mother

See also Diarrhoea, mother.

Irritable bowel syndrome (IBS) is a condition where the muscle in the wall of the intestine is hypersensitive (irritable) and contracts frequently, causing abdominal pain and diarrhoea, often associated with bloating and sometimes alternating with constipation. It is exacerbated by emotional upsets and/or by food allergy or intolerance. The condition usually predates pregnancy and often improves but may worsen in pregnancy. It does not affect your baby.

Nevertheless, it can be very upsetting and may be tiring for you if your symptoms persist. As a 'syndrome', IBS involves a number of symptoms and these vary from person to person. Your own symptoms probably vary depending on what's happening in your life (particularly levels of anxiety and stress) and what you are eating.

Action plan

It may be encouraging to have a range of support and advice as you address the triggers for your specific symptoms. A medical diagnosis is usually based on the symptoms and an absence of any signs that might indicate a more serious condition, such as INFLAMMATORY BOWEL DISEASE (IBD).

There may be many things you can do to ease your symptoms, chiefly by identifying triggers and avoiding them. For many women, the key is to reduce stress, and to redress the balance of exercise and rest.

Your body may hold several clues as to some of the triggers, and these may become evident with the skill and insight of one or more complementary therapists. Acupuncture, osteopathy and reflexology may be very helpful, both for unravelling your personal IBS and reducing the severity of your symptoms.

Nutrition is often a key factor. Taking note of what you eat and how you consequently feel, and/or performing a 'food challenge', as you might do when investigating a possible ALLERGY OR INTOLERANCE, may help you identify foods or food combinations that are affecting you. You may want help from a nutritional therapist (page 421) as you do this, and to advise you of ways you can continue to enjoy a fully nutritious diet.

Homeopathy is often very effective, but always needs to be prescribed on an individual basis by a homeopath.

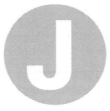

Jaundice, baby

Jaundice is yellowing of the skin and the whites of the eyes. It is caused by a build-up of a yellowish pigment, called bilirubin. In the womb, your developing baby has more red blood cells than he will need after birth. The haemoglobin that these cells contain enables your baby to obtain sufficient oxygen from the transfer across the placenta. After birth, the extra red blood cells are broken down and eliminated. In the process, bilirubin is produced. This is then processed by the liver, in preparation for excretion in the stools.

When bilirubin is produced more quickly than it can be excreted, the pigment is deposited in the skin, the whites of the eyes, and the mucous membranes (such as the inside of the mouth). If this happens, your baby will develop the characteristic yellow-brown colouring of jaundice. This is extremely common: approximately 60 per cent of babies born in the UK develop neonatal jaundice and it is more common among PREMATURE babies. It rarely needs to be treated.

What happens

Jaundice usually develops in the first few days following birth. This is because liver function is temporarily immature and bilirubin is processed slowly. This 'neonatal physiological jaundice' is completely normal. The yellow colour involves the entire skin, peaking after three or four days. It usually passes within seven to 10 days, with no complications, and does not recur. If your baby was premature, he may become jaundiced, and it may not clear for up to two months. Jaundice may be so mild that there is no obvious yellow coloration and it is harder to see in babies with darker skin tones.

Usually a baby is able to deal with the excess bilirubin, but occasionally the level will climb, resulting in hyperbilirubinaemia. If this happens it may lead to an extremely rare, but very serious condition called kernicterus that may affect the baby's brain function (page 329).

Breast milk jaundice

Around 5–10 per cent of breastfed babies remain jaundiced for up to 10 weeks after birth. It is unclear why, although it may be that hormones in breast milk interfere with the breakdown of bilirubin. Jaundice is usually mild, gives your baby a healthy suntanned appearance and does no harm. If you switch to bottle-feeding the jaundice will reduce rapidly, but this is not advisable nor is it necessary for a healthy thriving baby.

If your baby appears to have breast milk jaundice but it is prolonged beyond two weeks, your midwife, doctor or health visitor may request blood tests to confirm that your baby does not have abnormal liver function or biliary atresia (overleaf) or abnormal THYROID FUNCTION. If the condition is not serious enough to warrant treatment, nothing more needs to be done because providing your baby feeds regularly and frequently the bilirubin levels in the blood will fall.

Jaundice resulting from insufficient feeding

Some babies develop jaundice as a result of insufficient calorie and fluid intake, usually in the early days while feeding is being established.

If your baby loses an excessive amount of weight (more than 15 per cent) this may be associated with a high level of jaundice.

Less common causes of jaundice
Many factors can contribute and in the most severe cases, several causes may be present.

* *Blood group incompatibility.* If you and your baby have different blood types (ABO and/or Rhesus) you may produce antibodies capable of destroying your baby's red blood cells. This may overwhelm his ability to break down and excrete bilirubin. When the effect is severe, jaundice may be apparent within a day of birth. In the past, Rhesus incompatibility was a relatively common cause of the most severe form of jaundice but today it is usually prevented (page 67). ABO incompatability (page 67) is not preventable.
* *Premature birth.* If your baby is born before Week 37 he may become jaundiced if his liver is not sufficiently mature to process bilirubin.
* *Breakdown of blood.* Excessive amounts of blood released into muscles or the layers of the scalp from bruising during birth (page 53) may be associated with higher bilirubin levels as healing occurs. This is more common in premature babies.
* *Polycythaemia.* This is characterised by the presence of excessive red blood cells. There are usually no symptoms. Polycythaemia may be associated with INTRAUTERINE GROWTH RESTRICTION (IUGR), smoking in pregnancy and some chromosomal abnormalities. The polycythaemia does not need treatment but the jaundice does (see below).
* *Congenital hypothyroidism.* This one rare condition (page 513) affects approximately one in 4,000 white babies and one in 30,000 black babies and may cause prolonged jaundice because the thyroid gland fails to make thyroid hormone to assist excretion of bilirubin. Treatment focuses on replacement of the thyroid hormone. The diagnosis is based on testing your baby's blood and this is now routinely done on all babies at five days.
* *G6PD deficiency.* This is an inherited disorder more common in families of Asian or Mediterranean origin. The deficiency weakens the red blood cells and makes them break down more readily.

Late jaundice (after two weeks)
Although extremely rare, apparent jaundice in the first month may indicate **biliary atresia,** where the normal connection between the liver and the bowel needs to be surgically corrected. As well as jaundice, this may cause your baby to pass white or colourless stools. Another rare cause of late jaundice is neonatal liver inflammation (HEPATITIS). Both conditions require careful diagnosis and liver testing, and urgent medical treatment.

If your baby appears jaundiced after three months, it is unlikely to be due to bilirubin. A slight yellowy-orange tinge, particularly to the bridge of the nose and palms of the hands, is more often due to an excess of carotenes (naturally occurring red and yellow colours) in the diet. Organic varieties of carrots and peppers seem to have a more marked effect. If you are concerned do visit your doctor.

Action plan

If your baby is jaundiced in the two to four days after birth, ask your midwife to check his weight and arrange for his bilirubin levels to be measured. If the jaundice is due to insufficient calorie or fluid intake, help with latching on and positioning (page 83) may steadily bring your baby's weight up. Most babies clear excess bilirubin without needing treatment. If your baby is unable to eliminate bilirubin sufficiently, simple phototherapy (light therapy) treatment can help clear the excess.

The extent of jaundice is measured with a total serum bilirubin blood test, based on a drop of blood taken from your baby's heel. An alternative method is the transcutaneous bilirubin test that measures bilirubin non-invasively through the skin. This is only reliable in the 10 days after birth. After that time a blood test is required. Your doctor will also check your blood group for ABO and Rhesus incompatibility and assess any other risk factors in your family history or bruising during your baby's birth.

Phototherapy
The most frequently used treatment is phototherapy. This involves exposing your baby's skin to ultraviolet light that has the effect of altering the bilirubin in his bloodstream. The

altered bilirubin is then able to pass into your baby's urine and the level drops rapidly. Phototherapy may be administered through a fibre-optic blanket connected to an ultraviolet light source. If the bilirubin levels are very high, your doctor may feel more intensive phototherapy is required. In that case your baby will be exposed to overhead ultraviolet lights in a warm incubator. To protect his eyes from potential harm he will either wear an eye pad or a tinted head box will cover his head. Your baby's skin appears blotchy under the phototherapy lights because different areas absorb light at different rates.

While your baby is being treated you do not need to be separated: you can feed and care for him as usual. Even if you feed every hour, your baby can be away from the lights while he feeds. You may be advised to feed him more frequently to increase bilirubin excretion. Your baby's bilirubin levels will be measured every eight to 12 hours. When the level drops sufficiently, treatment is discontinued. Intensive or prolonged phototherapy may be needed for ABO incompatibility, prematurity and extensive bruising.

Exchange transfusion

If your baby has severe jaundice that does not respond to phototherapy, he may require an exchange transfusion to reduce the level of bilirubin and prevent the rare but serious complication of brain damage due to kernicterus (below). Exchange transfusion is very rarely needed and most exchanges are carried out for ABO blood group incompatibility problems. The procedure involves removing many small quantities of your baby's blood and replacing them with equal volumes of adult donor blood (not your own). The new blood cells will not break down easily and excess bilirubin production stops. The procedure may take up to six hours and will need to be carried out in the SPECIAL CARE BABY UNIT (SCBU). If bilirubin levels are very high, albumin may also be given to bind the bilirubin.

Homeopathy

There are a number of remedies for neonatal physiological jaundice. It is best to consult with your homeopath who can advise you on treatment for your baby.

▓ KERNICTERUS

Kernicterus is preventable and is thus extremely rare, but when present it may cause brain damage. It results from very high bilirubin levels and the risks rise if your baby is premature or has an infection. Kernicterus is almost unheard of in healthy term babies. Signs include: intense jaundice, sleepiness, weakness, limpness, high-pitched cry. Treatment involves extra fluids by IV infusion, phototherapy, and exchange transfusions.

Kangaroo care

See Touch, skin-to-skin contact.

Knees or elbows that click

If you feel your baby's knees or elbows clicking, don't worry – this is very common and is due to the loose ligaments sliding over the bones. During pregnancy, hormones from your body circulate around your baby's body and soften the ligaments, allowing movement without damage to joints or muscles, necessary for birth. Over six months his ligaments will firm up and the tendency to click will pass. Sometimes a few clicks persist. These are of no consequence at all and can be safely ignored.

Knock knees

When your baby begins to stand up, between eight and 12 months, or when walking begins, his knees may meet and knock together and his ankles may seem far apart. This is knock knees, the medical term for which is femoral anteversion. Children grow out of it except in rare instances. Treatment is very seldom required, but it is sometimes worth consulting an orthopaedic specialist with an interest in children. Osteopathy and physiotherapy may be very helpful if the knock knees are severe.

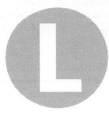

Labour and birth, baby
Being born

Your baby is exquisitely sensitive and aware. In the run-up to labour he prepares for the outside world and sends many signals to you. He plays an active role in helping your cervix to ripen and your uterus to contract and he influences the time of birth. In labour he moves and twists, wakes and sleeps, and experiences a wide range of physical and emotional feelings. Although you cannot control your own baby's experiences, you can offer him a gentle and loving environment for birth and a warm welcome when he arrives.

■ JOURNEY TO BIRTH

Position
Before labour commences, your baby adopts a position that feels comfortable to him. Most babies take a head-down position but there are variations (page 341).

Body feelings in labour
In labour your baby receives a vigorous and stimulating massage. He has been used to feeling your uterus contract for many months but in labour the contractions are more intense. The pressure on his skin awakens his body and prepares him for life outside the womb. It may be soothing but at times he may be alarmed.

Your baby's body plays an active role as he navigates your birth canal. His skull bones overlap to narrow the diameter of his head. His head can tilt and rotate and the neck is very flexible. The rest of the body may actively move

or he may be more passive and respond to your contractions. Typically, it is a combination of these factors.

As labour progresses, your baby feels the downward pressure of your uterus and upward pressure from your cervix and pelvic bones. This is unlikely to be painful for him. A cushion of amniotic fluid lies between his head and your cervix until the waters break and the top of his head is not very sensitive to pain. The skin on his scalp may become swollen with fluid (a 'caput') and this gives extra protection. The pressure from his head as he descends helps your cervix dilate. If the pressure is intense, your baby may have a cervix mark on his head when he is born, and he may feel some discomfort.

When your cervix has opened fully, contractions continue to urge your baby downwards. His head enters the soft space of your vagina. This may be comforting for him, or he may be disturbed by the pressure of the surrounding pelvic bones. It may take minutes or hours for his head to fully enter your vagina, and for his head to 'crown' and become visible as your vaginal lips part.

Hormones and emotional feelings
During labour, your baby produces many different hormones. Some of these facilitate labour and birth, while some are a reaction to what he is experiencing. He may feel invigorated, frightened or tired and his hormonal balance reflects this. Endorphins energise him, help to relieve pain and quell fear. The love hormone oxytocin (page 377) will help him feel good – and may flow most strongly at the moment of birth and straight afterwards when he feels your

skin. If he feels shocked or stressed he'll release adrenaline and cortisol, which help to stabilise his circulation. Babies react strongly to stress.

Your baby will be aware of your heartbeat and your voice, and how you feel – whether afraid, exhilarated, excited, happy, tired – is communicated to him by the hormones that filter to him from your blood. You also communicate by your body movements, the food you eat, the power and tone of your voice and how you feel emotionally. Many people believe babies are less anxious if their mothers are calm during pregnancy and labour. Your feelings do have an influence but your baby will not necessarily mimic you.

Waking, sleeping

During labour, your baby will spend some time asleep and some time awake and alert. Sometimes he may fall into a deep and pleasant sleep or wriggle and kick and try to move with the downward pressure he feels.

Birth

Your baby will feel the pressure of your uterus and of your bearing down. As his head is born your vaginal lips may feel tight, or soft. He will then sense the difference in temperature and feel air on his skin. This is a natural stimulus that causes him to take a breath, although this may not come instantly. He might remain quiet and calm, or open his mouth wide and cry. He will feel hands on his head if your midwife assists him. First one shoulder, then the other, and then the rest of his body emerge. If your baby is born in water he will sense a different feeling on his skin but the change in temperature occurs at the surface of the water. He will react to the air by drawing a breath.

▓ AFTER BIRTH

There is often an astounding shift in energy as mum and dad come out of the focused space of labour and birth and give their attention to their baby. The ideal for your baby is to feel the warm and loving contact of you, to feel welcomed and safe. Every birth is unique and you and your baby will come together after birth in the way that works best for you both. Some mums immediately bring their babies to their abdomen

or breast. Some gently explore their baby with their hands for some moments before getting closer. Your position for birth, the length of the umbilical cord and your baby's condition all influence how quickly you make close contact. Your midwives are important here: it is considered 'best practice' to help mum and baby be together, skin to skin, as soon as possible. The benefits of this intimacy are far reaching for your baby and for you (page 517).

At birth, some babies are calm and serene and begin to breathe with ease. Others cry and there are a small number who are shocked and require assistance to begin breathing. Once breathing is established, babies often stay awake and alert for an hour or two. This is precious time for exploration and bonding. Your baby is able to focus clearly at a distance of 25–30cm (10–12in), so she can watch your face as you hold her at your breast. It is comforting for her to smell, hear and see you, and within hours she will recognise your face. She already knows the sound of your voice and heartbeat.

Your newborn will be fully conscious and flooded by new feelings. You may be surprised that she is so present and communicative. The emotional energy that passes between babies and parents is usually intense. She may try to copy your facial expressions and you will also unconsciously mimic her by slowing your pace and mirroring her expression. Your baby can communicate expertly to get your attention and you are naturally programmed to focus on her from the moment of birth. The first hours of contact with you are very important for your baby and the ideal is for her to feel held and safe, with dim lights and soft touch, and to suckle at your breast if she wishes to. If contact between you is delayed for any reason, you can take the opportunity to be close and enjoy precious intimacy when one or both of you has received medical support and reassurance.

Breathing and crying

At birth, contact with the air stimulates the breathing reflex and your baby takes her first breath. Not all babies cry at birth. The lungs need to inflate but some babies do this without crying. Crying is also an expression of emotion and a vocal greeting. Your baby is so driven to connect with you she will begin a conversation as soon as you meet, and if she doesn't do this with her voice, she will do it through eye contact, touch and BREASTFEEDING.

As your baby's lungs expand, air displaces the liquid that filled them in the womb, the pressure changes and there is a release of prostaglandin hormones. This combination closes the channels from the umbilical cord and assists the circulation of oxygenated blood via the lungs around her body. Until the placenta separates from your uterus or the cord is clamped, your baby has a back-up system of oxygen. When she adapts to breathing air, her lips change from blue to pink. The midwives will be watching to see that the rest of her body takes on a pink colour within a few minutes. Her hands and feet may remain a little blue, not from lack of oxygen, but because her circulation there is naturally sluggish.

If you have given birth in an upright position, your baby will have been born head downwards, which helps mucus and amniotic fluid to drain naturally away and clear her passages for breathing. To help this process, your midwife may lie her face down on a towel immediately after birth, or you may lie her on your tummy and stroke her back gently. It is not necessary to routinely apply suction to the nose and mouth but if your baby needs assistance to establish breathing, it will be at hand (page 252).

Appearance

Your baby's skin will be covered or dabbed with vernix, a white creamy substance that protects and moisturises her in the womb, and there may be traces of blood. Her skin may be wrinkled and very pink. A few babies are born with spotty faces, a neo-natal acne resulting from blocked sebaceous glands. And because your baby's skull bones are soft and overlap during birth and the scalp skin may be swollen, her head may appear squeezed or even conical in shape.

If your baby's breasts seem a little puffy this is normal, minor stimulation resulting from hormones, and soon recedes. Your baby's genitals may also appear swollen. Again this is a hormonal effect, and in girls may result in a small amount of blood or vaginal discharge being passed during the first few days.

All these features will begin to recede in the first hours. Her spine will stretch and extend and her body will gradually unfurl. She will do this in her own time. If she enjoys stretching she may like to lie naked on you, with her body touching yours and her spine stretched out. Some babies prefer to flex and draw their hands and feet up and enjoy being held tightly.

Your baby's skin becomes less wrinkled, a process which may take some weeks, and you may notice peeling, which is a reaction to air. Gentle MASSAGE with pure vegetable oil can ease dryness. The head shape changes and although a baby's forehead always looks quite large, any cone-effect will be gone in two days.

Newborn check

Your midwife observes your baby's colour and breathing at birth according to criteria in the Apgar test (page 337), and again after five minutes. Later, usually within 72 hours, your baby will be given a more extensive examination by a paediatrician or a specially trained midwife. Part of the observation will include checking your baby's reflexes. These are listed on page 338.

Breastfeeding

Your baby has a powerful reflex to suckle and can locate your breast by its scent within minutes of birth. Your body responds by releasing rich, sweet colostrum (page 82). It is full of calories and is thought to be more powerful than morphine as a pain reliever and comforter.

Some babies turn very soon to the breast and others wait a while. If you are both well and relaxed, you can try the first feed within minutes of giving birth. This first feed is as much about contact as nutrition. It stimulates a flood of love hormones for you and your baby that help you feel loved and connected. First contact at the breast may last for an hour or more and after this you and your baby may fall into a deep sleep for several hours.

Washing and dressing

Your midwife may give your baby a light wash, if this is your wish. The wash can be gentle to remove traces of blood without removing the protective creamy vernix on her skin. The vernix is a natural moisturiser that you can gently rub into her body. Your midwife may offer to dress your baby. Most babies are warmest and most comfortable held skin to skin but it is also comforting to be held close in soft, natural fabric clothes. When you need to rest or wish to bathe, your baby's dad can hold her skin to skin or in her soft clothes.

If labour or birth is difficult
Every baby has a unique experience of birth.You cannot predict your baby's reaction. The entry on page 331 explores the range and gives advice if your baby finds the birth difficult. Whatever your baby's experience, loving care and frequent contact and feeding are some of the keys to helping her thrive and feel safe.

■ CUTTING THE UMBILICAL CORD

The umbilical cord that your baby has been touching and stroking in the womb pulsates after birth, giving a double lifeline and source of oxygen until he can breathe normally. When he is born, his umbilical cord remains attached to the placenta. Blood continues to flow through the cord for three minutes or more, and when this stops the cord stops pulsating and it becomes white and flaccid.

Late cutting and clamping of the cord is fine for your baby and is the most natural thing for him. It allows time for breathing to be established, and blood flow from the placenta to your baby is beneficial. It also delays separation of mother and baby after birth.

You may choose to cut the cord after it has stopped pulsating, or after the placenta has been born. It is safe for your baby to rest on your tummy, or in your arms and to feed before you clamp and cut the cord. The exception is if your baby has difficulty in establishing breathing. In this case, the cord will be cut and your baby taken to be given oxygen and resuscitation, if this is needed.

Delayed clamping and cutting
Delaying clamping and cutting of the cord allows blood to leave the placenta and enter your baby's circulation. His blood volume can rise by around 20 per cent if cord clamping is delayed by three minutes or more. This appears to be important in giving baby a store of red cells that can be broken down to release iron for future cell production and growth. Even in a newborn

needing medical care, there is often 60 seconds available for blood to flow before the cord is cut and clamped. This increases haemoglobin concentration, which reduces likelihood of ANAEMIA in the next six months.

The haemoglobin may give your baby ruddy coloured, healthy looking skin. While the cord is still pulsating it is best for your baby to be on your tummy or between your legs (less than 10cm (4in) above or below the placenta, which is still in your womb), as this encourages the blood to flow to his body from the placenta.

If you require an oxytocin injection to help you deliver the placenta (page 391) it is considered safe to delay the injection and clamping of the cord for one to three minutes, while the blood leaves the placenta. When the injection has been given it is safest to clamp the cord to prevent the drug entering your baby's circulation.

Early clamping
In some cases, it is preferable to clamp and cut the cord before it stops pulsating of its own accord. If the cord is wound tightly round the baby's neck or breathing does not begin and resuscitation is needed the cord will be clamped and cut soon so that he can be given extra oxygen. There are occasions when a baby is distressed and the birth team decides external oxygen under pressure is better than cord oxygen.

Prematurity
If your baby is born prematurely and does not need immediate assistance to breathe, delayed cord clamping is safe. Compared with immediate clamping it is associated with fewer blood transfusions in the first six weeks after birth.

Clamping and then cutting the cord
The cord is first clamped with a plastic clip and then cut about 2–3cm (1in) from your baby's body. He will be totally unaware of the process since there are no nerve endings in the cord. The site will heal naturally over the next 10 days – the old cord will drop off, and a neat belly button will remain. The shape of your baby's belly button and whether it faces inward or outward has nothing to do with the way the cord is cut. Many fathers enjoy the symbolism of releasing and welcoming the baby by cutting the cord after it has been clamped.

Special procedures

Sometimes the umbilical cord is used for special procedures if there are health concerns. The umbilical cord arteries or vein can be sampled to check the wellbeing of your baby after birth. Catheters can be inserted to allow samples to be taken and drugs and fluids to be administered.

■ EFFECTS OF BIRTH

Your baby may emerge with serenity and remain calm and relaxed; or he may cry and appear tense. After a difficult birth some babies appear calm and ready to take on the world with great energy; others are upset and find it difficult to settle. There is a greater likelihood of shock and stress if there has been FOETAL DISTRESS or intervention (such as FORCEPS), although there are no rules and many babies are extremely resilient. Some babies who have had an apparently easy birth may be fractious and irritable.

Your own baby's reaction will depend on his unique personality. This is partly due to what he experienced in pregnancy, but the way he feels with you and others after the birth is also significant. Being with you is important, and if your baby is separated from you after birth he may become anxious (page 220).

All babies have an intense need for loving care in the weeks after birth, and whatever feelings your baby expresses it is ideal for him to feel welcomed and accepted, fed when he asks, and reassuringly and lovingly held. If he has been put under stress, for whatever reason, levels of stress hormones rise. Yet he is able to pass from one state to another rapidly and feelings of stress may be replaced by feelings of safety, love, playfulness and bonding when he is in your arms. Kangaroo care, which allows prolonged and comfortable skin-to-skin contact (page 518), is known to reduce stress hormones in a baby's circulation, and your baby will feel reassured when you take his feelings seriously (page 209).

Some babies take time to let go of tension and need weeks or months of sensitivity and loving permission to express their feelings and let go. Your baby may do this most easily by spending time with you, and perhaps with extra care (such as osteopathy following forceps delivery). If your baby requires ongoing care after birth (page 497), he will benefit enormously from your attention and physical presence and the intimacy of skin-to-skin contact, if this is possible in your unique situation.

Labour and birth, baby
Breech baby

See Labour and birth, baby, position.

Labour and birth, baby
Checks during labour

The safety of your baby is a priority for your midwife, and there is a range of ways in which she will monitor him. She will check your baby's size and position, and the volume of AMNIOTIC FLUID when she examines you. If the membranes have ruptured, the volume and colour of the amniotic fluid are noted. She will also review your record of pregnancy and note previous scan and blood test results. If her assessment confirms your baby is healthy and at low risk, your midwife will re-assess the situation intermittently through labour. If there is an increased risk of problems, or a cause for concern arises, your baby will be monitored more intensively.

What happens

In labour, one of the main indicators of your baby's wellbeing is any alteration in his heart rate, as measured on an electronic foetal heart monitor, for example. This is because oxygen affects the sensitive heart muscle, as well as the HORMONES and nerves that originate in the brain and control the heart, and so any disruption in oxygen supply to the baby will be reflected in the heart rate.

Your midwife will check a number of features in the heart pattern:

- The average or baseline rate (normal: 110–160 per minute).
- The variation from one beat to the next (normal: greater than 10 per minute). If your baby is healthy, the heart rate varies from beat to beat. In distress, this variability reduces.
- Decelerations or drops in the rate, which are normally absent or may occur early in a contraction.
- Accelerations during foetal movements (normally greater than 10 beats per minute).

335

Variations from the normal rhythm may occur during baby's sleep or may suggest your baby is in FOETAL DISTRESS.

Electronic CTG monitoring

An electronic foetal heart monitor, also known as a cardiotocograph (CTG), assesses your baby's heartbeat and shows the pattern and intensity of your contractions. The monitor uses ultrasound. It gives a numerical read-out and traces a graph on paper. You can lie or sit or rest on all fours with the transducer strapped in place on your abdomen. The belt rarely causes discomfort and doesn't impede kneeling or squatting.

Initial monitoring may continue for around 20 minutes. Depending on the progress of your labour, you may be monitored in this way at intervals, or if there is concern or you have a full epidural, continuously. Alternatively, your midwife will assess your contractions by feeling your abdomen and watching your movements and your breathing, and she can listen to your baby's heart with a hand-held monitor.

Hand-held monitors

Small hand-held ultrasound monitors allow you to hear the heart rate without a graphic record. These are ideal during an active birth and can be used under water. Midwives usually check the heartbeat every 15 to 30 minutes early in labour. In the second stage, your midwife may listen more frequently, often after each contraction, because if the umbilical cord is around your baby's neck it may tighten. The tones of a normal heartbeat may be reassuring while you enjoy the natural force of labour; or you may not notice the monitor being placed on your body.

Internal monitoring

Very rarely, when an external monitor cannot detect the heartbeat accurately (usually in women with a thick abdominal wall), an electrode needs to be placed on the baby's scalp to obtain an electrical signal of the heartbeat. If the membranes have not already ruptured, they will have to be broken. The insertion probably causes a baby momentary pain similar to the discomfort from a blood test. Internal monitoring should not be done if you carry the HEPATITIS or HIV virus because viral particles may be transferred to your baby. Very

occasionally, a baby may develop a bacterial infection at the site of the puncture.

Accuracy of monitoring

Your baby's heart rate pattern provides an indication of health but it is only one index, so it is assessed in conjunction with the other clinical signs. Monitoring the heartbeat is not 100 per cent reliable. Sometimes there are variations but a baby is born fit and well. Occasionally a baby without variations requires breathing assistance after birth. Some women prefer to keep monitoring to a minimum to reduce distractions. Others are reassured to know all is well as labour progresses. Many advantages are offered by monitoring a baby's heartbeat, but there is a downside: some extra CAESAREAN SECTIONS are performed because of the pattern shown by the CTG trace. Newer computer-assisted monitors are being tested and show promise for more accuracy in the future.

Action plan

Your birth team will tell you if the heartbeat is normal. If there is a variation, they will make suggestions according to the pattern and your stage of labour.

No reading or very high and very low numbers

This usually indicates that the transducer placed on your abdomen has slipped. If this happens your midwife will adjust it and reassure you that your baby's heart is still beating normally.

Alterations in the CTG

If the baseline rate is above 160 or below 110 beats per minute, or there is less variation from beat to beat and few accelerations, this could indicate foetal distress.

Early deceleration occurs when the heart rate drops at the beginning of a contraction and rises by the end. It indicates pressure on the head of the baby and is not usually a sign of distress. Late deceleration occurring after a contraction or variable deceleration between contractions may indicate reduced flow of blood (and oxygen) to your baby.

In some hospitals, if there is a concern about foetal distress, you may be offered foetal scalp sampling to accurately assess your baby. The sample of your baby's blood is taken by inserting a speculum, similar to one used in taking a cervical smear, and pricking the scalp skin with a needle. The oxygen and acid–alkaline balance is then analysed on a machine. If the oxygen levels are normal, your baby does not have foetal distress at the time of sampling. This increases the accuracy of CTG monitoring of the foetal heart rate.

To correct the CTG pattern, it may be a simple case of getting you to move from your back to your side to increase blood flow to the placenta. In addition, your midwife may increase your fluids, particularly if you have been given an epidural, or reduce the dose of oxytocin if this is being administered to boost your contractions.

If the pattern indicates foetal distress, your medical team will take all factors into account, including the existing heart rate readings, your baby's condition in pregnancy, and your progress in labour. If your baby was healthy in pregnancy and birth is not delayed, the apparent foetal distress may have no effect. Alternatively, intervention may be needed to speed up the birth and reduce risks for your baby of reduced oxygen flow.

Labour and birth, baby
Checks following birth

As part of your baby's welcome into the world, a quick and simple examination is needed to assess her condition. Your midwife will be able to do this within the first minute of birth, while handing your baby to you.

■ THE APGAR TEST

The Apgar test is actually named after Dr Virginia Apgar and it also serves as a handy acronym: APGAR. The examination checks for **A**ppearance, **P**ulse, **G**rimace, **A**ctivity and **R**espiration. The result of the test is recorded with a number between 0 and 10. If your baby scores seven or more this indicates that she is off to a good start. If the result is below five extra attention and possibly breathing assistance will be needed. Traditionally, the Apgar test is carried out 60 seconds after birth and again five minutes later. Often babies needing breathing assistance or stimulation at birth may score low at 60 seconds but score eight or more after five minutes. If there is no improvement on a low initial score, your baby will need extra attention (page 250).

■ NEONATAL PAEDIATRIC CHECKS

After you and your partner have greeted and cuddled your baby, and she has suckled, the midwife will examine her and record weight, length and head measurements. This can wait up to one hour. The weighing process is very quick and you can hold your baby while her head and length are measured.

Within 24 hours, a more detailed check is carried out by a specially trained midwife or a paediatrician, or your GP if you have given birth at home. The midwife will check:

The APGAR Test			
Sign	**0 points**	**1 point**	**2 points**
Appearance (*Colour*)	pale or blue	body pink, extremities blue	pink
Pulse (per minute) (*Heartbeat*)	not detectable	below 100	over 100
Grimace (*Reflex irritability*)	no response to stimulation	grimace	lusty cry
Activity (*Muscle tone*)	flaccid (weak or no activity)	some movement of extremities	a lot of activity
Respiration (*Breathing*)	none	slow, irregular	good (crying)

- weight – and plot it on a chart;
- length of the body;
- head shape, size and circumference and fontanelles to ensure normal brain development;
- reflexes related to the nervous system, including stepping and placing (below);
- size, shape and movement of your baby's eyes and a check of the retina at the back of the eye;
- nose and ears, for size and shape, and mouth and palate;
- heart, circulation and breathing pattern;
- nipples and breasts;
- abdomen, for kidney or liver enlargement;
- genitals: in boys to ensure the testes are descended and the penis is normally formed, in girls to inspect the labia;
- hips, for congenital dislocation, and limb and muscle tone.

After six to eight days, a heel prick test is carried out. Also known as the Guthrie or PKU test, this involves removing a small sample of blood from the heel. The blood is tested to check for inherited problems, such as PHENYLKETONURIA and THYROID and haemoglobin function.

A second baby check is usually carried out by your GP at six weeks. This is particularly important to check the hips and weight gain.

▨ REFLEXES AT BIRTH

The 'primitive' reflexes with which your baby is born help him to communicate with you and to get his needs met, and to develop optimally, while his nervous system is developing. Each reflex will at some stage change or disappear when it is replaced by coordinated development, such as chewing and voluntary swallowing, rolling over, walking and fine balance. By observing the baby's reflexes a skilled paediatrician can monitor progress and detect problems early. Absent or weak reflexes can be caused by BIRTH TRAUMA, medications or illness. In babies with damage to the brain, the normal changes do not happen, or they are more pronounced on one side or the other. Some of your baby's reflexes – such as his reflex to breathe – are evident at birth, checked as part of her Apgar assessment (page 337).

Gasp reflex

This is the reflex to gasp for air and begin breathing. The triggers are the temperature change at birth and changes in cord blood oxygen, carbon dioxide or acid levels. Typically, the gasp reflex is triggered at birth. Rarely, and usually when there has been FOETAL DISTRESS, the reflex to gasp starts before birth, and may cause a baby to breathe in liquid in the womb. This can lead to breathing difficulties at birth which may necessitate extra care (page 253).

Rooting reflex

This is the reflex to turn to your breast and feed. You may notice it first when you hold your baby to your breast, and touch his cheek lightly with your nipple. It can also be triggered by the light touch of your hand on his cheek. Your baby may trigger it himself by brushing his face with his hands. He can relax easily when held close or kangarooed (page 518). This reflex is gone by about four months.

Sucking reflex

This reflex is strongly developed in the womb when your baby sucks on his hands and fists, and is important after birth for BREASTFEEDING. It is slowly replaced by voluntary sucking at roughly three months after birth. Babies who are tube-fed beyond this age may have problems making the transition to voluntary feeding, as the reflex persists.

Startle reflex

The startle reflex causes your baby to thrust his arms outward with his fingers extended, and then curl his fingers and draw his arms in towards his body when he is startled. It is also called the 'Moro reflex'. A paediatrician may check it by letting his head fall gently. You may see it if he is startled by a loud noise, a sudden movement, or if you let go of head support. The reflex slowly and progressively disappears by about three months of age. Persistence beyond four to six months is associated with nervous system disorders.

Palmar grasp

When you touch the palm of your baby's hand, his fingers will curl around your finger. This is the palmar grasp and it reflects your baby's primal need for safety and contact. Because of this reflex, it is often difficult to obtain handprints until about four to six months when it disappears.

Plantar grasp
When you stroke the sole of your baby's foot his toes will spread open and his foot will turn slightly inward with the big toe pointing upwards. This is the plantar grasp, also known as the 'Babinski reflex'. By the end of the first year this reflex is usually gone. Persistence beyond 12 months makes walking difficult.

Stepping reflex
If you hold your baby and place his feet on a flat surface, he will 'walk' by placing one foot in front of the other. This is also known as the 'crossed extensor response'. This isn't walking as such, as your newborn has neither the strength nor co-ordination to walk, and should disappear by about six months of age.

Tonic neck reflex
When you lay your baby on his back and his head turns to one side he will extend his arm and leg on that side while the opposite arm and leg bend, assuming a 'fencing' position – hence this is also called the 'fencing reflex'. This reflex is present until about the fourth month. In order to roll over, the reflex needs to disappear, and in babies with nervous system problems the persistence of the reflex can be an early clue to future difficulties.

Diving reflex
In the rare occurrence of even a single drop of water reaching the back of your baby's throat, receptors stimulate the 'dive reflex', which closes the airways and prevents breathing. This reflex also slows the heart rate and diverts blood away from the hands and feet, making your baby look a bit blue. It can also be triggered by water or cold air on the face. The reflex ensures safety during a water birth (page 351) but cannot ensure safety if a baby is submerged in water in the days, weeks or months after birth. A baby can drown in just 2cm (¾in) of water.

Labour and birth, baby
Cord compression and prolapse

See also Foetal distress and asphyxia.

Oxygen and other nutrients are passed from you through the placenta and the umbilical cord to your baby. If there is cord compression or it is prolapsed (displaced downwards), the blood flow is reduced and this may lead to foetal distress and asphyxia with low oxygen flow to your baby. With modern obstetric care and close monitoring (page 336), early warning signs help to increase safety for babies. The treatment of significant prolonged cord compression is to deliver the baby urgently.

What happens
The umbilical cord is well protected:
- The cord has two arteries wrapped around a vein and protected in a substance called Wharton's jelly, allowing the vessels to remain open. The cord is covered with a skin that allows it to slide and prevents it being trapped between the baby's head and your pelvis.
- The cord is usually long enough to prevent the vessels being stretched and narrowed if it is round the neck as your baby descends during the birth.
- Adequate amniotic fluid protects the cord from being compressed by your baby's head or shoulder.

If the umbilical cord is compressed and there is a reduction in blood flow to your baby this may be evident with a deceleration pattern on the foetal heart monitor.

The effect of the compression depends on a number of factors:
- The strength and maturity of your baby. A full term mature baby who has been well nourished in pregnancy can withstand reduced blood flow for longer.
- The duration and intensity of the cord compression. If the compression is intermittent and your baby has good stores of glycogen and glucose she can draw on these for cell nutrition while oxygen is reduced.

- A complete stoppage of oxygen for longer than 10 minutes, or less time for a baby with severe IUGR, may have long term effects from asphyxia.

Cord compression happens in roughly 10 per cent of deliveries and is usually intermittent, so that oxygen reduction does not cause foetal distress. If compression is not intermittent it is more dangerous.

A prolapsed umbilical cord is rare. This is when a loop of the umbilical cord is between the baby's body and the cervix before the head engages. If this is the case and the membranes rupture before the head has engaged the cord can slip ('prolapse') through the cervix. The main risk then is cord compression from the pressure of your baby's head as it descends, and this may reduce blood and oxygen flow. If the cord protrudes from your vagina, rough handling or exposure to air can cause spasm of the blood vessels and reduce blood flow to your baby, which is dangerous.

+ Red flag

If your waters break you need to contact your midwife immediately. If antenatal checks have discovered that your baby's head is high, she is in a breech position or you have an excess of amniotic fluid, or labour is premature, it is even more important that you are examined immediately.

If the cord does prolapse and it can be felt in your vagina this is an **emergency**.
- You need an ambulance to get you to hospital.
- Remain on all fours with your knees towards your chest to slow your baby's descent and reduce the pressure of his head on your cervix. Your midwife may hold your baby's head up by inserting her fingers into your vagina until a caesarean can be performed.
- If the cord is exposed she will replace it back into your vagina – you need to do this if it becomes exposed before medical help arrives.

Umbilical cord accidents are more likely to occur in late pregnancy and, particularly, in labour. A cord accident is more likely to cause foetal

distress and asphyxia for a baby who is already at increased risk. For example:
- If the umbilical cord is short or wound tightly around a baby's neck. Babies frequently have the cord around the neck, but if it is not pulled tight it is insignificant.
- If the amniotic fluid volume is low, particularly with growth restriction (IUGR) or POSTMATURITY. The risk rises after the membranes rupture and in labour.
- If the umbilical cord has prolapsed. Prolapse is more common if a baby is PREMATURE, breech or transverse lie (page 345) or if there is an excess of amniotic fluid.

Action plan

If your baby is at risk of cord prolapse, then intensive antenatal surveillance and early examination in labour are able to detect the problem early if it occurs. In labour, if your baby is at risk of cord compression, foetal heart monitoring will be intensified. Compression may occur in low risk pregnancies and this is the reason heartbeat is monitored routinely. As your contractions intensify and your baby moves down in the second stage the team will be alert to the risk of the cord tightening around your baby's neck.

If there are signs of compression from your baby's heart rate:
- A caesarean section may be needed if labour has not begun or birth is still a long way off.
- If you are in the second stage of labour the midwife may encourage you to squat and push or recommend the use of FORCEPS OR VENTOUSE to speed up the birth.
- Most babies recover easily, sometimes with resuscitation after birth. Some babies who are born with a tight cord around the neck can be red faced and this usually resolves over a few days. Your baby's reaction depends on the extent of oxygen deprivation and whether foetal distress was present (page 249).

Labour and birth, baby
Engaged and non-engaged head

Your baby's head will be engaged when the widest part (level with the ears) enters your pelvic brim. With your first baby this will probably happen some time after Week 36. In a second or subsequent pregnancy, engagement often does not occur until labour begins. If your baby's head is not engaged before labour, there is probably no cause for concern but non-engagement signifies the need for extra surveillance.

What happens

When your midwife or doctor feels your abdomen, if they can feel more than three-fifths of your baby's head above your pelvic brim, it is not engaged. You may be aware of this if you feel your baby pushing up under your ribs.

Your baby's head may not be engaged for a number of reasons:

* The most likely cause is that the ligaments supporting your uterus and cervix are attached high up to your pelvic bones and your baby's head will only be able to descend when your cervix has dilated fully. The head will then descend, unless your pelvis is too small disproportion.
* If your baby is large (page 396), or your pelvis is small, or both, the head cannot enter the pelvis (cephalo pelvic disproportion). In this instance 'five-fifths' of your baby's head may be felt when your abdomen is examined.
* Your baby may be in an awkward position, usually occipito posterior (page 344).
* Your baby may stay high if there is an excess of AMNIOTIC FLUID or PLACENTA PRAEVIA.

Action plan

In most pregnancies, the head will engage in labour and normal birth follows. Sometimes labour may need to be stimulated to assist progress. Each person is different and your midwife and obstetrician will advise you on the best course of action for your baby's safety.

* If your ligaments hold the cervix high, there is nothing to do but wait for labour. Contractions will probably encourage your baby's head to descend when your cervix is fully dilated.
* Excessive amniotic fluid is not treatable but if the membranes rupture before labour begins (page 391) you will need to be seen urgently, because these conditions increase the chance of umbilical cord prolapse (page 339), which may cause FOETAL DISTRESS.
* If your baby is large or if your pelvis is very small, you cannot do much to remedy the

situation. Depending on the extent of disproportion, you may be monitored closely and advised to have a CAESAREAN SECTION if labour is prolonged.

* If your baby is in an awkward position after Week 36, particularly occipito posterior, then attending to your POSTURE and doing YOGA may help optimal positioning. During labour, the power of contractions may help your baby's head to rotate and negotiate the birth canal. If the malpresentation continues, the birth may need assistance with FORCEPS OR VENTOUSE. A minority of women will require a caesarean section to give birth safely.
* If you are having your second or subsequent baby, your midwife will examine you to detect the size of your baby and the amniotic fluid volume. The head usually engages in labour.

Labour and birth, baby
Foetal distress and asphyxia

See Foetal distress and asphyxia.

Labour and birth, baby
Position

The way your baby is positioned in the womb has a major effect on the way labour progresses. Between Weeks 32 and 36 of pregnancy, most babies settle into the occipito anterior position (head down towards the cervix and back towards mum's belly – see page 344). Sometimes a baby may lie in a way that may make the birth process more difficult. Occasionally there is a clear reason for this, but often it seems a baby simply prefers the position he feels comfortable in. Your midwife will check your baby's position.

Optimal foetal positioning

Your posture and activity in pregnancy may affect your baby and there is a school of thought that suggests a mother's actions can encourage 'optimal foetal positioning' – that is the occipito anterior position. The main advice is to be mindful of your POSTURE. Avoid slouching. Sitting upright may encourage your baby's spine to face forwards. Exercise and good muscle tone also help, and if you attend a YOGA class your teacher may suggest several postures that are thought to assist good positioning. You are not solely responsible though, as your baby actively chooses which position feels best.

If your baby is not in the optimal occipito anterior position your doctor may refer to 'malpresentation'. A less usual position is not always a problem but it can contribute to difficulty in labour.

▨ BREECH POSITION

In around 3 per cent of pregnancies, the baby's buttocks are down and will be born before the head. This is a breech position. There are various types of breech:

- *Frank breech.* This is the most common, where both hips are flexed, the knees are at the level of the baby's nipples and the feet are by the head.
- *Complete breech.* Here the knees and feet are both flexed and the feet tucked under the buttocks as if the baby is squatting on the inlet to the mother's pelvis. At birth, the buttocks and feet emerge at the same time.
- *Footling breech.* In this case, one or two feet are lower than the buttocks, as if the baby is standing at the pelvic inlet and one or both legs are born before the buttocks. In this situation there is a risk of umbilical cord prolapse (downward displacement) alongside the leg when the membranes rupture.

What happens

It seems that some factors contribute in a minority of breech babies:

- Prematurity or a small growth restricted (IUGR) baby.
- TWINS.
- Excess AMNIOTIC FLUID (polyhydramnios) that allows the baby to move around freely.
- In placenta praevia (page 442), the placenta is low and prevents the baby's head from engaging in the pelvis.
- An unusually shaped uterus, usually a bicornute (heart shape), may make a baby's head more comfortable in the upper part.
- CONGENITAL ABNORMALITY of the baby's limbs or spine is a very rare cause. This is usually detected by a mid-pregnancy ultrasound scan.

Turning a baby

If your baby is still breech after Week 34, you will be given a clinical examination and an ultrasound scan may be suggested to exclude the above causes. Many babies turn in the last four weeks before labour, particularly in a second or third pregnancy, or where there is a lot of amniotic fluid. You may be happy to accept your baby's position and have no desire to influence it. If you are keen to have a vaginal birth without the risks associated with breech birth, there are several options that may encourage your baby to turn.

Exercises

There are exercises that can encourage a baby to turn and will do no harm. Kneel on the floor with your knees and legs wide apart and your buttocks in the air. Place your forearms on the floor with your hands on your elbows and rest your head on your forearms. Keep your buttocks in the air for three to five minutes with your pelvis higher than your head. This will encourage the breech (buttocks) to disengage from your pelvis and the head may turn. You may repeat the exercise twice a day.

Acupuncture

ACUPUNCTURE has been used with good effect for centuries. The treatment can begin from around Week 30. It involves moxibustion (page 14) applied to an acupuncture point on the outer side of the little toe with an acupuncture needle or by holding it 2cm (¾in) from the skin until the area is warm. The point may also be stimulated with acupressure by massaging the outer part of the little toe two or three times a day for a minute or two. The treatment is repeated on alternate days and you can even do it yourself. Professional treatment is preferable, however, and may involve stimulating additional points.

Homeopathy

Pulsatilla is one remedy used to turn breech babies. *Pulsatilla* is usually prescribed around Week 34 or 35. It is not advisable to self-prescribe so consult your homeopath who may advise using the remedy in conjunction with acupuncture and EXERCISE.

Medical care

Your obstetrician may attempt external cephalic version (ECV), which involves gentle manipulation and massage of your abdomen. The procedure is usually performed after Week 36, when the risks of prematurity have passed and the baby has had time to turn spontaneously. This technique is successful in over 60 per cent of cases.

* First, an ultrasound scan assesses the size and condition of your baby and the amniotic fluid volume. If there is a reduction in the volume of the amniotic fluid or any sign of intrauterine growth restriction (IUGR), then an ECV will not be recommended. If you have had a caesarean section in the past your doctor may not be keen to perform an ECV.
* The scan is often used during the turning and the obstetrician will be watching for changes in your baby's heart rate that may indicate tension on the umbilical cord or disturbance of the placenta that could lead to a placental abruption. These risks are very low but, if they occur, FOETAL DISTRESS may follow.
* In some hospitals, during ECV, a drug is given to relax the wall of the uterus. It is usually done on the labour ward.
* Your baby's heartbeat will be monitored immediately after the procedure using a cardiotocograph (CTG) in case there are signs of foetal distress. If this happens an immediate caesarean section is essential.
* Once turned, most babies remain in a head-down position. The baby may turn back into breech position if there is an excess of amniotic fluid or it is not the first pregnancy and there is more room in the uterus for the baby to move.

Giving birth

If your baby remains in a breech position at term, the risk of significant birth asphyxia or injury occurring in a vaginal birth is 3 per cent higher than for a caesarean section breech birth. It is for this reason that caesareans are generally recommended. Some women still elect to have a breech vaginal delivery in full knowledge of the risks. You may be able to have a vaginal delivery if hospital policy and your medical team support it.

If your obstetrician practises breech birth, he may agree if you have completed at least 36 weeks of pregnancy and you have not had a previous difficult birth. It is important that your pelvic capacity is large and your baby is under 3.8kg (8.3lb). This can be assessed through clinical and ultrasound measurements. There must be facilities for emergency caesarean delivery in case labour does not progress smoothly.

In a vaginal delivery, when the baby's body is born the umbilical cord may be compressed between the baby's chest and the vagina and the mother's pelvic bones while the head is waiting to emerge. When compression occurs, the baby receives less oxygen from the placenta and the head must be born within five to seven minutes after the umbilicus is visible. If birth is delayed it may result in severe foetal distress and asphyxia that could cause long-term effects on the baby's development.

If you plan to have a caesarean section a time will be set, usually after Week 38 to reduce the risks of prematurity and breathing difficulties after birth.

With a vaginal birth, close monitoring of your baby's heartbeat is absolutely essential.

First stage of labour

A vaginal examination will confirm that your baby's foot has not slipped into the cervix and that the umbilical cord has not prolapsed. Your baby's heartbeat is monitored to ensure that there is no foetal distress.

Second stage of labour

You must not bear down until your cervix is fully dilated because the buttocks may be born but the cervix could delay the birth of the head. A supported squatting position will help your pelvis to open maximally and allow you to push with optimal force when it is time, and gravity encourages your baby's head to engage after the birth of the body. Alternatively, you may use an epidural anaesthetic and be lying down but the mechanics of this position are less advantageous for birth. If there is a delay or difficulty in delivering the head, FORCEPS may be used.

An emergency caesarean can be performed at any time until the birth of the buttocks and umbilical cord: when these have passed the vaginal entrance there is a commitment to a vaginal birth. A caesarean birth is usually simple because there are no pelvic bones to impede the delivery of the baby's body and head.

Third stage of labour
After the birth the placenta will be delivered in the normal way.

After the birth
A baby who has been in a breech position will have different head moulding from a baby born head first – usually the back of the head is prominent. The head shape gradually normalises over a month or two. Breech babies have a higher incidence of dislocation of the hip joints because of the position of the legs in the womb. A clinical and ultrasound assessment of the hips is recommended after the birth to check for this.

■ BROW AND FACE POSITION

Occasionally in a head-down position, a baby may extend his head back so that his chin moves away from his chest. This occurs in about one in 500 births.

If the head is halfway back, this is known as a 'brow presentation' because the forehead comes first. This is an inefficient position for birth because the widest diameter of the baby's head usually does not succeed in passing through the pelvis unless the baby is premature and tiny. A caesarean section is usually needed for a safe birth.

In a 'face presentation', your baby's head will be fully thrown back and the diameter is smaller than in a brow presentation. This makes a vaginal birth possible unless the fit is too tight, in which case a caesarean section is safest. A baby born in this position often shows facial bruising that resolves in a few days.

■ OCCIPITO ANTERIOR POSITION: MOST COMMON

The majority of babies take the occipito anterior position, when the head is down towards the cervix and the chin is tucked onto the chest. Your baby's back faces your belly button and your baby's face looks towards your spine. When the head enters your pelvis the occiput (the bone at the back of the skull) faces anterior (forwards) towards your bladder. The widest diameter of the head is in line with the widest diameter of your pelvic outlet. This is the most helpful position, and allows your baby to negotiate the birth canal in the most effective way.

■ OCCIPITO POSTERIOR POSITION: BACK TO BACK

In an occipito posterior, or 'back-to-back' position, your baby's spine is towards your spine and his limbs and front face your abdominal wall. The occciput (back of the head) points posteriorly (backwards). If he is lying like this, you may feel kicks at the front rather than on the side. This occurs in 20 per cent of all labours.

There are a number of reasons your baby may choose this position:
- Some babies find it is more comfortable to face the placenta if it is implanted on the front wall of the uterus.
- If the shape of your pelvis is not oval but more triangular, with the widest space at the back, the angle between the bones at the front allows less space for your baby's head. In this case it is easier for your baby to be occipito posterior because the diameter of the head is widest at the back and this will fit better in the back part of your pelvis. If your pelvic capacity is large and your baby is normal in size labour is not affected, but if there is a tight fit labour may be prolonged.

There are a number of things you can do to help:
- In the first stage, labour may progress normally. However, your baby's chin may not tuck in and this means his head may press on your sacrum, giving you back pain. If your uterus contracts strongly, the power encourages the head to flex (tuck in).
- Water and massage may help relax the muscles surrounding your pelvis while movements such as rotating your hips and kneeling may encourage your baby to rotate.
- If your pelvic muscle tone is strong, an epidural will relax your muscles, and this may provide the space your baby needs for his head to rotate.
- In the second stage, staying upright in a supported squat maximises the opening of your pelvic bones and assists your baby's head to flex and rotate.
- Occasionally, assistance may be needed in the form of forceps or ventouse to rotate the head and help it to descend and be born.
- If your baby's head stays high, your obstetrician may judge that a caesarean section may be the safest option for you and for your baby.

▧ TRANSVERSE LIE

In fewer than one in 500 births a baby lies sideways (transverse) in the uterus, with a hand, shoulder or the umbilical cord nearest the cervix in a transverse lie. If diagnosed early, the position may be changed by external version (see page 342), but if the position cannot be altered and labour has started, a caesarean section is necessary.

* If the wall and cavity of your uterus is heart shaped (bicornute), a transverse lie is more likely because the shape encourages it.
* If there is an excess of amniotic fluid or twins there is more room for the baby to be in a transverse lie.
* Women who have had more than four babies have a higher chance of carrying a baby in transverse lie as the cavity of the uterus may have stretched and is larger.

Caution for labour and birth

* A baby in transverse lie needs to be born by caesarean.
* If your baby is in a transverse lie and your waters break there may be a risk of umbilical cord prolapse. This can be dangerous for your baby and so requires an ambulance and immediate medical attention.
* A few babies in a transverse lie do not need help because when labour contractions begin the baby turns and the head makes its way down into the pelvis.
* Your midwife will tell you your baby's presentation when you are examined – you need to contact your midwife as soon as labour starts or when your waters break, whichever occurs first.
* If your baby is in a transverse lie you may need to stay in hospital in the weeks leading to the birth to enable rapid attention if the waters break and the umbilical cord prolapses.

Labour and birth, baby
Shoulder dystocia

See also Birth trauma, baby; Large babies.

Shoulder dystocia is the failure of the shoulders to pass spontaneously through the pelvis in the second stage of labour. This happens in one in 200 vaginal births. Following the birth of the head, the shoulders may become wedged at the inlet to the pelvis and the baby can get stuck. This can be a very stressful experience for mum and baby although in most cases skilful assistance ensures birth without excessive trauma.

Risk factors for shoulder dystocia

Although half of all cases of shoulder dystocia involve babies weighing less than 4kg (8lb 12oz) at birth, the risk increases as the birth weight increases. At least one in 10 babies weighing more than 4.5kg (9lb 15oz) is affected. Large babies due to maternal diabetes are at even higher risk, because they have significantly greater shoulder-head ratios.

The risk of shoulder dystocia also rises in relation to the mother's size. If you are short or have a small pelvic capacity, the risk is higher. If you have had a previous baby with shoulder dystocia, you are more likely to have another. During labour, if the second stage is prolonged or difficult, or your team needs to assist your baby's descent with FORCEPS OR VENTOUSE, this may sometimes indicate that your pelvis is a tight fit for your baby and there is a risk of shoulder dystocia.

What happens

With shoulder dystocia, as your baby descends through the birth canal, the front or anterior shoulder remains behind your pubic bone, close to your bladder. This stops the shoulders from descending into the pelvic cavity. Once your baby's head has been born, her chin will be pressed against your perineum. At this time the umbilical cord may be compressed between your baby's chest and the side of your pelvis. This can rapidly lead to FOETAL DISTRESS AND ASPHYXIA, and is an emergency requiring specialist midwifery and obstetric skills. Your birth team needs to act quickly to ensure your baby's body is born because if asphyxia persists for longer than 10 minutes there is a risk of brain damage.

Action plan

If clinical and ultrasound measurements suggest that your baby is over 4.5kg (9lb 15oz), you may plan a CAESAREAN delivery.

If shoulder dystocia arises in labour, your team is trained to act quickly. There are a number of manoeuvres that can reduce the risk of asphyxia, and action needs to be swift – and careful. The use of inappropriate force to deliver the shoulders may cause birth injuries, such as a broken collarbone or damage to the nerves in the neck that control arm movement.

- The midwives may flex your thighs while you are on your back and apply pressure over your lower abdomen to nudge your baby's shoulder through the pelvic brim. This is usually sufficient to lead to birth.
- If this does not solve the problem, your obstetrician may need to put a hand into your vagina to ease round your baby's back shoulder. You may need an EPISIOTOMY (see LABOUR AND BIRTH, MOTHER) to help the process.

You will be asked to help by pushing and bearing down. If your knees are flexed, you will be able to summon maximal strength. The power of your pushes can be an important force helping your baby to be born.

After the birth, your baby may need resuscitation and will then be examined and observed during the first 24 hours to ensure there are no signs of clavicle (collarbone) or nerve injury (page 56) or asphyxia. Most babies who have had shoulder dystocia recover well with no long-term effects. Cranial OSTEOPATHY and MASSAGE may be very useful.

You may find the birth very stressful. Being with your baby will be the beginning of a healing process. Support and homeopathic remedies for shock (page 11) could be very useful. There is a possibility that the experience may not hit home for some time and you may require support to alleviate post traumatic stress (page 448).

Labour and birth, mother
Accessing energy and fear

The energy of life flows intensely during labour and birth. It allows women to be awake and powerful for many hours and spurs babies on to make the most incredible journey of a lifetime. You and your baby will ride the waves together. At times, the waves will be gentle; at times they will be strong and insistent.

You cannot predict in advance how you will respond in labour, but it is reasonable to expect that there will be times when the flow is

manageable, and times when it is more challenging, even overwhelming. If the going gets tough there are many ways to preserve your energy, to refresh yourself, and to draw on your reserves to progress and ride through the pain. You may also elect to use the help modern medical care has to offer.

Your tools
Each woman uses a different range of resources. You're unlikely to use all of the suggestions below and your needs will alter over the course of labour – something that helps you at one stage may be replaced later on.

▰ TRUSTING AND FEELING
The power of birth
Some women sense spiritual and instinctive physical forces. Arising from deep within the female body these forces have been felt by women for thousands of generations. They may surface and flow when conditions allow: when you feel safe, unthreatened and well supported. Accessing your own 'safe space' and working through your fears (page 212) in advance of labour may help you trust your inherent power and enjoy the journey.

One contraction at a time
The concept of taking one contraction at a time is very powerful. It helps you to be present rather than worrying about what is to come. Allow each contraction to take over, ride the wave as it rises and then relax as it recedes. If you don't fight the pain, it is easier to use the pain-free space between contractions to rest and find more strength.

Your feelings
Your feelings are part of the experience, and it's helpful to accept and express whatever you feel. Your sensations may include meditative calm, excitement, pain, fear, despair and the ecstasy of release.

Accessing fear
Anxiety is common, both before and during labour. You may, for instance, feel tense if you're worried about pain or about coping after birth or if you are afraid of hospitals or have had a previously difficult experience. With

support you will be free to focus on your baby and on the birth. There's more on fear on page 212 and its usefulness in the second stage on page 301.

Control and surrender
Pain may increase if you feel out of control. Sometimes labour demands surrender. You may need to trust and rely on your supporters.

■ ENVIRONMENT

During labour, deep parts of your brain are activated that heighten your mammalian instinct to give birth, affecting your physical, emotional and spiritual energy, your nerves, muscles and HORMONES. These parts of your brain are highly sensitive to feelings of fear and safety. If you feel safe and trust the people who are with you, the natural process of birth is encouraged. Knowing that your personal space is safe and respected often helps enormously. This may be a factor in your decision to give birth at home or in hospital (page 353).

Props
If you gather some props, you can create the option to choose what's comfortable at any given time, such as cushions, birth ball, chair, bed or stool. Familiar things may help you feel safe and confident. For example, you might have with you a cushion, a pillow from your bed, a blanket or a photo.

Lights and sounds
Dim lighting will help you feel private and supports your brain's release of birthing hormones. In hospital you may be able to use a lamp. Some hospitals also allow candles. You may be sensitive to noise and it is preferable if people knock before entering, and do not have general chit-chat around you. You might want to listen to music. If you have practised VISUALISATIONS or hypnosis, music may help you relax and enter your birthing space. Some odours might calm or boost your energy and you may want to have AROMATHERAPY oils or MASSAGE oils to hand.

Privacy
Feeling undisturbed is good for most women. This is possible with your birth partner or midwife present, watching out for you

unobtrusively. You do not need to be naked and you can ask to be sensitively covered. Some women feel embarrassed during examinations and are nervous of pooing in public. It is best to accept these as normal and welcome them as signs of birth: your inhibitions may hinder the flow of labour. The examinations help your midwife ensure you and baby are doing well, and as your baby's head pushes on your lower bowel the midwife knows that birth is imminent.

Water
Being in water may be deeply soothing. Even listening to flowing water can be relaxing. You may plan to use a birthing pool for labour and/or birth.

■ LOVING COMPANY
Who is with you
The flow of birthing HORMONES is optimal when you feel safe, loved and supported by the people with you. During labour it is okay to ask people to leave, except when their presence is essential for safety reasons.

Touch
The loving touch of skin on skin, perhaps during MASSAGE, can help: it is pleasurable and reduces the intensity of pain signals travelling to your brain.

Minimal disruption
New people coming into the room may affect your flow. You or your birth partner may ask for more privacy. If you require assistance from the medical team, having your birth partner close to you will help.

■ BREATHING AND VISUALISATION
Breathing
Your breath can be your anchor and keep you in touch with your strength and your safe space (page 105). Breathing deeply will help to oxygenate your body, energise your uterine muscle and reduce anxiety and pain. Your body tenses on the in-breath and relaxes on the out-breath. Breathing out to relax is a simple concept but it may be difficult to implement in the heat of labour and you may welcome guidance. For more information, see pages 362–3.

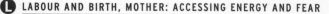

Visualising

Taking your awareness into your body and to
your baby may help you be in the moment and
feel the positive forces of birth. You can
visualise in whatever way you have practised
(page 549).

■ BODY POWER

Your body

Changing position, particularly moving and
being upright (page 350), can improve your
energy. If you are tired and your contractions are
not intense, resting can replenish your reserves.
Some women sleep for a while, and some go into
a meditative state between contractions. French
obstetrician Michel Odent calls this: 'Going to
another planet'.

Your voice

You may cry, sing, laugh, curse, moan or roar; or
remain quiet and focused internally. At the
moment of birth you will involuntarily utter the
'primal cry'. Free expression helps your
labouring rhythm flow well.

Warmth

Being too hot or too cold can increase tension
and pain. Your midwife and birth partner will
help you stay comfortable.

■ EATING AND DRINKING IN LABOUR

It is important to eat and drink in labour unless
you are likely to have an intervention that
requires a general anaesthetic. The advantages
of ensuring that you are well hydrated and that
you have food for energy are well known.
Labour is a long physical and emotional journey
and your emotions, your body and your uterus
function optimally if you are nourished and
hydrated. This applies particularly if labour goes
on for over 12 hours and even more if it exceeds
24 hours. Part of your birth plan (page 359)
may involve asking your hospital about its food
and drink policy and preparing your bag
accordingly.

If your blood sugar dips, adrenaline rises
and with it your anxiety, body tension and pain
perception. Dehydration reduces energy and
increases fear. Eat small amounts if you can,
and take frequent sips of water or sports drink.

Your midwife will ensure you do not drink too
much water because this can reduce the salt
content of your body and make you feel weak.
Water spray on your face may help.

Suggested drinks

* It is best to consume 1.5 to 2 litres (3–4 pints)
  per 24 hours, and more if the room is very hot.
  Sip small amounts every 15 minutes.
* If you drink a great deal of water, this can cause
  your mineral levels to be diluted and you can
  become hyponatraemic (low sodium), just like
  marathon runners. If this happens, it will
  interfere with the way your uterus contracts. It
  is preferable to use an electrolyte drink made
  for marathon runners and to ensure that you
  do not drink too much and become
  overhydrated. Your birth attendants can
  support you in this.
* Some sports drinks also have sugar or glucose
  added and this may help boost your energy
  levels.
* If you have an intravenous drip with an
  epidural your fluid levels will be maintained.
* If you are given a high dose of oxytocin to
  stimulate contractions, this may cause fluid
  retention and low sodium levels, and you may
  benefit from some sports drink.

Suggested foods

* It is not a good idea to eat a lot during labour,
  but a little every three to four hours will help
  to maintain your body's glucose (energy)
  reserves.
* Not all women want to eat, and some feel
  nauseous and are sick. Nausea may occur in
  early labour, when a small snack may give a
  useful energy boost.
* It is best to eat easily digestible foods. A
  banana, for example, will give you energy for 90
  minutes; a small bag of mixed dried fruit and
  nuts or a sports energy bar would give a balance
  of carb, protein and fat in easily digestible
  portions; or a simple sandwich made with
  wholemeal bread. You will have specific food
  preferences, but it is best to avoid very sugary
  snacks like chocolate.
* If you have an epidural or there is a possibility
  of a CAESAREAN or FORCEPS birth it is best to have
  an empty stomach, although it is not always
  possible (for instance, if the need for
  anaesthesia was unanticipated). The

recommendation is a precaution because anaesthesia can induce vomiting, which carries a risk of inhaling solid food.

* If your labour is prolonged or your midwife is concerned about FOETAL DISTRESS in your baby it is best to stop drinking and an intravenous drip can be used to provide fluid and nutrients. Alternative sources of energy include glucose tablets and drinks, but it is best to use them sparingly – too much may cause an exaggerated rise in blood sugar followed by a slump, which may make you feel weak and more sensitive to pain.

■ MEDICAL AND COMPLEMENTARY HELP

Energy boosts and pain relief
You may use complementary techniques (page 363) or consider medical pain relief (page 381) to increase your strength and/or help you rest.

Augmentation
If you become exhausted or your contractions lose their edge, medical augmentation (page 375) may give labour a boost and work well for you and your baby.

■ ON THE DAY: GOING WITH THE FLOW

During pregnancy you can prepare but when you enter labour you leave the preparation behind and enter the unknown. What's done is done: in labour it is time to let go and be in what is happening. It is best to have a broad view: if it is too rigid you are likely to be disappointed or even guilty that you did not provide the 'perfect' or 'only start' for your baby.

Labour involves your baby, his size and position and whether his head is tucked in. It also involves the efficiency of your uterus and the size of your pelvis, your mind and spirit and the free release of love hormones.

It is worth bearing in mind that the way we are born is very important but as babies we are resilient and our minds and brains adapt. What happened in pregnancy, and after the birth when you and your baby are together, are probably as or more important than the birth itself.

Labour and birth, mother
Active birth

Active birth is a term that can be applied to the whole of pregnancy and to the months beyond, involving active involvement in preparing for birth, active choices in labour and being present and responsive to your baby as a parent. There is a continuum from conception through the first months of your baby's life and an active birth has benefits for baby, mum and dad. In 1979, Janet Balaskas, who is a childbirth educator, coined the term 'active birth'. Yehudi Gordon was the obstetrician involved in the formation of the Active Birth Movement at that time.

What happens

In terms of labour, having an active birth implies that you will be physically active and also that you will take an active role in decisions about your care. This helps you to follow the rhythm of your contractions, choose comfortable positions and harness your natural power and the force of gravity to assist your contractions and the birth of your baby. Your supporting team are there to help you feel empowered and make choices. After an active birth, it is likely that you will go forward into the early days of parenting with positivity and confidence.

The opposite of active birth is 'managed' labour, where you lie on a bed throughout labour and an obstetric team makes decisions about when and how to intervene. Thankfully, managed labours are becoming less common, but some hospitals are still constrained by a lack of open-mindedness.

While active birth was once a reality for only a few women it is now accepted as a very real option for most mothers. With active birth your care team are able to do a great deal to ensure that both you and your baby are safe. Hand in hand with centuries of wisdom and experience, medical science is able to support the natural process and enhance the power and health of the birthing woman and her baby.

Natural birth
A 'natural birth' is one where no medical pain relief or intervention is used. Many women do manage without any medication: the female

body is designed to give birth and to cope with pain. There are many natural ways to encourage smooth progress, maintain energy and minimise discomfort. For some people, 'natural' represents the Holy Grail. If this is your ideal, on the day the safety net of medical pain relief or assistance may outweigh your commitment to natural birth. An integrated approach combining the benefit of modern medicine with the best of birthing wisdom is a very positive way to give you a fuller range of options and enjoyment. Your selection may combine the best of both worlds.

Action plan

You have months to read, chat to other parents, go to classes, watch videos or talk to your midwife to decide how and where you want to give birth. This time is a golden opportunity to gather information and prepare your body, mind and spirit so you can take an active role in your care.

On the day of labour, you and your baby may enjoy an active experience without intervention. There is no way you can guarantee a 'perfect' day, however, and part of being actively involved in your care is to be open to whatever happens on the day. This will help you greet and accept your baby, however she arrives, and avoid being upset if the unfolding of birth itself did not meet your expectations (page 434).

■ UPRIGHT POSITIONS

Being upright assists natural progress and allows you freedom to move and take positions that feel right. Mothers who have given birth in an active upright posture generally feel good – and this makes caring for a newborn easier. Lying down, in contrast, can slow progress, increase discomfort and raise the need for obstetric intervention.

While being upright is part of the active birth philosophy, there's no pressure to be upright all the time. The crucial element of remaining active is to listen to your body and do what feels right. There will be times when you wish to recline and rest. Being aware of different positions is useful preparation for whatever happens on the day.

What happens

Your uterine muscle contracts from the top downwards. In an upright position gravity is on your side and this natural contraction sequence is unimpeded. If you are lying on your back, your uterus has to work against gravity, which is much more difficult for you and for your baby.

When you give birth, being upright helps your pelvis to open and aids your baby through the birth canal. It helps your vaginal opening to stretch and at the same time helps your lungs expand fully as you breathe.

You can be upright in many different ways. In early labour, for instance, you may be comfortable standing and moving your hips, as if dancing, or leaning against a wall or chair. You may also kneel. When labour is more intense you may rely completely on your birthing partner or a midwife to hold you as you focus your energy on your baby and your uterus. It is possible to fully relax while being upright.

If you choose medical pain relief, you may still find it comfortable to stay upright. You will be able to use upright positions when using a mobile epidural and gas and air. You can also take upright positions in a water pool.

During labour

* Freely moving and expressing yourself can help you access your birthing instincts and reduce pain.
* Gravity helps your baby's head to be well applied to your cervix, and this enhances the efficiency of your contractions. This may result in faster dilation and a shorter labour.
* When you are upright, your uterus tilts forward, which helps to modify pain. It may reduce the need for an epidural.
* When you're upright, blood flow to the placenta is optimal, because there is no compression of your internal blood vessels (as there may be in a lying or semi-reclining position). This provides your baby with maximum oxygen flow and reduces the risk of FOETAL DISTRESS.

For your baby's birth

* Being upright maximises the natural pushing force of your body.
* When you're upright your pelvic capacity increases to give maximum space for your

baby's head to pass through. If you are lying down your pelvic joints are constricted and there is less space available for birth.

- The entire vaginal opening stretches more efficiently and tears are less likely.
- If being upright helps labour progress well, your baby will have a minimal risk of side effects from drugs or interventions and is likely to be born in an optimal condition.
- If your partner is physically supporting you he will be intimately involved in the power and magic of birth.

For the birth of the placenta

- When you are sitting upright, it is easier to hold and welcome your baby.
- If you are holding and perhaps feeding your baby, your body produces HORMONES that enhance your contractions and precipitate birth of the placenta. These hormones include love hormones that help you feel good and encourage bonding.
- With gravity in your favour, your contractions work optimally for the birth of the placenta.

Active parenting

The philosophy of active birth is underpinned by an attitude of active involvement and loving acceptance. Many women and men find that when these are strong during labour and birth, there is a flow into the hours, days and weeks beyond. Active birth extends to lovingly accepting your child, being with her, and responding to her needs. This active parenting is likely to help her feel secure and content and bring richness and enjoyment to family life, and follows the principles of infant-led parenting, outlined on page 432.

Action plan

If you are keen to remain active it is worth practising with your partner while you are pregnant. You may have a chance to do this at antenatal classes and/or follow advice in books.

When you are in labour it may not be easy to mentally recall all the positions you 'learnt' or the advice you received. But your body has its own power and memory: your muscles and joints know instinctively what to do and practice will pay off. Many women enter a trance-like state during labour which helps them go into their 'birthing space' and move freely.

The options for being upright include:
- Using a birthing stool.
- Using a birthing ball.
- Standing with your arms and head resting on the wall.
- Standing with your arms around your partner's shoulders.
- Kneeling with your forearms and head resting on a chair or bed.
- Kneeling over a pile of pillows so your upper body is completely supported.
- Resting on all fours.
- Squatting with your partner supporting you from the front or from behind.
- Sitting semi-upright with pillows behind your back and under your buttocks.

The importance of resting

You may need to rest between contractions and it is important to preserve energy. This is particularly true in the first stage of labour, which may be very long. If you wish to lie down it is preferable to lie on your side or in propped up sitting, with your upper body supported on a bank of pillows. Kneeling can be very relaxing. You may want an extra pillow between your legs or beneath your buttocks.

Labour and birth, mother
Active birth in water

For many women, the flowing, warming and nurturing properties of water fit well with labour and birth, offering comfort, security, privacy and pain relief. It gives a sense of gentleness and peace for mum and baby, and for dad too. Although it is a minority of women who actually give birth in water, many thousands enjoy a bath or time in the pool during labour: water has a natural draw and is relaxing and revitalising. Even though a minority of women give birth in a pool, this still accounts for tens of thousands of babies who have been born into water since the 1970s. After a water birth, 95 per cent of women say that they are delighted and would not want to give birth any other way.

Water for labour and birth was introduced by Michel Odent in France and by Igor Tcharkovsky in Russia. Yehudi Gordon was one of the first obstetricians in the UK to use water in this context. It is now fully supported for mothers who have no complications in pregnancy, and more and more hospitals have one or more pools and midwives who are experienced as practitioners of active birth in water. Many families choose to hire a pool for use at home.

What happens: how water can help

Water may simply feel good for you. Since its increasingly widespread use, research has revealed many of its powerful properties. Water has many known benefits:

* Being in water can feel cosy and private, helping you relax, focus and feel confident.
* As water caresses your skin it occupies nervous pathways to your brain, reducing anxiety and weakening the intensity of pain signals caused by your contractions.
* It encourages the release of pain-relieving endorphins and birthing hormones including oxytocin that help your cervix dilate and give power to contractions. It also lowers the production of stress hormones.
* You are less likely to require synthetic oxytocin to augment contractions (page 377) or epidural anaesthesia for pain relief.
* Water can help muscles in your body to relax so your energy can be focused on the flow of birth.
* Immersion in water can assist maximum stretching of your vaginal opening for birth.
* Many women are more easily able to 'go off to another planet' while in water.
* For your baby, birth into water offers a smooth transition, where warmth and water continue to caress the skin and offer protection in the sensitive minutes after birth. Being held to your breast without leaving the water minimises feelings of separation and any anxiety this causes. Babies born into water often appear calm and very relaxed.

Safety issues

Sterility

Your baby is protected from organisms that pass from your body into the water by your antibodies that cross the placenta. To reduce the risk of infection, the birth pool in a hospital will be cleansed thoroughly before you use it. You or your partner will ensure the pool is sterile if you hire one for use at home. Your baby is brought to the surface soon after his body is born underwater so the infection risk is minimal.

Temperature

Your baby uses your blood to maintain his temperature. If your core temperature rises his will also rise and his metabolic rate and his oxygen needs will increase. Your midwife will maintain the water below your body temperature (37°C/98.4°F). If you choose to stay in the pool with your baby after the birth, your midwife will adjust the temperature of the water to ensure that he does not become cold.

Monitoring

Your midwife can intermittently monitor your baby's heartbeat with a handheld monitor designed for use in water. If your baby requires closer or continuous monitoring it will be necessary to leave the pool.

Risk of inhalation

A baby born into water won't draw breath until there's contact with the air. In the rare occurrence of even a single drop of water reaching the back of the throat, receptors stimulate the 'dive reflex' to prevent breathing in water. A tiny risk of inhaling water occurs only if a baby has had foetal distress (page 249). If he has lacked oxygen during labour there is a reflex to gasp that overrides the dive reflex. This is where midwifery skills come into play and by listening to your baby's heartbeat your midwife will be able to detect signs of foetal distress. If this occurs you will be asked to leave the pool.

Pain relief

You can use gas and air (page 386) while in the pool. An epidural or injections of pethidine or morphine are not permitted in the pool.

Prolonged or difficult labour

Water often helps the progress of labour. If labour is slow, you and your midwife will discuss leaving the pool. It may be okay to take time out of the water, and re-enter later in labour, if you feel like it.

Using water at home

It is vital to hire a pool from a reputable company, and to be sure that the midwife attending your birth is experienced with water pools. A bath is not an acceptable substitute. It's a good idea to get familiar with the pool. Practise filling it so you know how long it takes, and try sitting, lying, kneeling, squatting and floating. You could practise with your partner so that he feels at ease about being with you during labour and birth.

Action plan

You may plan to use a water pool, or be unexpectedly drawn to water on the day. Whatever your intentions, it is useful to go with what feels right – and what is safest – for you and your baby.

Using a pool in labour

* It is best to use the pool after your cervix has dilated to 6cm. Before this, the relaxing effect of water may reduce the power of your contractions.
* The key is to be comfortable. You can use all kinds of props, including plastic stools, rolled up towels or a plastic pillow. There will be room to sit, kneel, squat, or float with your legs straight out. Water helps to support your body and take your weight.
* The pool sides are strong and easy to grip. Your partner can give you maximum support either in or outside the pool.
* You may use gas and air (page 386) while in the pool.
* Immersion in water at 37°C (98°F) tends to aid labour for a limited period of time, and this varies from woman to women. Depending on the woman, this may be 30 minutes to two hours: longer than this and progress may be slowed.

When to leave the pool

In spite of being in strong labour, it is very simple to leave the pool within 20 seconds between contractions. It is the same as stepping out of a bath. It is advisable to leave the pool:
* If you do not feel comfortable or happy.
* If you choose to have an epidural anaesthetic.
* If your contractions are ineffective: harnessing gravity and being active on dry land may help them pick up.
* If your baby's heart rate suggests foetal distress.
* If your midwife is concerned about you or your baby and needs to monitor you more closely.
* If labour is prolonged or complicated and you or your baby need or may need help.

After birth on dry land you may want to return to the pool with your newborn baby resting against your skin and supported by the warm, soothing water.

Water for birth

When you begin to push, you can use the pool side and/or your companions for support. When your baby's head has crowned, the water will take the edge off the stinging around your vaginal entrance and adds some lubrication to encourage stretching, making tears less likely.

Your midwife will gently help the birth of your baby's head if this is needed, and his body will follow with the next contraction. Your baby will not be stimulated to take a breath until he senses air on his skin. In less than 30 seconds, your midwife will lift him out of the water and onto your tummy or chest, depending on the length of the umbilical cord. You may then gently blow on your baby's skin to stimulate breathing. Water babies are often calm at birth but many still cry in greeting, expressing their reaction to their birth and expanding their lungs for the first time.

The transition of birth in water is usually smooth and beautiful, an unbroken continuum from your womb into your arms. The water will take the weight of your baby, and as he feels your skin, he will explore the world and look for your eyes: in this intimate space mums often feel as if the world has disappeared, and all that exists is their baby. This is a wonderful way for your baby to be greeted and will be a time you will never forget. Your partner may have similar feelings. Provided your baby is breathing well, it is okay for you all to stay there: your midwife will help to ensure your baby doesn't get cold. You can begin to feed in the pool.

It is safe for you to deliver the placenta in the pool. If you prefer to leave the pool, your midwife will ensure that you and your baby are dry and warm. You can then hold, greet and feed your baby as you await the placenta.

Labour and birth, mother
At home or hospital

As recently as 40 years ago, most babies were born at home. In 2005 only 2.4 per cent of babies in the UK were born at home. However, these figures are now rising as more women are offered midwifery support to give birth at home, if this is their wish and there are no reasons why mum or baby may need extra medical care.

The more relaxed, safe and comfortable you feel, the less likely complications will arise. For you, feeling safe may mean being in a hospital or it may mean being at home. Your choice will depend on your pain relief preferences, how active you wish to be, whether you want medical support on site, and whether you have a low- or high-risk pregnancy. Your partner will also have a view.

For pregnancies without complications, termed 'low-risk pregnancy', there is no statistical difference in safety between home births and hospital births.

At home

Women who give birth at home tend to feel more in control of their choices, less inhibited and freer to be mobile and use upright positions. You may hire a birthing pool. At a home birth, intervention is less likely than in a hospital setting. Partly this is because your birthing hormones flow more effectively when the environment is familiar and you feel relaxed and undisturbed. Welcoming your baby and savouring the sacred hours after birth in your own space can be a powerful reason for choosing to give birth at home.

You need to be aware that birth does have risks and there is a chance that a complication may arise that necessitates the move to hospital. This happens in a minority of home births. One of the most important safety issues to consider is the distance to hospital. A home birth is usually only sanctioned when mother and baby are known to be low risk.

At home your midwife will monitor you and your baby, but not as closely as is possible in hospital. Your midwife can offer gas and air as PAIN RELIEF, and pain-relieving injections, but not an epidural, and can perform an EPISIOTOMY but not use FORCEPS OR VENTOUSE.

Organising a home birth
The first people to talk to are your midwife and your GP. In most areas there is a team of community midwives who can attend home births. You may prefer to hire an independent midwife who will care for you throughout

pregnancy and birth, and you may invite a DOULA. Having a midwife present who is like a family friend is highly rated by many couples.

If you choose to be at home, nesting takes on a new meaning as towels and sheets are washed, furniture is moved and the bathroom cleaned to welcome the baby. You decide who will be with you or you may create a quiet space to be alone. Your other children may enjoy being part of the experience.

Home labour, hospital delivery
While the environment at home and the loving support of your family increase the likelihood that birth will go smoothly, there may be unforeseen events that interrupt the flow. A midwife may have several reasons to believe that transfer to hospital is the safest option.

In a small number of cases, labour and birth proceed without cause for concern but the baby needs assistance after birth. Midwives carry equipment to encourage breathing and are trained to administer neonatal resuscitation until a transfer can be arranged. They also carry equipment and medication to stop bleeding from the uterus and to prevent or treat blood loss. In an emergency, a midwife will summon help from the local ambulance service and from the nearest hospital maternity unit.

If your midwife recommends a transfer, she arranges this. You will go directly to the labour ward and your midwife may accompany you. When you arrive, your care will be taken over by a hospital midwife and doctor who will assess you and your baby and suggest a course of action.

In hospital

Most women opt to give birth in hospital, particularly in the first pregnancy. The main reason is safety. Some women also enjoy the company of other women and babies and are pleased to have the space to relax and settle with their babies while professionals are at hand.

Hospitals vary, and so do individual experiences depending on how busy a unit is on any given day, and who is on the staff. Some women do not feel they receive personal attention and lack privacy. Others praise the hospital and its staff and love the experience.

It's important to explore your options. You can visit to get a feel for a place with your antenatal group or arrange it personally. You may check records of statistics including intervention, water births, use of epidural and neonatal transfer.

You may be advised that hospital is the safest place for you to be, for instance if your baby is in the breech position, you have had a previous CAESAREAN or for other reasons (page 302). Planning ahead to make the space comfortable (page 347) may help you enjoy labour and progress without complications.

Midwifery and GP units

Midwifery and GP units are homely and their equipment is limited because they are designed for low-risk pregnancies. Women who give birth in these units are usually very happy that the atmosphere was close to having a baby at home. The choice is becoming more popular among women who like a homely environment and want the safety net of modern medical care at hand. An increasing number of hospitals have midwifery units on site and in the unlikely event that extra support is needed for mum or baby, the disruption will be minimal. Alternatively, an ambulance journey may be necessary to a larger hospital.

Consultant led units

If you have a high-risk pregnancy (page 302) or you wish to have epidural anaesthetic and operative facilities at hand, you need to give birth in a consultant-led unit in hospital. It is not always the case, but intervention is more likely in an environment where high-tech anaesthetics and obstetric care are available.

Labour and birth, mother
Beginnings of labour

See also Labour and birth, mother, contractions; spontaneous and premature rupture of membranes.

The onset of labour is influenced by your baby and by you. What is happening hormonally is not the only factor: your own wellbeing, your confidence and state of mind, your nutrition and your fitness have an impact, and your baby's physical wellbeing and emotional state are also influential.

For a small number of women, labour begins with contractions at maximum intensity and comes with very little warning. It's more common to have advance notice, maybe over a few hours or days before contractions begin. You may experience one or more common signs.

Early signs of labour

In the days leading up to labour, you may notice many changes in your emotional, mental and physical state that indicate that the long-awaited birth may be imminent. For example:

State of mind

Your moods and energy may become internally focused. This is a natural state of mind for labour, when the chemical balance and activity in your brain incline you to ignore external events and focus inwards. Some women feel quiet and calm and become thoughtful or meditative.

Change in energy

Some women are highly energetic, others sleep more than usual. If your energy varies from the norm, your body and mind may be preparing.

Nesting

Don't be surprised if you have powerful urges to clean and tidy, to ready your baby's environment and even to bake. You may have your most vigorous tidy-out hours before labour commences.

Dreams

Your body knows at an unconscious level what is happening, and is able to pick up signs from your baby and your uterus. Dreams are one way in which the unconscious allows messages to surface into awareness. You may also access your unconscious through meditation or VISUALISATION.

Bowel movements

Prostaglandin, the hormone-like chemical released by your baby and the lining of your uterus to instigate labour, may stimulate your bowels to empty more frequently. It's common for movements to become loose when labour is imminent.

Backache and period pains

Other common signs are backache, abdominal pain or period-like pains, and twinges in your lower back or tummy. You can check if you are having uterine CONTRACTIONS: place your hand on your uterus, which will harden as you feel pain.

Contractions

Regular painful contractions are the most common sign that labour is actually beginning. The range of contraction sensations through labour is described on page 367.

What to do when you think labour has started

- If you have not been advised otherwise, it is fine to wait to call your midwife until contractions are roughly five minutes apart and each lasts for over 30 seconds.
- If your midwife or obstetrician has concerns about you or your baby, or you live a long way from hospital, you may need to call sooner – perhaps when contractions are 10 minutes apart.
- If your pain is severe or there is no let up between contractions, it's important to talk to your midwife immediately.
- Unless you don't want to talk, it's more helpful for your midwife to listen to you than to your partner. Your tone of voice or the length of your silences as you breathe can reveal a lot.
- If you are having a hospital birth, you need to call to let your midwife know when you are coming in. Your midwife will then advise you.
- If you are planning to give birth at home, your midwife will decide when to come and see you.

Breaking waters

The membranes around your baby protect her in pregnancy. Usually, the membranes break in the first stage of labour and release the AMNIOTIC FLUID. Less commonly, the membranes break before labour contractions begin (see page 392). You might want to plan ahead and cover your mattress with a waterproof undersheet in case your waters break at night.

The experience

- Sometimes the membranes break and release a gush of fluid.
- If your baby's head is snug in your pelvic inlet, the amniotic fluid is contained above and below her head and will be released in a dribble.
- Amniotic fluid is urine coloured, but the smell is distinctively sweet.
- Some women think they have wet themselves. Some women are embarrassed about urinary incontinence if the waters are dribbling. You can tell the difference from the smell.
- Usually, contractions begin within 24 hours of the waters breaking but the leak can continue for longer.

What to do

- Let your midwife know.
- She will advise you, depending on recent measurements of amniotic fluid volume and your personal medical history. If your baby's head is very high and not engaged in your pelvis, it is important to be examined to ensure the UMBILICAL cord has not prolapsed into the VAGINA below the head.

+ Red flag

- If you have been told you have a reduction (page 25) or an excess (page 24) of amniotic fluid, an urgent examination by your midwife is essential.
- If the fluid is greenish, your baby has had a bowel movement in the womb. This can be a sign of FOETAL DISTRESS. Your birth team will want to monitor your baby.

- Amniotic fluid is constantly replenished by your baby and placenta. Unless there is another factor interfering with this, your baby is not at risk of becoming dry, nor will birth be affected.
- Your baby and the volume of amniotic fluid may be assessed using ultrasound.
- You need to abstain from sexual intercourse.
- It is safe to bathe because your vaginal walls prevent the entry of water to the level of the CERVIX.
- If you are known to carry GROUP B STREP (GBS) in your vagina or bladder, INDUCTION of labour using oxytocin is essential to prevent the bacteria from infecting your baby and your uterus. You will also be advised to begin antibiotics to reduce the infection risk. If your GBS status has not been tested you will be advised to have a vaginal swab taken when your waters break.

- If there are no other recognised risk factors and labour hasn't started within 24 to 48 hours, it may be safest for your baby for labour to be induced.

A show

As your cervix ripens and effaces it changes shape and may release the plug of mucus that acts as a barrier between the uterine membranes and the vagina. This is known as 'a show'.

The experience
- The mucus is a jelly-like substance, and may be brown, pink or stained with blood because tiny blood vessels in your cervix may bleed as it opens.
- You may notice it in your pants or when you urinate.
- A show may occur hours or days before labour, or not at all.

What to do if there is a show
- Ring your midwife immediately if a show is accompanied by heavy bleeding or blood clots. It may be a sign of haemorrhage (page 360).
- You do not need to ring your midwife if you have a show without additional blood loss.
- Provided the membranes have not ruptured, your baby is not at higher risk of infection because the membranes act as a barrier.
- It is safe to bathe because your vaginal walls prevent the entry of water to the level of the cervix.
- Sexual intercourse is also safe. In fact, the prostaglandin in semen may stimulate your uterus to contract and expedite labour.
- Remember that there may be a delay of many days before the onset of labour.
- If the discharge persists, the symptoms may indicate a vaginal infection and it is worth consulting your midwife.

▨ PRE- AND FALSE LABOUR

Prior to true labour itself, most women experience a form of contraction known as 'practice' or Braxton-Hicks contractions. They can occur from early pregnancy but are usually not felt by the woman until later in pregnancy. For some women, these contractions can seem very strong, perhaps from as early on as Week 25. If you are sensitive to the activity of your uterus, you may have the feeling that labour is beginning, although there is no dilation of the CERVIX. It happens more often in second or subsequent pregnancies. This is known as 'pre-' or 'false labour'. Usually the contractions are irregular.

The term 'false labour' is also used medically to describe apparent labour where the cervix remains below 3cm dilation. This can be called the 'latent phase' of the first stage (page 387). It can last for days. Many women who feel a lot of pain at this stage would class this as true labour. Medically speaking, 'true labour' begins when dilation progresses beyond 3cm: this is the 'active phase' of the first stage.

What happens

Each person's sensitivity is different and you may experience Braxton-Hicks as painless tightenings, or there may be considerable pain. As your uterus contracts, other organs in your abdomen may also contract. This applies to your bowel if you have CONSTIPATION or irritable bowel syndrome (page 326), either of which may be brought on if you are anxious. It may apply to your bladder from pressure or if you have CYSTITIS, or to the muscles in your abdominal wall.

The way to distinguish uterine contractions is to sit quietly and place your hand flat on your abdomen over your belly button. With a contraction, you will feel your uterus hardening when you feel discomfort. Hardening from a contraction comes and goes within 60 seconds. This will guide you to detect a contraction (practice or otherwise) as distinct from intestinal, bladder or abdominal muscle pain.

Action plan

If you are concerned, contact your birth team, particularly if you have been told you are at increased risk of premature labour, perhaps because you have previously had a PREMATURE BIRTH.

Medical care
- A midwife will monitor your baby's heartbeat and your contractions.
- She will assess the extent of your cervical dilation with an internal examination. If your cervix is shortened and softened and at least 3cm dilated you are in established labour.
- If needed, your cervix can be measured accurately on ultrasound scan.

What you can do in pre- or false labour

- If you are still a long way from your due date it is worth taking it easy. Resting and nourishing yourself are important. You may consider taking time off work and enlisting help and support at home.
- HOMEOPATHY or ACUPUNCTURE may be helpful.
- If you are close to the due date and are having runs of painful Braxton-Hicks contractions it is best to maintain your energy and rest and nourish yourself for when true labour begins.
- There may be a gentle gradation between pre-labour and the first stage of true labour, so keep in touch with your birth team. If you are at term but becoming tired and unable to sleep, they may suggest inducing or augmenting labour (page 374).

Labour and birth, mother
Birth partner

Being a birth partner – usually the role for dad-to-be – can be a very intense physical and emotional experience with feelings ranging from incredible energy and joy to exhaustion and concern. You will bring your unique energy into the birthing room and be there to offer support, encouragement and acceptance. During pregnancy, focusing on the birth together will be very useful. On the day, it may be your role to ensure that your partner has what she needs, and to be emotionally present for her. It may be reassuring to know that just being there with a loving heart is fine. Having someone else to relieve you so that you can keep up energy and enthusiasm is helpful.

General tips

- Be there and listen: at times may be needed nothing more than your quiet presence.
- You could choose appropriate music, make drinks, ensure there are snacks for both of you.
- You can help your partner stay calm by being calm yourself.
- She may ask you to hold her hand, MASSAGE her gently, stroke her back, and generally help her relax.
- Your partner's requests may change and so if she decides she doesn't want you to touch her,

or even to be near her, don't take it personally. Her focus is on the birth.
- In labour, your partner's attention is likely to become focused inwardly. It is best not to bring her out of the 'zone' by asking detailed questions. Stimulating thought can suppress the flow of birthing hormones.

Breathing and contractions

- Breathing and movement will be most effective when they are natural and instinctive. If your partner loses her rhythm, you can gently guide her back. You may want to demonstrate it for her – say 'breathe with me...' and then inhale fully and exhale long and slow, until she begins to mirror your rhythm. Establish eye contact if you can.
- Affirmations – positive statements – spoken in time with her breathing can encourage her. Talk to her by name: 'You are doing fine, you are doing well ... our baby is coming down gently, everything's going well ... I'm with you, I'm here.'
- If you have practised VISUALISATIONS use hypnotic language as you guide her.

Active support

- You may give a lot of physical support, helping with upright positions to enhance labour and help to reduce pain.
- You may need a lot of stamina and energy so remember to care for yourself, too, with drinks, snacks and good POSTURE.

What you can do for yourself

- Do whatever you need to stay calm.
- Rest, because the first stage can be up to 20 hours long.
- Going for a walk or doing light exercise may boost your energy and lift your spirits.
- If you are feeling anxious or afraid you can help to calm yourself by taking slow, deep breaths.
- If you do not like to see blood and body fluids you don't need to: you can stay at your partner's head – midwives are adept at being discreet.
- If you have concerns, you may wish to talk to a midwife or doctor. It is usually best to do this outside the birthing room. You can then return feeling better informed.
- It may be difficult to just be there to support your partner but your presence, love and commitment are immensely powerful.

When birth is imminent: the second stage

The rhythm of labour changes in the second stage, when your partner begins to push.

* She may be empowered by your encouragement and presence. At this stage she may feel strong and excited, or overwhelmed and fearful.
* If you don't want to witness the actual birth, you could stay close to her head. You may be supporting her from behind, depending on the position she chooses.
* Even if you are tired, you will feel a surge of energy when you meet your baby.
* Once your baby is born, if there is no need for medical support the best place for him is on mum's body, and he may start to feed soon. You can begin communicating through touch, talking and eye contact in the first minutes of life. If your partner is exhausted she may ask you to cuddle your baby in the minutes after birth.
* You may wish to cut the umbilical cord.
* If there's room in the bed or in the water pool, you could all rest together.
* When the time is right, you can phone around with the good news.

If intervention is needed

* If any difficulties arise during labour, your love and support will mean a lot. You may be a valuable go-between for your partner and the midwives.
* If the midwife or doctor suggests intervention, your partner may look to you for support as she considers the options.
* It is worth reading about intervention in advance so you feel prepared should it happen.
* If a CAESAREAN delivery is needed you will be able to stay in the operating theatre unless there is an emergency and a general anaesthetic is given.
* If your partner needs extra medical attention after birth, an important role for you is to rest calmly with your baby. It is best to be in close contact, preferably skin to skin.

Labour and birth, mother
Birth plan

Making a birth plan focuses your mind and may help you make important decisions in labour. Your plan also tells your birth team what you want – an important issue if you are cared for by a number of different people. It can include looking ahead to the time beyond birth as you plan to enjoy time with your baby, and offer her the best possible welcome into your family.

It's a good idea to create your birth plan with your partner and in consultation with your midwife or other supporters. The feeling of being in a partnership, where your wishes are known and respected, will increase your confidence. You can alter your plan if your views change before labour.

Please remember that many things affect labour and you might want to have a backup – 'Plan B'. It is best to be flexible and regard a birth plan as a set of options rather than a strict order of play.

You can use the suggestions below as a guide – add or omit sections depending on your needs. It is important to discuss whether your preferences fit with the protocol and availability of equipment at your chosen maternity unit. For instance, if you want soft lighting and the hospital doesn't have lamps, can you bring your own and plug it in?

Labour

* I'll call my midwife when …
* I want [name] and [name] to be with me …
* I wish to bring things into the room (such as a CD player, birth ball) …
* We will prepare the following snacks and drinks …
* My preference for monitoring is …
* For pain relief I would like to begin with …
* If I need further relief, my preference is …
* My feelings about internal examinations are …
* My feelings about being clothed in labour are …
* I am keen/not keen to use the water pool for labour/for birth …
* My preferences concerning being active and upright are …
* My partner wishes to take breaks, if appropriate, every [x] hours …

Birth

* My feelings about intervention (FORCEPS OR VENTOUSE or caesarean) are …
* My feelings about oxytocin stimulation of contractions are …
* I'm keen/not keen that the lights are dimmed and the room is quiet …

* I wish the cord to be cut after it stops pulsating/after the third stage ... by [name]
* I want to hold my baby straight away/or after she has been washed ...
* My feelings about BREASTFEEDING in the delivery room are ...
* I want/don't want oxytocin to speed up the delivery of the placenta (page 391).

In the first few days

Although your focus may be on your labour and the birth, it is worth planning a few things that will help to make the period after birth comfortable and hassle-free, maximising the time you have to rest and bond with your baby. This may involve asking friends and family to help out, for example, by cooking, shopping, cleaning or other simple errands.

Labour and birth, mother
Bleeding during labour

See also Bleeding, mother, during pregnancy.

One of the fundamental principles of modern midwifery care is to prevent and treat bleeding early. There are a number of reasons bleeding may occur in labour.

A show – mild, bright red bleeding
Labour is usually accompanied by bright red bleeding in the form of a 'show' that heralds the onset of regular contractions. This bleeding is not usually profuse and there is often mucus with the blood.

Significant or profuse bright red bleeding
If bleeding is significant your medical team will assess whether it is arising from a low-lying placenta (page 442) or there has been placental abruption where the placenta has separated from the wall of your uterus. If either is occurring, bleeding is usually profuse. Praevia is often suspected from ultrasound scans carried out in pregnancy. Abruption is accompanied by pain.

Blood loss from a clotting disorder
On rare occasions, bleeding may be excessive because of a blood clotting disorder in the

mother. Usually, affected women are aware of the problem, but childbirth may be the first time it becomes apparent.

Bleeding coming from baby (vasa praevia)
On extremely rare occasions bleeding in labour comes from the baby's blood vessels. This is known as vasa praevia and occurs when blood vessels from the UMBILICAL CORD are not inserted directly into the placenta but run along the amniotic membranes that line the uterus between the baby and the placenta. The vessels may tear when the membranes rupture. If birth follows rapidly, the baby will not lose much blood and may be unaffected but if not there may be FOETAL DISTRESS, so urgent delivery is essential.

Action plan

* You will be given a drip to replace lost fluids and blood if the loss is heavy.
* Your blood clotting factors can be tested and replaced if they are low.
* If bleeding is profuse and/or if your baby shows signs of foetal distress, immediate delivery may be recommended, usually by CAESAREAN SECTION.
* Rarely (with vasa praevia), the baby may require a BLOOD TRANSFUSION after birth.

+ Red flag

If you are not already in hospital it is essential to call for medical help and get to hospital as soon as possible, particularly if the bleeding is profuse. You and your baby can be closely monitored and treatment can begin as soon as you are examined. Time is of the essence, particularly if you are bleeding heavily or experiencing significant pain. Early treatment and, perhaps, birth without delay can be life saving for your baby.

Labour and birth, mother
Bleeding following birth

▇ EXCESSIVE EARLY BLOOD LOSS

The birth of the placenta – the third stage of labour – is always accompanied by bleeding. The loss is usually less than 500ml (around 1 pint). After birth the muscle in the wall of the uterus contracts, retracts and shortens, compressing the blood vessels that supplied the placenta and slowing bleeding to a trickle. Natural blood clotting also reduces bleeding. On average, the blood loss with a caesarean birth is greater than after normal birth.

Excessive bleeding in the 24 hours following birth, known as primary postpartum haemorrhage, occurs in fewer than 10 per cent of births. Very heavy bleeding after birth can be an acute emergency requiring urgent attention.

What happens

Heavy bleeding is more common in a first labour, particularly if labour is long and oxytocin has been used. It may happen if you have had more than four children. Infection in labour, or giving birth to a LARGE BABY or TWINS, increases the risk, as do FIBROIDS in the wall of your uterus or a heart-shaped (bicornute) uterus. If you have experienced postpartum haemorrhage (bleeding after birth) once, the risk of it occurring again increases slightly in the next pregnancy.

After your baby is born your midwife will check the flow of blood from your vagina and assess how well your uterus has contracted. If labour has been long or difficult and you needed oxytocin, the power of contractions may be reduced.

Sometimes the uterus is unable to contract fully because the placenta has not detached completely from the uterine wall. This is called a retained placenta (overleaf).

Bleeding originating from an injury such as a tear or episiotomy is usually slight but it may be profuse and stop spontaneously or after the area has been stitched.

Action plan

If you are bleeding excessively after your baby's birth, your midwife will want to speed up the birth of the placenta. She may massage your uterus as a first step. It is good to begin breastfeeding your baby because this releases oxytocin from your pituitary gland and boosts contractions.

Medical care

- Contractions can be boosted with an injection of synthetic oxytocin into your thigh. Some hospitals do this routinely, and it is discussed on page 377. If this does not keep your uterus contracted, prostaglandin may be used to provide a more powerful boost, but this is infrequently needed. You may feel your uterus contract strongly from the medication but discomfort and heavy blood flow usually stop within a few hours.
- If the birth of the placenta is delayed, manual removal may be needed. This may be because the muscle of the uterus has clamped down and the placenta is trapped or, occasionally, the placenta is deeply embedded in the wall of the uterus (placenta accreta). Manual removal is discussed on page 442).
- If bleeding is excessively heavy after the birth of the placenta, an intravenous drip can be used to administer oxytocic drugs and keep your uterus contracted, and to replace lost fluid. Very rarely, a BLOOD TRANSFUSION may be needed.
- If there is an indication that levels of blood-clotting factors may be low they will be checked and replaced as part of the blood transfusion.
- A tear that is bleeding excessively will be stitched as a matter of urgency.

Preventing bleeding after your next labour

- Eat well and take supplements.
- Let your midwife know that you bled after birth; she is likely to recommend active management of the third stage (drug assistance for the birth of your placenta), particularly if you have fibroids, a heart-shaped uterus or a clotting problem.

■ EXCESSIVE BLEEDING IN THE DAYS FOLLOWING BIRTH

After the birth, your uterus retracts to its pre-pregnant state and sheds its lining, the decidua, together with any remaining fragments of placenta or membrane. This causes blood loss (called lochia), whether birth was vaginal or CAESAREAN. The flow normally lasts for between two and eight weeks. Frequent BREASTFEEDING will help your uterus to contract and expel the remaining fragments. Very heavy blood loss after birth (secondary postpartum haemorrhage) may be a sign of retained placental tissue, which needs to be removed to prevent infection and stop the bleeding.

What happens

Offensive smelling or heavy bleeding may be a sign of infection. A vaginal swab may be needed to check for bacteria.

If blood loss is still excessive or clots appear after the fifth day, an ultrasound scan can check for retained tissue. If there is retained placental tissue you may feel discomfort and bleeding will continue. If you bleed heavily you may feel weak, tired and light-headed when you stand or walk.

Action plan

If you do lose an excessive amount of blood you need to return to hospital for emergency treatment.

Lifestyle

You will need to rest and you may need extra help at home so you can use your energy to recover, care for your baby and establish breastfeeding. After heavy blood loss you may have ANAEMIA and will need to treat this with good nutrition and appropriate mineral and iron supplements. Your levels may return to normal over a few weeks but the supplements need to be taken for six months to replace your body's stores of iron.

Medical care

- If an infection is identified, you will be offered antibiotics. A low level of the antibiotics will be passed in your breast milk with minimal effect to your baby.
- A BLOOD TRANSFUSION is needed if your haemoglobin is below 8–9 gm/dl, but this is rare.

Retained placental tissue and dilatation and curettage (D&C)

If there is retained placental tissue this will be visible on an ultrasound scan. If large placental fragments have been retained these may need to be removed under anaesthesia with an operative DILATATION AND CURETTAGE (D&C), usually within six weeks of birth. D&C involves the following:

- Under a short general or epidural anaesthetic, the placental fragments are gently scraped from the uterine wall with an instrument called a curette.
- The procedure lasts roughly 20 minutes and need not interfere with breastfeeding.
- Within four hours of the operation you will feel little pain and the bleeding will have greatly reduced. If bleeding is excessive, a balloon may be inserted via your vagina and cervix and left in your uterus for two to three hours to apply pressure. It is then simply removed.
- Antibiotics after surgery reduce the risk of infection.

Labour and birth, mother
Breathing

Breathing is a powerful tool in labour. Slow, deep breathing may help you to access and preserve your energy, rest when you need to, and harness your maximum power for giving birth at the end of the second stage. Your muscles need oxygen to work, and deep breathing also nourishes your baby with oxygen. And when you feel anxious, breathing slowly and deeply will help to restore you to a state of calm.

You will have a strong instinct to breathe deeply, and if you have practised during pregnancy your learned response will kick in. If you breathe well while contractions are mild you will be in the swing of things and automatically keep your mind on your breathing when your contractions intensify. Singing or sighing with the out-breath is a powerful way to prolong the breath and relax. A long outbreath is a relaxed breath.

If you become tired or panic, or lose touch with the rhythm of your contractions, your birth partner and midwives can help you come back to yourself and breathe gently. Don't worry – you are never more than a few seconds from the next breath.

Breathing through your contractions

- Begin to inhale as you feel the first tension: relax your shoulders and breathe slowly and deeply. The slow inhalation keeps you steady and supple. Imagine the breath carrying energy throughout your body, to your uterus and to your baby. Your exhalation is a long, continuous release of tension. Think of sending the pain out of your body. Let all the air out before you take the next in-breath.
- Keep breathing deep slow breaths, one after another, until the end of the contraction. When your contractions get stronger you may need to pay more attention to your out-breath, as this is likely to be short if you are tense. It is easier to control than the reflexive in-breath.
- Don't hold your breath.
- Rapid breathing is called hyperventilation. If you do this, you will feel light-headed, weak and afraid, with tingling lips; your muscles lose their power and twitch out of your control. If this happens you can counteract it by slowing your breathing: your birth partner and midwives will help.

Talking yourself through your breath

It can help to focus or meditate on a positive thought, like a mantra that you say to yourself with a rhythm that matches your breath. Use one phrase for each set of breaths through a contraction. Try declaring, 'I am fine, I am fine, I am fine' … 'My body knows how to give birth to my baby, my body knows what to do' … 'My baby knows what to do' …

Transition and birth

Moving and making a noise might help you breathe steadily. Counting or talking silently to yourself may help you stay with your breath in the intensity of transition. A partner or midwife may need to accompany you, as it is difficult to switch from deep breathing to panting.

Many women find it extremely helpful to have their partner by their head, and to breathe calmly together. In the final stages your midwife can help you use your breath to maximum efficiency as you bear down. Once the birth is over, your breathing is likely to be easy and no longer any concern, as you focus on your baby. You may need to take a few deep breaths as you give birth to the placenta.

Labour and birth, mother
Caesarean section

For some mothers and babies, birth by caesarean section is recommended for safety reasons. Occasionally, a mum chooses a caesarean for personal reasons that do not reflect medical risks to her or her baby. Caesarean is covered on pages 108–16.

Labour and birth, mother
Complementary care

See also Complementary therapies.

You may choose one or more complementary therapies through pregnancy and to support you during labour. Your partner or birth attendant may play an important role, and some midwives train in one or more techniques. The benefits range from improving your energy and emotional state to enhancing progress and the strength of contractions and relieving pain. It is best to become familiar with them in advance. Commonly used methods include REFLEXOLOGY, ACUPUNCTURE and MASSAGE.

Specific suggestions for using aromatherapy follow, and a range of homeopathic support remedies, which are often surprising in their power, is given below.

▓ AROMATHERAPY

Aromatherapy oils can influence your mental and physical state in labour. If you are familiar with them and enjoy the scents, you may want to plan ahead to use one or more.

Aromatherapy oils can be blended with a carrier oil, such as almond or grapeseed, and used for MASSAGE. Use a blend of 10 drops of aromatherapy oil to 100ml (¼ pint) of carrier oil. Or you could put two drops of aromatherapy oil in water and heat it gently in a burner or vaporiser or in a bowl placed on a radiator so that its scent fills the room. The scent may also have a calming influence on others who are with you. If you need a stronger boost you could put a few drops on a tissue and sniff it whenever you like.

* *Lavender* is a good all-rounder that calms and stimulates circulation and healing. It is also a good painkiller and can reduce headaches and feelings of faintness. It is the oil most commonly used in labour.
* *Clary sage* can be euphoric – good in times of stress and anxiety. It may act as a mild painkiller that relaxes and aids breathing, and can boost contractions.
* *Neroli* is good for calming the nerves, reducing anxiety and tension, alleviating shock and as an antidepressant and antispasmodic.
* *Marjoram* helps with breathing and acts as a mild sedative. It can help to lower BLOOD PRESSURE. It has a warming effect and helps with pain relief, particularly for muscular pain, for example in the back. It has antispasmodic properties, aids blood flow and is a uterine tonic.
* *Jasmine* is known as the king of oils. It is a uterine tonic and its relaxing properties help to relieve pain and cramps. It also helps to strengthen contractions.
* *Frankincense* may help you to overcome fear. It has the power to cut links with the past and quash memories of bad experiences. It also encourages slow and regular breathing.
* *Camomile* reduces sensitivity and calms.

A herbal mix to aid healing after tears or episiotomy is detailed on page 372.

▓ HOMEOPATHY

HOMEOPATHY can offer powerful support in labour, assisting progress, reducing physical tension and lifting your spirits. The remedies work in labour to support your natural ability. A homeopathic remedy may help you overcome fear and relax into a natural rhythm. For you and your birth partner to meet with your homeopath, prior to labour to discuss which remedies to use, will achieve best results. An increasing number of midwives and obstetricians are now training in the use of homeopathy in labour and birth.

As a general guideline to choosing a remedy, you or your partner, who may have a more objective view, need to focus on the way labour is progressing, any pain you feel, your energy and your emotional state. The symptom pictures for each remedy include all these aspects.

The usual remedy dose for use in labour is a single tablet of 200 potency (200c) (page 306). If the remedy you take suits your needs at that particular moment, it should take effect within a matter of minutes. It is only advisable to repeat the remedy if the same symptoms re-appear. If there has been no change within 10 minutes, it's best to re-assess and choose a different remedy.

Labour and birth

If your birth partner or midwife can pinpoint the reason for difficulties this will help enormously in finding the correct remedy. The cause could include being afraid, uncomfortable or cold, contractions weakening or your baby being in an awkward position. As examples, the following remedies may help when you are experiencing:

Fear, with strong contractions, but slow dilation or extremely fast labour
Aconite, particularly if you are panicky, and are worrying that you or your baby will die, you do not want to be examined or touched and feel better for fresh air.

Exhaustion, and contractions slow down or stop
Caulophyllum, if contractions are short, irregular, feeble or feel sharp and move from place to place or you feel them low in your pelvis or groin, you

are shaking and trembling, perhaps irritable, and you feel chilly but want fresh air.

Note It is not advisable to take this remedy routinely in the last few weeks of pregnancy with the intention of promoting a faster labour. This is a question asked by many pregnant women.

Changeability, with a stop-start labour and weak contractions

Pulsatilla when the rhythm of contractions is interrupted (for example, on the move to hospital), contractions are feeble, irregular or short, with no cervical dilation, your feelings and physical symptoms are changeable, you are clingy and apologetic, have a dry mouth but don't want to drink, feel hot and want fresh air and feel better for sympathy and encouragement. Pulsatilla may kick-start your labour.

Fatigue and exhaustion

Kali Phos is useful at any stage, particularly when there are very few other symptoms. It is best to give the remedy between contractions until energy picks up. This is useful for partners or attendants whose energy is also flagging

Changeability, a lack of rhythm and intense contractions

Cimicifuga for a lack of rhythm, changeable emotional and physical symptoms, strong contractions, some feeling like electric shocks or as a movement from side to side, but your cervix is not dilating. You may be excitable, cry out in agony or claim you cannot go on, become mistrusting and gloomy (worse from noise) and feel cold.

Backache and slow progress

Kali Carb, particularly if your baby is in posterior position, you have back pain and sharp pains radiating into the buttocks that is relieved with pressure or massage, you are over-sensitive, obstinate, bossy and irritable and feel bloated, possibly flatulent and sweaty.

Hypersensitivity and irritability

Chamomilla if you are sensitive to pain, light and/or noise, irritable and irrational, contractions are irregular and there's slow dilation, you're frustrated and become rude, feel dizzy, faint and nauseous and need to urinate frequently, you look hot and want to strip off.

Physical weakness, progressing slowly, and for transition

Gelsemium if you doubt your ability to carry on, have anticipatory anxiety, feel exhausted, dizzy and faint, you tremble, have pains in your joints and muscles, contractions hurt your back, with pain that travels up so that it seems your baby is ascending rather than descending, you don't want to be examined and feel better for moving around. Gelsemium may work well when *Caulophyllum* seems appropriate but fails to act.

A need for privacy, or feeling exposed

Natrum Mur if you feel stuck, self conscious, claustrophobic, vulnerable and want to be left alone, have a headache, crave fresh air and feel thirsty for gulps of water. You may be holding back emotionally. This remedy often 'flicks the switch' and labour begins to progress rhythmically.

Terrified or spaced out feelings

Opium when you are upset and look dazed (like a rabbit caught in the headlights), your face looks red and puffy, your breathing is irregular, your skin is clammy and sweaty, and contractions may slow down or cease.

A need to be in control, but can't be

Nux vomica for pains that are in your back, exhausting and violent, that give you the urge to pass a stool or urinate (although nothing comes), you are not making progress, you feel sick and may retch, with no result, if you become irritable and rude and feel worse from cool air. Nux vomica can help you let go of the desire to be in the driving seat.

Nausea and vomiting

Ipecac for hot-cold feelings, pale appearance with blue-black rings under your eyes.

Birthing the placenta

Once your baby is born you may feel calm and not distracted about the third stage, the birth of the placenta. Homeopathic remedies may aid this last stage to progress smoothly and effectively, leaving you to rest and concentrate on your baby. If you react well to a remedy but your symptoms return after a short time, it may be helpful to repeat the dose (200c potency). If there is no change, then try a different remedy.

To boost contractions and energy
Caulophyllum, particularly after a long labour.

After a long tiring labour
Arnica, particularly if there are no other characteristic symptoms.

For encouragement and relief from feeling upset
Pulsatilla, when the placenta seems to be high, contractions seem ineffective, you have urine retention, your lower abdomen feels hot and tender and you are tearful, hot and bothered. This is best taken very soon after your baby is born.

If you are afraid and in pain
Cimifuga if you have tearing pains but your contractions are absent or lazy, you are very afraid or slightly hysterical, feel chilly and tremble.

If you feel unable to respond to your baby, and you're in pain
Sepia for bearing down pains, but the placenta is slow to descend, pains in your cervix and rectum.

When an oxytocin drug has been given
Secale helps to counter side effects and if you feel excessively hot and distressed and have strong, constant contractions.

Afterpains

In the hours and days following birth, most women get 'afterpains' as the uterus contracts. This tends to be strongest with BREASTFEEDING. You may take one of the following in 30c potency, every four hours for the first 12 hours after delivery and if pains persists you may take the most indicated remedy twice a day for two days, and re-assess.

- *Arnica*, particularly after a long, arduous labour.
- *Sepia* for pains with a strong bearing-down sensation, often after a second or subsequent birth.
- *Cimicifuga* for violent spasms low in the pelvis moving to the abdomen and groin.
- *Pulsatilla* for protracted and changeable pains,

worse during breastfeeding, particularly if you feel weepy, miserable and not thirsty.
- *Chamomilla* for unbearable pains making you feel irritable and difficult to please.

Postnatal support remedies

Many women find the following remedies are invaluable after birth. Each one may be taken in the indicated potency three times per day for five to seven days.

- *Arnica* 30c is the main remedy for trauma – it reduces swelling, encourages healing and eases aching and soreness.
- *Hypericum* 30c for nerve pain and trauma and shooting and tearing pains that radiate from the site of the trauma.
- *Bellis Perennis* 30c for deep tissue healing and for soreness, aching and sensitivity.
- *Calendula* 30c for speedy healing.

In addition, *Hypercal* tincture (10–15 drops) in the bath promotes healing.

If you are feeling emotionally and physically battered after labour, you may take *Staphysagria* 200c – three doses over a 12 hour period.

For your baby

You may give *Aconite* 30c if she is shocked after the birth – one dose may settle her. You may follow this with *Arnica* 30c, which may ease any bruising and trauma to her head, cheek or jaw. It is preferable to use a soft tablet, which absorbs almost instantly on contact with the mouth. If your baby remains unsettled or appears to be in pain, consult a homeopath.

▓ SELF-HYPNOSIS AND HYPNO BIRTHING

Hypno-birthing requires preparation before labour. You may be guided in self-hypnosis. Part of the preparation is to learn how to go into a deep state of relaxation. You will learn triggers for relaxation that your 'bodymind' unconsciously responds to during labour. These may include music, touch on certain parts of your body, breathing patterns or words you say out loud or to yourself. VISUALISATION may be an important element in this.

Labour and birth, mother
Contractions

Your experience of contractions is unique to you. Contractions vary from woman to woman, and from one labour to the next, if you have more than one baby. The power of contractions tends to build up through labour, reaching a peak during birth, but it is also normal for contractions to become weaker and more widely spaced, and then speed up and become more intense again. Sometimes labour can begin with full intensity. You may feel a dull backache, or something like a period pain. You may feel waves of pain in your uterus, following one another with a gentle rhythm that is easy to go with. You may feel forceful pressure and almost overwhelming pain. The power of contractions may take over your body and transform you as you go fully into the birth.

Usually, the pain of a contraction lasts while the uterus tightens, and then there is a completely pain-free interval until the next wave rises. Occasionally, there is no respite. At the other end of the scale, some women feel very few contractions and no pain as the cervix ripens and dilates, though this is rare. In second and subsequent births, contractions tend to build up faster and be more intense, but this isn't always the case.

What happens

Many women like to know what is happening with contractions: if you know they have a purpose it can be helpful as you breathe through each pain as it rises and passes.

Tightening and discomfort
- With each contraction, the muscle wall of your uterus tightens from the top (fundus) down to the bottom (cervix).
- The sensation usually begins when the uterus has begun to tighten and reaches a peak at the height of a contraction. It lasts from 30 to 60 seconds.
- The interval between contractions is often completely pain free.
- Pain perception varies widely, and the intensity of pain you feel is likely to alter from stage to

stage. If you are sensitive to pain, or have a low pain threshold, you may have experienced pre-labour Braxton-Hicks contractions (below) as painful and labour may be acutely painful for you. If you are less sensitive to pain or have a higher pain threshold, the pain of your contractions may be relatively easy to bear.
- If you feel anxious, this may increase the risk that you will feel pain and also the level of pain you feel.
- Occasionally pain is constant and it is difficult to relax between contractions, particularly if oxytocin or prostaglandin has been used to boost labour. Sometimes pain-relieving medication makes it difficult to relax and let go between tightenings.
- Contractions may make you feel nauseous.
- Your bowel may contract, causing pain during or after a uterine contraction.

Your baby
- As your uterus contracts and the muscle fibres shorten, the blood flowing to the placenta is reduced. The rest period between tightenings allows the blood to flow strongly to nourish your baby with oxygen. Healthy babies are well equipped to cope with this temporary reduction of oxygen.
- Contractions probably feel like a massage in early labour, and a forceful push later on. Your baby's experience is not the same as yours and it is unlikely that the contractions feel painful.

Braxton-Hicks contractions
Braxton-Hicks contractions are the tightenings most women feel in mid- to late-pregnancy. They may also be a feature of pre-labour (page 357). While everyone feels them differently they are not often painful. Your abdomen will feel tight during each contraction, which lasts 30 to 60 seconds, and then relaxes. The contractions come in runs but do not continue regularly for more than 60 minutes. In true labour, the runs of contractions continue and the time between each one diminishes to less than five minutes and discomfort increases. If you are in doubt, you are probably not in labour – you may want to check with your midwife. Occasionally Braxton-Hicks contractions may be painful and then it is difficult to distinguish them from labour.

Timing and regularity of contractions in labour

Timing contractions is a way of gauging how labour is progressing. The time is measured from the beginning of one contraction to the beginning of next. It's useful for your midwife to be aware of the timing, and it isn't necessary for you to analyse what's happening: being too preoccupied with timings could impede the progress of labour. Your midwife or your birth partner may keep an eye on this so you can focus on your body and baby.

Contractions in early labour

In early labour it may be difficult to see a pattern. Contractions are usually spaced between 10 and 30 minutes apart. It is common but not universal for them to come forcefully in runs and then to have times when they are slight or even disappear. If your contractions are not close together it's okay to relax or move gently. Some women feel happy to get on with simple tasks, such as cooking or light cleaning, or go for a short walk, while things are relatively calm, or get some sleep. Sometimes labour starts with contractions at full intensity and this continues until the birth.

Contractions in established labour

As the cervix opens wider, contractions tend to get more frequent and powerful. They may begin at 10 minute intervals. In the active phase of labour, in most women they become more frequent and often occur every two to three minutes. Each contraction is over within 30 to 60 seconds and then you relax. The pattern varies from woman to woman, and is also likely to vary over the course of your own labour with maximum intensity for birth. If the power of your contractions is not optimal, there may be slow progress (page 387).

Contractions and the birth of the placenta

The contractions encouraging your uterus to expel the placenta begin between two and 15 minutes after your baby is born, or sooner if oxytocin hormone has been used to speed the process. If you have given birth two or three times before, these may be intense but they are typically gentler than the forceful contractions of late labour.

Contractions during breastfeeding

BREASTFEEDING stimulates the hormone oxytocin, which acts on your uterus, helping it to contract. You will feel it contracting as it shrinks after birth, and the pain usually lasts about a week. These 'afterpains' can be uncomfortable, and tend to be more painful in subsequent pregnancies.

Action plan

On page 346 you'll find an overview of ways to enhance the power of your contractions, to follow their rhythm, keep your energy up, reduce pain and continue through discomfort. Options for pain relief are discussed on pages 381–6.

Labour and birth, mother
Disproportion (tight fit)

See also Labour and birth, mother, progress, slow; Large babies.

The position your baby chooses will largely depend on her, and to a lesser extent on the size and shape of your pelvis. The term 'birth disproportion' means that the fit between your baby's head and your pelvis is tight. This will make it more difficult for her to advance through the birth canal. Depending on the nature of disproportion, labour may progress normally, progress may be slow, or a CAESAREAN SECTION may be recommended. Your midwife and obstetrician will advise you on the best plan of action. Disproportion occurs more often with large babies, but cannot always be predicted in advance of labour.

What happens

Disproportion occurs if your baby is large or your pelvis is small or its shape is not optimal for birth. Your pelvis is fully grown by the time you are 17 years of age and its adult size reflects your nutrition as a child and teenager. Good nutrition in teenage years may increase pelvic size and capacity. If you are shorter than average height, your pelvis may be small.

In some women the pelvis is shaped with the pubic bones in front of the bladder forming a narrow triangular-shaped arch rather than a round arch. This leaves less space for the round baby's head to fit and engage in the pelvis. In a small number of women, an accident may have caused a fractured pelvis. If this has happened to you your obstetrician will assess whether this will interfere with birth. Pelvic X-ray (pelvimetry) to determine the exact size of your pelvic bones is not recommended in pregnancy because of the radiation risks.

Action plan

It may be possible to prevent your baby from growing too large by attending to your nutrition during pregnancy and, if you have DIABETES, close management of your blood glucose levels. Her size is not entirely in your control, however.

Pregnancy and birth

* Your midwife or obstetrician may anticipate disproportion if your baby appears large in pregnancy, or if there is a non-engaged head in late pregnancy (although disproportion is only one possible cause).
* If labour progress is slow (page 386) your midwife or doctor will check the cause. They can assess the shape of your pelvis and the extent to which your baby's head is engaged via an internal vaginal examination. If there is a tight fit, your baby's head is more likely to be positioned awkwardly (page 344).
* Your baby may need help to be born if progress is slow.
* If your birth team decides there is sufficient space for your baby to be born, you may be offered an oxytocin infusion to boost contractions (page 377).
* If disproportion is mild, your baby may be born without intervention if your uterus contracts well and you are able to bear down strongly. Being upright will maximise your power to push and open your pelvic cavity as wide as possible.
* Your baby may need intervention with FORCEPS OR VENTOUSE if the second (pushing) stage is long.
* If your birth team decide it would be safer for your baby not to be born vaginally, they may advise a caesarean section.

Labour and birth, mother
Episiotomy and tears

See also Labour and birth, mother, forceps and ventouse.

■ ADVICE AND PREVENTION

Your vagina is designed to stretch at birth and there are some measures you can take to prepare it. Nevertheless, the vaginal opening may tear so that it becomes wide enough for your baby's head to pass through. This sounds worse than it usually is – with the pressure and the force of birth, few women notice they have torn, and tears typically heal relatively quickly. Many tears need to be stitched.

Some women need extra help to widen their vaginal opening, and this can be done with an episiotomy. This is an incision in the perineum, the area of tissue between the vagina and the anus. The cut needs to be stitched after birth.

Some women feel an episiotomy is an acceptable part of having a baby. Some are upset if an episiotomy is performed and would prefer to have torn or to have had no tear. Others choose to have an episiotomy because they fear tearing.

Arguments against routine use of episiotomy

Episiotomy is used frequently in some countries, with a variation in rates: from 8 per cent in the Netherlands, to over 90 per cent in Eastern Europe. Episiotomy is used in 14–20 per cent of births in the UK.

Research evidence suggests that a rate above 20 per cent is not medically justified. Obstetricians tend to be more convinced than midwives that an episiotomy is an integral part of managing a first birth. Tears and episiotomy are less common in second and subsequent vaginal births.

Episiotomies became popularised by Dr Lee in the USA in the 1920s. They were thought to prevent damage to the perineum as well as a prolapse of the vaginal and pelvic floor. It was also thought to protect the baby from birth injury or FOETAL DISTRESS by reducing the pressure of birth. These theoretical benefits have since been disproved and there is little justification for its routine use. But it is accepted that when episiotomy is used selectively it is an effective way to widen the vaginal entrance and allow a baby's head to emerge. This may be necessary when birth needs to be speeded up because there is evidence of foetal distress, the tissues are too tight to stretch, particularly if a baby is large, or when an extra pulling force is needed in some FORCEPS OR VENTOUSE deliveries.

* Even if a woman chooses not have an episiotomy, she may still tear, but with rare exceptions the tear will be smaller than an episiotomy cut would have been. Many women do not tear at all. An episiotomy does not prevent deep tears into the vagina or into the anal muscle.
* An episiotomy does not prevent baby's birth injuries.
* It can increase the amount of maternal blood loss (page 361).
* Pain in the stitches after birth is likely to be greater with an episiotomy, as is persistent pain during intercourse.
* An episiotomy does not heal more quickly or more efficiently than a tear, nor is it easier to repair.
* Tears of the anal sphincter muscle are more common with episiotomy and may lead to flatulence or anal incontinence (page 317). Yet an episiotomy does not reduce the chance of urinary incontinence, nor reduce laxity of pelvic floor muscles, nor promise better sex after birth.

Preparing your vagina to stretch

Preparation and care during labour reduces the likelihood of tearing or the need for an episiotomy, but cannot be a guarantee.

* During pregnancy, perineal massage and pelvic floor exercises are helpful (page 438).
* During labour, your position and your birth team's skill and assistance can help.
* Giving birth in a supported upright position may help your vagina to stretch to its maximum.
* You may use focused breathing and VISUALISATION to concentrate your energy in your vaginal area at the moment of birth. Deep breathing helps your tissues stretch.
* Your midwife may ease pressure on your vagina by facilitating slow delivery of the head while

supporting your perineum, delivering the shoulders one at a time.

* Giving birth in water may help to maximise the stretch in your vaginal tissues.
* Some midwives gently massage the perineum to encourage stretching when birth is drawing near.

What happens

Tears

If you tear, this is because your baby needed more space to emerge from your vagina. The most common place to tear is backwards along the perineum, between the vagina and the anus, but a tear may involve the front of the vagina and the labia and may go towards the clitoris. If you are on your back, tears tend to involve the back wall of the vagina whereas if you are upright or leaning forwards, the tear may be more superficial towards the front of the labia. Every woman is different and some have more elasticity in their vaginal tissues than others.

* A superficial tear in the vaginal or labial skin is classed as first degree.
* If the underlying muscles are involved, which is less common, this is a second-degree tear.
* On very rare occasions, the tear is third degree and extends into the anus. The likelihood of a third-degree tear increases with episiotomy and forceps delivery, and with LARGE BABIES and a prolonged second stage of labour.
* Extremely rare fourth-degree tears involve complete disruption of the anal sphincter muscle and the lining of the anus.

Episiotomy

If you and your team decide to go ahead with an episiotomy, your vaginal area will be numbed with a local anaesthetic injection, unless you already have an epidural in place. The injection will give a small, stinging sensation and the anaesthetic will become effective immediately. Your midwife or obstetrician will then perform the cut and you will not feel anything. An episiotomy cut extends from the back wall of the vaginal opening to the side of the anus along the perineum, and includes the vaginal and perineal skin and the underlying muscles.

* A midline episiotomy runs straight down toward the rectum and is the preferred method in the USA and Canada.

- A mediolateral episiotomy runs down and off to one side and is the preferred method in Europe.
- A midline episiotomy is less painful, heals better, is less likely to cause pain during sex and causes less blood loss, but there is a risk that the incision may extend during the birth and the anus may tear. The opposite is the case in a mediolateral episiotomy.

◼ POSTNATAL COMFORT AND CARE

When the birth is over and your baby's placenta has been born, your midwife or obstetrician will assess the need for stitches. Reading this before birth may be scary but when stitches are needed the process is usually straightforward and being with your baby is a wonderful distraction.

Minor, first-degree tears of the skin heal spontaneously and often do not require stitching. Second-degree tears of the skin and muscle, if long or deep, are usually stitched. Third- and fourth-degree tears need to be stitched and a senior member of the obstetric medical team usually does this. An episiotomy is always stitched.

Stitching

You will be asked to lie on your back and the head of the bed may be raised so you can hold your baby. You may breastfeed. The area is numbed and the stitching process usually takes 15–30 minutes. Depending on the area involved, the stitches are in three layers: the vaginal lining, the muscles and the external skin. Skin sutures dissolve in four to six days while muscle sutures take a few weeks.

Discomfort

Unstitched tears or a stitched tear or episiotomy may be uncomfortable. The degree of discomfort and the rapidity of healing depend on the length and depth of your tear or cut, the skill of the obstetrician or midwife, and the quality of suture material. While the area is healing you can care for your vagina and perineum and keep pain to a minimum. A tear or an episiotomy may contribute to blood loss immediately after birth.

Pain may arise from a number of areas.

- *Healing skin.* This may be tender for the first week. The discomfort will be increased if the healing area is inflamed or infected. Your pelvic muscles may be under tension from the stitches.
- *Swelling and bruising.* Your vaginal tissues are able to expand and swelling may be caused by fluid passing into the tissues from the pressure of birth. This usually settles in a few days but if the area is infected or there has been bruising, swelling may last longer. Bruises are from bleeding in the area of the tear and usually heal in seven to 10 days.
- *Muscle spasm.* Spasm in your back muscles and from pelvic joints and ligaments that may have stretched during the birth can be very painful. Your pelvic muscles may be in spasm as a reaction to the stitching. Discomfort usually recedes in one to two weeks but some women have pain for months.
- *Haemorrhoids* (PILES). These can add to painful spasms after birth.
- *Scar tissue* may form around the stitches, and is more likely after a large tear or episiotomy or if there has been infection. Scarring is rare but it may cause discomfort for months after the birth: sex may be painful and the vaginal opening may even be narrowed. The usual site for scars is on the back wall of the vagina at the junction of the perineum.

Pain relief and other treatment

- Pain from skin or muscle sutures usually passes in 10 to 14 days and can be relieved with painkillers (page 408).
- Pain from the pelvic joints or ligaments, or from muscle spasm, may respond well to physiotherapy or OSTEOPATHY.
- An infection may require antibiotic treatment.
- For scar tissue, pelvic floor exercises and perineal massage are very helpful.
- For around 5 per cent of women, discomfort takes months to settle because of muscle spasm and scar tissue forming in the deep tissues. In a tiny number of women, an operation is needed to remove the scarred area.

Posture and movement

- You may find it helps to lie on your side instead of sitting, or to sit on a rubber ring.
- From the first day it is good to walk around. Later you may do postnatal pelvic floor exercises and begin gentle YOGA stretches. The exercises may heighten discomfort in your vaginal area but they will increase the blood

flow to the muscles and help healing. Modern sutures are very strong and will not break if you contract your muscles.

Urination and opening your bowels

If there is stinging or burning, it may be from superficial tears in your vagina. Try pouring lukewarm water over your labia as you urinate. Initially you may find it easier to urinate in the bath or the shower. If your urine continues to burn after a few days, you may have infection of the bladder (page 170), particularly after a long labour or if your midwife used a catheter to empty your bladder.

Although it is rare, you may experience urinary incontinence (page 317) or flatulence (page 64). This may be linked with stretching of your tissues at birth and usually passes in a few days. Sometimes, it persists for longer. Pelvic floor exercises may help you build up tone.

Many women feel sore after birth and are nervous about pooing. Modern sutures last for weeks and will not break with a bowel action. For some women, discomfort from stitches or piles may reduce awareness of needing to poo. To reduce the chance of CONSTIPATION it is best to eat a high-fibre diet, consider taking lactulose and drink lots of fluid for the first few days: this will help you go, and helps to prevent your stools getting hard. Some women need a suppository to help their bowels to open.

Homeopathy

After birth these remedies are commonly used to speed up healing and ease discomfort, each may be taken three times a day for five-seven days.
* *Arnica* (30c) reduces swelling, promotes healing of bruised tissue and reduces aching and soreness.
* *Hypericum* (30c) works particularly on nerve pain and damage and is good for shooting or tearing pains.
* *Bellis Perennis* (30c) helps to heal deep tissue, relieves soreness and sensitivity and throbbing pains, and is good in conjunction with *Arnica*.
* *Calendula* (30c) speeds up the healing of tears and wounds.

Hypercal tincture may be applied externally in conjunction with the above. Add 10–15 drops to the bath or bidet or soak a sanitary towel or cotton wool in diluted tincture (10 drops in 250ml/½ pint water) and bathe the area. If it stings when you urinate you can pour this diluted tincture over yourself as you sit on the toilet.

If bowel movements are a struggle, you may take *Nux Vomica* (30c) three times per day for two days (or try another of the remedies in the constipation entry).

Staphysagria may be helpful if you feel emotionally bashed and raw after an episiotomy or tearing badly. You may take three 200c tablets within 12 hours.

Herbs and aromatherapy

A few drops of tincture of *comfrey*, *calendula* and *hypericum*, or a decoction of the herbs themselves in a warm bath will soothe and help the healing process. You can make the decoction by placing a handful each of *Calendula Officinalis* flowers, *Hypericum Perforatum* (St John's wort) leaves and some *Symphytum Officinale* (comfrey) in a large stock pot of water. Bring these to the boil with two whole bulbs (not cloves) of fresh garlic, simmer for 30 minutes and then crush the garlic with a potato masher into the 'soup' and strain the whole mixture into a bowl. Save the liquor and discard the herbs. You should have enough for three baths.

You can also add it to a warm sitz bath (a small tub in which you can sit to ease vaginal/anal pain – some people may use a bidet).

Making love again

Within four weeks, the site of an episiotomy cut or tear will probably be completely healed and sexual intercourse will be safe. Your muscles may take time to regain normal strength and, because the oestrogen output from your ovaries will be low after birth, your vaginal skin will be thinner and particularly sensitive. This effect lasts longer if you are breastfeeding and occurs even without stitches. Your emotions following birth, and while you focus on your child, will also affect your libido. There is more on sex after birth on page 474.

Your emotions

The emotional impact will become clear with time when you have your baby with you, and when you have had time to rest and recuperate.

Some women are so pleased to have a baby that they are unaffected by tears or cuts. Less commonly, women experience a long-term effect on their self-confidence, body image and sex life. This is more likely if you feel pain or if you have a degree of incontinence.

If you have pain after the first week, show signs of urinary incontinence, excessive wind or faecal incontinence, or feel emotionally vulnerable and upset, do talk to your doctor, midwife or health visitor. Sometimes a difficult birth may have repercussions in weeks or months and it is worth seeking support as early as possible (page 395). If there is an underlying physical problem that needs attention, it is best to have it treated sooner rather than later.

Labour and birth, mother
False and pre-labour

See Labour and birth, mother, beginnings of labour.

Labour and birth, mother
Forceps and ventouse

Two important medical devices used to aid the delivery of the baby are forceps, a traditional tool that dates back over 400 years, and the ventouse, or vacuum extractor, which was first introduced over 40 years ago. Forceps or ventouse are used in 3–11 per cent of births, and are more commonly used in first births.

Forceps
Forceps consist of two metal blades shaped like salad spoons that are put into the vagina and placed on either side of a baby's head. Their introduction in 1598 was a milestone in obstetric history, allowing intervention in difficult births when the lives of mother and baby might otherwise have been lost. Forceps are now much less commonly used than ventouse.

Ventouse
The ventouse, invented in 1957, is a plastic cup that is placed on a baby's scalp and connected to a vacuum pump. The cup is held on the baby's head by suction and the obstetrician pulls to give an extra downward force (traction) while the mother pushes. Modern cups fit well to a baby's head and cause minimal trauma. The ventouse is used more frequently because it occupies less space and there is less risk of tearing (an episiotomy is not always essential). Ventouse includes a safety feature that ensures the cup will automatically detach from the baby's head if too much pressure is applied during traction.

Why assistance may be needed
Antenatal preparation and active upright birth positions (page 350) may reduce the chances that your baby will need assistance, although circumstances cannot always be in your control. Your baby may need help for one of several reasons:
* The second stage of labour may be prolonged (page 389) or you may lack energy to continue.
* Your baby's head might be large in relation to your pelvis (although a very LARGE BABY will need to be born by CAESAREAN SECTION).
* Your baby may be in an occipito posterior position (page 344). His head can be rotated with forceps or ventouse, after which delivery follows easily.
* If your baby has FOETAL DISTRESS, assistance helps speed up the birth and maximises safety.
* If you have had an epidural (page 383) this can reduce your pushing force (a mobile epidural is preferable to enable you to change position and increase the downward force of your contractions).
* If you are afraid of pushing or tearing you may require help.
* Your baby may be in the breech position (page 342) and the assistance helps his head to be born.
* You may have a medical condition (such as high BLOOD PRESSURE) that makes bearing down unsafe.

Safety is the key issue and if the force of assistance needed is excessive, and the obstetrician feels it may be too traumatic for you or your baby, an emergency caesarean section is preferable.

What happens

Forceps or ventouse can only be used when your baby's head has fully entered and engaged in your pelvis. Your CERVIX must be fully dilated and open. Before the procedure, priority will be given to effective pain relief. You may have the option of an epidural if an anaesthetist is present. Alternatively you may be offered a pudendal or perineal block given by injection (page 383). If you already have an epidural in place, it can be topped up.

You will be asked to lie on your back with your legs supported by stirrups. This position helps the obstetrician to feel and deliver your baby as safely and as quickly as possible. A catheter tube may be passed into your bladder to empty it and protect it from damage during delivery. Your partner will probably be welcome to stay. He may sit by your head during the procedure, and be there to hold your baby. Alternatively he may not feel comfortable and choose to leave the birth room.

The forceps or ventouse is applied to your baby's head and pulled with carefully controlled pressure with each contraction. The pulling force will combine with your pushing force to help your baby descend. Many women feel as if they are doing a lot of the work to help the baby out. If your medical team believe that an EPISIOTOMY is necessary (less common with ventouse) it will be done as you push. Birth usually occurs within three contractions after the application of the instrument.

Action plan for recovery

Your reaction and your baby's response will reflect the wider context of your labour and birth and the degree of ease or trauma involved (page 393). For both of you, skin-to-skin contact and frequent BREASTFEEDING will help your body's release of pain-relieving and feel-good HORMONES.

You

After the birth, you may feel sore and bruised in the front and back pelvic joints, which may open more than usual. The pelvic muscles may also have stretched, giving a sensation of bruising. Ventouse is less likely to cause muscle tears or excess stretching. You may feel uncomfortable if you have had stitches from an episiotomy or a tear and healing may take a few weeks (page 371).

Your baby after forceps or ventouse

Your baby feels the pulling force of forceps during the contractions, each lasting less than one minute. He may feel a strong tug and it may be painful. After birth there may be marks on his cheeks or jaw for a few days. If a ventouse has been used he will feel suction on his scalp for some minutes and this might be uncomfortable. His scalp may be swollen and red (page 54). This settles in a day or two.

Some babies are irritable and cry a lot and they appear to have a headache. Frequent sucking at the breast or bottle is a good remedy, and is reassuring because of the warmth of a loving embrace. Cranial OSTEOPATHY can be effective in reducing the tension that builds up in reaction to the force on your baby's head. Osteopathy is also useful to treat the tension in your own pelvic joints and muscles.

Homeopathy after the procedure

HOMEOPATHY may help your own healing. The advice on page 372 for healing after episiotomy or tears applies.

For your baby, *Aconite* 30c potency may be useful if he is shocked after birth – one dose may settle him. You may follow this with *Arnica* 30c potency, which may ease any bruising and trauma to his head, cheek or jaw. If he remains unsettled or appears to be in pain, consult a homeopath.

Labour and birth, mother
Induction and augmentation

See also Labour and birth, mother, overdue (post maturity); progress, slow.

Induction is the name given to the process of artificially starting labour. In the UK, this occurs in 10 to 20 per cent of labours but the rate varies from hospital to hospital. It is more usual to induce a first baby. There are a number of traditional methods of inducing labour (page 377). There are also complementary methods including HOMEOPATHY and ACUPUNCTURE. Medical methods that rely on administration of synthetic versions of natural hormone-like chemicals, such as prostaglandin and oxytocin, are commonly used in the UK (below).

Augmentation

In some cases, whether labour is induced or begins spontaneously, dilation is slow or contractions become ineffective. If this happens labour can be supported by using the same medical methods that are used for induction. This is called augmentation of labour.

Why induce?

Induction of labour is usually considered for one of the following reasons:

* OVERDUE. Going beyond the due date is the most common reason for induction of labour. Sometimes induction is preferred by a mum who is keen to give birth. Sometimes it is recommended by the birth team because the placenta can become less efficient as pregnancy continues.
* IUGR (INTRAUTERINE GROWTH RESTRICTION). This may occur at any time during pregnancy. If there is evidence that your baby is not thriving it may be preferable to induce labour, particularly if you are more than 37 weeks pregnant. The effects of IUGR are more marked in late pregnancy because placental function may naturally decline at this time and your baby may be better nourished outside the womb.
* Premature rupture of the membranes (page 391). After the membranes have ruptured, bacteria in the vagina can infect your baby. If there are signs of infection, an induction is essential.
* Placental function. If you have a condition that may affect placental function, such as pre-eclampsia/high BLOOD PRESSURE or kidney disease, induction may be needed if tests show that you or your baby may be at risk. If you have DIABETES, labour may be induced if your baby is growing too large or if your obstetrician is concerned about how your placenta is functioning.
* Patient choice. Labour is sometimes induced because it suits the family to have the birth on a particular day. This is not an option in all hospitals. It is essential to be sure of the dating of pregnancy to prevent PREMATURE BIRTH.

To induce or not to induce?

Induction of labour is a very emotional issue and women are divided in their views. Some like to be certain that labour will not be prolonged beyond a set date. Others feel ready and are looking forward to the birth. Many prefer to wait for labour to begin spontaneously. You will probably want to talk through the pros and cons with your midwife, obstetrician and partner. If there are any concerns that it is safer for a baby to be born than to remain in the womb, the vast majority of women are content to accept induction.

Some hospitals are happy to let women who have been induced use the birth pool providing there is no suggestion of foetal distress. On rare occasions, foetal distress may come about if contractions are very intense. If induction fails, which happens in a minority of cases, your baby will need to be born by caesarean. Because there are risks involved in caesarean delivery, it is best to ensure that there are sufficient reasons to believe it is best for your baby to be induced. Induction undertaken for convenience may lead to a caesarean.

Enhancing labour

* If you have been having runs of contractions that are not associated with dilation of your CERVIX, you may be in 'false labour'. If you are at or past full-term, you and your birth team may consider augmenting labour because there is a chance that you will become increasingly tired. The process is similar to induction and it boosts your existing contractions and encourages the cervix to dilate. Augmentation is not compulsory and it will be done when you feel the timing is right.
* If you are established in labour but your cervix is dilating slowly, or your contractions lose their intensity, your midwife and obstetrician will assess the cause of slow progress. She may recommend oxytocin, which is also used for induction to boost the power of your contractions.

▓ MEDICAL METHODS

Medical induction may be the preferred choice if your birth team has advised you that it is safest for you and your baby, or you have chosen to induce labour. There are two main ways in which labour may be induced. The medical team may induce labour chemically, by giving vaginal prostaglandin, or they may break the waters manually by rupturing the membranes and also give oxytocin by intravenous drip. This may also be done to augment labour if progress is slow. Modern induction of labour is usually successful.

What happens

Before deciding on induction, any relevant medical aspects of your pregnancy will have to be considered. There may be reasons why induction may not be appropriate, such as disproportion (page 368) or transverse lie (page 345). Your baby's size and position in relation to your pelvic capacity will be checked. Many hospitals do not induce if women have had previous surgery, such as a CAESAREAN SECTION or myomectomy (operation to remove fibroids from the uterus). It is also important to consider your baby's age in the womb so that issues of premature birth can be taken into account. If you are not full term, your uterus may not be responsive to induction.

Your doctor will examine the ripeness (softness) of your cervix (called a Bishop score), because induction is more successful if it is ripe. If your cervix shows no signs of ripening and an ultrasound scan shows your baby is growing well and the placenta is providing adequate nutrition, you may decide to delay induction. If there is concern about the wellbeing of your baby, induction will go ahead. You will be given synthetic prostaglandin hormones in hospital to ripen your cervix and induce labour.

Most women experience gentle contractions that gradually become stronger and more closely spaced and then go into labour that progresses well. If contractions are very painful you may also need PAIN RELIEF.

Prostaglandin

The majority of inductions are now undertaken using synthetic prostaglandin dinoprostone (Prostin). This is a synthetic form of prostaglandin, the hormone-like chemical produced by the lining of the uterus that stimulates contractions and helps the cervix to ripen.

- The Prostin is inserted as a vaginal gel, with an applicator the thickness of a pencil. Your

midwife may perform a gentle 'stretch and sweep' (page 378) at the same time.
- The dosage needs to be carefully controlled. It is lower if you have had ASTHMA, more than four babies, are carrying TWINS or have an excessive volume of AMNIOTIC FLUID.
- After insertion, it is best to rest in bed for an hour or two. Your baby's heartbeat and your contractions will be monitored regularly.
- Your uterus may respond rapidly and contractions could begin within an hour or two. If your cervix is dilating, the second dose will be delayed. Sometimes feelings of discomfort come from 'Prostin pain' and there is no dilation. If your cervix is not ripe, the initial doses of prostaglandin help it to soften and ripen. The following doses stimulate labour as the cervix dilates.
- Every six hours, your midwife will check your cervix and may insert Prostin every six hours until labour begins. There is a recommended maximum dosage that is higher in a first birth.

Side effects of prostaglandin

Possible side effects of prostaglandin include nausea, vomiting and diarrhoea, which affect 5 per cent of women and usually disappear in a few hours. Vaginal sensitivity and soreness may occur after 12 hours. In about 5 per cent of women, the uterus may respond by contracting excessively (hyperstimulation), which may lead to intense discomfort and sometimes to FOETAL DISTRESS. Close foetal heart monitoring is essential after Prostin has been inserted, particularly if your contractions are very frequent.

In a small number of women, labour does not begin within 24 hours. The next option is to rupture the membranes and use artificial oxytocin to further stimulate contractions.

Artificial rupture of the membranes (ARM)

Some birth teams choose to break the waters manually to augment slow progress or to induce labour. This is done if prostaglandin has not stimulated labour within 24 hours; or it may be the first choice if the cervix is ripe and partly dilated (usually in second and subsequent pregnancies). In response to the membranes breaking, the lining of your uterus releases natural prostaglandin and labour usually begins.

Artificial rupture of membranes may not be the preferred choice if your baby is in an awkward position or you have a vaginal infection, particularly GROUP B STREP. Once the membranes have been ruptured they no longer protect against bacterial organisms in the vagina. Most hospitals are keen that birth follows no more than 24 hours after the rupture. If contractions do not begin within a few hours an oxytocin hormonal infusion is usually started to boost contractions.

- During a vaginal examination, the doctor or midwife inserts a thin plastic instrument into the cervix and punctures the membranes. The procedure can be uncomfortable.
- If your waters are broken to augment the first stage of labour because progress is slow, your baby's head may descend onto your cervix and the efficiency of contractions may improve. For your baby's safety, your midwife will ensure that the head is sufficiently low to prevent a cord prolapse (downward displacement) before rupturing the membranes, and she will monitor your baby's heart rate afterwards.

Oxytocin

- Synthetic oxytocin (also called Syntocinon) stimulates uterine contractions in the same way as the natural hormone produced by your and your baby's pituitary glands. It may be used if prostaglandin and rupturing the membranes do not induce labour. It is used to augment a slow labour. Oxytocin is administered using an intravenous drip.
- In most hospitals oxytocin is administered at a slow rate and the rate is gradually increased using a pump while the baby's heartbeat and uterine contractions are continuously monitored. The rate depends on whether or not this is your first labour and on the intensity of your contractions. It is very carefully regulated if you have high blood pressure or fluid retention, or if you have a heart problem.
- Oxytocin is a very effective way to improve progress in the first or second stage of labour. It tends to boost the strength of contractions and can improve their co-ordination. If your baby is in a slightly awkward position, oxytocin may boost your uterus enough to help her negotiate the birth canal in readiness for the birth. It may also encourage a baby in an occipito posterior position to turn and move down. If you are given oxytocin to augment your labour, contractions will probably take 15 to 30 minutes to reach maximum power.
- With the drip in place you may also receive intravenous fluids. If you are dehydrated, this will improve your energy levels.

Side effects of oxytocin

Unwanted side effects occur in a minority of women:

- Oxytocin may make contractions less co-ordinated.
- Oxytocin occasionally stimulates excessive contractions (hyperstimulation of the uterus) and this may reduce the flow of blood in the placenta and lead to foetal distress. The amount of oxytocin administered in second and subsequent pregnancies is lower because the sensitivity of the uterus may be greater. The rate of oxytocin flow can be safely controlled or stopped if necessary. The oxytocin effect begins to diminish within five minutes and the levels are close to normal in 60 minutes. Oxytocin will not be given if there are any signs of foetal distress.
- Oxytocin may, in extremely rare circumstances, lead to rupture of the uterus. This is usually in women who have many children or have had a previous caesarean section.

On balance, when potential side effects are weighed against the benefits, oxytocin is an important drug for use in induction and in labour. Its use needs careful supervision to maintain safety.

■ SELF-HELP, TRADITIONAL METHODS AND COMPLEMENTARY THERAPIES

You may want to try one or more methods to encourage labour to begin, and there are some suggestions below. There are also a number of things you can do to augment labour, once it has begun. Suggestions are listed below.

Methods for inducing labour

There are several self-help techniques that have been used for many years to induce labour, with effects that vary from woman to woman. For example, you or your partner could stimulate your nipples because this releases oxytocin, which in turn stimulates your uterus to contract. If your cervix is ripe, sexual intercourse may trigger labour because the semen contains prostaglandin to stimulate the uterus. These approaches will only work if labour is about to happen within a few days. They cannot cause premature labour.

Castor oil is an old-fashioned, sometimes effective remedy. It can be made more palatable by mixing with orange juice. It often brings on DIARRHOEA and theoretically could cause your baby to pass a bowel movement (meconium) in the womb: it is best to check with your midwife if you wish to take it.

If tension is hindering the start of labour or prolonging pre-labour, gentle MASSAGE or a soak in the bath with a soothing AROMATHERAPY oil, such as lavender, may help you relax. Jasmine and frankincense can help to boost contractions if you are in pre-labour.

There are many myths about foods that induce labour, and these include hot curry. There is no scientific proof that they work but you may hear a number of anecdotal stories in their favour. Curries are not dangerous.

A stretch and sweep

Your midwife is able to use the centuries-old technique of 'stretching the cervix and sweeping the membranes' that may bring on contractions if your cervix is ripe.

- Your midwife will insert her finger into your vagina and reach up to the cervix, then sweep the membranes gently away from the lower part of the uterus. This releases prostaglandin from the uterus and may lead to the onset of regular uterine contractions. If labour does not begin, the sweep may be repeated on one or two other occasions in the days that follow.
- Most women find the procedure slightly uncomfortable. A minority do experience pain and if you let your midwife know it's uncomfortable, it's easy for her to stop.
- Sweeping the membranes may cause BLEEDING, similar to a show (page 357), from tiny blood vessels in the internal lining of the cervix.
- Provided you do not have a placenta praevia or low-lying placenta, which will be clearly marked in your medical records, there is no risk to your baby.

Acupuncture

ACUPUNCTURE can be very effective in triggering labour. Treatments may be needed over a few days. It is also helpful during labour if progress is slow.

Homeopathy

Because your symptoms will be so individual and may be quite subtle, it is preferable to consult your homeopath. You may be offered a remedy that helps you to relax and let go of anxieties or kick-start the process. Some of the remedy suggestions on pages 364–6 may be very helpful if your labour is slow or delayed.

Labour and birth, mother
Monitoring in labour

See Labour and birth, baby, checks during labour.

Labour and birth, mother
Non-engaged head

See Labour and birth, baby, engaged and non-engaged head.

Labour and birth, mother
Overdue (post maturity)

The majority of babies are born between Weeks 37 and 42. A pregnancy that lasts more than 42 weeks (or 294 days since the first day of the last menstrual period) is considered overdue or post mature. A first pregnancy is more likely to go beyond the due date. Fewer than 10 per cent of babies are overdue.

Your midwife will estimate the delivery date of your baby based on the date of your last period, or the date of conception if you know it. A due date is only a guide, however, and most babies do not arrive on the expected day. Labour is triggered by a combination of HORMONES released by your baby and the placenta and hormones released by you. Post maturity is more likely if you have had two previous overdue pregnancies.

One reason for going beyond your expected date of delivery (EDD) may be inaccurate calculation. Using the last menstrual period as a starting point for calculations, 7.4 per cent of babies are regarded as post mature. According to calculations using early ultrasound scans for dating, around 3 per cent of babies are post mature. The difference arises because the last menstrual period calculation is based on a four week (28 day) cycle. If your menstrual cycle is five weeks then ovulation and conception are later, and your expected date of delivery will be one week later. Ultrasound scans calculate the due date by measuring the length of your baby's body and are not dependent on the length of your cycle.

What happens

Generally, being late is not dangerous. Despite knowing this you may feel anxious and anxiety may be compounded if you are uncomfortable and do not sleep well. You might feel under pressure from your family or friends and/or your hospital if they want to discuss induction (page 374). While some couples enjoy the extra days, this can be a very vulnerable time. If you are desperate for labour to start, you might be able to request induction. Alternatively, you may want labour to start spontaneously and you may need to defend your wishes.

The small risks associated with post maturity increase as pregnancy continues, particularly after Week 42. In a prolonged pregnancy, a baby is likely to be large and his size may contribute to a longer labour and the need for birth assistance (page 373). Though the placenta will probably continue to function well, its efficiency may fall after Week 40.

Placental function will be of particular concern if there have been signs of INTRAUTERINE GROWTH RESTRICTION (IUGR) in the third trimester because your baby has stopped gaining weight. Placental function can be assessed using ultrasound (page 33).

The AMNIOTIC FLUID volume can be similarly assessed: it naturally decreases at the end of pregnancy but if the decrease is significant there may be an increased chance of umbilical cord compression during labour, which may contribute to FOETAL DISTRESS. The rate of stillbirth (page 501), although still very rare, rises after 42 weeks (14 days after due date).

Action plan

If your pregnancy is prolonged according to accurate ultrasound dating, the main priority will be to prevent complications for your baby. Policies regarding post maturity and the need to induce labour vary from hospital to hospital and country to country. You could choose from a number of COMPLEMENTARY THERAPIES to encourage labour to start and for relaxation while you wait you might use MASSAGE, AROMATHERAPY, meditation or VISUALISATION.

Medical care

- In many hospitals, an ultrasound scan is performed after the due date to check the condition of the baby and the function of the placenta. Signs of placental insufficiency are a reduction in the volume of amniotic fluid, a slowing of the growth rate of the baby and reduced umbilical blood flow that can be seen on a Doppler ultrasound scan. If there are signs of reduced placental function, the birth may be induced.

- If your care team is concerned about your baby's wellbeing or if you have high BLOOD PRESSURE (pre-eclampsia) they may be keen for the birth to be induced after Week 40.

- If all has gone well in pregnancy, you may be asked to note your baby's movements and return for another check-up at Week 41. You may be checked frequently and scans are often done twice a week after Week 41. If you feel fewer than 10 kicks a day, this could indicate that your baby is under stress and it is important to report this.

- If your baby is large, you may be tempted to induce labour rather than wait until your baby grows bigger. The medical information is that induction on the basis of foetal size does not reduce difficulties in labour and the CAESAREAN SECTION rate is not decreased.

- After 42 weeks, it is advisable to have your baby's heartbeat monitored daily or on alternate days. At the same time, your midwife will examine your abdomen and check the amniotic fluid volume. Amniotic fluid and foetal wellbeing can also be monitored by frequent ultrasound scans. Overdue babies are more likely to have a bowel movement and pass meconium into the amniotic fluid before birth. If the amniotic fluid volume is reduced then foetal distress becomes more likely because the umbilical cord may be compressed in labour and meconium may be breathed in by the baby (page 253) causing breathing difficulties after birth.

- During labour, your baby will be closely monitored and the team will be aware that post maturity is associated with potential difficulties. If your doctor is worried that foetal distress has occurred or is concerned that your baby is too large to navigate your pelvis, then a caesarean section may be recommended.

If your labour begins spontaneously or you are happy to be induced and all goes well, once your baby is born the lateness will seem irrelevant. If you accepted induction with reluctance or there was a complication in labour arising from post maturity you may feel upset – some women feel guilty that they made the wrong choice or could have prevented a problem in some way. You may need time, support and a listening ear to help you to let go and enjoy your baby. If it has been difficult for you, or your baby seems upset, the advice on page 395 may be useful.

Labour and birth, mother
Pain

See also Labour and birth, mother, accessing energy and fear; contractions; pain relief.

Your 'bodymind' can act as its own natural painkiller. The pain you feel can be much reduced if you remain mobile and feel safe, loved and supported – which is part of accessing energy. There are no rules about how much or how little pain you *should* feel. Some women who are highly sensitive to pain and/or have a low pain threshold may go through labour without needing any additional pain relief. Others who ordinarily have a high pain

threshold may need extra pain relief on the day. There is no 'best' way.

It is difficult to know how you'll feel on the day but you will be able to choose from a broad range of pain relief at each stage. If you are aware of what is available (it is not the same in every hospital) you may feel more at ease. For most women, pain disappears almost instantly following the birth but some women find the contractions after birth very painful. It is well established that being prepared, feeling confident and in control, and using whatever techniques work best for you to manage stress and ease anxiety and tension, are likely to reduce the pain you experience.

What happens

Pain is a gift from your body: a way of communicating what's going on. Midwives and obstetricians use pain as an indicator, along with other factors, to gauge what's happening for you and your baby.

The experience of pain is a combination of what is happening physically in your body combined with how your mind interprets the sensation; so the experience can change from hour to hour and depends on many factors. The normal process of labour may demand maximum effort from you emotionally and from your muscles, nerves, bones, ligaments, breath and stamina. In a first labour, the newness of the sensation can cause your body and brain to perceive the pain intensely. Occasionally, pain signals a problem such as awkward positioning. At other times intense pain indicates anxiety about whether what is happening is normal.

Pain and anxiety

If your pain is manageable it may spur you on and reassure you that things are going well. If you become anxious, your sensitivity to pain might be heightened and you may become physically more tense. These and other factors may slow your progress. Each woman is different and for some using medical pain relief helps. Others prefer calming techniques or VISUALISATIONS to reduce their anxiety so that the pain becomes more manageable.

Action plan

- The list of suggestions for accessing energy (page 346) may help to relieve your pain.
- You can do more than one thing at a time. For instance, you can be in water, move around freely, express your feelings and focus on your breath while your midwife gives you a massage. One thing, like moving, may help you do another, like voicing your feelings or accessing your power and courage.
- You can use a range of techniques in conjunction with medical and complementary pain relief.

Labour and birth, mother
Pain relief

Pain plays a central role in labour, as discussed opposite, and so pain relief has always been an important aspect. Before anaesthetics became widely available, pain relief ranged from emotional support and plant medicine to touch, MASSAGE and moving, singing and chanting. With the advent of safer anaesthesia, women now have more options, many of which do not interfere much with a normal vaginal birth. It is easy now to incorporate natural and complementary methods alongside medical technology. The combined approach can often work well.

In early labour you will probably have time to talk over your options. When you are in strong labour if you have 'gone off to another planet' it will not be appropriate to have a long discussion. The key is to trust in your birthing partner and the birth team so that you know your needs are heard and you do not feel coerced. If you are in very advanced labour and the birth is likely to occur soon, your midwife may encourage you to wait, breathe and take contractions one at a time as you enter the intense stage that culminates in birth.

You may request pain relief, or your midwife or obstetrician may suggest it. It is always your choice and the birth team can advise but not insist if:
- Pain is distressing you.
- Pain is reducing the efficiency of your contractions.
- Progress is slow (page 386) and you need a rest

to relax your muscles and reduce resistance to your baby's descent. You might then let the pain relief wear off before giving birth.
- You have an uncontrollable urge to bear down and your cervix is not fully dilated.
- Your pain is so intense that you are inhibited from pushing in the second stage.
- You require assistance with the delivery such as forceps or ventouse.
- Your baby needs to be delivered by CAESAREAN SECTION.

Natural, complementary or medical?

It is difficult to anticipate how you will feel in labour, and what you will ask for. You may plan ahead to use natural means to harness positive energy, and find you need different, additional or stronger pain relief on the day. The general principle is to use the option or options that ensure you have a rewarding experience and your baby has a safe birth. You may need to discuss your views with your medical team in advance of birth.

A brief history of medical pain relief

1847: Chloroform used for the first time during birth.
1950s: First use of epidural anaesthesia.
1950s: Suspicion that anaesthetics may have an adverse effect on the baby before and after birth.
1960s and 1970s: Evidence that anaesthetics increased the number of forceps and caesarean deliveries.
1970s: Introduction of water births.
1980s: Natural childbirth proponents claim labour without pain relief is 'the best way to give birth and to bond optimally with the baby'.
1990s: ACTIVE BIRTH and being mobile found to reduce the need for medical pain relief for many women. Epidurals also become widely available.
2000s: Safer low-dose mobile epidurals become more commonplace. Water pools introduced in many hospitals.

Your reaction to pain relief

Most women are happy with the pain relief they need and receive, even if it was not planned, and are elated to give birth and finally meet their baby. Often relief makes way for renewed energy and a positive feeling of involvement.

For others, there is a compromise between relinquishing control and being in pain. Some feel disappointed if the presiding memories of labour and birth are of pain and distress, and may be upset or feel that their body let them down and that somehow pain relief could have been avoided. Others are upset if they 'opt out' of experiencing all the sensations of birth.

If you have set your heart on a natural birth you may be disappointed or feel that you did not try hard enough. You may be annoyed that your baby's position meant you couldn't manage without relief. There are many possible reactions (page 395). It helps to be open to the possibility that your need for pain relief may be much stronger than you had originally planned for.

Optimally, your BIRTH PLAN should be flexible to welcome pain relief if it is needed. If you feel some resentment because the birth didn't go as you had planned, it's important to talk about your feelings with your partner and with a midwife or doctor who was at your birth. If you tried pain relief that didn't have the desired effect or you experienced a complication, discussing it may be reassuring.

■ ACUPUNCTURE

For full ACUPUNCTURE support through labour you will need a qualified practitioner, but your midwife may have acupuncture training. You may also try a self-help technique to relieve pain. While contractions are relatively mild in the passive first stage of labour, you or your birth partner can use finger pressure to reduce pain.

- Locate the acupuncture point Bladder 60, midway between your Achilles tendon and your outer ankle bone.
- Press the point quite firmly with the thumb at the beginning of each contraction, and continue with this pressure until the contraction has finished. Repeat with each contraction for as long as it remains effective.

As labour progresses and contractions become stronger, the relief provided by finger pressure alone on Bladder 60 will diminish. Advanced acupuncture can alleviate labour pain considerably but this can only be done by a fully trained acupuncturist.

■ ANAESTHETIC

An anaesthetic is any drug that numbs sensation in the nerves. It can be used in many ways to provide pain relief, and can be targeted to specific areas or have more general effects. There are three main types of anaesthesia. Local anaesthetic drugs are applied around the site of a wound or incision and numb sensation in that specific area only. Regional anaesthetic drugs can be injected alongside nerves to block the nerve fibres that conduct pain impulses travelling to your spinal cord and brain. These agents were originally derived from cocaine, a morphine derivative. As the agents improve they become more effective at selectively blocking pain fibres without interfering with the motor fibres that control the muscles and internal organs so that mobility and bladder function are less affected. General anaesthetic drugs are inhaled or injected to put you to sleep, reduce pain and relax your muscles.

Local anaesthesia

Local anaesthesia is often used before an EPISIOTOMY is performed or before a tear is stitched after the birth. The anaesthetic is injected using a fine needle into the tissues around the tear so the repair is pain free. Most women feel the injection as a sharp sensation that lasts for 20–30 seconds before the area is numbed.

Regional anaesthesia

Epidural, spinal and pudendal anaesthetics are examples of regional anaesthesia. The sensation from a region of the body is blocked by numbing the nerve fibres that carry pain sensation from the area to the spinal cord and from there to the pain centres in the brain. Modern anaesthetic agents that block the pain fibres may be used with analgesic agents that reduce pain sensations in the spinal cord and the brain. These combinations are safer and the dose of both anaesthetic and analgesic is lower because they are synergistic – more powerful together than separately – and so each one bolsters the effect of the other.

Epidural and spinal block
An epidural or a spinal block may be used for pain relief in labour and for operative (caesarean or forceps) delivery. In an emergency, a spinal block is quicker to administer. Epidural and spinal anaesthesia are discussed below.

Pudendal block
The pudendal nerves transmit pain signals from the lower half of your vagina to your spine, from where they travel to your brain. They can be blocked if you need a forceps or ventouse delivery or stitching to repair an episiotomy. The pain relief is less reliable than with an epidural anaesthetic and because a pudendal block does not affect the sensation of contractions from the uterus, it is only useful to assist birth at the end of the second stage of labour. While you lie on your back, your obstetrician inserts a needle via your vagina to inject the local anaesthetic into the pudendal nerves. You feel a short-lasting sting as the needle is inserted. In some women the pudendal nerves may be difficult to anaesthetise. This form of regional anaesthesia is useful if an anaesthetist is not immediately available to administer an epidural or spinal anaesthetic.

General anaesthesia

General anaesthesia is now used much less often as regional anaesthetic techniques improve. Its main advantages are speed in an acute emergency or when the mother wants to be asleep during a caesarean section.

Sleep is induced by injecting the anaesthetic intravenously (into a vein) and it is maintained with muscle relaxing injections. Analgesic gases are administered via an endotracheal tube, inserted into the mother's airway (trachea), to give pain relief. If you have a general anaesthetic you will be able to see and hold your baby within half to one hour of birth, and will be supported to breastfeed as soon as you wish. Until you wake, your partner may hold your baby, preferably skin to skin.

Possible side effects of general anaesthesia
* The major side effect for a baby is that she may receive gases or drugs via the placenta and become sluggish and sleepy. The effects are more likely if she is PREMATURE. Modern anaesthetic agents and a skilled anaesthetist

ensure that the baby receives the minimum amount of anaesthetic agents.
* You may feel groggy and nauseous and may have a sore throat from the endotracheal tube.
* The most serious complication of general anaesthesia is inhaling vomit into the lungs, which has the potential to trigger severe aspiration pneumonia due to the acidity of gastric juices. This is called Mendelson's syndrome. This risk is minimised with the use of a fluid-tight endotracheal tube to prevent fluid from tracking into the lungs. It helps if the anaesthetic is given on an empty stomach. However, an antacid is given to neutralise the acidity of the stomach contents before the operation.

▪ EPIDURAL

An epidural is a form of pain relief in which anaesthetic and analgesic drugs are injected between the vertebrae (spinal bones) into the epidural space surrounding the membranes that enclose the spinal cord. The experience of birth has been transformed for many women since the availability of epidural anaesthesia. It's not the preferred choice of all women. But as the anaesthetic agents used become more sophisticated, an epidural presents an opportunity to feel in control without feeling in pain.

You may request an epidural at any time in labour. Some women begin very early in labour but the majority wait to see if pain is too difficult to bear. Sometimes an epidural can be given if there is delay in the second stage of labour or a forceps or ventouse birth is needed. Many women use an epidural for a respite during labour. It lets them have a sleep and then they allow it to wear off in order to summon maximum power to give birth. Alternatively, it can be left to work during the birth. An epidural can be left in place for 36 hours for pain relief after an operative delivery.

The incidence of side effects with epidural is reduced as the skill of the anaesthetist and anaesthetic agents improve. However, epidurals are linked with a higher rate of medical intervention for the birth.

How epidurals work
Epidural anaesthesia alters the conduction of pain impulses from the uterus, abdomen and vagina to the spinal cord. It uses a combination

of a local anaesthetic to block nerve fibres and an analgesic to reduce the pain sensation in the spinal cord.

When an epidural is working effectively you will not feel pain, but can still feel touch and feel your baby being born as the nerve fibres transmitting touch and pressure sensations are not affected.

Mobile epidural

Many hospitals prefer to use mobile epidurals, which do not block the motor nerves supplying the bladder, abdominal and leg muscles and allow movement and upright positions for labour and birth. A mobile epidural:

- uses low doses of the anaesthetic agent combined with an analgesic to reduce pain.
- is less likely to hinder a normal vaginal birth than a full epidural.
- has other advantages: you are less likely to need oxytocin (page 377) to stimulate uterine contractions, and it is less likely to distress your baby.
- takes 20–30 minutes to become effective.
- can be topped up with anaesthetic solution every one or two hours by your midwife.
- is less likely to cause bladder numbness, but a catheter may occasionally be needed to pass urine while the anaesthetic is in place.

Full epidural

The full epidural is the favoured choice when medical intervention such as a caesarean section or a forceps or ventouse delivery is needed. If a full epidural is used routinely, it may increase the need for assistance such as forceps because there is less freedom to use the power of gravity or movement to assist birth.

- A full epidural uses a more concentrated anaesthetic that usually inhibits abdominal and leg muscle movement and sensation from the waist down. It often affects bladder control so a catheter is typically used. It does not affect the smooth muscle of your uterus from contracting.
- You'll be supported on your side or sitting up in bed to maximise blood flow to the placenta.
- The anaesthetic remains effective for between two and six hours.

Positive effects of epidural

- Pain is relieved without altering consciousness or inducing drowsiness.
- An epidural may help you rest or sleep and assist dilation of the cervix.
- It is helpful if intervention is needed (ventouse, forceps or caesarean) and allows you to remain awake and alert to greet your baby.
- It is much safer than general anaesthesia for both mother and baby.
- It reduces high BLOOD PRESSURE.
- It counteracts the fear of pain and may relax pelvic muscles and encourage your baby's descent.
- It can transform a traumatic experience into one of pleasure and joy.

Side effects of epidural

The incidence of side effects is low and epidurals have become progressively safer as the dose of local anaesthetic is reduced. Side effects are less likely to happen when skilled anaesthetists, obstetricians and midwives are present.

Blood pressure fall

The anaesthetic relaxes the blood vessels in your legs and the blood flowing back to your heart is reduced and may cause a fall in blood pressure. Levels normalise within five to 30 minutes. There may be temporary feelings of faintness and this may cause anxiety if you are not prepared for it. Blood pressure can be maintained if intravenous fluid is given to fill the extra space in the vessels. Rarely, blood pressure does not rise easily and intravenous fluids and medication to contract the blood vessels may be needed. Lying on your side may help to reduce pressure and compression of the blood vessels behind your uterus. Low blood pressure may cause foetal distress (opposite).

Continuing pain and contractions

Occasionally, one of the nerves leaving the spinal cord is not fully blocked and pain can still be felt in one area. This may be due to the anatomy of the nerve in the epidural space. If the pain is too intense the anaesthetist can re-site the epidural. Contractions may become less powerful, particularly if you are lying flat. It may then be necessary to use oxytocin to stimulate contractions and the likelihood of foetal distress and intervention rises.

Baby's position

With a full epidural, your pelvic muscles may be paralysed and your baby's head is then less likely to rotate forward (occipito-posterior) so that a forceps or ventouse delivery may be needed. If there is no sign of foetal distress it is preferable to wait until your baby's head rotates and descends through your pelvis before you begin to bear down. This will increase the likelihood of a normal birth.

Risks of foetal distress

The epidural may cause your baby's heartbeat to drop significantly leading to foetal distress, and urgent delivery may be essential. The changes in heart rate are partly the effect of the anaesthetic entering your bloodstream and then passing to your baby, and partly a result of a lower blood pressure and less blood flow to the placenta. If you are repositioned on your side and the fluid from the drip is increased that is usually sufficient to bring the heartbeat back to normal. Foetal distress is less common with a mobile epidural.

Lower back pain

Occasionally, lower back pain may arise from the needle puncture site or from the muscle activity in your lower back during labour and the birth. Resting will help and you may need physiotherapy or OSTEOPATHY in the weeks after birth to relieve the discomfort.

Headache and spinal block

When the epidural is set up, the needle may enter the dural space inside the membranes surrounding the spinal cord itself, which could cause a drop in cerebrospinal fluid pressure, leading to a low-pressure headache that can persist for days. This is a spinal block. The anaesthetist may take some blood from your arm and insert it into the epidural space to form a patch – the blood clots to seal the hole in the dural membrane. Lying flat in bed for two to four days until the fluid pressure readjusts is the treatment. You will gradually be able to sit upright and move around. You will be able to breastfeed if you lie on your side.

Nerve damage

Occasional serious and dangerous side effects have been reported. Nerve damage from the needle to one of the lumbar nerve trunks is an exceedingly rare complication. With a high dose of anaesthetic the nerves that control chest movement and breathing and blood pressure may be affected and you may need artificial ventilation for a few hours until the nerves recover. Fortunately, with the low-dose mobile epidurals this is now exceedingly rare.

When to avoid epidural

An epidural is not recommended if the mother has:
* A clotting problem and is more likely to bleed, for example due to low platelet levels/thrombocytopaenia (page 57).
* Previous spinal surgery with fusion of the lumbar spine so that the anaesthetist has difficulty injecting into the epidural space.
* Fear or phobia of an injection needle in her spine, leading to intense anxiety.
* Acute emergency (mainly when there is foetal distress) where immediate birth is essential and there would not be time for the epidural to take effect.

Administering the epidural

* A drip is inserted into a vein in your arm to provide extra fluid and keep your blood pressure stable.
* You will be asked to lie on your side while the skin on your back is numbed with local anaesthetic.
* A needle is placed into the epidural space in the lumbar vertebra of your spine and a fine polythene tube is inserted before the needle is withdrawn. The tube is taped to your back so the anaesthetic solution can be topped up painlessly when needed.
* Your wellbeing, blood pressure and your baby's heartbeat are monitored frequently.

After care

* After the birth, the catheter in your lower back is removed when you no longer need top ups.
* If you have had a caesarean or forceps with episiotomy, you will need top ups. You may need the intravenous drip and the urinary catheter in place for 12 to 24 hours as you recover.
* Numbness of your legs may be pronounced for the first few hours after a caesarean and you

will be encouraged to turn in bed to prevent excess pressure on your skin causing blistering or an ulcer.

- Occasionally there may be a low pressure headache or lower back pain (see above).
- Unless you baby had foetal distress an epidural has no effect on her.
- It is easy to fully breastfeed your baby in bed with an epidural still being topped up.

Spinal block

Pain relief in labour is mainly with an epidural. A spinal block alone or combined with an epidural may be used for operative (caesarean or forceps) delivery. In an emergency a spinal block is quicker to administer.

A very fine needle is inserted between vertebrae in the same way as for an epidural but the cerebrospinal fluid is entered and a mixture of local anaesthetic and analgesic painkilling solution is injected. The needle is withdrawn so the anaesthetic cannot be topped up unless an epidural catheter is inserted at the same time. The pain relief is usually excellent and lasts four to six hours. The main disadvantage is that a low-pressure headache is more likely.

▓ GAS AND AIR (ENTONOX)

'Gas and air' – also known as Entonox – is the most common form of pain relief used routinely in hospitals and for home birth. Entonox is a mixture of 50 per cent nitrous oxide (an anaesthetic gas) and 50 per cent oxygen (30 per cent more than in normal air). The gas is inhaled from a mouthpiece linked to a cylinder on a mobile support so you can breathe it in whether you're sitting, kneeling, standing, walking or in a birthing pool. Your midwife will help you to combine inhalation with effective breathing. Rather than relieve pain completely, it takes the edge off, or takes your mind away from, the pain. Some women find it very helpful; others find it less useful than focusing on breathing or being in water.

Although gas and air does cross the placental barrier to the baby, any effects are very short lived and there are not known to be any serious side effects for a baby. Entonox may make you nauseous but has no long-term side effects on you.

The gas is most useful when contractions become more insistent in the active first stage of

labour. You may enjoy feeling light-headed and even laughing (nitrous oxide is also called 'laughing gas') but it could take a few moments to regain control so you have less time to relax between contractions. During the second stage, using the mouthpiece may hinder you while you bear down and you may have to stop the inhalation to find your full power to push. The nice thing about gas and air is that you control it so you can simply choose not to use it anymore if you do find it unhelpful.

▓ TENS

TENS stands for transcutaneaous electrical nerve stimulation and it is an electrical device that helps to alleviate pain in a similar way to acupuncture. It is attached to your skin and does not affect your baby.

A TENS set contains adhesive pads (usually four), each containing electrodes linked to a battery-powered unit. You place the pads over specific spots in your lower back and switch on the unit. Electrical impulses stimulate the nerve endings in your skin and help to prevent pain signals travelling from your uterus to your brain. You can adjust the level of electrical impulse yourself, for example with a hand held button, as a contraction begins. In this way you can maximise the TENS stimulation during the contraction.

TENS is best used in early labour. It's a good idea to try it out before you go into labour. TENS is available at some birth units and can be hired for use at home from a range of chemists and suppliers. It cannot be used in water. It may be sufficient to control your pain throughout labour and has the advantage of being very safe.

Labour and birth, mother
Premature labour

See Premature birth.

Labour and birth, mother
Progress, slow

Every labour is different and there is a wide variation in the overall time that elapses from the onset of labour to the culmination of the birthing process when the placenta emerges. This variation makes it difficult to give a simple definition of 'normal' or 'slow' labour. Most mothers and babies are healthy and well even after a long labour. However, slow progress can indicate that things are not going as well as they might. It therefore prompts midwives and doctors to monitor mother and baby closely, at all times making safety the top priority. Sometimes a helping hand is needed to assist progress.

With modern care, slow progress is approached with the safety of mother and baby as the highest concern. Slow progress (or dystocia) may be difficult for women and for their birth attendants. It may lead to tiredness and anxiety. Most women are pleased to be helped if they feel that there has been sufficient time given for them to progress and the intervention was in their interests and that of their baby.

What happens

Labour can be divided into pre-labour and the three stages of labour and birth. The estimated time for each stage refers to a first labour. Second and subsequent labours are usually – but not always – shorter.

* During pre-labour, the cervix dilates (the opening widens) from 0 to 3cm. This may take up to three days. (This is also called first stage – latent phase.)
* During the first stage, the cervix dilates from 3cm to 10cm. This takes from two to 20 hours. (This is also called the active phase of the first stage.)
* During the second stage, you bear down and push and your baby is born. This takes from five minutes to two hours.
* During the third and final stage, you have your first contact with your baby and the placenta is born. The placenta usually emerges after five minutes to one hour.

Dystocia applies to women in established labour: progress is slow if you exceed the upper limit of the timings in stages one, two or three.

Your doctor or midwife will probably use a form of graph called a partogram to evaluate your progress. This charts the dilation of your cervix and the descent of your baby's head and defines progress in relation to the slope of a line on the graph. Many hospitals use the graph to practise active management of labour and intervene if the cervix does not dilate at a defined rate within four hours. Others take their lead from the mother and observe the baby's heartbeat readings, and suggest assistance if there is any indication that labour needs to be speeded up because it is safer for mum or baby. Most women prefer the individual approach. You may wish to discuss your preferences with your midwife.

Action plan

Your midwife will ask about your progress in pre-labour. She will suggest monitoring the timing of each stage to observe your energy and emotions and the strength of your contractions. She will also assess your baby's wellbeing.

If your progress is slow, you may draw on techniques on page 346 to boost your energy and improve the power of your contractions. Depending on the causes affecting your progress, something as simple as dimming the lights, altering your breathing, or using a homeopathic remedy (page 364) may be all the assistance needed for you to progress. There are also options for midwifery and medical assistance. The range of choices for each stage is covered in the following entries.

▓ FIRST STAGE

See also Labour and birth, mother, induction and augmentation.

The active phase of the first stage of labour, when your cervix dilates (opens) from 3cm to full dilation, is the longest stage of all. It may take under two hours, but more commonly lasts longer, although usually less than 20 hours in a first birth. If your cervix is less than 3cm dilated you are still in 'pre-labour' (or in the latent phase of the first stage).

If the first stage (active phase) is lasting for more than 20 hours, or less time than this but your cervix is not dilating, your birth team will assess whether you need assistance.

What happens

A diagnosis of slow progress is only made when labour is truly established: this is during the first stage – active phase (when your cervix is 3cm or more dilated). If pre-labour (latent phase) is difficult or extended you may want assistance to help you move into the active phase.

At the end of the first stage there will be a period when you will be in transition before you have the urge to bear down and give birth. Transition may take anything from five minutes to two hours, and even longer with an epidural anaesthetic.

A lengthy first stage can be emotionally exhausting as well as physically draining. Some women, and their birth team, choose to augment labour because they feel so tired, and indeed tiredness can itself hinder progress. Others are able to rest and sleep intermittently and keep their energy up. When the first stage is prolonged the risk of FOETAL DISTRESS increases and if there are signs of this your medical team will be keen to speed up birth.

There are a number of factors that may prolong the first stage. Your progress reflects an intricate mix of emotions and physical changes and the close partnership between you and your baby. Factors that affect your energy (see page 346) also influence your progress.

When progress is slow, contractions may not be optimum.

Slow activity of the uterus (hypotonic labour)

This involves infrequent contractions that are accompanied by slow but progressive dilation of the cervix. Although this low-intensity labour takes a long time there is an opportunity to rest between contractions. With patience, it is relatively easy to handle because you can keep yourself nourished and energised. If labour has been progressing well and uterine activity slows in the first stage (active phase), it may indicate that your baby's position or size does not fit your pelvis optimally. It may also happen with an epidural anaesthetic.

Uncoordinated uterine activity (hypertonic labour)

This involves strong and painful contractions but slow dilation because there is not good co-ordination between the upper half of the uterus pulling upwards and the lower half stretching as the cervix dilates. It may be due to your baby's size or position, or may occur if your cervix is not ripe when contractions begin. Hypertonic labour is more common with medical induction of labour and it may be the way your uterus responds to prostaglandin or oxytocin drugs used for induction.

The size and shape of your pelvis

Labour may be slow if your pelvis is small and your baby is large.

The size and position of your baby

Your baby's position may make the birth difficult for him (malpresentation). If his size is not the best 'fit' for your pelvis (disproportion), this may also affect labour. In both cases, contractions may become uncoordinated or slow.

Action plan in the first stage

Your midwife will check the position, size and descent of your baby, the quality and tone of your contractions and the size of your pelvis and note whether the membranes have ruptured. Initially, she will check dilation of your cervix and with ongoing examinations she will know whether dilation is progressing.

Your birth team will discuss what might be causing the slow progress and you will be involved in the plan of action. You may welcome regular examinations or if your midwife agrees it may be preferable to keep them to a minimum, to maintain the flow of your birthing hormones.

If your midwife decides you are having a long latent phase and/or false labour (page 357), you may be encouraged to go home. If you have been having days of false labour and you feel tired you and the team may decide that induction is a good option.

What you may do

* The advice for keeping yourself energised and relieving pain (page 346) may help your birthing hormones to flow and improve your confidence.
* Sometimes it is enough just to move around a little, for instance, changing into an upright position.
* Feeling well supported by your birth team may

help reduce your anxiety, so that progress picks up again.

- Having a snack may raise your blood sugar levels; and continuing to drink regular sips of water or a power drink will help if you are dehydrated.
- If you are tired, having a rest may allow you to preserve your energy and refresh yourself.
- It is common for contractions to reduce in power if you move from home to hospital, or from the ward to the labour suite. They may pick up again once you feel settled. A change of scene or a new burst of energy can help things move on remarkably quickly.
- PAIN RELIEF may be very helpful.

What your partner and birth attendants may do
The people with you may be able to make your environment more comfortable, perhaps by dimming the lights or reducing interruptions. They may also help by supporting you, encouraging you, massaging or holding and comforting you.

The benefits of water
Being in water can be wonderfully relaxing and helps to reduce pain. Moving to the birthing pool may boost your contractions. It is best, though, to wait to use the pool until you are 6cm dilated because earlier immersion may slow contractions.

Medical options for augmenting labour
If labour is progressing slowly, your midwife may suggest augmentation, as discussed on page 374. If your waters have not broken spontaneously, she may recommend artificially rupturing them to help your baby's head descend and enhance the power of your contractions. If this does not have an effect, or your waters have already broken, the next step is usually to use synthetic oxytocin (page 377) to boost contractions. This is usually very effective.

Complementary options
REFLEXOLOGY and ACUPUNCTURE can both help to augment labour. In combination with movement and breathing techniques, and with medical augmentation, if this has been recommended, homeopathy (page 364) may also be very powerful.

Caesarean section
If, in spite of using oxytocin, the rate of dilation of your cervix does not improve, or if your baby appears to be distressed, a caesarean section (page 108) may be the best option. One of the commonest reasons for caesarean is failure to progress in the first stage of labour.

SECOND STAGE
The second stage of labour runs from full dilation of your cervix until your baby is born. Although this stage can take as little as five minutes, many hospitals regard 120 minutes as acceptable for a first birth and up to 90 minutes for subsequent births.

This stage is typically intense, with very powerful contractions. Many women enjoy this stage and have a rise in confidence, knowing that birth is imminent. You may be unaware of time passing as you take each contraction, one at a time. Or you may find each minute difficult, even though progress is going well.

Your medical team will keep an eye on you and your baby and will reduce the time if you or your baby are distressed. If you have had an epidural the second stage is often longer.

What happens
Often the most relevant factors slowing progress in the second stage are low energy after a demanding first stage, and fear.

If you have had a large dose of pain-relieving opiates or a dense epidural anaesthetic, the reflex to push may not be strong. Many women feel more capable of pushing once the effects have worn off. It is safe to wait for this, provided your baby's heartbeat is giving no signs for concern.

If your contractions are infrequent and lack power, this is a 'low intensity' labour. This may be compounded if your baby is in an awkward position (page 344) or there is disproportion and a tight fit through your pelvis.

Action plan
Your midwife will continue to monitor the progress of your labour and your baby's condition. If there is no cause for concern, with

encouragement and support you may find the energy and stamina to continue.

What you may do

- If your baby is healthy, it is best to delay pushing until the head descends and presses on your pelvic floor and you have the urge to bear down. Your midwife will guide you.
- Getting into an upright position may help considerably. Try to relax your pelvic floor while bearing down.
- If you are in pain, it may be hard to change position and you will need to rely on your supporters who can also guide you and help you to push. The people with you may be able to help by gently massaging you or putting slightly firmer pressure on your lower back, if you would like them to.
- Your breath will be very useful to you now, and your midwife may help you use it effectively as you bear down.
- The force of birth and the accompanying adrenaline surge may cause you to moan or scream. Being expressive may help you to go with the flow of your labour and harness your power. If the energy of vocal expression is distracting, though, your midwife may encourage you to bring your focus back to your baby in your pelvis. Some women find it is better to be quieter and direct their energy downwards.
- Being in water may prolong the second stage and if you need maximal energy it is preferable to leave the pool and to be upright on land.
- Homeopathic remedies may help shift your mood and increase your urge to push (page 364).

If you are afraid

Fear when you are bearing down to give birth is normal, and it is positive. It is linked with a flow of adrenaline that will help your baby to emerge. If you feel overwhelmed you may be able to draw on advance preparation – breathing, being upright or moving may help you to enter your safe internal space and feel grounded and powerful, able to trust that you and your baby know what to do. Being in this space will help you to bear down powerfully, help the birthing hormones to flow strongly, keep you energised and increase your confidence to move on.

Fluids for energy

If your labour has been very prolonged and you are exhausted, an intravenous drip to provide fluids and minerals is likely to improve your energy.

Pain relief

It is often best to let an epidural wear off because this inhibits pushing power. Rarely, an epidural is administered when birth is delayed if assistance with VENTOUSE OR FORCEPS is needed.

Augmentation

If your contractions lack power, an oxytocin infusion (page 377) may help. This will be an option if your midwife believes that your baby is able to pass through your pelvis safely and is not in distress.

Assistance with birth

If your baby's head is engaged in your pelvis but there is no advance after you have been pushing and you are very tired, your obstetrician may decide that your baby needs to be born using forceps or ventouse (page 373). Once the instrument is in place your baby will be born with two to four pushes. If your baby's head is not deeply engaged in your pelvis and the second stage is significantly prolonged, your obstetrician may advise a caesarean section. The decision may also be taken if there are signs of foetal distress or of disproportion or malpresentation where a vaginal birth could put your baby under too much pressure.

■ THIRD STAGE

This third stage of labour is usually a joyous time when the baby is welcomed and the placenta emerges. It is prolonged if it takes longer than 60 minutes. The placenta won't be born immediately after your baby, so you have time to change position. You may want to be sitting so that you can be skin to skin with your baby. If there is a pool, you can relax in the water with your baby and wait.

What happens

After giving birth to your baby, your uterus will begin to contract within five to 15 minutes. The contractions are typically gentler than previous contractions, although in a third or fourth birth they can be as strong. They encourage separation of the placenta and it is usually born within five to 30 minutes.

In some hospitals, midwives recommend the routine injection of oxytocin hormone with ergometrine to encourage the birth of the placenta and as a precaution against excessive blood loss. This is called active management of the third stage and the placenta usually emerges within five minutes.

On balance, if your pregnancy has been normal and your baby is not excessively large then there is no need to speed up the third stage. If your hospital routinely uses an injection you may be able to request oxytocin without ergometrine (see below), or request that the injection is delayed to give the placenta a chance to emerge spontaneously. Some hospitals have a selective policy and use drugs only when there is a risk of extra bleeding.

The placenta typically emerges with very little effort. There is no stretching, just a warm, slippery feeling. You can see and touch the placenta and the attached membranes that have nourished your baby if you like, and you may choose to keep it. Your midwives will examine it closely to see whether any part of it has not come away. Your uterus will continue to contract as the muscle fibres shorten and constrict the blood vessels that fed the placenta, and this helps to stem the bleeding.

If your placenta does not appear after 30–60 minutes, your midwife will consider assistance.

The main risk associated with a prolonged third stage of labour is excessive BLEEDING (post partum haemorrhage).

What you can do

You can encourage the natural delivery of the placenta if you hold your baby and begin to feed, because this will stimulate the release of oxytocin into your system, which encourages your uterus to contract. Resting in a supported sitting position will also help because gravity will be in your favour. If the room is quiet and dimly lit this may help you focus on your baby. Some midwives gently massage the abdomen to encourage the uterus to contract and the placenta to separate.

Medical assistance

* If your progress is slow, or if you are losing an excessive amount of blood, a synthetic oxytocin hormone, such as Syntocinon, may be used. Sometimes Syntometrine is used. This consists of the hormone oxytocin and the drug ergometrine. Many units use Syntocinon alone because of the side effects of ergometrine (nausea and vomiting, raised BLOOD PRESSURE and headache) and only use ergometrine if excess bleeding occurs.

* When the injection is given, it is usual for the midwife to clamp the cord soon after the injection to prevent the drug from entering your baby's circulation. It is considered safe to delay clamping for one to three minutes, allowing beneficial blood flow from the placenta to your baby (page 334).

* After the injection, your midwife needs to deliver the placenta within three to five minutes before the muscle of the uterus clamps down and may trap it. She will apply a gentle pulling force on the umbilical cord to help the placenta to separate.

* If you have been given an oxytocin injection and the umbilical cord tears while the midwife applies gentle traction you then have a retained placenta. This occurs in fewer than 5 per cent of births. Then an obstetrician manually removes the placenta under an epidural or general anaesthetic. This is covered on page 442. Sometimes fragments of the placenta remain attached to the uterine wall. This usually becomes apparent if there is excess bleeding after birth. If so, the fragments may need to be surgically removed.

Labour and birth, mother
Spontaneous and premature rupture of membranes

See also Labour and birth, mother, beginnings of labour; Premature birth.

Spontaneous rupture of the membranes (SROM) occurs when the chorion and amniotic membranes surrounding your baby in the womb start to leak, releasing AMNIOTIC FLUID into the VAGINA. When this happens before

Week 36, it is referred to as premature rupture of the membranes. After 36 weeks it is called pre-labour rupture or spontaneous rupture of membranes (SROM). Premature rupture affects 3–5 per cent of all pregnancies. It accounts for over one-third of all premature births.

The membranes confine the amniotic fluid and protect your baby, allowing for growth and development and providing a barrier against infection. The earlier the membranes rupture, the greater the effect on your baby.

Possible causes of SROM

* In most instances the cause of SROM is unknown.
* There may be an increased risk if there is a vaginal infection, such as bacterial VAGINOSIS (gardnerella), GROUP B STREP (GBS) or CHLAMYDIA. The organisms may reduce the strength of the membranes and stimulate the release of prostaglandin hormones that encourage uterine contractions.
* The incidence rises if there is increased intrauterine pressure due to excessive amniotic fluid or if you are carrying TWINS.
* The risk increases for women who work with physically demanding industrial machines in late pregnancy.
* Good maternal nutrition and health can reduce the risk of prematurity.

What happens

If your membranes rupture a large volume of clear amniotic fluid with a distinctive sweet smell may gush out of your vagina. There may be a little blood mixed in with it. If the rupture occurs behind your baby near the top of the uterus in a 'hind water leak', the fluid may trickle out from your vagina and you may mistake it for a vaginal discharge or urinary leakage. Amniotic fluid is light urine coloured and has a distinctive sweet smell, totally unlike urine. A vaginal discharge is thicker. To be sure, ask your midwife or doctor to examine you and confirm the diagnosis.

In a minority of cases the leak may seal and the flow of amniotic fluid then ceases.

The most serious risk to your baby is prematurity. Complications are related to your baby's age and become less common after Week

34. If there is a risk of infection entering the uterus via your cervix (chorioamnionitis), labour will need to be induced. This risk is increased if you carry Group B strep (GBS) in your vagina. Other less common complications may include UMBILICAL CORD COMPRESSION OR PROLAPSE.

Amniotic fluid is constantly being produced. If there is a slow leak, the fluid is soon replaced and the volume remains stable in late pregnancy. If the leak begins in mid-pregnancy, the amniotic fluid volume may drop (oligohydramnios). The risks to the baby from premature birth or INTRAUTERINE GROWTH RESTRICTION (IUGR) and compression effects on the baby's body are then very significant, particularly before 26 weeks. Significantly low fluid levels usually lead to the early onset of labour.

Action plan

If you think your membranes have ruptured, at whatever stage of pregnancy, call your doctor or midwife, who will examine you as soon as possible.
* A diagnosis can be made using a speculum (like the one used for a smear test) to look at the cervix and view the fluid that is emerging.
* The fluid can then be tested with Nitrazine, a dye that changes colour in amniotic fluid. It is 90 per cent reliable and so may give an incorrect result (false positive) in 10 per cent of cases. Therefore actually seeing the fluid is optimal.
* Your baby's wellbeing will be assessed on an ongoing basis by foetal heart monitoring and by ultrasound scan to check the amniotic fluid volume, foetal growth and placental blood flow.

SROM after Week 37

* A swab is usually taken from the vagina to detect infection. This is repeated every few days until birth. This means that if an infection is detected in the amniotic fluid, and is therefore putting your baby at risk, antibiotic therapy can begin immediately. Preventive (prophylactic) antibiotics are used in some hospitals even when no infection is detected, but this is less important than for SROM earlier in pregnancy.
* Labour may begin spontaneously. It is safe to wait for this provided there is no sign of infection and the amniotic fluid volume remains normal. Opinions vary: in some hospitals induction is advised within eight hours of the rupture of the membranes; others

wait 48 hours. It is rare to wait longer than 48 hours for labour to begin.

- If there is a sign of infection or concern about your baby's health, labour may be induced using prostaglandin gel or an oxytocin injection (page 376). You may elect to be induced if you are close to or past your due date.
- If there is major concern about your baby's wellbeing, a CAESAREAN SECTION may be the best option.

SROM before Week 37
The medical approach to rupture of the membranes has changed considerably since techniques to delay labour were introduced. The aim is to avoid infection and to delay premature birth.

- You will be given frequent clinical examinations to check for infection, your baby's heart rate will be monitored and her wellbeing and growth and the volume of amniotic fluid assessed through ultrasound scan. After the initial assessment, it is best to avoid internal vaginal examinations, which may increase the chance of infection and early birth. It is best to discuss the frequency of examinations with your midwife.
- In pregnancies under 32 weeks, monitoring and treatment may be in hospital and you may need to stay in.
- You may be given antibiotics that help to reduce infections. The antibiotics used will cover the most common infections such as Group B Strep and bacterial VAGINOSIS (gardnerella). Further treatment will depend on the infection.
- Prolonged rupture may reduce the risk of breathing problems, more likely if your baby is premature, by stimulating the lungs to mature early. If your pregnancy is less than 34 weeks you may be given corticosteroids, to further help your baby's lungs to mature, and reduce BREATHING DIFFICULTIES after birth. This is standard procedure during premature labour.
- If there are any signs of infection, you will be offered intensive antibiotic therapy and advised to deliver your baby without delay.
- If your baby is born before Week 37 (premature birth), she may need to be cared for in a SPECIAL CARE BABY UNIT (SCBU). She is likely to grow and recover well, although the precise outlook does depend on her age in the womb and whether there has been infection.

Labour and birth, mother
Water birth

See Labour and birth, mother, active birth in water.

Labour and birth, mother
Your 'bodymind' after birth

Your body undergoes huge changes as it reverts to its pre-pregnancy state. Your uterus needs to contract, which may be painful for many days; your muscles and ligaments alter, and your balance, spine, vagina and skin all change. It may take many weeks before you feel fully recovered and until BLEEDING from your vagina (lochia) stops. Your breasts will get larger and feeding will take a considerable amount of time and energy.

The natural processes of transition, healing and feeding will work most effectively when you are well cared for. If you overdo things or do not get enough sleep you will feel the effects physically and emotionally. The tips in the entry CARING FOR YOU are intended to help you care for yourself and be cared for by others. If you listen to your body, allow time to rest, eat well, exercise gently and sensibly, and accept your feelings as they rise and fall, you are doing the best you can to look after yourself and give your new family the best start.

You may find a number of COMPLEMENTARY THERAPIES useful, such as OSTEOPATHY to rebalance your body after pregnancy and labour; HOMEOPATHY to assist postnatal healing and address any problems; and/or ACUPUNCTURE, AROMATHERAPY, MASSAGE and YOGA for relaxation.

Normal postnatal 'bodymind' and signs of possible complications

Afterpains
You are likely to experience afterpains as your uterus contracts. These can be worse when breastfeeding and may continue for up to three weeks (page 1). If the pain becomes sharp, either in your uterus or abdomen, especially if you also

have a raised temperature, a vaginal discharge (page 541) or you are passing clots (page 362), visit your doctor for a check.

Bladder

You may experience reduced bladder control for two to three days after the birth. This is more likely if you have had a catheter fitted (e.g. during a caesarean) and/or an epidural. If a lack of control continues and you experience incontinence (page 317) or cannot feel your bladder emptying, it's important to discuss this with your doctor.

Blood loss

After birth, you will have blood loss from your vagina, lasting for two to nine weeks. Use maternity or super-absorbent sanitary towels at first, down-sizing as your flow decreases. If you are passing clots (page 362) or have a smelly discharge (page 541) let your doctor know.

Bowels

After birth you may be nervous of passing a poo, and you might have increased flatulence. Typically, bowel movements return to normal within one or two days. Seek advice if you feel constipated and do not pass a stool for three or more days (page 152); if you experience faecal incontinence (page 318); and/or there is any blood loss from your anus.

Breasts

Although breastfeeding is often straightforward and comfortable, many women find it takes a while to feel comfortable. It's normal for your breasts to be tender, swollen and sometimes sore as your milk comes in and they adjust to feeding. If they are hard with redness and painful to touch, particularly with lumps that have well-defined edges, this may be a sign of blocked ducts (page 91) or mastitis (page 95), so do seek advice and take action promptly so that any problems can be treated, and you and your baby can continue breastfeeding. Tender nipples are also normal when you start BREASTFEEDING but if they are painful, cracked or bleeding (page 97) you need to take steps to reduce discomfort and address the cause of the problem.

Emotions and feelings

Having a baby is often a time of euphoria. The range of normal emotions that parents and babies experience are discussed opposite. It is always useful to listen to your feelings as emotional signs are just as important as physical symptoms as indicators that something needs extra care. If you are unable to stop crying, you need additional emotional support and practical help to ensure you are well cared for and can relax with your baby. The entries on sadness (page 218) and depression (page 174) may be useful for you. If you are frequently or constantly worried your anxiety may reduce with loving support from others. If you have little or no interest in your baby and you do not feel as if you are bonding, there are a number of ways to support yourself and your baby (page 210).

Energy levels

It's normal to feel generally tired and to have muscular aches and pains for a few days after labour and birth. The length of time it takes your energy levels to pick up depends on what happened in labour, on your baby's personality and how you both settle in after birth, and on your energy and fitness levels in pregnancy. If you feel weak and exhausted a week or more after the birth please remember how important it is to eat well (page 253) and rest. You may need advice to exclude or diagnose and address anaemia (page 26); and/or extra support so that you can sleep better (page 495). If low energy is combined with a raised temperature it's vital to get your doctor's advice in case you have an infection that needs treatment.

Vagina

Vaginal pain with feelings of bruising is normal after birth. You may experience stinging pain on urination if the skin was grazed, torn, cut or stitched. If you have had vaginal tears or an episiotomy, there is advice on page 369. Talk to your midwife or doctor if you have the sensation of your vaginal walls dropping down (page 317), intense itching (page 117) or severe pain before and when passing urine (page 170).

Labour and birth, mother
Your unique reactions to birth

See also Emotions.

Every mum, dad and baby reacts in a unique way to labour and birth. The majority of parents feel happy that their baby has arrived safely and the overriding feeling is euphoria. This is true even though it is usual to feel tired, since labour is demanding for everyone. It is also normal to feel upset, and blues may occur at any time. If the birth did not go as you had hoped, and if there were difficulties, particularly if you feel sore or unwell, you may feel shocked, upset, angry or confused. Sometimes labour and birth go smoothly but the reaction is not joy. Your emotions will reflect your experience of birth as well as your experience of parenting, and it is completely normal to have fluctuating emotions, just as your body will sometimes feel energized and comfortable, and at other times you may be tired or uncomfortable. Grief – at losing the intimacy of pregnancy for example, or following difficulties at birth – may at times be just as powerful as the joy of nurturing and being a family.

Sharing your story
The experience of birth is almost always intense and talking is helpful. Your family and friends are probably interested – and attentive – listeners. Dads often feel reluctant to tell their side of the story, as the spotlight is on mum and baby, but feeling heard is very important. Your baby will express his reactions honestly in his own way, and will feel good if he is heard. He will be in tune with you, and when you talk honestly with a loving tone he is likely to feel welcomed and secure.

Your baby
Your baby will immediately reveal his personality and will express a range of feelings in response to his experience of birth, pregnancy and being with you now. An overview of babies' reactions is given on page 335.

If there were difficulties
Fortunately, difficulties are usually mild and midwifery and obstetric skill ensures safety. When a difficulty arises, the priority is to act in your own interests and those of your baby. You may have received reassurance while the action was taken, but usually attention is focused on the baby. Parents often feel helpless, and after the birth it is common to feel numb, angry or confused. Sometimes dads feel greater stress because they could do nothing except stay and watch events unfolding. The weeks following birth could be an emotional roller-coaster; and it may take weeks or months before some feelings become apparent. Even with a safe outcome, the experience may be difficult emotionally.

It is okay and you are allowed:
- To feel grateful that help was offered and delivered.
- To feel sad that your perfect fantasy birth did not come to pass.
- To be disappointed that despite all that preparation you still needed help.

If you are not sure why assistance was needed, or you feel the situation was badly managed, it is best to talk with your care team, perhaps the obstetrician or paediatrician who was involved. The procedure for gathering information and making complaints is discussed on page 45. You and your baby play important roles in the birth process and there are many factors involved: you were not in control and you may need reminding of this if you are blaming yourself.

If the birth was traumatic for you, you may be at risk of developing POST TRAUMATIC STRESS DISORDER (PTSD). Symptoms include tension, nightmares, inability to concentrate, unrelenting anxiety and feelings of DEPRESSION. In a severe form, PTSD affects a minority of women, but mild forms are more common. Acting early if you have these feelings could prevent the disorder from disrupting your life.

Being honest
Even if you are tearful or in pain, your baby can sense your love and acceptance if you let him know. Some parents find it helpful to say something along the lines of:

'That was really hard for me and I think it may have been hard for you too. I feel upset, but I am not upset about you, I am so pleased to see and hold

395

you. Whatever you are feeling is okay, I am here for you.'

Although babies do not understand words, they are extremely sensitive to emotional energy and body language, and know when they are welcomed with love and acceptance.

Being honest is also important between you as parents. One or both of you may hold back from saying you're upset or angry because you don't want to upset the other; but your body will express any anger, resentment or upset you are feeling. If you are not being honest with one another, and this is causing friction or distance between you, the active listening tips on page 462 might be useful.

Emotional healing

Your baby is very loving and being in skin-to-skin contact is incredibly healing for both of you. Your senses will be filled by one another and your bonding, love and feel-good hormone levels increase. Love and companionship from other adults is also important, and with them you may be able to talk at length and express some of your more intense feelings, maybe shout and cry if you need to.

Many people integrate the emotional impact of the birth relatively easily, but sometimes it is delayed and the impact is initially expressed with physical symptoms (such as appetite changes, sleep difficulties, headaches). This is true for dads as well as mums: if you have unexplained symptoms it may be useful to take some time out where you can relax and allow your emotions to surface. Professional emotional support (such as counselling, page 162) might help and some maternity units offer postnatal counselling to mothers and couples. If your baby is not well, you will benefit from a great deal of support, from your friends and family and from the medical and nursing team.

Family time

Life quickly becomes very busy when the family unit grows. For the majority of people time flows seamlessly on, and everything feels good. Memories of the birth, even if stressful, may fade into the past while you focus on the present. Your reactions to birth (perhaps the most profoundly moving experience of your life) are an important element of your journeys as individuals and as a family. Acknowledging your

feelings is a powerful way of easing the transition into active parenting. If difficult feelings are ignored, there is a risk they may surface in the future through conflict in your relationships and/or with anxiety or depression.

The precious days after the birth, when you may all rest together in bed and release the cares of the world, offer a wonderful time to do this. If it takes a while for you to feel settled, you may be able to arrange special holiday or paternity leave and delay tasks that take you away from the place or people that matter to you: your baby, your new family, your extended family, and your friends.

Large babies

Your baby's birth weight can never be known for certain before birth, but during antenatal tests your midwife, obstetrician or ultrasonographer may suspect that a baby is larger than usual for the stage of pregnancy. A large (macrosomic) baby generally weighs more than 4kg (8lb 12oz) at birth. Some 10 per cent of all babies fall within this weight range. Some 2 per cent weigh more than 4.5kg (9lb 15oz). These babies are unusually large and this increases their susceptibility to a number of problems.

Not all large babies have a difficulty during birth but there is an increased risk of problems, such as difficulty passing through the pelvic cavity (page 368), birth injuries, and difficulty delivering the shoulders (page 345).

A mother is also at risk of third- and fourth-degree vaginal tears (page 370). If you know your baby is very large or you have had problems with a large baby previously, a vaginal birth will be closely monitored and a CAESAREAN SECTION may be recommended.

What happens

Birth weight often relates to a mother's size and body build, and her own weight at birth. Size also relates to ethnicity. While one-third of large babies are born to mothers with no apparent risk factors, and genes do play a role, there are some factors that may contribute. These include:

- Maternal diabetes.
- Previous pregnancy with a large baby.
- High weight before pregnancy.
- Excessive weight gain in pregnancy.
- Pregnancy lasting more than 42 weeks (page 378).

Antenatal care

During antenatal checks, your baby's size will be assessed by feeling your abdomen and with ultrasound scans. Both of these methods allow baby's size and amniotic fluid volume to be calculated. Neither method is wholly accurate, however.

Feeling the abdomen gives an average error of around 330g (11oz). Accuracy is more difficult if you are overweight or tall. Ultrasound scans have a similar margin of error, although accuracy is increasing with more sophisticated measuring techniques.

If you are at risk you may be able to take preventive measures. For example:
- Manage diabetes and blood sugar because high sugar levels in your blood pass to your baby, causing her body to produce excess growth hormone.
- Keep to a nutritious diet and avoid sweets, biscuits, colas, white pasta, white bread and other fast-burning foods (page 261).

Birth

Suspected high birth weight alone is not sufficient to prompt an elective caesarean section. If your baby's weight is estimated to be 4.5kg (10lb 12oz), you may be encouraged to give birth vaginally, depending on hospital policy. The decision will also rest on your experience in any previous births, and your own stature – if you are small, the risks of complications during birth increase.
If your baby might weigh more than 4.5kg (10lb 12oz), a caesarean section is probably the safest option.

After Week 37, a baby's weight gain usually slows but inducing labour before term has not been shown to prevent the complications associated with large babies or reduce the rate of caesarean deliveries. The risks of induction outweigh the benefits of early birth.

If you go ahead with a vaginal delivery you will be monitored closely. It is worth familiarising yourself with upright positions (page 350) because these will assist your baby's descent.

- If the first stage is prolonged (page 387) you may be offered oxytocin to boost contractions. If your baby appears to be having difficulty descending through your pelvis, a caesarean section is safer than a difficult FORCEPS OR VENTOUSE delivery (see LABOUR AND BIRTH, MOTHER).
- If you have previously had a caesarean section and this labour is prolonged, another caesarean will be advised.
- If you have already given birth vaginally but the birth was complicated by shoulder dystocia, your team will consider whether your current baby appears to be smaller. If so, the problem is unlikely to recur. But if your baby is as big or labour is prolonged, a caesarean may be the safest option.

Large babies who have had an uncomplicated birth are usually robust and adapt well to being born, and usually feed well and gain weight normally. Some may behave like infants of diabetic mothers. These babies may need to be closely monitored for low blood sugar (HYPOGLYCAEMIA) and BREATHING DIFFICULTIES (more likely if you have DIABETES). The size and weight of your baby in adulthood depends more on her genetic mix than on the birth weight.

Potential complications at birth
Sometimes being a large baby does lead to some other complications, usually related to the trauma of delivery. This can range from extra bruising (page 54), which may result in jaundice (yellowing of the skin) as the blood in the bruise is broken down, to fractures of bones (page 53) as a result of the massive forces required for birth. Any bone injury will heal within two to three weeks. However, there is a possibility that a bone injury may not be picked up early on and your baby may be very irritable until the cause is found and pain relief and treatment are given.

Large babies, especially the biggest babies with a birth weight of over 4kg (8lb 12oz), can have many of the problems associated with smaller premature or intrauterine growth restricted (IUGR) babies. These include problems with regulating blood glucose levels, body temperature control, and establishing feeds.

After birth: catch down growth

Some babies of 4–5kg may not put on much weight for a few weeks after delivery and may draw energy from the stored fat they have laid down before birth. This is called catch down growth and is not unusual. As long as your baby is well this should not be a cause of concern. As soon as your baby reaches her growth line, or centile, the growth rate will follow the normal rate of increase. Occasionally apparent catch down growth reflects an underlying health problem, such as urinary infection, so it is important to carry out simple tests to exclude this.

Laryngomalacia

See Breathing difficulties, baby, noisy breathing.

Leg pain and cramps

See also Pain, mother.

Leg cramps caused by tightness and spasm in the calf muscles are more common in the second half of pregnancy. If you are getting cramps you can prevent and treat them.

✚ Red flag

If you get a pain in your calf that does not go away within 12 hours or if there is swelling in one calf, consult your doctor to exclude the very small chance that you have a blood clot (thrombosis) in a deep vein in your calf (page 545).

What happens

If you frequently wear high-heeled shoes and do not stretch your Achilles tendons and calves, over time the muscle fibres shorten and your muscles may become tight. Short muscles are more liable to go into spasm. Doing aerobic exercise without stretching also increases the likelihood of cramp. Another cause is inadequate nutrition. Reduced intake of minerals in your diet may lead to the muscle being more irritable and contracting.

Action plan

In addition to the guidelines for easing general pain (page 431), the following techniques may reduce the occurrence of cramp and/or relieve it when it occurs.

Exercise and rest

- Try this gentle stretch. Stand facing the wall, 60cm (2ft) away, and rest your elbows, forearms and wrists on the wall. Now leave one knee bent and the foot stationary and move the other away from the wall with the knee straight until there is a feeling of tightness in that calf muscle. Maintain the stretch for one to two minutes and then change legs. Try to repeat the exercise four times a day. It is a very successful way to reduce pain. It is usually very effective at reducing restless leg syndrome, too.
- There are yoga postures that stretch the muscles of your lower back and thighs, calves and feet and cure cramps.
- Stretch all your main muscle groups before walking or exercise and again when you finish.

Diet and lifestyle

- Eat foods rich in minerals, and especially calcium (see page 263), but reduce your intake of phosphorus by avoiding fizzy drinks and pre-prepared instant soups because phosphorus competes with calcium and renders muscles more sensitive.
- Vitamin and mineral supplements with additional magnesium help to provide the background nutrients that help muscles to contract.
- Wear comfortable shoes with a flat heel. Trainers or walking shoes are preferable.

Massage

- Lightly rubbing or massaging the cramped area can help. To break the spasm, straighten your knee and flex your toes towards your knee.

* In massage, in the bath or as a compress, try a base oil mixed with the essential oils tangerine, orange or lemon and, from Week 24, lavender or geranium.

Homeopathy

One of the following remedies may match your symptoms, and may be effective in 30c potency, taken three times per day for one week; then re-assess.

* *Sepia* helps to improve circulation and relieves cramp that is usually felt in the calf, toes and soles of the feet, is worse at night and while walking and leaves you irritable, snappy and worn out.
* *Nux Vomica* for cramp felt in toes, calf, soles of feet, numbness or pins and needles in arms and hands with pains that can radiate over the whole body and you are hypersensitive and quarrelsome, feel chilly and better from rest and warmth.
* *Ledum* if your legs and feet feel cold and numb and yet are relieved by cold applications.
* *Cuprum Met* for severe cramps in the feet and legs that begin with twitching in the muscles.

You may take *Mag Phos* (6x potency) as a tissue salt, morning and night for one to two weeks alongside one of the remedies above.

Listeria

Listeria is a food-borne bacterium (*Listeria monocytogenes*) that may be carried in the intestine without causing infection. It is not common and is usually fought off by the body's natural defences. Sometimes it may exist without causing illness. When symptoms occur they may include fatigue, DIARRHOEA, nausea and VOMITING, FEVER and flu-like feelings. Very rarely, the illness may be more serious, with septicaemia (blood poisoning), MENINGITIS or pneumonia.

During pregnancy, women have a lower resistance to the bacteria. Few women become infected, but along with infection there is a very small chance of the infection crossing the placenta, possibly leading to late MISCARRIAGE or stillbirth. An infected baby may remain well or develop problems, ranging from conjunctivitis to neonatal meningitis and neonatal pneumonia. Infection of a healthy baby after delivery is rare, and usually due to the baby being fed infected foods.

Listeria is not routinely tested for. The main aim of medical care is to highlight the risks and the possibility of prevention. Chiefly, this involves food hygiene and avoiding foods that could carry the bacteria.

Action plan

Prevention: avoidance

The bacterium *Listeria monocytogenes* is found in soil and water and may enter your digestive system via contaminated food and drinks. This is why your midwife or doctor will advise you to pay scrupulous attention to hygiene and keep all fresh food refrigerated. You will also be advised to avoid:

* Unwashed vegetables.
* Unpasteurised dairy products.
* Soft cheeses such as feta, Brie and Camembert, and blue-veined cheese. (Hard cheese, processed cheeses, cream cheese, cottage cheese, or yoghurt made from pasteurised milk need not be avoided.)
* Raw or undercooked meats, undercooked eggs, and left-over foods or ready-to-eat foods that are not thoroughly reheated.
* Very rarely, pre-processed food carries the bacteria if manufacturing processes are not hygienic.

Treatment

* If you contract listeria, you will need antibiotics in high dosage, usually a combination including ampicillin or penicillin, that are safe for use in pregnancy. If treatment begins early enough, it can prevent your baby from becoming infected.
* You can safely breastfeed without passing on the infection.
* If your baby is infected she can also be given antibiotics (ampicillin and penicillin), usually for 14 days.

Loss of a baby

See also Miscarriage; Neonatal death; Stillbirth; Sudden Infant Death Syndrome.

Losing a baby, at any stage of pregnancy, at or after the birth, is one of the most devastating and traumatic experiences in any person's life. When things do not go as planned, hope of new life is taken away. Fortunately, only a minority of pregnancies do not result in the birth of a live baby, and death during or soon after birth is rare. Miscarriage is the most common cause of loss in pregnancy and it is most likely to happen early on but may occur up to the end of Week 23. If a baby dies in the womb between Week 24 and birth, this is defined as a stillbirth (page 501). Death within 28 days of birth is a neonatal death (page 420), irrespective of the period of gestation (period of time in the womb). Death of a child between 28 days and one year is an infant death. Sudden infant death syndrome (page 503) was previously referred to as a 'cot death' and affects one in 1,600 babies.

What happens

Every parent's reaction to losing a baby is unique. You and your partner may be surprised that you respond very differently to your loss. One of you may cry more than the other, one may be quiet and feel cut off, some days one of you may be angry, and there may be a difference in how intimate you wish to be with one another. You may each be overwhelmed by your own feelings and questions. It is important to recognise that what you are going through is a period of grieving. You may feel shock, anger, disbelief, despair, guilt, confusion and the need to lay blame. Powerful feelings can linger for a long time and fluctuate in intensity.

The loss of a baby can sometimes be anticipated if a problem has been diagnosed. Knowing that you may lose your baby does not reduce the impact of the loss, but gives some time for you to begin to gather a team of loving and supportive people. If your baby was unwell at birth, you may have spent time in a SPECIAL CARE BABY UNIT (SCBU). You will need a lot of support as you move on to the next stage and begin to grieve for your lost baby and a lost future. Accepting the reality and grieving are often made more difficult if a cause for death cannot be found or the death is sudden, or if there has been a miscarriage and the baby felt part of you but you have not seen him.

In many ways, living with loss follows a pattern similar to that related to receiving bad news (page 45), as you feel shocked by what has happened, react to the reality, adapt and begin

to orientate yourself. Many parents feel completely numb.

Fortunately, most hospitals offer support and counselling to parents but the need for support continues, perhaps for years. Less fortunately, some women and men do not feel they received sympathetic care and are deeply scarred, not only by their grief, but also by the way physical procedures were carried out. This may be the case during examinations at a miscarriage, if a baby has died in the womb and birth is induced, or if a baby is unwell at birth and is taken away before the mother and father have had a chance to greet him.

Grieving

While every person is different, grief brings on a number of common symptoms: crying, feelings of intense loneliness and isolation, the need to talk, anger, guilt, an urge to allocate blame, anxiety, insomnia, a lost appetite or compulsive overeating or taking drugs or alcohol. You may find it hard to concentrate or to remember events and facts, lose sight of your goals and all hope or enthusiasm for the future. Physically, you may feel tense, achy or breathless and there may be secondary symptoms, such as digestive problems.

Grieving, mourning and healing are long processes and you will have ups and downs. It is common to have thoughts that are painful and may not have answers, such as: 'Why did this happen to my baby?', 'Why did it happen to us? To me? To our family?', 'Why didn't I do something better/differently to stop this?', 'Could I have acted sooner?', 'Why didn't the medical team stop it from happening?' 'If only...'

You may find support among your family and friends, your medical team, other parents who have had similar experiences, and/or local or national help groups. It may be some time before you find the right person to talk to about your experience. Don't forget the team who cared for you. Talking may enable you to come to terms with the fact that the loss is real. Some people find writing things down helps. Over time, as troubling thoughts become less frequent you may find it easier to move on.

What you may do

Most parents need to say goodbye. Some choose to be with their baby for a couple of hours or days, and this is often possible in the hospital.

Although it is very painful to see your baby, this short time is precious and can provide a chance for you and your partner to welcome your baby, bid him farewell, and share your feelings with each other. The time together can be a crucial part of the grieving process. You may take the opportunity to name your baby and there may be comforting memories of seeing, holding, loving and caring for him. Many parents choose to have a photograph or keep a footprint or a lock of hair. Some people find these keepsakes too emotive and choose instead to keep some blankets or a nursery toy, hospital records, sympathy cards and perhaps scan pictures or photographs taken during pregnancy.

Practicalities

If your baby's death was unexpected, your doctors may ask you to consider a post-mortem examination. A post-mortem cannot be carried out without your permission, except when a death occurs unexpectedly and your health-carers cannot give a cause of death. In such circumstances, such as occurs in Sudden Unexpected Death in Infancy, the coroner will take responsibility and request the necessary examination by an expert pathologist. The tests cannot be guaranteed to identify a cause but it is important that any information arising from the examination is shared with you, if you wish. You may want to talk to your midwife, obstetrician or a genetic counsellor about the pros and cons. If you are considering another pregnancy, it might be helpful to know whether any future babies may be at risk.

Parents who have lost a baby after Week 24 are given a medical certificate of stillbirth. This needs to be taken to a registrar before a certificate stating the cause of death is given, and permission given for burial or cremation can be issued. Some hospitals can undertake burial or cremation on parents' behalf if you wish. Alternatively, you may make your own arrangements. Some parents find that organising the ceremony helps them feel more involved in their baby's short life, while others prefer not to face this. In the event of a late miscarriage, having a funeral or cremation may be an important way of saying goodbye. Some people find actions and ritual assist mourning, while others put all their energy into practicalities and only feel the intensity of their grief when things are quieter. Some delay a memorial service.

Depression, anxiety and healing

Feeling depressed and anxious is very common after losing a baby and is a natural part of bereavement. As time passes you will notice the feelings lift but this may take many months. If you have a history of DEPRESSION, or your feelings do not lift, you may need additional support. Depression and useful practical and emotional support are discussed on pages 174–7; and homeopathic remedy suggestions for grief are listed on page 224.

Consider asking your friends and family to care for you in a practical way, to ensure you eat well and rest enough. It will be helpful to get out of the house regularly, perhaps doing some exercise. Remember that you need to take care of yourself as your body adapts and heals after pregnancy and birth, and the period of recovering from the loss may be long. You may need to put major plans, such as moving house or changing jobs, on hold.

Other people

Other people may be unsure about what to say or how to act. You might come across a number of 'stock' phrases that may seem like platitudes but are, probably, uttered because those who love you are trying to say something that might lessen your pain. For instance: 'Don't worry, you will have more children', 'You were lucky that it was so early in pregnancy', 'It is a good thing you never brought your baby home from hospital', 'At least you are fit and well.' Let those who are close to you know how important your baby was and is to you. Sometimes it may help to ask them simply to listen. It may be up to you to keep in contact. This is often worthwhile – with your encouragement others may soon feel more comfortable listening to you and feel better about sharing their own grief, and about sharing joy and laughter as well. Letting them know what they can do to help you and being honest about the way you feel may reduce their feelings of helplessness.

As the days and weeks pass – some more easily than others – you will continue to benefit from support. You may meet other parents who have been similarly affected through your hospital or a support group. They may make good listeners, may become close friends, and help you to believe that pain can soften over time.

Your partnership
Couples often come together in a time of loss but it is also fairly common for anger and frustration to affect a partnership and underlying relationship problems might surface at this vulnerable time. Sometimes mothers and fathers blame one another for the event, or for everything else that seems wrong. It is common for the mother to be blamed as if it was her fault and she had let the baby down. It can be helpful to know that people may react in this way.

If your relationship is feeling the shock waves, try to acknowledge the difficulties and, with appropriate support, listen to one another and work through areas of conflict. You need to take things one step at a time while you are both physically, mentally and emotionally exhausted. Sex can sometimes create conflict, as one partner needs closeness, or reassurance that some aspects of life remain the same, while another cannot even consider sex in the light of what has happened. Trying 'active listening' (page 462) may help you appreciate one another's needs and feelings, and work together to face each day, make plans for the future, and nourish your partnership.

There is no set timetable for recovery, no goals that you 'should' reach, either together or separately. You cannot change what has happened, yet you can move forwards without belittling your feelings or the life that you lost. Your relationship may be uncomfortable for some time – this does not mean that it will always be uncomfortable.

Breastfeeding and lactation
If you have lost your baby in late pregnancy or after birth, your breasts may produce or continue to produce milk for a short while. This might be extremely upsetting and it is best to take practical steps to reduce and stop the flow (page 92) and ease discomfort from a build-up of milk.

Surviving siblings
If you have other children they will feel the impact of the loss, even if there has been an early miscarriage. When you are with your other children, give them space to express their feelings. Every child powerfully expresses themselves. With younger children, the feelings are often expressed most strongly in actions and

behaviour. As language develops words can be straightforward, with an honesty and directness that is sometimes lost in adult conversations. If your child talks about the death, let him continue and give your full attention to him while he does. If he does not express his reaction through words, you may decide to encourage him to tell you. Many bereavement organisations have support groups and reading material especially for children and there are special groups for children who have experienced the death of a brother or sister.

Anniversaries
Your feelings may be very intense on anniversaries of the loss, of conception or of your baby's birth or due date. These dates may remain embedded in your mind. You may like to do something special on the given day and acknowledge how you feel now and how you felt at the time. Even five minutes of quiet time can be useful.

Looking ahead to another baby
The decision to have or not have another baby belongs to you and your partner. There is no 'appropriate' waiting period. No matter what decision you make it will probably not change your grief for your baby who died. Conceiving again is not a quick-fix way to fill the gap in your life. Grieving takes a lot of energy and enjoying pregnancy while you are still mourning may be challenging.

Although most parents who lose a baby are unlikely to lose another, you may want to talk to an obstetrician, paediatrician or a genetic counsellor about possible causes. In another pregnancy it is also important to remember that you may be more emotionally stressed. Your support network will be extremely important: this begins with your partner and includes the medical team. You will be helping yourself if you ask as many questions as you need to regarding the safety of your pregnancy and the wellbeing of your baby and request extra antenatal testing. Hearing your baby's heartbeat or seeing the ultrasound scan will be reassuring.

You may choose to involve people who can help you towards optimum health with a balance of relaxation, exercise and work, optimum nutrition and emotionally supportive friends and groups. There are also organisations, such as the Stillbirth and Neonatal Death Society (SANDS), that offer support for women who are expecting a baby having previously lost a child. Success stories are often encouraging. Other women who have made it through a subsequent pregnancy are living proof that it is possible to give birth to a healthy baby after a traumatic loss.

Love

See Emotions, love.

Low blood pressure

See Blood pressure, low and fainting.

Low milk flow

See Breastfeeding, difficulties, low milk flow.

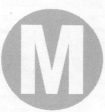

Malpresentation

See Labour and birth, baby, position.

Massage

See also Touch, skin-to-skin contact.

Every baby has a profound need to feel touched and lovingly held. Massage extends the normal mother-baby and father-baby skin-to-skin contact and, in addition to loving closeness, helps your baby develop her spine, posture and muscle tone optimally. The great thing about massage for babies is that parents can do it – often better than any massage therapist – with a moderate amount of guidance, and there are plenty of classes and DVDs available today.

The soothing and nurturing benefits of massage are also on offer to you – you may enjoy massage with your partner or friend, or visit a specialist who is trained to ease aches and pains and improve wellbeing. There are many types of massage available including Swedish, Thai, Shiatsu, sports and deep tissue. Massage is more common in some countries and cultures than in others, and western parents may not be used to massaging one another and being touched. Beginning in pregnancy may form a new habit for you and your family.

▨ HOW MASSAGE WORKS

The skin and brain develop from the same area in the foetus, and every touch on the skin initiates a mental response. Internal feelings and health directly affect your skin. For example, exhaustion leads to dark areas under the eyes. Likewise, sensations on your skin can affect your mood. Massage stimulates points along the meridian lines of the body to balance energy and affect internal organs.

For adults and babies, massage:
* brings emotional pleasure,
* relaxes,
* promotes growth and development,
* stimulates the skin and boosts the immune system,
* promotes optimum muscular and joint activity,
* reduces pain perception,
* lowers the circulation of stress hormones, reducing anxiety and tension,
* aids digestion,
* eases aches and tensions.

▨ MASSAGING YOUR BABY

In the womb, your baby is massaged by contractions that reach their height during labour and birth, stimulating her nervous system and awakening her survival mechanisms. After the birth, massage continues when she is caressed and held by loving hands, and breastfeeds, preferably with skin-to-skin contact. A mother's touch is instinctive. Fathers are usually just as sensitive. Regular massage brings peaceful togetherness, increases your confidence and is a chance to share in your baby's beautiful energy.

When to massage

You can massage your baby as often as you and she enjoy it. At first, your newborn baby may only enjoy massage for a few minutes. In time, sessions will get longer. A good time may be after a bath, or an hour or two before your baby's usual crying time (often in the evening), or before usual sleeping time. When your baby is lying or sitting quietly, or feeding, you could massage her feet or hands or stroke her face or her body. Choose times when you are both relaxed. If she cries, stop.

How to massage

Massage for a baby involves very gentle touching and stroking. It is most effective when your baby is naked, but some very young babies don't like this.

Choose pure oil such as grape seed, sweet almond or sunflower oil. If you want to add some essential oil, always do a skin test on your baby first by applying it and leaving for 30 minutes, then checking for an adverse reaction. You could use one of the following, putting five drops in 100ml (¼ pint) of carrier oil or lotion:
* *Camomile* – calming.
* *Lavender* – clears airways, relaxes, and good after immunisations (but wait 48 hours after injection).
* *Tea tree* – antiseptic healer, good for minor skin infections (such as nappy rash) if your doctor agrees.
* *Rose* – for dry skin, though it is expensive.
* *Frankincense* – relaxing, encourages steady breathing.
* *Myrrh* – for clear breathing and to encourage the elimination of mucus.

Find a warm place where you will not be disturbed and unplug/switch off your phone. Take a few minutes to ease the tension from your face, neck, shoulders, arms and hands and focus on your breathing (page 105). Make sure your hands are warm. When you feel ready ask your baby if she would like a massage.

Newborn massage
A good way to introduce massage is to lie on your side facing your baby and, with a well-oiled hand, stroke her upper back in a clockwise circular motion for about a minute. Then massage her hips and the base of her spine for another minute. Now lie on your back and lift your baby onto your abdomen (preferably skin-to-skin) and stroke hand-over-hand down her back on both sides of her spine.

Massage from six weeks
When your baby is about six weeks old or when she is ready, she will happily lie on her back and you can introduce a simple routine of all-over body massage, stroking and stimulating her legs and arms, and gently massaging her abdomen and back. Lying her on her front and massaging her back is an important part of any massage routine and will help her gain strong head control and upper arm strength, and strengthen her spine. It is preferable to have guidance – a book, DVD or class. Most parents get into an easy rhythm with their baby within days or weeks.

When you feel ready – from three months onwards – you can make massage more dynamic and help your baby to bend, flex, strengthen and move in a balanced way. If you have a baby massage or exercise class near you, you will be able to learn a number of postures together.

Points to remember
* Relax and enjoy this time with your baby.
* Always keep your hands well oiled.
* Repeat each stroke several times.
* Never force your baby's limbs into positions.
* Stop if your baby cries and give her what she wants. Sometimes stopping and resting your hands on your baby will give enough reassurance to allow the massage to continue, sometimes she'll want a short feed, sometimes it's best to stop altogether.
* Always keep your baby warm. When it's cold, you may need to massage through clothes and without oil, or after a warm bath.
* Be aware of your own posture and ensure your back is not under any strain.
* Don't wake your baby for a massage.

Do not massage:
* If your baby has a high temperature or is otherwise unwell.
* If your baby has any cuts.
* At all in the 48 hours following immunisation.
* If your baby has had surgery.

Conditions that respond well to skilled massage include COLIC, reflux, constipation and digestive difficulties, sleep disorders and excessive CRYING, muscle tension and irritability.

405

Mastitis

See Breastfeeding, difficulties, mastitis and abscesses.

Measles

See also Vaccinations, baby.

It's rare for a child in the UK to come down with measles (also known as rubeola) these days, following the introduction of the MMR vaccine in 1988 (1963 in the USA). The vaccine is 95 per cent effective and its widespread use has reduced the infection rate by 99 per cent.

If you have had measles or have yourself been vaccinated, you will pass protective antibodies to your baby in pregnancy. The protective effect begins to disappear from six months onwards, with maximum vulnerability from 12 months after birth, after which time immunisation is recommended. Measles is highly contagious and infants over 12 months of age who have not been immunised have a 90 per cent chance of developing the illness if they come into contact with it.

Measles is caused by a type of virus called a paramyxovirus, which can be passed through sneezing and coughing. Infectious droplets stay active for two hours in the air or on a surface. A baby who breathes in these droplets or comes into contact with them can become infected. It usually takes seven to 18 days for a child exposed to the virus to become ill. A person with measles is contagious for four days before and four days after developing the telltale rash. Measles usually passes within a week, but is an unpleasant illness that does carry a risk of complications. Rarely, it may be fatal.

What happens

- If your baby has measles, he'll start out with a fever, an extremely runny nose, a cough, and red, runny eyes.
- A few days later, he may develop characteristic spots in his mouth, particularly on the mucous membranes that line his cheeks. The rash starts out as flat red patches but eventually develops tiny white dots (Koplik's spots) like grains of salt or sand on reddish bumps. The rash tends to begin on the face and neck and progress down the back and trunk, then arms and hands, and finally legs and feet.
- As the rash appears, your baby will develop a fever that may reach as high as 40°c (104°F). The rash may be itchy.
- He may also feel nauseous and vomit and may have DIARRHOEA, and his lymph nodes may be swollen. He may get an irritating cough.
- The rash usually lasts about five days, and as it fades, it turns a brownish colour. It will fade in the order it appeared on your child's body and may leave his skin dry and flaky.

Most healthy children recover from measles with no problems. Twenty to 30 per cent of children develop some kind of complication, like diarrhoea or an ear infection.

Other less common difficulties include pneumonia, MENINGITIS, encephalitis (inflammation of the brain), and, very rarely, other serious brain complications, some of which can be fatal. World-wide, measles accounts for 745,000 deaths (out of 30–40 million infections) per year. Complications are more likely in children under five years old and adults over 20.

Action plan

If you suspect that your baby has measles, call your doctor right away.

Once the doctor has confirmed the infection, you cannot treat it. Your priority is to keep your baby comfortable. Stay with him, ensure he drinks plenty of fluids, and give him an appropriate dose of paracetamol or ibuprofen (page 429) to ease discomfort and bring down his fever. If your baby is younger than three months, check with your doctor before giving him any medication, even over-the-counter pain relief.

If your baby has just been exposed to the measles virus and hasn't yet been immunised, talk to your doctor. If it's been six days or less since exposure, your doctor may suggest an immunoglobulin injection, which can help prevent measles from developing or at least make the symptoms less severe if they do show up. This may be required for some vulnerable babies, such as those of HIV positive mothers, or where the mother has not had the MMR vaccine or a measles infection.

If your baby is six months or older and it's

within 72 hours of exposure, your doctor may also recommend that he receive one dose of MMR vaccine. He will still need to receive two more doses of the vaccine: one at 12 to 15 months and another at four to six years. Typically, the first vaccination is offered as part of the MMR vaccine (page 539) between 12 and 15 months of age.

If you wish to use HOMEOPATHY, you may use remedies to bring down your baby's fever (page 240). It is best to consult a homeopath for specific measles remedies.

Medications

It is always sensible to restrict the use of any medicine to a minimum, particularly during the first 13 weeks and the last four weeks of pregnancy. Do not be lulled into a false sense of security in taking non-prescription items during pregnancy. Medication use is only recommended if the expected benefit to the mother is greater than any potential risk to the baby. As a general rule, drugs that have been extensively used in pregnancy and appear to be safe should be used in preference to new or untried preparations.

Research into the effects of drug use in pregnancy is limited, for obvious reasons. Your baby is particularly vulnerable between Days 17 and 57 of pregnancy while crucial organ development is taking place. If you take a drug that affects your baby, there is a chance of a birth defect. Before Day 17 the effect may be total (causing MISCARRIAGE) or absent. After Day 57, if a drug has an effect it is more likely to interfere with growth of the organs (leading to INTRAUTERINE GROWTH RESTRICTION), although the brain and nervous system can also be affected.

+ Red flag

If you require medication you need to consult your doctor who will try to recommend a safe dose or an alternative. Over-the-counter drugs are usually labelled clearly if they should not be taken in pregnancy, but to be safe it is always best to consult a doctor or ask your pharmacist for advice.

This list gives guidelines. There are details for specific health conditions within the A–Z.

Anti-anxiety drugs and antidepressants
These can carry implications for a growing baby and can be passed on in breast milk. The options are outlined on page 176.

Antibiotics
Penicillins such as amoxicillin, erythromycin and a number of other antibiotics appear to be safe. Your doctor will advise you depending on the treatment you require. There are antibiotics that should not be taken in pregnancy including tetracyclines (which affect bone and teeth), streptomycin (affects hearing) and trimethoprim (affects cell development). Chloramphenicol can cause a serious illness in the newborn. There are usually alternatives available from your doctor.

Anticancer drugs
The cells in a growing baby's tissues multiply rapidly and are very vulnerable to anticancer drugs. It is essential to consult a doctor before conception.

Anti-clotting drugs
Warfarin may cause birth defects. Heparin is a safe option and does not cross the placenta to a baby, yet needs to be taken under supervision (page 546). Low dose aspirin may be recommended, see below.

Anticonvulsant drugs
Some drugs to reduce FITS may cause an increased risk of CONGENITAL ABNORMALITY (7 per cent). It is preferable to use single medications rather than a combination. The drugs may reduce a baby's blood-clotting ability and this is minimised with injection of vitamin K at birth. It is essential to consult a doctor before conception.

Sex hormones
These are used to treat hormone disorders, excessive body hair and endometriosis, and can affect a baby's genital organs. The contraceptive pill has not been shown to affect foetal development if it is taken in pregnancy.

Skin treatments
The retinoid (vitamin A) type of skin treatment can cause birth defects and it is important to stop use for up to one year before starting a family. It is best to consult your doctor if you are considering taking the medication.

Sleeping pills

Zopiclone is a sleeping pill that is claimed to cause less risk of physical dependence than traditional benzodiazepine drugs. In practice, physical dependence and withdrawal syndromes similar to benzodiazepine (below) have been described so this medication is best avoided.

Steroids

Taking corticosteroids (for ASTHMA or INFLAMMATORY BOWEL DISEASE) carries a small risk to a baby but this is often smaller than the risk of complications if drug use is stopped. The exposure is minimised when corticosteroids are taken as inhalations or enemas and the doses are kept low.

Tranquillisers

The risk of benzodiazepines (a range of preparations including temazepam and Valium) outweighs their benefit so it is best not to use them. There may be an increased risk of your baby developing cleft lip and palate in the first trimester. Benzodiazepine withdrawal occurs in newborns after use in pregnancy (page 192), although the symptoms can be reduced by using low doses and tapering the medication weeks before the birth date. In you, stopping the medication (page 189) may cause withdrawal symptoms including anxiety, tremor, sweats, flushes, palpitations, and insomnia.

Vaccines

Except under special circumstances, vaccines made with a live virus are not given to women who are or might be pregnant.

▦ ANALGESIC OR PAIN RELIEVING MEDICATION

If you are in pain, you may consider taking pain relief (analgesic) medication. In pregnancy, paracetamol (below) is considered safe to use as directed. Bear in mind, though, that there may be a number of non-drug options that will relieve your pain such as OSTEOPATHY for muscular-skeletal pain and HOMEOPATHY for headaches. There is advice in the PAIN entries that may provide alternatives to medication if you prefer to avoid it.

Paracetamol

It is safe to use paracetamol in low doses to control temperature symptoms or as pain relief. If you require a stronger painkiller, morphine and codeine are options that can be taken, under close medical supervision.

The recommended dose for pain relief is one to two 500mg tablets every four hours, with a maximum of eight tablets in 24 hours. It is best to take the smallest effective dose and to restrict use to the minimum.

Side effects are rare with paracetamol when it is taken at the recommended doses. Skin rashes, blood disorders and acute inflammation of the pancreas have occasionally occurred in people taking the drug on a regular basis for a long time. One advantage of paracetamol over aspirin and other NSAIDs is that it doesn't irritate the stomach or cause it to bleed. An overdose of paracetamol, however, is very dangerous because it causes severe liver damage and can be fatal.

Paracetamol does not appear to increase the risk of a miscarriage. In late pregnancy women involved in a UK study who took paracetamol 'on most days' were more likely to have a baby who had wheezing. It is still the safest of the painkillers but the lower the dose and the less often it is taken the safer it is.

▦ NON-STEROIDAL ANTI-INFLAMMATORY DRUGS (NSAIDS)

Unless your doctor prescribes it, you should avoid taking a non-steroidal anti-inflammatory drug (NSAID), particularly in the last four weeks of pregnancy. This group includes aspirin, ibuprofen and naproxen. If you buy over-the-counter medicines, make sure they don't contain aspirin or other NSAIDs: the ingredients are on the labels, but do ask the pharmacist so that you are sure.

Aspirin

If you need to take aspirin for an underlying medical condition, your doctor will advise you. Low-dose treatment is unlikely to have a significant effect on your baby. Taking large doses during pregnancy may delay labour and may also cause early closing of the ductus arteriosus in the heart. This blood vessel channel closes after birth when a baby's body adjusts to breathing in air, rather than receiving oxygen via the umbilical cord. Premature closure can overload the baby's circulatory system. The NSAID drugs in large doses could cause BLEEDING problems in the mother or the newborn around the time of birth and contribute to JAUNDICE in the baby. If you are taking them under the advice of your doctor, it is best to stop them at 36 weeks to allow time for your clotting system to recover. Aspirin intake during a viral infection has been associated with Reye's syndrome in babies, a rare condition that causes brain and liver damage and death.

When to avoid aspirin

* Taking aspirin around the time of conception and in early pregnancy may be associated with an increased risk of MISCARRIAGE.
* Taking full-dose aspirin late in pregnancy might delay labour.
* Aspirin is avoided during the third trimester due to an increase in heart and lung problems in a newborn. It may affect the physiological changes that allow a baby to breathe in air, and increase pressure in the lungs. This applies to all NSAIDs.
* It is also advisable to avoid aspirin when BREASTFEEDING. Aspirin is transferred to breast milk and a nursing baby receives 4–8 per cent of the dose a mother takes. The World Health Organization considers this to be unsafe for a baby. Continued exposure to small doses of aspirin may be harmful because aspirin builds up in your baby's body.

Low-dose aspirin (75-150mg daily)

If you have a blood clotting disorder (page 58) that can cause miscarriage, pre-eclampsia or growth restriction in your baby your doctor may advise you to take a small dose of aspirin each day. It is sometimes used with heparin. Aspirin may improve the outcome but it is only taken when advised by an obstetrician. The other exception is when travelling by plane when a single low dose (75 mg) taken at the beginning of the flight may reduce the risk of deep vein thrombosis (page 545).

Other NSAIDs

All other NSAIDs are best avoided during pregnancy and when breastfeeding. Like aspirin, they may affect your baby's heart and lungs.

There may also be side effects for you, which can include: INDIGESTION, HEARTBURN, feeling or being sick and DIARRHOEA. Ibuprofen is among the NSAIDS least likely to cause these problems. Occasionally, serious bleeding and ulceration in the stomach can also occur. Other less common side effects include ankle swelling, headache, dizziness, vertigo (a sensation of spinning), tinnitus (ringing in the ears) and unusual bruising or internal bleeding. NSAIDs can also cause allergic reactions such as skin rashes and wheezing. NSAID preparations applied to the skin can cause reddening, smarting, itching and skin rashes.

Meningitis, baby

Meningitis is infection of the meninges, the membranes that cover the brain. It is a very rare disease in babies under nine months, although for the small number affected, the infection may be severe. Usually meningitis is viral and is not serious. But because the illness can develop suddenly and there is a small risk of a serious infection, it is helpful to be aware of the symptoms that denote an emergency.

What happens

When the meninges are infected, the virus or bacterium causes inflammation with swelling of the membranes and an increase in the volume of cerebrospinal fluid that surrounds and protects the brain. These effects give classic symptoms of fever and headache and neck stiffness.

Viral meningitis

This may be caused by one of many different viruses. It can be a mild illness, where your baby has a high fever, is off feeds and has a headache. There are no long-term problems for the vast majority of infected babies. A very small number, however, have a severe illness with long-term effects.

Bacterial meningitis

More rarely, in a newborn baby, Group B streptococcal (GBS) meningitis is the usual bacterial form. PREMATURE babies are at greatest risk. The infection may occur in labour if the mother is a carrier of GBS.

In babies older than three months, the three most common bacteria that cause meningitis are:

- *Haemophilus influenzae* Type B (Hib), which has nearly been wiped out in the UK since the Hib vaccine was introduced in 1992.
- *Pneumococcus*, for which a vaccine has been introduced for all babies since September 2006.
- *Meningococcus* Groups A, B and C. *Meningococcus* Group B is the most common infection, but Group C is more severe and can be fatal. Group C vaccination is very effective and is offered to all babies (page 538).

About 1,500 cases of Group C meningitis were reported in the UK each year up to 1999. Since then there has been a 90 per cent reduction in cases in 15- to 17-year-olds and an 82 per cent reduction in cases among babies under one year old. This is one of the most significantly beneficial vaccines ever introduced. Unfortunately, there is no safe and effective vaccine against *Meningococcus* Group B.

The majority of children with viral illnesses recover from meningitis quickly and completely without long-term effects. In some children, particularly with bacterial infection, meningitis may lead to FITS (seizures) and damage to the brain. This may result in mild to severe learning difficulties, with deafness being the most common complication. As a result of widespread vaccination, the once-common bacterial meningitis is now very rare indeed.

Symptoms

Meningitis can develop very quickly. A baby can seem perfectly well then, just a few hours later, be extremely ill. The symptoms of meningitis are difficult to distinguish from symptoms connected with many other common childhood illnesses. The Meningitis Trust produces an excellent leaflet about diagnosing meningococcal diseases and your health visitor or midwife may have an easy-to-view card. Things to look out for include the following – which may not all occur at the same time:

- Altered level of consciousness.
- Vomiting and/or refusing feeds.
- Fever and a blank, staring expression.
- Fretfulness, seeming unsettled with a high-pitched cry, particularly when picked up.
- Pale skin and cool limbs with toes and fingers

that are cold and appear blue despite high temperature.
- Doziness and reluctance to wake.
- Tense or bulging fontanelles.
- The neck may be arched backwards.

✚ Red flag

Call your doctor immediately if your baby:

- has a fever: temperature of or above 38°C (100.4°F).
- has a rash that does not fade when a glass is pressed against it (see below).
- develops a sudden rash or bruising beneath the skin.
- has a stiff neck with fever.
- is having difficulty breathing.
- appears to be having a convulsion, with stiffened body followed by shaking.

Meningococcal rash

Some bacteria that cause meningitis can also cause infection of the blood (septicaemia). Meningococcal septicaemia causes a rash to appear under the skin that starts as a cluster of tiny spots of blood, like pin-pricks. Without treatment, these grow larger and look like bruises, with bleeding under the skin. The rash can appear anywhere on the body and is difficult to see on dark skin.

The classic way to test for this is to use the glass test. If a glass tumbler is pressed firmly against a septicaemic rash, the spots/bruises do not turn white and will show through the glass – the glass test is positive. Call your doctor immediately. Most children with rashes do not have meningococcal disease, but it is best to be sure so that medical investigation and treatment can begin urgently if required.

Action plan

If your doctor suspects meningitis infection, a lumbar puncture test can be carried out in order to analyse the cerebrospinal fluid. An excess of white blood cells, which are produced by the immune system, indicates infection. Hospital admission is usually necessary for the first 24 or 48 hours while the bacterial test results come back.

- Your baby may be given antibiotics straightaway in case the infection is bacterial – tests for bacteria (bacterial culture) take 48 hours to produce a result. If the infection is viral, antibiotics will not be effective. If no bacteria are found, the infection is more likely to be viral and your baby is likely to recover within 3–5 days.
- If bacterial meningitis is confirmed, intravenous antibiotics can be given at home by a specialist nurse or by daily visits to hospital. The course will be completed in seven to 10 days, depending on the nature of the bacterium.
- After treatment has been completed, some doctors carry out a second lumbar puncture to test the cerebrospinal fluid to make sure all bacteria have been killed.
- A hearing test is usually performed after about four weeks, as deafness is the most common complication of bacterial meningitis.
- If your baby has meningitis, it may take months to get completely back to normal sleeping and behaviour. By about three months after the infection, it is usually possible to check for evidence of damage to the brain. Sometimes, however, minor degrees affecting learning skills do not become apparent until the age of five to seven years.
- HOMEOPATHY can be an effective adjunctive treatment but in the case of meningitis always needs to be prescribed by your homeopath.

Miscarriage

See also Loss of a baby.

If a pregnancy ends spontaneously before the end of Week 23 it is termed a miscarriage or a 'spontaneous abortion'. After Week 23 (from Week 24), the loss is called a 'stillbirth' (page 501).

Many pregnancies end without a woman even being aware she is pregnant when an embryo is lost before implanting in the uterus. Of the pregnancies that are recognised, 20–25 per cent end in miscarriage. The most vulnerable time is between Weeks 4 and 12. Miscarriage is less common after this. With each week that passes, the risks decrease rapidly.

The rate of clinically evident miscarriages increases with maternal age. This is related to the age of an egg and to low progesterone release from the ovary after conception, see below. The rates are:

- Age 20–29: 10 per cent.
- Age 30–39: 15 per cent.
- Age 40–45: 33 per cent.
- Age 45+: over 50 per cent.

The most common reason for early loss is because the embryo has not developed normally. A small number of pregnancies are lost because there is low progesterone produced by the ovary, which is needed to keep the pregnancy going until 8–10 weeks.

Miscarrying or experiencing bleeding is frightening and upsetting. The experience is usually deeply emotional for women and their partners (page 399). In the event of miscarriage, practical concerns initially take priority and it is important to seek medical advice and treatment. Coming to terms with what has happened may take weeks or months.

What happens

The earliest sign of miscarriage is bleeding. However, not all bleeding during pregnancy signifies miscarriage (page 63). The greater the volume of blood loss, the higher the chance the pregnancy will miscarry, particularly if there is pain and blood clots are being passed.

Threatened miscarriage
If there is light bleeding with no pain, you may be having a threatened miscarriage. The chances are high that your baby is alive and your pregnancy will continue. Over 70 per cent of all mothers diagnosed as having a threatened miscarriage in the first 12 weeks carry their pregnancies to term.

Missed miscarriage and blighted ovum
In a missed miscarriage, the embryo is visible but it has stopped developing. A blighted ovum occurs when the embryo does not develop but the placenta forms and continues to grow. A pregnancy may continue for as long as 14 weeks because the placenta continues to produce

hormones that show up as positive in pregnancy tests, even though the baby is not viable. An ultrasound scan will show the placenta but the embryo is absent or has no heartbeat. Miscarriage occurs eventually but many women prefer to have the placenta removed in hospital instead of waiting.

Action plan

If you bleed heavily, it is important to get someone to take you to hospital urgently.

Medical diagnosis

If you have bleeding, an ultrasound scan will be performed to observe the placenta, amniotic sac and the embryo's heartbeat. In very early pregnancy it may take an extra week to detect the heartbeat on scan. An obstetrician or midwife may perform a gentle vaginal examination. If your cervix is dilated, a miscarriage is inevitable. Early bleeding is common and it is often related to the placenta implanting in your uterus. This is your own blood. It is not an indication of a developmental problem with the baby.

The experience

Every woman's experience is of course unique and involves both the physical symptoms and intense emotions. There are some universal physical features.

* If you have a miscarriage early in pregnancy, you may pass blood and clots. It is best to keep the clots so that they can be inspected by your doctor or nurse.
* If you have had a 'threatened miscarriage' with bleeding but the scan shows everything is okay, you will be advised to take it easy, stay at home, avoid strenuous exercise and cut down on work. Strict bed rest is not advisable because of the risk of blood clots forming in your veins. It is best to avoid sexual intercourse until bleeding has stopped. This is an anxious time so support and tranquil surroundings will help you to relax.
* If you have a missed miscarriage that is diagnosed with ultrasound but you have not been bleeding before week nine, you may be offered medication to induce a miscarriage at home. The initial pills stop progesterone output from your ovary and these are followed a few days later by prostaglandins to

stimulate your uterus to contract. The sensation is like an intensely painful and heavy period.

* If you begin bleeding before Week 9 and an ultrasound scan confirms the embryo is not viable, you will miscarry with blood loss similar to a very heavy menstrual period. The miscarriage is usually complete within a week of the initial bleeding. If it has not occurred in this time you may need to go to hospital for a D&C (below). A week after you miscarry, it is wise to have an ultrasound to confirm your uterus is empty of placenta.
* A miscarriage after Week 9 is like labour and there may be a lot of pain and bleeding. It is best to come into hospital so that a surgical procedure called a D&C – dilatation of the cervix and curettage of the uterus – can be performed under general anaesthetic. This is to remove the placenta if it does not separate completely and ensures your uterus is clear of all placental and membrane fragments, to avoid infection. The decision to do a D&C is usually based on a scan. If you have not miscarried yet but your uterus is larger than nine weeks or if there is retained placental tissue after you miscarry a D&C is advisable.

Following miscarriage

* After a miscarriage, bleeding usually stops within 14 days as the lining of the uterus sheds. If you bleed for longer or if your temperature is elevated at any time, you may have retained tissue or an infection. Prompt medical diagnosis and care are important to ensure that you recover completely.
* You will be given a blood group test: if you are Rhesus negative (page 67) you will be given an anti-Rh D injection to protect future pregnancies.
* The placental tissue may be sent for microscopic examination but the cause of miscarriage is not usually identified. You may choose to have the chromosomes from the placenta cultured to discover the gender and chromosome count of the foetus.
* It will take time for your body to return to normal – the process takes longer the later in pregnancy you miscarry. Periods usually return within four to six weeks, but could take a few months. For advice on preparing for your next pregnancy, see opposite.

Emotional journey

Your emotions and feelings are unique to you, and will change frequently. Many women feel bereft and have intense feelings of loss, often with a sense that they have lost part of themselves. You may be surprised by the intensity of your grief, although the degree varies and it can take time to surface. A ceremony or funeral may be important to help you and your partner to grieve. As well as grief you may feel guilty or feel it is your fault. It is helpful to remember that miscarriage is usually a chance occurrence and no one is responsible. However, women often feel they are to blame, or feel blamed by others, and this can increase a sense of upset and loss. You may need courage to accept your feelings and to reach out for help (page 400).

Sometimes a miscarriage comes as a relief if you had not wanted a baby or your life circumstances were not appropriate for welcoming a new baby.

If you are able to express your feelings with someone who is loving and supportive, this is part of your healing. Professional support, ranging from homeopathy to psychotherapy, can also be helpful if you feel overwhelmed, or find it difficult to feel the loss and grieve. With professional support you can go at your own pace, whether you seek professional help at once, or months or years after the event.

Healing is a step-by-step process, and feelings in your unconscious 'bodymind' may surface later as DEPRESSION or anxiety or with bodily symptoms like abdominal pain or headaches. Men often experience deep sadness, anger and despair. On a positive note, healing is possible and many women (and men) grieve, let go, and feel renewed for the future.

▓ PREGNANCY AFTER MISCARRIAGE OR TERMINATION

If you have had a miscarriage, the chance of losing another baby in the next pregnancy is not increased, unless you have had more than two miscarriages in the past. If you have had an uncomplicated termination of pregnancy, your next pregnancy is likely to be normal.

Planning for another conception

* It is wise for you and your partner to take pregnancy-formulated vitamins and minerals, including folic acid and zinc, and essential fatty acids (page 263) to provide optimal nutrition for your egg and his sperm. It is best to do this for three months prior to conception.
* Medically, it is best to wait for two normal periods before trying for another baby, to allow your uterus to recover from a miscarriage. Emotionally, however, you may need longer than this.
* If you have had more than two miscarriages in the past, your doctor will give you advice according to your unique situation. Recurrent miscarriage is discussed overleaf.

Pregnancy

* Once you are pregnant, an early ultrasound scan will let you know that your baby is developing normally.
* If you had a late miscarriage (after 13 weeks) it is best to have a vaginal examination and a scan in this pregnancy to check that the valve mechanism in your cervix is competent or functioning correctly (page 127).
* If there was evidence of low progesterone output from your ovary last time then supplementary progesterone may reduce the risk of miscarriage in this pregnancy (overleaf).
* You may feel nervous about this pregnancy continuing normally. If anxiety is a problem, the suggestions on page 176 may be useful.

Following a termination

* Most pregnancies are unaffected by prior terminations.
* It is wise to follow the nutritional advice above, and to wait for at least two cycles before you conceive. Depending on the reason for the termination you may wish to consult with your doctor or specialist before trying to conceive.
* If you have had multiple terminations involving surgical dilation your doctor may recommend a check for cervical competence (see above).

Emotions

If uncomfortable and intense feelings arise in a pregnancy following a previous loss, emotional support may be very useful for you and for your baby. This may come from friends, family, your medical support team or a counsellor or psychotherapist. Emotions are discussed in more detail on pages 206–25.

▓ RECURRENT MISCARRIAGE

It is natural for any woman who has miscarried to be worried she may do so again. Yet in most cases miscarriage is a chance occurrence. Only 1 per cent of all women experience three or more miscarriages, and of these up to 75 per cent go on to have a successful pregnancy. Recurrent miscarriage is diagnosed after the third successive miscarriage – two miscarriages may be unlucky chance.

If you have recurrent miscarriage, your medical team may look into the possible causes. You and your partner will be offered blood tests and you may be given an ultrasound scan to examine your pelvic area and assess the condition of your ovaries, uterus and cervix.

Recurrent miscarriage leaves parents upset and in conflict between hope and despair. With improving medical care and ever-advancing technology the underlying causes are more frequently diagnosed and recurrent miscarriage can often be prevented. If you have had recurrent losses and are going through a process of investigation this is likely to be challenging and potentially stressful. You may both wish to have emotional support (page 46).

Possible causes and treatment options

Genetic factors

About 3–5 per cent of couples who experience recurrent pregnancy loss carry a chromosomal abnormality. Often this is a translocation, when one part of a chromosome attaches itself to another chromosome (page 187). Depending on the maternal and paternal genes in an individual embryo, the baby may have the translocation but still grow and develop normally. Sometimes the embryo may not be viable.

Low progesterone levels

Some early miscarriages are a result of insufficient levels of progesterone, which is produced by the ovaries for the first 10–12 weeks before the placenta takes over production. Low levels are more common among women over 38 years old or those with polycystic ovaries. It is possible to supplement progesterone levels with medication. Treatment gives a promising outlook for future pregnancies.

Blood-clotting disorders (thrombophilia)

These may lead to miscarriage if untreated. Around 15 per cent of women with recurrent miscarriage test positive for thrombophilia (page 59) where the blood clots excessively, leading to a reduction in placental blood flow and foetal nutrition. Your blood clotting can be tested. If there is an abnormality, treatment that begins in early pregnancy using aspirin or heparin to thin the blood is usually effective.

Drugs

Intensive medications prescribed for malignancy and diseases of the immune system can increase the risk of miscarriage. Other DRUGS, including alcohol and recreational drugs, may cause miscarriage if used in high dosage for a long period of time.

Infections and illnesses

A tiny fraction of miscarriages are caused by infections, but recurrent miscarriage is not.

Cervical weakness

The medical term for this problem is cervical incompetence (page 127). It can cause miscarriage after 12 weeks, in the second trimester (three-month period). A stitch can strengthen the cervix in future pregnancies.

Psychological factors

Although there is a link between hormones and anxiety (page 310), many women across the world have borne children in extremely stressful situations. Believing that stress can influence miscarriage may incline a mother to blame herself for an event that was not within her control. Some women also blame themselves for exercising too much or even for flying in an aeroplane, but there is no evidence that these cause recurrent loss.

Poor nutrition

Supplements taken by both partners before conception along with avoidance of alcohol, drugs and smoking may reduce the overall incidence of miscarriage. This is easy and safe to do.

Occupational exposure

Little reliable evidence exists that exposure to herbicide spraying, electromagnetic fields, chemical inhalation, anaesthetic gases or computer screens causes recurrent miscarriage.

MMR (Measles, Mumps, Rubella)

See Vaccinations, baby, MMR.

Money

Finances are central to the running of family life and having a new baby is likely to affect the family budget – your outgoings will probably go up while your ability to make money may be temporarily or permanently reduced. It is common for many couples to have a fall in income for months or years after the birth of a child. Some people accept this and take the view that time with their children in infancy is more precious than money. Others begrudge it, and some find it very difficult to make ends meet. If you are in a partnership, it is useful to talk about finances during pregnancy. You cannot always predict how your family situation will pan out, but you can take some factors into account.

How much does it cost to have a baby?

The cost of pregnancy and baby care varies widely from family to family. Babies can be expensive but they needn't cost a fortune. If you would like to budget:

- Start by estimating the expenses of your daily essentials (rent/mortgage, food, taxes, car and clothes, for example).
- Then add on the cost of what your baby will

need. You can decide whether to buy new or secondhand items, and you may be given many useful items. Bear in mind that babies quickly grow out of their early clothes and most people enjoy handing on good-quality clothes.

- Grandparents can be very generous and if you have friends who have had babies you may be offered equipment that suits you well.
- One of the greatest expenses is nappy provision (page 418).
- The cost of washing increases.
- Food costs need not go up while your baby is very young, although if you decide to buy organic, expenses will rise.
- Many families move home or refurbish their homes as part of the nesting instinct and budgeting for this will involve a lot of skill.

Against your outgoings you will need to calculate your income, including benefits. You will be entitled to maternity benefit – either from your employer or via the government. You may be offered paternity benefit. Your health visitor or local social security office, or the human resources department at work, will advise you on the details and on your entitlement to any other family benefits (or you can browse the internet).

If and when you return to work your plans will include valuing the cost of CHILDCARE. Many parents find that almost all of one partner's salary goes on childcare. In the short term this may put you under considerable financial pressure, but being at work may bring new energy for you and your family. Only you can weigh up the pros and cons, now and for your long-term career prospects.

Money and stress

Money is often a source of stress. It is common for couples to struggle financially. A mum and dad may alternate working and childcare and rarely have time together. One or both partners may feel forced to stay in a job that is unpleasant or stressful in order to make ends meet. Debts can mount. It is common for resentment to build if one person works longer hours, and/or if one person spends money inappropriately or when there has not been agreement.

Although many more women go to work after having children than was the case 50 years ago, it is still more common for mums to stay at home and for dads to work, and this may bring its own set of difficulties. For example, dad may be absent from the family for much of the time, mum may miss the mental stimulation and friendships of work, and resentment may build between them. When the opposite is true and dad stays at home, mothers sometimes feel confused or guilty (page 213). Most babies enjoy consistency of care and if the necessity to work takes one or both parents away for much of the time or contributes to family stress, having a loving carer (page 134) may make a big difference to your baby's contentment.

Attitudes to money are typically part of family culture and you and your partner may have very different views. Spending time together to discuss your budget and being honest about your dreams and your anxieties may help you meet your immediate needs and avoid some potential causes of stress (page 462). It is usual for couples to put holidays and big purchases on hold until the youngest of their children has reached school age, or later, when the reduced need for hands-on childcare allows more time to earn money, or to retrain or change job.

Morning sickness

See Vomiting and nausea, mother.

Mouth ulcers, mother

Mouth ulcers may be cold sores, resulting from HERPES infection. These normally appear around the lips but can occur in the mouth. Alternatively, they may be an apthous or canker ulcer, which may occur when the body's immune cells attack the lining of the mouth. These ulcers are caused by dysfunction in the immune system, not by a virus, and tend to be less of a problem in pregnancy.

Action plan

* If you have ulcers resulting from cold sores, keep fit and healthy to boost your resistance. They can be treated with creams (acyclovir) and remedies for herpes infection.
* To reduce apthous ulcers, eliminating certain triggers may help. Common allergens are wheat

and dairy, as well as toothpastes containing sodium lauryl sulphate.
* Good dental hygiene and a balanced diet may help. Deficiencies in certain vitamins and minerals – principally B9, B12 (cobalamin) and iron – may increase susceptibility to ulcers.
* A gargle of warm sage tea to which is added two drops of tea tree oil may help – but do not swallow the tea.

Homeopathy
* *Hypercal* homeopathic tincture is a useful mouth rinse to use two to three times a day. Dilute five drops tincture in 250ml (½ pint) of boiled, cooled water. In addition, you may use the most appropriate remedy from the list below in 30c potency three times per day for three days and then re-assess.
* *Mercurius* for ulcers mainly appearing on the tongue, that tend to sting, particularly on contact with food, and where there is increased salivation, often a metallic taste, smelly breath and a coated tongue.
* *Nitric Acid* for ulcers that give splinter-like pains and may be on the side of the tongue or on the soft palate.
* *Borax* when your mouth feels hot and tender; ulcers may bleed on contact, particularly after eating; and your tongue looks coated.
* *Arsenicum* if your mouth is dry and ulcers burn although warm drinks alleviate.

Movements of baby in pregnancy

Every baby has a different pattern and rhythm of movements. You may begin feeling your baby move inside you from as early as Week 16, or as late as Week 22, but usually it's around Week 20. It is often later in a first pregnancy.

What happens

At first, movements feel like butterfly flutters or small bubbles of wind. As your baby grows, they become stronger and more definite. If you are very busy during the day you may not notice movements until the evening. This is usually not because your baby is moving more at this time but because you are more aware of it. Towards the end of pregnancy, you may notice your baby has formed rhythms of waking, sleeping and moving.

Movements are a sign of good health, and your midwife may ask you to remain aware of them. The minimum normal number you are advised to note is 10 per day. These may come in a quick flutter lasting less than an hour or may be spread over the day.

Action plan

If your midwife tells you that your baby is growing normally and the amniotic fluid is of normal volume, then it is wise to report a change in pattern, particularly if your baby stops moving for longer than six to eight hours.

If there is a concern about your baby's growth and your midwife feels your baby may be small (page 323) or there is a reduced amount of amniotic fluid, it is even more important to focus on your baby's movement pattern. Again, the recommendation is to note more than 10 movements per day. At or after 40 weeks there is often relatively less amniotic fluid, particularly if you go past your dates. The number of movements may reduce but more than 10 movements in 24 hours is still considered normal.

If you feel your baby slows downs significantly, or stops moving for longer than eight hours, then report to your midwife who may examine you and monitor your baby's heartbeat. She may also ask you to have an ultrasound scan to check your baby and the function of your placenta. Usually the findings from the ultrasound scan show that everything is normal. The benefit of doing an early ultrasound scan is that, in the unlikely event that there is a problem, early action can be taken.

Mumps

See also Vaccinations, baby.

Mumps is a viral infection that causes the salivary glands in front of the ears (the parotid glands) to swell. It is very rare in children below the age of 12 months and since the introduction of the MMR vaccine it has become very uncommon after this age.

The condition can be very painful and is infectious for up to 10 days. It usually passes of its own accord, but rarely may cause complications. Occasionally, mumps can cause swelling of the testicles in boys and the ovaries in girls, and rarely this may cause infertility. Another concerning complication, although rare, is associated inflammation of the lining membrane of the nervous system, extending to the brain. This is called meningo-encephalitis (and has symptoms similar to MENINGITIS) and carries a risk of hearing loss.

What happens

Your child will complain of tenderness and pain when chewing and will find swallowing uncomfortable. She may develop a temperature, dribble and may appear to have hamster cheeks, due to the enlarged salivary glands. The symptoms may last for three to five days – getting better within a week.

Action plan

You must contact your GP if you think your child has mumps. Your GP will be able to give an accurate diagnosis, and detect and treat any complications that develop along with the infection.

* The infection will run its course, and treatment is simply to make your child more comfortable.
* If she has a temperature, you may use child paracetamol in appropriate doses (page 429).
* Your child is unlikely to want to eat solids, but it's important for her to drink plenty of fluids, and breast milk if still breastfeeding.
* Avoid fruit juices as they are acidic and may cause more pain by encouraging saliva production.
* A warm water bottle (placed under the cheek) may also help.

Most children recover with no long-lasting problems. You should call for urgent medical help if your child remains unwell or you are concerned by symptoms. If your child shows any signs of meningo-encephalitis, with high fever, confusion, headache and excessive sleepiness, it is extremely important to take her to the doctor. Antiviral medicines may be needed.

Nappies

You will make your choice of nappy depending on your circumstances. Many parents use a combination of washable and disposable for home and away. Increasingly, biodegradable nappies are chosen to reduce long-term pollution.

Many parents' concern is nappy rash. Your baby is susceptible but the risk is reduced by avoiding a plastic outer nappy. The other thing to do is not to allow your baby's skin to be in prolonged contact with urine or faeces. There are tips on prevention below.

Nappy rash

Almost every baby gets a rash in the nappy area at some point. Contrary to popular belief, this is not exclusively caused by the contact of urine and faeces with the skin, or by the nappy itself. A rash may also occur as a result of something your baby has eaten or it may be due to a fungal infection. The term nappy rash actually covers a variety of rashes, each of which looks different. Some rashes do not seem to irritate, others itch or sting, and may become inflamed or raw, and might cause extended or distressed crying. Once you have identified the cause, your baby's nappy rash can almost always be treated quickly and simply.

Preventing rashes
* Complete prevention is not possible but extra care will help. Caring for your baby's nappy area, and for the rest of her skin, is a matter of keeping her clean and dry, and being observant about what she eats.

* Every day let your baby spend some time without a nappy on.
* Moisturise the nappy area with a light, natural carrier oil (grapeseed or almond). This allows the skin to breathe and improves its resilience.
* Use water to clean your baby's bottom at each nappy change, saving baby wipes for changes away from home.
* Change your baby's nappy roughly every three hours, and straightaway if she has passed a stool.
* At night you needn't change her nappy if she has no rash; but when she has a nappy rash one or two changes will help her feel more comfortable.
* Soap triggers an alkaline reaction in the skin and removes its natural acid protection, which may aggravate eczema and rashes. Bacteria are more likely to grow and cause infection in an alkaline medium. Your baby's skin may only need washing with water at bathtime, except when it is soiled, in which case a mild soap is best. Wherever possible, use mild washing powder if you are using washable nappies – the effect of detergent can be very significant.
* Don't give your baby full-fat cow's milk to drink before she is one year old.
* If you are breastfeeding, reduce spicy or acidic foods if these seem to irritate your baby.
* Antibiotic use can be linked with the development of a fungal infection, such as candida. If your baby (or you while you are breastfeeding) has a condition for which antibiotic treatment is recommended, following the supportive suggestions on page 34 may be useful. Some mothers are keen to pursue alternative methods (such as homeopathy) that may eliminate the need for antibiotic treatment; if you choose to do this it

is vital that you seek professional advice (see page 147).

A rash may arise or become worse:

- If your baby becomes dehydrated, for example, in hot weather or in an overheated home.
- When your baby is teething or has a cough or cold, or another mild illness.
- If your baby is emotionally stressed.
- If your baby cries a lot and becomes hot.
- If your baby is red-headed as she may be more susceptible, with an altered skin pH.
- If you are using washable nappies with plastic over-pants, as these may trap heat.
- If you do not change her nappies frequently enough.
- If any nappy you use is too tight or has abrasive sections that rub her skin.

Action plan

When your baby gets a rash, the priority is to keep her comfortable – often this is as simple as leaving the nappy off whenever you can – and to treat the cause. There are general steps to take for any rash.

- Clean your baby's bottom gently with water, and allow it to dry completely – drying in air is best.
- There are many conventional creams that may be soothing, such as Sudocrem, Morhulin, Vaseline, zinc cream, zinc and castor oil ointment or Metanium. These are usually effective, but use only a small amount because if you use too much the cream will trap moisture on the skin and worsen the rash.
- Gentler creams include calendula-based creams.
- Acupuncture or acupressure applied to the legs correctly can be very helpful.

Homeopathy for nappy rash

You may choose a remedy according to your baby's symptoms and give it in the 6c potency, three times per day for up to three days and re-assess.

- *Apis* for a rash that is shiny, looks sore and slightly puffy and is bright red, makes your baby restless, agitated and fidgety, but he is better with few or no clothes and in cooler conditions.
- *Cantharis* for a rash with inflammation and burning heat, that is markedly worse when your baby urinates, makes him distressed and unable to sleep, but when he feels generally better in a warm environment.
- *Rhus Tox* for a spotty, itchy rash that is worse

from exposure to heat and when your baby cannot get comfortable, particularly at night.

- *Graphites* for nappy rash that is most severe in the creases of skin in the buttocks and genital area. The skin may crack and is worse for heat.
- *Sulphur* for a red, raw-looking rash that is obviously itchy and worse from scratching and after any form of heat.
- *Calendula tincture* may also be effective – 10 drops diluted in 250ml (½ pint) boiled, cooled water for a light wash with a sponge, or 10 drops in a bath.

Types of nappy rash, and specific treatments

While the general prevention and treatment advice, above, applies to all nappy rashes, if you can identify which type of rash your baby has and target the treatment, it is likely to clear up very soon. Complementary therapies combined with chemical or over-the counter treatments are very powerful healers.

Ammoniacal dermatitis

Faeces contain bacteria that may act on urine, breaking it down to release ammonia. This burns the skin, producing a moist rash of inflamed patches around the genitals, although it seldom affects the skin creases. The skin gradually thickens and wrinkles and then peels and becomes raw. The burn may be aggravated by cow's milk, acid water mixed with formula milk, or plastic pants. The most common cause is leaving wet and soiled nappies on for too long, so the first line of treatment is to change your baby's nappies frequently and to expose her skin to air as often as possible. As a guide, don't keep a wet nappy on for longer than half an hour, and change a soiled nappy straightaway. Wash with water, dry and then apply a small amount of barrier cream over the rash.

Candida albicans (thrush)

The fungal infection thrush is a frequent cause of nappy rash, and may not clear easily in babies. Its characteristic appearance is white patches surrounded by reddened skin, usually starting around the anus and spreading across the buttocks. It may be worse in the skin creases where it is warm and moist, the perfect environment for the candida fungus. If the rash causes cracking, there may be small points of bleeding on the skin. Thrush can also cause redness and small white spots inside the mouth and on the tongue, and may make feeding uncomfortable for your baby.

If your baby gets thrush, she will have caught the infection from you and you both need to be treated. In addition to the general advice above, specific treatment for candida will help – see page 117 for treating your baby, and page 118 for treating yourself.

Seborrhoeic dermatitis (napkin psoriasis or cradle cap)
If the rash consists of dry, scaly and brownish-red skin, it may be the same as cradle cap. Treatments for this are discussed on page 164.

Eczema (allergic or atopic dermatitis)
If a rash begins as a red area that becomes raised and itchy, and perhaps dry, it may be eczema, which is usually a symptom of an allergic response. This is covered on page 204.

Nasal congestion

See Blocked nose, baby.

Nausea

See Vomiting and nausea, mother; Vomiting, baby.

Neonatal death

Neonatal death is the term given to death within 28 days of birth. During this period, around one in 300 babies dies, most commonly within the first week (defined as early neonatal deaths). Around 25 per cent of neonatal deaths occur because babies have severe genetic or chromosomal abnormalities (page 148) or developmental problems, most commonly affecting the heart. Usually when this is the case, pregnancy ends in an early miscarriage, but some pregnancies continue to full term. Early death is also associated with very early PREMATURE BIRTH. Rarely, death follows infection in pregnancy or FOETAL DISTRESS AND ASPHYXIA during labour.

When a problem is detected after the birth, parents may be able to prepare for the short time they will have with their babies. Often, however, parents anticipate the birth of a healthy baby and are shocked when their baby is born very ill and is not expected to survive.

If your baby is born very prematurely or is very sick, he may be transferred into the neonatal intensive care unit or the special care baby unit. If he needs to be transferred to another hospital it may be extremely traumatic for you and your partner to be separated from him. Soon after the initial shock, you may find yourself watching your baby fight for life in an unfamiliar setting that may feel intimidating. It is common to feel helpless, frightened, angry and emotionally overwhelmed and you will need a great deal of support from your family, friends and medical team. Even if your baby survives for only a short time, being with him and being involved in his care in whatever way is possible may be very important for you. Losing your baby is likely to affect you in many ways. The emotional impact and the practical steps you may take are covered on pages 400–3.

Neonatal intensive care unit (NICU)

See Special baby care unit (SBCU) and neonatal intensive care unit (NICU).

Nipples, cracked

See Breastfeeding, difficulties, nipples, cracked.

Nipples, inverted

See Breastfeeding, difficulties, nipples, flat or inverted.

Nutrition, baby

See also Bottle-feeding; Breastfeeding; Weaning.

How, when and what babies eat, and their reaction to eating, is a very common concern for parents. If you are in any doubt, don't hesitate to talk to your health visitor, GP, feeding counsellor or nutritionist.

The best nutrition for your baby is breast milk, and you will be giving her a great start if you establish feeding after birth, and for as long as you both enjoy it. While you breastfeed, you are your baby's sole source of nutrition, and what you consume, she consumes. If you are unable to breastfeed you may be able to express milk for your baby. If this is not an option, bottle-feeding with formula milk is a good alternative.

Your baby's digestive system is immature at birth and the sensation of digesting food is new, so your baby may sometimes have discomfort (such as wind or constipation). It's also common for babies to 'posset' – bring up small amounts of milk after a feed – and to vomit occasionally. As the months pass, your baby's digestive system matures and by around six months of age she will be able to cope with solid food. There are guidelines for weaning on page 557.

Enjoying food

Food is about physical nourishment and also about love. The emotions linked with food and eating (page 258) can have roots in childhood, and you will be offering your baby a good start if she is regularly able to eat in a relaxed and calm environment, and if eating is fun. Being together while you breast- or bottle-feed is a wonderful opportunity to explore one another and to play, and once your baby is eating solid food mealtimes can become increasingly sociable.

If you are concerned

If you suspect your baby has discomfort, ask for advice and address the cause. This will help eating remain an enjoyable part of her life. Common feeding-related difficulties include gastro-oesophageal reflux (page 554), COLIC, food intolerances (page 19), CONSTIPATION and DIARRHOEA, all of which are covered in this A–Z. There is also a risk of babies developing deficiencies, despite a range of fortified foods. The most common deficiency is inadequate calorie intake resulting in slow growth. Routine health and growth checks ensure this will be spotted early. Rickets is also becoming more common, due to prolonged exclusive breastfeeding for over 12 months, and the use of organic feeds that do not contain sufficient calcium.

Nutrition, mother

See Food and eating, mother.

Nutritional therapy

See also Food and eating, mother; Weight, mother.

Nutritional therapy is a practical tool for enjoying food and eating well, ensuring that you get the nutrients you need. Suggestions for easy ways to achieve good nutrition are listed on pages 253–5. You may also wish to seek further advice for yourself or for your whole family from a registered nutritional therapist.

At a consultation you will discuss your lifestyle, eating habits and medical history and any concerns about your health. Some nutritional therapists offer tests such as hair analysis (to assess levels of helpful and harmful minerals in your system), and stool tests (to learn more about the condition of your gut). If you have strong reactions to one or more types of food, or combinations of foods, you may ask to be tested for ALLERGY AND INTOLERANCE.

The therapist helps you create an eating plan that is abundant in wonderful foods and avoids foods or drinks that are not suitable for you. Vitamin and mineral supplements, antioxidants and essential fatty acids are often recommended, and some therapists are also qualified to prescribe HERBAL MEDICINE.

Eating foods that suit your personal constitution and metabolism is likely to boost your daily energy, keep your weight within the limits you are happy with, improve sleep, boost immunity, ease digestion, help to balance your moods and your hormones and is, of course, important if you are nurturing a growing baby. You may focus on what you are eating if you are troubled by symptoms such as HEARTBURN, nausea or CONSTIPATION.

You may want to connect with a therapist at intervals as your child grows to help you combine healthy eating with other aspects of busy family life.

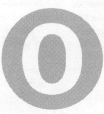

Obesity, baby

See Weight, baby, overweight and obesity.

Obesity, mother

See Weight, mother, overweight and obesity.

Oedema

See Swelling (oedema), mother.

Oesophageal atresia and tracheo-oesophageal fistula

See also Congenital abnormalities; Genes and genetics.

Oesophageal atresia affects around one in 1,800 babies. It refers to malformations present at birth that affect the oesophagus, the muscular tube that connects the mouth to the stomach. Most babies with this condition have a connection between the trachea (windpipe) and the oesophagus, a tracheo-oesophageal fistula (TOF).

What happens

Instead of attaching to the stomach, the oesophagus may end in a closed sac, or join with the trachea leading to the lungs (TOF). The oesophagus may be narrow. A third of babies with TOF have defects of the vertebrae, heart, anus, kidney and the limbs.

Symptoms include excessive dribbling, inability to feed properly and VOMITING. With tracheo-oesophageal fistula, swallowed food can get into the lungs leading to coughing and choking when feeding, and there may be a blue tinge to the skin due to lack of oxygen (cyanosis).

Action plan

The condition may be diagnosed before birth. If so, arrangements may be made for the baby to be born in a specialised centre, where surgery is available. An alternative is to give birth in a local unit with arrangements in place for transfer after birth.

After the birth, oesophageal atresia can be diagnosed with X-rays or by threading a slender feeding tube down the oesophagus to see if the stomach can be reached. The condition requires urgent surgery, usually carried out within a day or two of birth, providing there are no other serious problems, such as abnormalities of the heart, which may need more urgent attention.

After surgery, feeding may be quickly established. Sometimes there may be more difficulties in establishing feeds, and surgery may be more complex. For some babies this results in a prolonged hospital stay, often of many months, and possibly multiple operations follow. Your baby may have to be tube fed for much of the first year, and the time in a special care baby unit (SCBU) may be very difficult for you and your family. TOF is a serious disorder and requires intensive treatment and care. Most babies come through the operations and do well yet there may sometimes be feeding difficulties for months or years. Long-term care of you and your baby involves a team of nurses, surgeons, paediatricians and nutritionists. In the long term the surgery is curative.

Older parents

The concept of an 'older parent' is not the same now as it was a few decades ago. In the 1960s, most women had babies in their early 20s and 'middle age' began at 40. Today, the average age for an adult to have their first baby is almost 30, and the 40s are regarded as the upper range of 'youth'. Many doctors and midwives would not consider you to be 'old' for a first baby – 'elderly prima gravida' – until the age of around 37 years.

There are pros and cons of a later pregnancy. Some risks increase but there are additional benefits and most women who have a baby after the age of 40 thrive, as do older fathers. Few of these 'older' parents feel 'old'.

Being an 'older' mother

Whether planned or not, on the road to parenthood you will face the same issues that are faced by parents who are younger than you. Later in life, though, you may have the advantage of being financially more stable and have an established network of support. You may also feel better about giving up less healthy aspects of your lifestyle, such as smoking, late nights and parties, to focus on your baby and your family's wellbeing.

This could reduce anxiety or depression that can arise if you feel conflict between responsibility and independence. Another advantage is that you may feel emotionally more prepared – research suggests that older mothers tend to be more patient and relaxed. A number of older parents also feel fulfilled in their careers, perhaps ready to cut down or stop work, or very well established and able to negotiate suitable timetables. Waiting for pregnancy later in life may be the best thing for some people who had a difficult childhood and needed time to live comfortably with past experiences.

The slightly increased risk of complications in pregnancy is often overstated, but is worth acknowledging. Some are less significant than they were a few decades ago because of advances in medical technology and because more women are physically active, fit and healthy. After an uncomplicated pregnancy and delivery, your baby is as likely to thrive as a baby of a younger mother.

- Some women conceive soon after they decide to start their family, others have to wait for up to two years. Fertility reduces progressively after 35 years of age.
- There is a higher risk of miscarriage if you're 40 or over (page 411). This is partly because of the age of your eggs and partly because your ovaries produce less progesterone (treatment with additional progesterone may prevent miscarriage).
- The risk of your baby having Down's syndrome rises progressively to 1 per cent after age 40 (page 187).
- You are more likely to conceive two or more babies because multiple ovulation is more common.
- You have a higher likelihood of developing medical conditions such as DIABETES, FIBROIDS and high BLOOD PRESSURE with pre-eclampsia, but seen in context the majority of women over 40 do not have these problems.
- Many women have perfectly normal and natural births over 40 but a higher proportion have a caesarean section, sometimes through choice, sometimes because of complications such as high blood pressure and sometimes because an attending obstetrician is more wary of potential complications. Sometimes an older uterus may be less efficient but the majority contract normally.
- You may find the physical and emotional demands of parenting harder than you might have earlier. This depends on many things, including your baby's health and character, your fitness, your relationship, your support network and time management. Some women find it easier because they are more relaxed.

'Older' fathers

Many men may be even keener than their partners to begin a family later in life, or to extend an existing family. This is often the case in a second or third marriage when a child can cement a relationship. Some feel ambivalent and can become distanced – often when a pregnancy comes as a surprise. This is no different from the range of reactions among fathers of any age, although an older man may be more 'set in his ways' and could take longer to adjust to the idea of a baby.

Your partner may feel less pressurised about financial issues and be able to afford more help. If he is retired he might have plenty of time and energy and enjoy this new beginning. An older man will probably have a wide network of male friends who can offer advice and encouraging stories based on their experiences of bringing up children. In fact, this is more likely than when he was younger and most of his friends were still without children.

Emotions and feelings

Although pregnancy in later life is becoming more commonplace, many men and women feel distanced from friends their own age who have grown-up children or have declared themselves child-free. It may be difficult to feel at ease at antenatal and postnatal groups where most other women are younger than you. If you already have grown-up children, you may feel sad that you had regained your independence and will be putting this on hold while you bring up your baby.

It's more common for older parents to have ageing mothers and fathers who may need care, and this can increase practical and emotional challenges in the family. Some have lost their own parents. It might be difficult at times if you do not have your mum or dad around to share the joy your baby brings.

If you give birth at or after 40 you might be anxious that you will be pushing 60 when your children are in their teens, and wonder what implications this will have. Remember that if you feel happy at 40 you are likely to be happy at 60. Your age may improve your ability to love and care for your children, and to bring them up feeling wanted and adored.

Action plan

If you take care of yourself with a balanced nutritious diet and regular exercise balanced with rest, you are doing the best for yourself and your baby, whether you are 18 or 45 years old. It

helps to think about the balance between time for your baby, time for you, time for your partnership and time at work, if you stay on. Organisation can reduce tiredness and low energy and improve your relationships.

* Obstetricians and midwives sometimes treat older women differently but the prejudice is quickly disappearing. Different treatment reflects the concern for a good outcome, particularly in a first pregnancy after fertility treatment. You will be monitored as usual and the team will bear in mind any risk factors. They may be more keen to induce birth if labour is delayed, because of the risks associated with postmaturity (page 379).
* After the birth, there is no difference between an older woman and a younger woman in terms of the care they may benefit from, including practical help and loving support.
* BREASTFEEDING is usually successful in older mothers. If you have other children who are also young, you will need a lot of energy to keep on top of things. If you have children who are grown, you may have extra help from them.
* You may take longer to get your figure back after birth – this depends on keeping fit and exercising regularly, and eating well. Some older mothers need to pay more attention to pelvic floor exercises to regain strength (page 438), especially if they have had children before.

Osteopathy and cranial osteopathy

Osteopathy is a very powerful way to reduce areas of tension and relieve pain by the physical manipulation of muscles and joints. It can also release emotional stress that underlies or accompanies a physical complaint. Qualified osteopaths are accredited with a diploma, and osteopathy is a central part of treatment programmes in many healthcare settings. The discipline was founded in 1874 and is officially recognised by the Osteopathic Council.

An osteopath uses his or her hands to feel your body and locate and release areas of tension. Osteopaths are trained to assess the severity and longevity of strain patterns in the body. Some problems may date back to very early life (such as a forceps birth) or may have been forgotten (perhaps an accident in childhood).

Structural osteopathy involves manipulation to correct the alignment of bones and joints. Cranial osteopathy does not involve manipulation to the same degree. A cranial osteopath senses the rhythm of flow of body fluids. These include the cerebro-spinal fluid, which flows in and around your spine and brain, and other fluids that pass through your body's web of connective tissue. The flow influences your health and also reveals a lot about your life story. A cranial osteopath gently holds your head or back and follows and guides the rhythmic flow of the fluid. It is extremely safe for adults and babies and can have far reaching positive effects, particularly for newborns.

Babies respond rapidly because their tissues are supple and symptoms usually improve within five or six treatments. In adults, treatment may be needed over a number of months to release patterns that have been present for years as deep tension is encouraged to rise to the surface and the body slowly adapts. If your ligaments cause discomfort while they are naturally softening in pregnancy, you may feel better after treatment. Releasing tension also encourages your baby to engage in your pelvis and take an optimal position for birth.

Osteopathy is extremely valuable after birth, for both mothers and babies. The physical and emotional experience of even the gentlest birth can result in strain. Treatment is most effective in the weeks after delivery while the body tissues are still soft and malleable and you are emotionally open. Colic, excessive crying and disordered sleep in babies usually responds well to cranial osteopathy.

Osteoporosis

Bone is constantly being broken down by the body and rebuilt again. Osteoporosis happens when this breakdown occurs faster than new bone is formed, leading to a decrease in bone density. Osteoporosis can lead to back or hip pain and spine or hip fractures. Except in very rare instances, pregnancy does not cause osteoporosis and may even increase bone density. Breastfeeding may decrease bone density but the effect is temporary, and there are many ways to improve your bone strength before, during and after pregnancy.

What happens

A diet low in calcium-rich foods and lack of bone-building exercise, especially during childhood and adolescence, can sow the seeds of osteoporosis in later life. This is because most bone-building occurs when you are young. From the age of 35 onwards, the bones tend to become less dense, so the less dense they are to start with, the more fragile they will become, possibly leading to osteoporosis.

During pregnancy, your baby needs plenty of calcium and other minerals for bone development. Your body actually increases its absorption of calcium from foods and supplements and at the same time, high oestrogen levels give protection to your bones. The load-bearing exercise of carrying your baby in a sling after birth encourages bone strengthening. If you do not ingest sufficient minerals at this time, your bone density may reduce with an increased number of births.

Bone loss can occur during BREASTFEEDING because the calcium demands on your body increase, and the prolactin breastfeeding hormone reduces oestrogen in your system. The increased calcium demand depends on the amount of milk produced and on how long you continue to breastfeed. Any loss of bone tends to be temporary, with full recovery of density six months after stopping feeding: so there's no reason to avoid breastfeeding to protect your bones.

Very rarely, and for reasons that are not well understood, some women develop osteoporosis during pregnancy. Although pregnancy-associated osteoporosis is rare, it is worth being aware of how to protect your bones, particularly if:

- You have a family history of osteoporosis.
- You do not exercise sufficiently, as this may leads to reduced bone density resulting in osteoporosis in later life.
- You did not eat well as a child, so you may have had reduced bone density before you became pregnant.
- You have coeliac disease or other intestinal absorption difficulties.
- You have had anorexia and/or your periods

have stopped for a few months.
- You have taken long-term corticosteroids or heparin or thyroxin.
- You smoke or drink alcohol heavily.
- You are still in your teens, which means you are still building up your bone density and you and your baby may compete for the available minerals in your system.

Action plan

If you have osteoporosis you will need to be treated by a doctor who is an expert on the condition.

Preventive measures

There are many ways to prevent osteoporosis and these will also help to reverse any bone loss that might occur during pregnancy or breastfeeding. These are lifestyle issues and are just as important for men.
- Eat well, with a regular, balanced intake of minerals including calcium, magnesium, zinc and boron. Women who are pregnant or breastfeeding require 1,000mg of calcium each day and other minerals, including magnesium, zinc and boron, are equally important. The calcium requirement is higher for teenage mums (1,300mg per day). Good sources of minerals include: dark green, leafy vegetables, tofu, nuts and seeds, dairy products and corn. You do not have to eat dairy foods to have a good intake of calcium.
- Consider vitamin and mineral supplements during and after pregnancy (page 263).
- Avoiding fizzy drinks and tinned foods that contain phosphates is very important, as these interfere with calcium absorption.
- Carry your baby in a sling or papoose – the added weight encourages your bones to deposit calcium and increase density (and it's good for your baby's bones too).
- EXERCISE regularly, including weight-bearing exercises, such as walking with a back pack or carrying your baby, dancing, tennis and lifting weights, and YOGA postures where your bones carry the weight of your body.
- If you are on corticosteroids (cortisone), heparin or thyroid medication, or you have a bowel absorption problem, ask for regular bone-density monitoring.

Overactive thyroid

See Thyroid, baby; Thyroid, mother.

Overdue

See Labour and birth, mother, overdue.

Overweight, baby

See Weight, baby, overweight and obesity.

Overweight, mother

See Weight, mother, overweight and obesity.

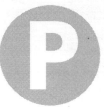

Pain relief, mother

See Labour and birth, mother, pain relief;
Medications.

Pain, baby

Babies are highly sensitive to both pleasure and pain from very early on. From birth, especially among premature babies, pain sensitivity is acute. It is much higher than an adult's. Inhibitory mechanisms that block incoming pain do not develop until after birth.

Babies are also able to feel emotional pain, whatever the trigger. This may include separation from mum, intense rage, being neglected or insensitively handled, and being denied food, warmth or love. The parts of the brain and body involved in emotional experience are well developed early on in foetal life.

Why does it hurt?

Your baby may experience pain for many reasons, and not just because he is ill, is having treatment, or has had an accident. Your baby may be uncomfortable because of pain following labour and birth, and digestion, excretion or hunger may be uncomfortable. Seemingly simple things such as feeling overwhelmed, or having a nappy change when he is tense and cold, may cause discomfort.

Intense or prolonged pain early in life that is not relieved, and/or is suffered in isolation, may predispose a person to hypersensitivity or chronic pain in the future. This is part of a patterning sequence that affects the way your baby develops through childhood and beyond. If your baby does experience pain, there is much that you and others can do to offer relief, and to help him feel safe while he is in pain and as it passes.

What happens

The perception of physical pain depends on messages travelling along nerve pathways from the source of pain, through the spinal cord, and to the brain. These pathways have already begun to form by the eighth week of pregnancy, and by Week 28 the wiring of pathways is more or less complete. By this time, if a baby senses pain he may grimace and draw his legs and arms into his body.

The perception of emotional pain is less clearly understood but is in part dependent on activity in ancient parts of the brain that enable a baby to react to the environment, and to express his feelings. You may also believe that spiritual energy – the soul, spirit or essence of a person that cannot be described in scientific terms – is involved in pain perception.

Physical or emotional pain is accompanied by the release of stress hormones (page 310). These assist survival but some of the effects are not helpful if the stress is prolonged. For instance, pain and accompanying hormone release can raise a baby's heart rate and disrupt natural body cycles (including appetite, digestion and sleep-wake cycles). It may lead to the baby becoming an anxious adult.

How your baby may indicate pain

Any pain may be unpleasant and frightening. Depending on your baby's unique personality and the nature of the pain, he may fight and complain with gusto, or he may withdraw and become self-protective. There are many possible ways to indicate pain:

* Crying – ranging from moaning (whiny) to a high-pitched scream (red alert), or crying with tears where usually there are none.
* Grimacing.
* Hitting his head with his hand(s), or leaning his head to one side (indicating head pain or ear pain).
* Banging his hand or fist on the part of the body that's hurting.
* Banging his head on the ground, wall or side of the cot.
* Dribbling from his mouth or opening his mouth wide (mouth pain).
* Reluctance to feed (could be mouth pain, head, ear, tummy, general).
* Drawing his knees into his chest (a common sign of COLIC pain).
* Arching his back (may be digestive discomfort).
* Closing his eyes tight or squinting (eye pain, such as a scratch on the cornea).
* Shutting down – averting his gaze, being very still, sleeping a lot.
* Irregular breathing or grunting.
* Reduced movements (a painful limb or joint).
* Being less active or very quiet.

Action plan

Fortunately, there are many sources of pain relief and there is a lot that can make your baby more comfortable.

* BREASTFEEDING is soothing. The action relieves pain and releases strain around the head, ears and face. Breast milk contains powerful pain-relieving substances and love hormones.
* Skin-to-skin touch will stimulate your baby's body to produce natural pain relievers and feel-good endorphins.
* Eye contact with a loving adult (preferably mum and dad) triggers the brain to stabilise the 'bodymind' and induce feelings of pleasure and comfort.
* Your voice can be very soothing. Your baby will be familiar with mum's voice from pregnancy and soon becomes accustomed to dad's voice. Gentle loving and melodic tones are soothing.
* The smell of you or another familiar person can make your baby feel safer and more comfortable. Pleasurable smells can activate pleasure systems in your baby's brain, together with the release of love hormones.
* Going at your baby's pace can help to avoid

overwhelming and extremely intense experiences. This includes telling your baby when something is about to change, taking care to avoid sudden noise, light or movements, or going to your baby to comfort him when he is crying. It doesn't mean being excessively cautious, but it does mean respecting your baby's sensitivity.
* Pain relief medication could help. (See guidelines, below.)

Complementary therapies

OSTEOPATHY is probably the most popular therapy used to relieve babies' pain, particularly following birth when there has been intervention or assistance with FORCEPS (see LABOUR AND BIRTH, MOTHER). Gentle cranial osteopathy can be extremely effective in relieving current pain and colic, and correcting patterns of strain so they do not become established and cause discomfort in later life.

MASSAGE is also very effective, and this is something you may want to do yourself. There are many benefits and pain relief is just one of them.

Homeopathic remedies for specific causes of pain are listed in the relevant entries. While you consider what might be at the root of your baby's discomfort, one of the following remedies may help calm him down and you may try one dose in 30c potency, and re-assess after half an hour.

* *Chamomilla* if your baby is crying pitifully, is irritable, doesn't know what he wants but clearly doesn't want to be put down.
* *Aconite* for acute anxiety and fear with pain.
* *Arnica* if you suspect your baby is in physical pain and you are not sure where it is.

Your baby may respond to a number of other COMPLEMENTARY THERAPIES.

▓ MEDICAL PAIN RELIEF

Until conclusive scientific proof that babies feel pain became available in the last 10 years, medical diagnostic and treatment procedures were carried out without administering any form of pain relief. Thankfully, there is now greater awareness and a range of pain relief is available. Breastfeeding may be possible while you visit a doctor and during some medical procedures, offering a source of security and comfort. If it is not possible during a procedure, it is likely to be comforting for your baby afterwards. Touch provides emotional and physical comfort and is an option even if your baby requires an anaesthetic.

General anaesthetic

This is commonly given to children for a wide range of surgical treatments and examinations. These days the procedure is straightforward and the risks are minimal. Usually the anaesthetist will allow your child home that day, following several hours of observation. Some hospitals inject a drug called ketamine, a safe and effective alternative to anaesthesia, for quick procedures where the child needs to keep still, such as stitching or removing foreign bodies.

Ibuprofen

Ibuprofen is a nonsteroidal anti-inflammatory drug (NSAID) that is used to relieve pain and reduce fever and inflammation. It is an optional medication for pain relief for children aged over one year old. Ibuprofen is only recommended if your child's fever or pain has not reduced in response to paracetamol or your health professional recommends it. Ibuprofen is available in various branded forms, including Nurofen Paediatric and Junifen.

For safe use, a child should weigh over 7kg. Ibuprofen should not be given if a child has a history of asthma, heart problems, kidney problems, stomach ulcers or indigestion. Speak to your GP or pharmacist if you are not sure, if your child has any other recognised medical condition, or if he is on any other medication.

Taking care with ibuprofen

* Before giving ibuprofen, review your use of paracetamol and ensure you are giving the correct dosage.
* Do not alternate ibuprofen and paracetamol. This is not recommended and does not appear to have any advantage over ibuprofen alone.
* It is important to read the instructions carefully. The correct dose and timing are important for the medication to work well and the dose is measured according to weight. The maximum recommendation is four doses in a 24-hour period.
* It is only appropriate to give ibuprofen to your baby under six months (or weighing less than 7kg) when the medication has been prescribed by your doctor.

Local anaesthetic gel

This reduces pain sensitivity at a specific site and may be used if a painful procedure is being carried out.

Opioid drugs

Morphine and similar opium-based drugs are used in hospitals where pain is persistent and severe, such as after an operation or during a painful procedure. Morphine can be used under supervision at home, but only with chronic cancer pain. It is also used to control withdrawal symptoms following maternal drug abuse in pregnancy.

Paracetamol

Paracetamol is the medicine most commonly prescribed to reduce a fever and relieve pain in babies. When working effectively, a single dose may reduce a fever (page 240) by 1–1.5 degrees Centigrade, for up to four hours. It is gentle on the stomach and is less likely than anti-inflammatories (such as ibuprofen) to cause worsening of ASTHMA or an asthma attack.

Paracetamol works by blocking the manufacture of prostaglandins, which arise when there is infection or injury and can cause pain, fever and swelling. It is available for children in liquid forms ('oral suspension'). It may also be administered in a suppository, which is extremely effective and fast acting for children who cannot take medicines by mouth, usually because of vomiting.

Paracetamol doses

There are different brands of paracetamol for children. In the UK, the most popular one is Calpol. It's important to check the strength of the brand you buy and ensure it's appropriate for your child's current age.

The clearest advice is to follow the instructions that come with the medication you choose. It is important to use the spoon or syringe provided to ensure you do not give too much. The amount in each dose depends on the strength of the preparation but is usually 120mg per 5ml for children aged three months to six years, and 250mg per 5ml for children aged over six.

Two to three months: On a doctor's recommendation only, you may give paracetamol following immunisation, in a single dose of 2.5ml at a strength of 120mg per 5ml.

Three months to one year: Give 2.5–5ml at a strength of 120mg/5ml every four to six hours, as needed, to a maximum of four doses in 24 hours.

One to five years: Give 5–10ml at a strength of 120mg/5ml every four to six hours, as needed, to a maximum of four doses in 24 hours.

Six to 12 years: Give 5–10ml at a strength of 250mg/5ml every four to six hours, as needed, to a maximum of four doses in 24 hours.

Taking care with paracetamol

* It is crucial not to exceed the recommended dosage – giving more will not provide extra pain relief, but may be dangerous.
* Paracetamol can be taken on an empty stomach.
* Once you have given paracetamol, you can expect it to take around 20 minutes to lower your baby's temperature and/or ease his pain.
* If your child still has pain or fever after using the correct dose of paracetamol, check with your doctor.
* If you are giving your baby any other medication – including cough mixture or a night sedative – take care that you do not exceed the recommended dose of paracetamol.
* You may be advised to avoid paracetamol or use a reduced dose if your child has liver or kidney disease.
* Side effects are rare and include skin rashes and other allergy symptoms.

✚ Red flag

If your baby has more than the recommended dose:

An overdose of paracetamol can cause liver damage. Seek emergency medical treatment immediately, even if there are no symptoms.

Sugar solutions

The sweet taste of these solutions is thought to activate opioid pathways that stimulate the production of natural pain relievers in the brain. The act of sucking can be soothing. These simple, inexpensive, non-invasive methods can be very helpful, although if your baby is premature it is important to take advice if he needs frequent pain relief. Routine use of sucrose as an analgesic for preterm babies may be linked to poorer mental development. Talk to the care team looking after your baby.

Pain, mother

See also Labour and birth, mother, pain relief.

✚ Red flag

Medical disorders

Although pain often does not indicate a serious issue, during and after pregnancy pain may signal a serious underlying medical disorder and it is important to report it to your midwife or doctor. This is especially crucial if you have other symptoms in addition to the pain such as fever, vomiting, fatigue or feeling unwell.

During and after pregnancy, your body undergoes many changes, and some may be uncomfortable. Most aches and pains do not point to a significant problem. Occasionally, however, pain may signal abnormality and if it is severe or continues for a long time, or you have other symptoms in addition to the pain, it is essential to be examined. Even when there is no significant medical problem, there are usually ways of reducing pain.

Pregnant women are usually most concerned by pain in the abdomen and pelvic region. Most times pain in these areas indicates muscle or ligament strain and does not signal a problem with the pregnancy.

A problem in one area may result in discomfort in another. For instance, an imbalance or strain in your pelvis may bring on a headache or a pain in your lower back.

■ CAUSES

The majority of pregnancy and postnatal pain relates to normal pregnancy changes; or to normal physiological events in the bowel, bladder and other organs, and some of these are listed below. Details of causes relating to each specific body area are listed under the relevant entries. Remember, though, it is vital to consult your midwife or doctor, particularly if you have other symptoms.

After birth

During birth the pelvic joints open and the ligaments and muscles in your pelvic area and lumbar spine may be stretched.

Bowel, bladder and other organs

In pregnancy, your bowel or bladder or your other abdominal organs may not function optimally and this can cause pain. Each organ is discussed in other sections of the book.

Daily baby care

Feeding and carrying your baby may impose additional tension on your spine.

Fatigue

Tiredness exaggerates poor posture and strain, and increases pain sensitivity.

Ligament and joint laxity

The production of the hormone relaxin increases through pregnancy, allowing your pelvic joints to expand. Aches and pains associated with muscle and ligament changes settle down after birth, and may take six months to return to normal. Your joints may feel more lax in second and subsequent pregnancies.

Posture

In pregnancy, the normal curve of your spine alters, your abdomen becomes heavier and your abdominal muscles are stretched, so there is more strain on your back. The way you sit and stand, the layout of your work area, your footwear, sofa and bed may all accentuate strains.

Previous back problem

Old areas of discomfort may be resolved in pregnancy, but in some cases an underlying tension pattern gets worse or causes new or increased discomfort. If you have had pain in a previous pregnancy, or are carrying more than one baby, you are more likely to have discomfort.

▓ EMOTIONS AND PAIN

Emotional issues may underlie or exacerbate your pain. Being in pain may cause you to feel down or anxious; and feeling emotionally depressed may manifest in physical pain. In some families it is acceptable to be in pain but not to feel depressed. This may apply to you. If you get anxious easily, you may feel pain more acutely. Your body and mind are interconnected – your 'bodymind' (page 73).

▓ SELF-HELP AND TREATMENT OPTIONS

There is a huge range in individual pain thresholds, and there is no 'right' way of responding to pain.

The most important thing is to take your pain seriously and seek medical advice if you have

- Upper abdominal pain in late pregnancy (pre-eclampsia).
- Pain in the area of the uterus, especially with bleeding and if the pain increases in intensity, spreads, or is severe to begin with.
- Pain associated with feeling faint or ill.
- Pain with a rise in temperature.
- Pain that is severe or lasts for longer than two hours.

The first step is to consider the cause(s) of your pain, preferably in consultation with your midwife or doctor. You may also seek advice from other healthcare professionals. If you require medical treatment this will be a key part of your care.

- The basic measures you can take to relieve or avoid discomfort include EXERCISE, YOGA, attending to your posture (including the back support your bed and chairs offer), rest, eating well, spending time in loving company and seeking emotional support when you need it. These are part of caring for you (page 121).
- You may wish to take pain relief medication (page 408).
- Complementary therapies offer numerous ways to relieve pain (e.g. osteopathy is often very effective for headaches or back pain).
- Time is often a great healer and when discomfort is associated with pregnancy, it tends to pass after birth.

Depending on the area and type of pain you are experiencing, you will find suggestions of possible causes and advice for easing discomfort under the relevant entries: abdomen, back and pelvis, breasts, hands, head, legs and vagina.

Palpitations

See Heart rhythms and murmurs, mother.

Parenting

See also Caring for baby; Caring for you; Relationships.

Parenting is about being there for your baby and also being there for you. You and your baby dance together. Parenting is something you learn on the job and the rewards and demands alter from day to day and week to week. There is no rule book and no 'right' or 'wrong'. You bring your talents, instincts and skills, and your own unique dance pattern evolves as you respond to your baby and listen to your feelings. Your style and how things go for you all also depend on your baby's unique personality. When you are in tune with your baby, you are likely to be 'infant-led' (see below) and this is usually a great recipe for family life. You will also benefit from advice and practical and emotional support.

The way you parent will be based on your experiences as a child. Even though you may not remember what happened in your infancy, your unconscious holds memories and feelings that affect you now. The way you felt as a baby, in childhood and in adolescence, as well as your family's belief systems and ways of communicating, have had a tremendous impact on you: these constitute your family of origin (page 207), which will profoundly affect the way you are with your baby today. Your approach will also be influenced by your current beliefs, your peer group and the media. In some areas, you and your partner will inevitably have different views, or you may not be in agreement with your parents. It may take time and honest discussion to reach agreement that suits your baby and family.

▓ A LOVE AFFAIR

There is something exquisite about the love between mother and baby, or father and baby. This special relationship can be one of life's most intimate love affairs.

When you parent from the heart, rather than from the head, you are on track. When your heart is open, you let your baby feel loved, wanted, welcomed and adored for who she is rather than what she does. This is infinitely more important than whether your baby sleeps 'well', and so on. At the same time, loving and accepting yourself – on good days and on bad days – will help. You and

your baby may be separated by years, but your emotional drives to feel loved and to express yourselves are equally strong. When you dance together and love flows between you, you are both likely to feel good and enjoy yourselves.

Infant-led parenting

Many people once believed, and still believe, that babies do not know what they need and parents must be in control. When your baby is encouraged to lead, however, and you respond to her, she will feel safe. She will express her needs and when you respond, she is reassured. This will not 'spoil' her; rather it helps her feel secure, to bond with you, to feel joy and to build a foundation of self-belief that is likely to remain in place for life.

Allowing your baby to guide you is known as 'infant-led parenting'. This is not the same as infant-*dominated* parenting, where a child controls the family or when parents' needs go unmet. With infant-led care, you provide boundaries (see below), your baby is acknowledged and allowed to lead, and your own needs are valued. When this is in place, your baby feels safe, nurtured and welcome, and the family is also nourished. Although life seldom goes according to expectations, a foundation like this offers a stable ground for you all amid life's opportunities and challenges.

▓ BOUNDARIES

We all have boundaries. Within our boundaries we feel comfortable. Outside of them we do not. Mostly boundaries are not written or spoken, yet they are central to happiness and also to conflict and feeling upset. Suitable boundaries are part of a loving, friendly relationship or environment. When there are too few, you or your baby may feel unsettled. When boundaries are too rigid and/or do not suit you or your baby, you may feel upset or angry. It can therefore be helpful to acknowledge these feelings because this creates the possibility of change.

Physical boundaries begin in the womb and continue after birth in the safety of a loving person's arms. They extend to a cot, a room and a house. Boundaries also reflect beliefs and wishes and time. They may apply to behaviour, finances, childcare, sleeping, crying, and so on.

Many boundaries form early in life and you may notice some that are part of your family culture – for instance, something your mum or dad believed; the way a nursery 'should' look; how babies 'should' sleep; or whether it is acceptable to express anger. Some may still appeal; others may no longer feel right. You and your partner are bound to have different ideas about some boundaries.

Positive boundaries

Positive boundaries can increase a sense of freedom. For instance, a boundary that aims for '30 minutes with my baby when I do not answer the phone or do any domestic chores', allows you and your baby to freely play and focus on one another. Creating definite time to exercise will similarly be helpful for you all.

When boundaries are crossed

There will be many times when boundaries are crossed – this is reality. Your baby's needs and desires develop and alter with incredible rapidity in the first year. Sometimes when this happens you, and others, may feel upset. Then it is time to review your boundaries. They may remain valid, or may need to shift because circumstances have changed.

For instance, you may have boundaries relating to your eating habits – perhaps preferring to dine at the table rather than in front of the television. If your partner disagrees you may feel resentful or upset. Another example is how often you are happy to have your mum/dad/in-laws in your house. For new parents, sleep (how, when and where) is a very common boundary issue. For babies, boundaries begin with the need to feel loved, held and cared for. When these boundaries are not respected all babies feel upset.

If your boundaries are being crossed you have a choice – you can say why you are upset, and then discuss either reinforcing or altering the boundary. Alternatively, you may not acknowledge the boundary. Some people decide to make do, put up with a difficult situation, or ignore their own needs. When boundaries are crossed, however, this is uncomfortable and resentment may build, trigger arguments and reduce family unity.

When boundaries become barriers

Boundaries work best when they are loving and fluid. Your baby needs to feel boundaries around her and to push against something – both physically and emotionally. This is part of her

growth. When boundaries are flexible they can alter to meet her changing needs.

Inflexible boundaries seldom reflect the needs of each person and become barriers. Barriers tend to be uncomfortable and can make adults as well as babies grumpy, argumentative, frustrated and 'rebellious'. Behaviours like these are useful signals for you to consider changes. When parental discipline is excessive, barriers frequently suppress a child and can cause relationship problems and/or upset, in the present or in later life.

Assessing your boundaries

Many boundaries will concern your family and your partnership; others may involve your extended family, work colleagues or the medical team. Creating and reviewing boundaries is a skill that will set you, your partner and your children in good stead for the rest of your lives together. Many people develop this skill first as parents and apply it in other areas of life with great effect. There are countless examples:

> 'It's not okay to shout at my baby.'

> 'I would like to have X hours sleep each night.'

> 'It's not okay for my toddler to hit my baby.'

> 'It's okay for us to have sex while our baby is in the room.'

> 'It's important for both of us to make time to exercise each week.'

> 'It's nice to have one or two takeaways a month, but not more.'

> 'It's okay/not okay for you to work weekends.'

> 'I'd like to arrange childcare so we can go out every week.'

If you have crossed a valid boundary (for example, you shout at your baby or you/your partner spend more time away from the house than you agreed) it is best to acknowledge it and discuss possible changes.

> 'I am sorry I shouted at you, it wasn't anything you did. I was irritable about something else, and there is nothing you did wrong.'

> 'You are spending a lot of time outside the house, more than we thought was reasonable, and I'd like to talk about this.'

Assessing and adjusting boundaries is an ongoing task. Trying things out to see what works can lighten up your everyday experience of parenting. It does get easier with attention and time. There may be conflict between your values regarding parenting and those of your partner, family or peer group. See if you can acknowledge areas where opinions differ as the first step. Active listening (page 462) may help if there is an impasse.

DISCIPLINE

Discipline is not appropriate for babies. There is no such thing as a naughty baby. In the first year your baby's brain is not developed sufficiently to allow her to consciously disregard a rule. Her behaviour, even when it is challenging for you, is simply an expression of what she is feeling: she is not able to purposefully annoy or contradict you and she is not trying to make life difficult for you.

Discipline is the opposite of nurturing, and suppresses your baby's spirit, whether through:
* hitting;
* enforcing sleeping/feeding schedules that do not meet your baby's individual needs;
* leaving her in isolation; or
* ignoring her cries.

If there is physical abuse (page 131) the effect is particularly devastating.

Various forms of 'discipline' give a baby the message that her needs are not important or are wrong, and that she is not valuable or good enough. With perceptions like these, a baby may feel anger, confusion, pain and sorrow, and question her natural impulses so that she carries self-doubt through life. Early experiences are like the architects of her brain. The feelings she has and her experience of your response become part of her neural patterning. Discipline is not appropriate, whereas meeting her emotional and physical needs and creating good boundaries are likely to give her a great start that will bring benefits throughout her life.

PERFECT PARENTING?

The desire to give your baby the best is universal, but there is no such thing as a perfect parent – or a perfect baby. It is commendable to aim for high standards but it is important to remember that there is no 'right' or 'wrong' way to parent.

Getting it right as often as possible is most definitely good enough. It's definitely okay for your baby to have good and bad times, be quiet and noisy and feel angry or sad – all her feelings are natural and important (page 206). The same applies to you.

Many parents feel torn between the needs of their baby and other aspects of their lives. Returning to work, for instance, often brings conflict and maybe guilt or sadness. In reality, being a parent encompasses caring for your baby and caring for yourself and your family: all need attention. Trying out different ways to meet everyone's needs is part of the learning curve you're on. Be gentle with yourself, and honest with your baby: even if she cannot understand your words she will feel your integrity and love.

Expectations and upsets

It's common to feel upset when reality falls short of your expectations. Some examples include:
* Birth didn't go as you'd hoped.
* Your baby doesn't sleep for as long as you'd like.
* Breastfeeding is a challenge.
* You feel that you are doing more than your fair share of housework.
* You and your partner do not agree about something.
* Your sex life isn't great.
* Your mum isn't around.
* You are working hard all day and get back to a grumpy baby and partner.

When you are upset you may expect your partner, and your baby, to behave differently, or expect yourself to cope better. Yet there is a positive note here – the chance to take the opportunity presented by a difficult situation.

Take a moment to consider your expectations. You could talk with your partner, your midwife, a friend or a counsellor. You can also talk to your baby. She will appreciate your honesty, although it is important to take responsibility for your feelings and not to blame her for what you feel. She may influence or trigger your moods but she is not the cause of them.

Over time, it will be easier to distinguish between expectations that echo the needs you had as a baby, or your parents' ideals, and the expectations that help you meet the needs of your baby and family today. Remember, your baby does not think or behave like a mini adult, nor is she a mini version of you; just as you are not a clone of your mother or a 'perfect' friend or sibling. It may take courage to acknowledge the reality of your life and to decide when and how things need to be changed.

What do you expect of yourself?
Sometimes your expectations are appropriate and offer helpful guidelines. At other times they are not suitable. You can get an idea of your expectations by completing the following sentences. It is also useful to look at the expectations you have of other people and other areas in your life.

* A good birth entails ...
* A good mother never...
* A good father never ...
* My mother would ...
* My father would ...
* Fathers nowadays ...
* Mothers I admire do ...
* My generation believe that a baby is ...
* I should be able to ...
* My sister/friend should ...
* I believe that ...

Your answers reveal the view you have inherited from your family (page 207) as well as what your heart tells you. You may have an inner voice that encourages you. An inner voice that makes you doubt is your inner critic that says, 'I am not good enough, they will not approve.' The two voices tend to co-exist and may sometimes make it hard to trust your feelings and make appropriate choices.

What do you expect of your baby?
Do you have thoughts such as, 'Babies should sleep through the night from six weeks,' or, 'Babies should have at least one tooth by the age of five months'? If you think in terms of, 'Babies do ... babies should ... they always do ...', try turning the words around: 'My baby does x, y and z and that is fine even though my sister's baby does a, b and c.' 'This is the way my baby behaves in this situation ...'

Every baby behaves differently, has a unique personality, and develops at her own rate. When a baby is young the need to be good or best belongs only to the parent. Children can tell from a very young age if they meet, surpass or fall short of their parents' expectations by the encouragement they receive and the energy of

pride or disappointment conveyed in tone of voice and body language.

Babies are driven to connect with their carers and they adapt to feel safe and to get love and attention. At a very early age, a baby can learn to please. If this happens, a baby begins to rate her own needs and feelings below other people's – this is compliance (page 121) and suppresses personal expression. When a baby is loved and listened to and accepted for who she is, regardless of expectations, she learns to value herself, and express herself joyfully.

Perfectionism
Perfectionism often arises from fear, from not feeling good enough and having a low self-image. These feelings, in turn, may stem from disapproval, neglect or even abuse in childhood. Many people who strive for perfection did not feel listened to, and/or felt controlled and restricted by their (often strict) parents, and seldom felt their needs were important. Some parents are afraid that if they do not repeat the pattern and their baby is not controlled she will be wild. Many developmental biologists believe the opposite and the guidelines in this book reflect this view. If you are a perfectionist it will be a challenge – and a pleasure – to let go of tight control and learn from your child while you put in place flexible, appropriate boundaries. Being playful may be a good place to start.

▇ RHYTHM AND ROUTINE
Most babies and adults feel more secure when days and nights have a structure. In most parent-baby partnerships this becomes established naturally. Sometimes a structure falls into place early, but usually it takes weeks or even months. Your rhythms will continue to alter as your baby's and your own needs change – for instance, as your baby's appetite changes, feeding times need to alter. The same applies to her sleeping rhythms. It will be easiest for you and your baby if you do not rush into a schedule and if you spend quality time together, so that you tune into one another. It is optimal to follow your baby's lead and at the same time put appropriate boundaries in place: it is entirely possible for your baby's rhythm to guide a structure that is predictable and suitable for you, too. This takes love and acceptance, and flexibility so that your boundaries (page 433) are supportive rather than restrictive.

Routine

A routine is more rigidly defined than a rhythm. Generally speaking, having a routine demands that a baby's natural behaviours (crucially eating and sleeping) need to fit into specified time slots through each day. This is not the same as responding to a rhythm where the activities of each day fit around a baby.

Structure can be very reassuring for a baby, yet it is important to be led by your baby rather than by your need to keep within a defined regime. If you are keen to set up a routine, it will help to keep a high degree of flexibility rather than being coercive or expecting your baby to conform; and it is important not to aim for a routine before your baby is ready. (It takes time, for instance, for her brain to respond to light/dark cycles with an altered sleep pattern, and for her stomach to grow sufficiently for her feeds to be widely spaced.) This may not be at the same time as other babies – either your previous children or other children in your family or community. When your baby feels comfortable and is able to flow in her natural rhythm, she will feel good. This tends to make day-to-day family life more relaxed and enjoyable.

If a routine feels crucial for you but when you try to establish it your baby is upset or stressed (or you are), these are signs that what you are doing isn't in your best joint interests. Consider your need to be in control. How do you feel about being in charge? How do you feel when you let your baby guide you? How do you feel about your ability to understand and be there for her?

Often, the pressing need to install a routine is based on fear, including one or more of the following parental anxieties:

- I am afraid I will not get enough sleep (consider co-sleeping, page 487, and resting during the day).
- I am afraid my baby will be grumpy if she doesn't have a routine (more likely to be grumpy if her needs are not met as they arise).
- I am afraid I'll make a rod for my own back if I am not in control (being controlling is more likely to make your life feel rigid).
- I'm afraid I will spoil my baby if I follow her lead (babies cannot be spoilt, page 47).
- I am worried my mum will disapprove of what I am doing (your mum's feelings are her issue and your choices as a parent are your issue).

- My partner thinks differently, I don't want to upset her/him (it is better to communicate with your partner about the importance of your baby's need for security).
- I am afraid I will never have time away from my baby (you may feel better if you and your baby spend time with other adults. Trust that being there for your baby is incredibly valuable, and remember, she is only dependent on you for a short time. The more secure she feels now, the less dependent she will be on you in the long term).

Loving and trusting

The need to have a routine tends to be led by the head (anxiety/control), rather than the heart (love and trust). You may want to listen to your heart, and see what it feels like to let go of your attachment to having a routine. It is okay to take it day by day, or week by week, and without anxiety over timings. This may enable you to enjoy more 'quality' time with your baby. Your baby invites you to slow down to be in harmony with her. She is a great teacher. When she feels you're there for her, she will feel safe. From this place of security she knows she can relax into her own rhythms; and the chances are that these rhythms will soon feel comfortable and predictable for you too. She will also mirror the rhythms of you and your family, and in time you will fall into synchronicity. One of her great teachings for you is to slow down and be present for what is happening here and now.

▓ TIME AND SPACE

When you have a baby, she becomes the focus. Yet this is not to the exclusion of everything else, and aspects of your life that nourish you deserve quality time: food, rest, exercise and time with your partner. A new style of organisation might help you ensure these are not neglected.

Getting a balance doesn't demand that you become a highly organised goddess overnight. Just a few simple steps can make a huge difference. For most people, it's a combination of adjusting personal goals and adopting new techniques, with help from your baby, your family, friends and other people.

Fitting it all in

It is difficult to overestimate the change of lifestyle that comes with parenthood. Sleep patterns change, domestic chores multiply and your responsibility to your baby limits what you can do. This may leave you feeling, at times, under pressure and restricted, particularly if you are tired or your energy is low, or you have too little support. When there is time and space for you and for your relationships, though, the positive aspects of parenting can predominate, such as adventure, a growing family and community, love and bonding, and the magic of being with your baby.

Each person has different commitments and demands, and you will adapt in a way that suits your family and your lifestyle. The tips below offer suggestions for making life easy.

- Being well rested and getting enough sleep will help you avoid becoming overwhelmed. Eating well and exercising are core elements of your wellbeing. All of these will give you more energy and time.
- You could cook double quantities (or more) and freeze meals. Consider internet shopping.
- Consider enrolling help (page 123).
- Review your diary: booking time to exercise, to rest and to be with your partner can ensure you don't leave these important elements until everything else is done (which, in reality, seldom happens).
- Remember the importance of fun time to play.
- Having a 'cosy corner' in each room where you keep a spare set of baby clothes, a soft blanket and nappy equipment means you can stay with your baby and spend less time running around.
- Consider buying a large bed so you can all sleep and/or rest together, and have at least one really comfortable chair for feeding.
- There may be possibilities for change at work to reduce pressure and allow you more time at home.
- Sharing can be the best way of reducing your load: with other mums, with your sisters, through groups and so on.
- Set realistic goals as this will reduce a build-up of unfinished tasks.
- Many people underestimate how long tasks can take – even leaving the house to go to the local shop may take 40 minutes with a baby, compared to two or three minutes when you were on your own. Consider over-estimating

and using phrases such as 'morning' and 'afternoon' rather than specific times until you are used to the new pace of life.

Quality time

Quality time is time when you are focused on what you're doing and feeling and who you are with right now – free from anxiety about what you're not doing, didn't do or still have to do. Your baby has a slow rhythm. She will entice you into her space and when you are there with her, her energy will make it easier for you to let go, enjoy and simply be.

Parvovirus (slapped cheek disease)

Parvovirus B19 is a virus that lives in red blood cells. It is sometimes called 'fifth disease' or 'slapped cheek disease' because one of its characteristic signs is a facial rash, resembling the reddening of a slap. It most commonly infects children and is often present in day-care settings during winter and spring. If you have been infected in childhood you will be immune as an adult. There is no vaccine against the disease but most adults are unaware of their immunity status. If you are not immune and come into contact with an infected person, you have a 30 per cent chance of catching the virus through inhalation. Most babies of infected pregnant mothers do not become infected themselves.

What happens

The parvovirus B19 rash, with red cheeks, pale lips and a generalised rash on the trunk, is more common among children. In adults, symptoms usually involve joint pains and stiffness in the hands and knees. Symptoms begin four to 14 days after infection and commonly pass within a couple of weeks. Around 20 per cent of infected adults have no symptoms at all. The rash is similar to RUBELLA (German measles) infection.

If you are infected with parvovirus during the first 20 weeks of pregnancy, there is a small chance of your baby being infected (less than 10 per cent). For most of the babies who do become infected, the infection is mild. There is a 3 per cent risk that the infection can depress the bone marrow and as a result may cause ANAEMIA. Infection in the womb does not cause CONGENITAL ABNORMALITY but anaemia in the womb may result in heart failure and fluid retention, a condition called HYDROPS. This may require treatment by transfusion in pregnancy (intrauterine) or after birth and sometimes early delivery. Recovery of the bone marrow, with or without transfusion, will be complete with no long-lasting damage to the bone marrow, or any genetic damage to the baby.

Action plan

Prevention
Your best precaution is to avoid close contact, as you would to guard against CYTOMEGALOVIRUS (CMV) infection, particularly if you work with children.

Treatment and medical care
If you develop parvovirus B19 in pregnancy there is no effective treatment, except for relief of symptoms. Your body naturally forms antibodies to tackle the infection. Your medical team will, however, closely monitor your baby's wellbeing.
- Because the parvovirus rash mimics rubella, a sample of your blood will be tested in a laboratory to confirm or exclude the diagnosis of a recent infection.
- You will be offered ultrasound scans to detect whether your baby has developed anaemia and swelling from fluid retention.
- If your baby has foetal anaemia your medical team will monitor pregnancy and labour closely, because your baby is at a higher risk of FOETAL DISTRESS.
- Treatment depends on the degree of anaemia and the stage of pregnancy. If foetal anaemia is severe and may lead to hydrops, an intrauterine blood transfusion improves your baby's health.
- After birth your baby's blood will be checked for anaemia and a transfusion may be needed if the haemoglobin level is very low. The effects of the virus disappear over the following few weeks.

Pelvic floor exercises (Kegel)

When you give birth to your baby, there is pressure on your vagina and perineum (the area of skin and muscle stretching between your

vaginal opening and your anus). Your body prepares for this as hormones soften muscles and ligaments to encourage stretching; you may notice the effect of this during pregnancy if your vagina feels 'loose' or you experience slight incontinence (page 317). Active preparation of your vaginal area can improve strength and increase flexibility, reducing the likelihood that an episiotomy (page 369) may be needed to widen the entrance or that you may tear when you give birth. It also has long-term benefits that may improve urinary continence, sex and body image. In addition, attention to perineal strength in your first pregnancy can reduce feelings of looseness in your next. A few simple exercises practised each day can have huge results.

■ PELVIC TUCK-INS

You may repeat the following exercises in sets of five to 10, at least five times a day. You can do them anywhere at any time – no one will know what you're up to. Think of a trigger to remind you: perhaps you could do a set each time you are in the car or waiting at traffic lights or when you watch a regular television programme. After the birth a useful connection is to do a set each time you feed your baby. Walking and exercising are powerful ways to strengthen the pelvic floor as are some yoga postures.

Tighten your pelvic floor muscles as if you are stopping the flow of urine or tightening your vagina around a penis. To begin with you might find it easier to start at the anus and tighten the area gradually, moving towards your vagina.

Tighten, count to five, and consciously release and relax. Do this five times and then do five sets of tightening without holding the tension.

As you build up strength and control, practise on your partner during intercourse and see how many tightenings he can count – the extra squeeze for him is guaranteed to thrill.

■ PERINEAL MASSAGE

A light and gentle massage of your perineum can improve its ability to stretch. From six weeks before birth you may begin to massage your perineum three to four times a week, for around two to four minutes at a time. Massage after a bath or shower, ensure your bladder is empty and relax your pelvic floor as you do so. In the beginning you will feel tight, but with time and practice the tissues will relax and stretch. The massage shouldn't hurt.

Lubricate your thumb or fingers with olive, almond or grapeseed oil and squat or rest one foot on a chair or bath.

Place two fingers or a thumb about 5cm (2in) into your vagina (up to the second knuckle) and move rhythmically from 3 o'clock to 9 o'clock and back again, using a sweeping motion with downward pressure.

If there is a tender area, breathe in, hold the pressure lightly on the area and breathe out very slowly while relaxing your abdominal and back muscles and your pelvic floor. You may repeat this two or three times and you will feel the area relax.

You can also massage the perineal skin between your fingers and thumb. Apply steady pressure downwards towards the back passage until you feel a tingling sensation, which is in fact like the feeling of your baby's head crowning before birth.

Pelvic pain

See Back and pelvic pain.

Penis, baby, hypospadias and chordee

Hypospadias is a congenital condition involving the position of the urethra, the tube and opening through which urine passes out of the body. The defect may occur anywhere along the underside of the penis down to the scrotum, but most commonly it is close to the normal opening site. Males with hypospadias usually have normal testes and fertility is unaffected. It occurs in roughly one in 350 boys born each year.

Another condition, chordee – downward curve of the penis, especially when erect – is associated with hypospadias. Boys with uncorrected chordee must often sit to urinate, and in adult life it can make intercourse impossible. Fortunately, treatment for both conditions is usually successful.

What happens

Around Week 10, the urethra begins to fold and close and the penis grows. If the folding is incomplete, hypospadias occurs. The actual cause is unknown but it is more common when the mother is aged over 35. If two people in a family have hypospadias, the chance of recurrence is about 20 per cent.

Action plan

Hypospadias and chordee are looked for during normal checks at birth. Treatment of hypospadias requires specialist surgery. CIRCUMCISION must not take place, as surgical treatment may use some of the foreskin to reconstruct the opening back to its normal position.

The best age to have corrective surgery depends on the size of the penis and degree of the defect. It is usually performed at six to 12 months on an outpatient basis. Some 90 per cent of corrections are completed in one operation. The operation corrects the chordee so that the penis straightens with an erection, and extends the urethra to the tip of the penis. Corrective surgery usually results in a penis that looks and functions as normal.

Phenylketonuria (PKU)

Phenylketonuria is a rare disease occurring in about one in 125,000 newborns. It is caused by a defective gene that results in a deficiency of the enzyme needed to convert the amino acid phenylalanine into another amino acid, tyrosine. As a result of the defect, harmful chemicals called phenyl ketones build up in the bloodstream. When they reach high levels, they are toxic to the baby's developing brain. The condition is detected by a blood test, called the Guthrie test. This is done on the heel prick blood spot (page 338) obtained when your baby is about one week old and feeding well. Treatment beginning in the first few weeks can prevent the build-up of toxins. Without early treatment, a child would suffer irreversible brain damage and develop learning disability.

Action plan

Treatment involves a special diet low in phenylalanine, including special milk. To maintain normal growth and intellectual development a child needs to keep to the diet for the rest of her life. All food labels must now state whether a food contains a source of phenylalanine (such as the sweetener, aspartame). For girls with PKU not on the special diet, there is a risk of damage to their babies in pregnancy through high levels of phenylalanine, which can affect foetal brain development in the womb.

Pilates

See also Exercise, mother.

Pilates is becoming a popular choice of exercise, before, during and after pregnancy. Pilates began as a set of remedial exercises for dancers. Like YOGA, pilates is designed to improve balance, strength and flexibility through a series of exercises and postures. The focus is awareness of the core of your body (around your lower back, abdomen and pelvis) coupled with awareness of breath. You may already find pilates relaxing and energising. Alternatively you may want to begin during pregnancy, or after the birth. Some of the exercises are physically demanding so it is important to go at a pace that suits you and always stay within your comfort zone: The ideal is to attend a class designed specifically for pregnancy and, postnatally, to be sure not to over-stretch or over-exert yourself. Your body will be very flexible at this time but needs time to regain pre-pregnancy strength.

Some pilates practitioners say that with core strength and with concentration, you can tap into your 'belly brain', a focus for physical and emotional stability and strength. This may be a good resource, particularly after the birth when pilates exercises may help you to rest and replenish your energy in a few minutes. Many people experiencing pain in the back, head or shoulder do pilates to ease the discomfort and to improve their strength.

Piles (haemorrhoids) and anal fissure

Piles (haemorrhoids) are small, blood-filled swellings caused by dilated veins. Initially, they are located just inside the anus (internal haemorrhoids) but can sometimes protrude

(external haemorrhoids). Haemorrhoids are not dangerous. During pregnancy, increased blood flow to the pelvic area may cause the veins to swell and this effect increases if you are passing hard stools or you have CONSTIPATION. Pressure in the veins increases as pregnancy advances and is at its height during and immediately after birth, then as pressure decreases the piles typically resolve. Piles often coexist with varicose veins (page 544). Small piles affect many pregnant women and usually pass after birth. Large piles may very occasionally prolapse out of the anus.

What happens

Small piles – pea size – can exist without giving any symptoms. If they reach the size of a grape, or larger, the anal muscle may go into spasm. This causes burning on passing a stool, particularly if the stool is hard. You may notice a mucous discharge and if the lining of your anus has become inflamed, this may be sore. Often, there is bright red bleeding during a bowel movement.

If the piles are small you may not be able to feel them, as they won't protrude. Your doctor may perform a gentle examination with a finger to confirm their presence, and may use a proctoscope, a small instrument that enables the doctor to visualise the lining of your anus.

Piles are biggest following the pushing force of birth and they may get larger if your pelvic muscles go into spasm following a vaginal tear with stitches, because when this happens the blood may not drain freely from the veins.

Action plan

You can expect your piles to get better over a six to 12 week period, and you can help this process with a few simple measures. Even large ones may disappear completely.

Diet and lifestyle
- Follow the advice for avoiding constipation (page 153). This will help you avoid straining, which will stop the piles from getting worse.
- To reduce pressure on your rectal veins, avoid standing for long periods of time.
- If you have large piles, and they are causing pain, you could sit on an inflatable ring or lie on your side.

Medical care

* It is best for your doctor to check your piles after the birth.
* Your doctor may recommend glycerine suppositories for lubrication, or a suppository or cream containing a local anaesthetic and a mild corticosteroid (cortisone) which helps to prevent irritation and muscle spasm pain. An alternative is to lubricate your anus with a pure vegetable oil (such as almond or grapeseed) with your finger after each bowel movement.
* Ice packs, cold compresses (page 36) or cabbage leaves kept in the fridge and applied to the area for 20 minutes every three to four hours bring relief and can reduce swelling.
* Piles tend to recur in subsequent pregnancies, or if you are constipated after birth and strain to pass stools.
* Occasionally an operation may be required to remove the swollen veins.
* Extremely rarely, where anal bleeding does not stop, there may be a rectal polyp or cancer and further examinations will be needed.

Exercise and aromatherapy

* Don't forget to do regular pelvic floor exercises (page 438). They increase circulation and may reduce swelling. Begin by tightening your anus.
* A compress with cypress oil applied to the piles for 20 minutes, three times a day, may help, but the anal skin may crack and cause a fissure if the compress is left on too long. Alternatively, you could apply one to two drops of oil diluted in a carrier oil (almond or grapeseed) to the piles every eight hours. If you have had stitches be sure not to get cypress oil on them.

Homeopathy

A suitable remedy may be taken in 30c potency three times a day for five to seven days, then re-assess.

* *Hamamelis* if your piles protrude, feel tight, are bluish in colour and can bleed profusely. Pains are pulsating, pricking and stinging, accompanied by pains in your back.
* *Collinsonia* for chronic internal or protruding piles with itching, burning and tightness in the anus, intermittent bleeding with splinter-like pain, worse at night and better in the mornings.
* *Aesculus* relieves prolapsed, purple, bleeding piles that give a constricted feeling in the anus with burning, itching and sharp splinter-like

pains. There is a tendency for discomfort to linger for a long time after passing a stool, worse in the morning and better for bathing with cool water.

* *Nux Vomica* for sensitive, inflamed piles that bleed easily with stitching pains that can be felt up the spine, there is constipation with much ineffectual straining, your rectum feels constricted and the piles feel large and inflamed. It is worse at night and when you're stressed, better later in the day and from resting.
* *Sepia* may give relief when there is a strong bearing down sensation with large, hard and protruding piles that can bleed. There is the feeling of a ball in the rectum and you generally may feel run down, miserable and exhausted, with mood swings.

Creams are available from the homeopathic pharmacies which can be applied externally to bring relief.

Prolapsed piles

If the rectal muscles go into intense spasm, pressure in already swollen veins increases and piles may swell further and protrude in a painful condition known as prolapsed piles. It usually occurs after birth and is treated with:

* rest in bed;
* painkillers; and
* application of a local anaesthetic cream a few times a day.

Ice packs, cold compresses or cabbage leaves kept in the fridge and applied to the area for 20 minutes every three to four hours bring relief and can reduce swelling.

The piles usually recede within a few days and even large piles may not be visible six months later. Very rarely, surgery is needed after the birth.

▓ ANAL FISSURE

A fissure or crack in the anal skin may mimic piles (opposite) by causing bleeding and pain. It may also cause a yellow discharge. Fissures are most common after birth. They are usually caused by constipation and heal when stools become softer. Rarely, a fissure may signal an underlying ulcerative colitis (page 320).

- Softening stools and avoiding constipation (page 153) is very effective.
- Keep the anal area clean with plain warm water, several times a day. Use a hair dryer to dry the area.
- Most fissures heal with the use of a cream or suppository to protect the anal lining. An alternative is to lubricate your anus with a pure vegetable oil (such as almond or grapeseed) with your finger after each bowel movement.
- A small number of anal fissures do not heal rapidly and an operation may be needed to close the skin crack.
- *Homeopathy.* You may soak the anal area using a combination tincture of *Paeonia, Ratanhia* and *Calendula* – put 15 drops in a shallow bath several times per day.

Placenta accreta

See also Labour and birth, mother, bleeding following birth.

When you become pregnant, the internal cavity of your uterus becomes lined with a spongy membrane, or decidua, into which the placenta embeds. After your baby has been born, the placenta separates by shearing off at the decidua. In placenta accreta, the placenta grows through the decidual layer and into the muscle of the wall of the uterus, becoming so firmly attached it will not separate in the third stage of labour. The condition is rare and is more likely to occur in women who have had surgery to the uterus or a prior CAESAREAN SECTION. It may accompany a placenta praevia (low-lying placenta, see below).

What happens

In the third stage of labour, after the baby has been born, the uterus continues to contract to assist the separation and birth of the placenta, but a placenta accreta does not separate. This stops the uterus from contracting and retracting and carries a risk of heavy bleeding.

Placenta accreta may sometimes be suspected on ultrasound scan using Doppler colour flow in late pregnancy.

Action plan

After the birth of your baby, the birth of the placenta will not follow. Almost always, a placenta accreta requires surgical removal in the operating theatre. An epidural or a general anaesthetic will be used, and an obstetrician will manually separate the placenta. While you are in theatre your baby will appreciate the closeness of another adult so your partner may want to hold him.

After the placenta has been removed, you can expect a normal amount of postnatal bleeding. It is usual to administer antibiotics after surgery to prevent or treat infection. The operation is over soon and you can breastfeed your baby within four hours.

On exceptionally rare occasions, the placenta penetrates the wall of the uterus completely and a hysterectomy to remove the uterus may be needed to stem the bleeding.

If ultrasound scans lead your team to suspect placenta accreta during pregnancy, particularly if you also have placenta praevia, a caesarean section birth is essential to minimise the risk of life-threatening bleeding. Senior members of the obstetric, surgical and anaesthetic team will be with you to ensure that the placenta is completely removed and excess bleeding is prevented.

Next pregnancy

After one placenta accreta, there is a higher risk of the problem recurring in a future pregnancy, particularly if your baby was born by caesarean. Your care in pregnancy with frequent ultrasound scans to detect the problem and during labour and birth will reflect this.

Placenta praevia

When the placenta implants in the lower half of the uterus (the lower segment) and it extends to partially or completely cover the internal opening of the cervix, it is called a low-lying placenta or placenta praevia. In early pregnancy, the placenta covers most of the cavity of the uterus but as pregnancy progresses and the uterus enlarges the placenta becomes confined to one portion of the uterus. Usually this is the upper half, clear of the cervix. Placenta praevia is a common finding on ultrasound at 12 weeks, but it is less common at

20 weeks and by Week 32 fewer than 1 per cent of pregnancies are praevia. With a placenta praevia, delivery by caesarean is the safest option. There are two main forms:

- 'Minor' placenta praevia – when the placenta partially covers the internal opening of the cervix.
- 'Major' placenta praevia – when the cervix is completely covered. In this case there is likely to be bleeding.

What happens

Sometimes the placenta praevia is detected on routine ultrasound scans before any symptoms occur. The main symptom is painless bleeding. This may occur at any time but is more common after Week 30. The bleeding is usually bright red, can be light or heavy, may occur with no obvious reason or might follow sexual intercourse or straining. The first bleeds are usually light but later on the blood flow may increase and become heavier. Bleeding usually stops and then often starts again.

Bleeding occurs because the lower part of the uterus normally stretches during pregnancy as the cervix ripens before labour. This stretched area is called the lower segment. The placenta, though, cannot stretch, so as the uterus stretches a small area of placenta separates and there is bleeding from your blood vessels in the uterus. This bleeding does not interfere with the placental function or the supply of blood and oxygen to your baby.

Some women with a placenta praevia don't experience bleeding in pregnancy and bleeding only occurs as the cervix dilates in labour. Major placenta praevia tends to cause bleeding earlier. It may begin before Week 20, when it is defined as a threatened MISCARRIAGE.

A low-lying placenta keeps your baby's head high, stopping it from engaging in your pelvis. Occasionally it is the reason behind a breech or transverse lie position.

Diagnosis

Modern ultrasound scans are usually reliable in detecting a placenta praevia. A vaginal scan is more accurate than an abdominal scan. However, a vaginal examination by your doctor is not recommended as it may provoke dangerous further bleeding.

When a placenta praevia is diagnosed in late pregnancy, a ceaesarean will be planned. In addition, Doppler blood flow ultrasound scans are recommended to exclude placenta accreta (where the placenta is deeply embedded in the muscle wall of the uterus, see above). If there is a combined praevia and accreta, considerable skill is needed during the Caesarean section to prevent excess bleeding during surgery.

Causes

There is usually no obvious cause. The risk is increased when there has been a previous caesarean section or uterine surgery or previous pregnancies have been followed by gynaecological DILATATION AND CURETTAGE operations. The chance of placenta praevia rises with twins because the placenta is larger. Placenta praevia is unlikely to recur in a subsequent pregnancy but the chances do increase slightly.

Action plan

Your placenta will probably function normally even though it is praevia, and your baby is likely to develop and grow normally. His growth and wellbeing will be checked regularly. The main health risk is to you, from heavy bleeding.

Before delivery, take time to talk to your medical team about the risks associated with a placenta praevia, delivery by caesarean section and possible additional operative steps and the possibility of a blood transfusion, which may be necessary if you bleed heavily. If you have an unusual blood group your team will need to ensure that appropriate blood is available for you. It is best to air your queries so that you can be fully informed and make choices to suit your unique circumstances. It is important to strongly request that senior members of the obstetric team are present to deliver your baby to reduce the risk of bleeding.

Placenta praevia with light bleeding

- If bleeding is light or stops completely you may be allowed home and advised to take it easy.
- You may have to stop working and must avoid sexual intercourse and heavy exercise.
- It is essential to have access to a hospital that can be reached within 15 minutes and to have an adult available 24 hours a day who can contact the emergency services and admit you

to hospital if bleeding recurs or you have contractions or pain.

- You need to be booked into a hospital with facilities to perform emergency caesarean sections and to administer urgent blood transfusions.
- You will need to give birth by caesarean and your recovery will be closely monitored after the birth to detect excess bleeding.

Placenta praevia with significant bleeding

- If bleeding is significant, you will have to remain in hospital until your baby is mature enough to be born. The aim of your medical team will be to keep pregnancy going until your baby is no longer premature, around Week 36.
- Depending on the blood loss and your haemoglobin level, you will need iron and vitamin supplements. Rarely, a blood transfusion is necessary.
- If you are in bed for more than a day, reduce the risk of deep vein thrombosis by wearing support stockings and walking around every few hours.
- If you have a major placenta praevia, your baby will need to be born by caesarean section before labour starts because the risk of bleeding as the cervix dilates makes labour dangerous. Often caesarean section can be done under epidural anaesthesia unless there are any factors that indicate the need for a general anaesthetic.
- If bleeding becomes life threatening at any time your baby will be born immediately by caesarean section and you may need a blood transfusion. The obstetrician needs to deliver the placenta carefully. The main concern is your blood loss during and after the operation – you need to be attended by an experienced obstetrician and anaesthetist, and possibly additional surgical and anaesthetic support staff. This is very important if you have a higher risk of very heavy bleeding because of previous uterine scars or associated placenta accreta.
- If your baby is PREMATURE he will need to be cared for in a SPECIAL CARE BABY UNIT (SCBU).
- Intense monitoring is essential after birth to ensure your uterus is well contracted and to prevent or treat excessive bleeding from the placental site.

Having a placenta praevia is taxing emotionally because you will need to alter your lifestyle, you may have to give up work early and there may be the threat of haemorrhage until your baby is born. You may need to stay in hospital for the final stage of your pregnancy. It is natural to feel anxious and upset, and it is common to have a false alarm or two before your baby needs to be born. Very rarely, a placenta praevia is not diagnosed until labour has begun. In this case a caesarean will be performed as an emergency.

Placental abruption

See also Bleeding, mother, during pregnancy.

In placental abruption bleeding occurs between the normally positioned placenta and the wall of the uterus and the placenta starts to separate. The usual sign is bleeding and pain, although minor abruption may not cause symptoms. Fewer than one in 100 pregnant women are affected, usually in the second half of pregnancy. Abruption carries risks for mother and baby and although the outlook is improving with modern obstetric care, it is essential to act quickly and get medical help if you have bleeding or pain.

What happens

An abruption may be 'revealed' when blood escapes from the uterus into the vagina or it may be 'concealed' when blood loss becomes

+ Red flag

A large degree of separation usually causes intense bleeding and severe abdominal pain, and your uterus will feel tender and hard. Blood is usually dark in colour, and may contain clots. If bleeding is heavy you may go into shock and feel faint and cold. Internal bleeding may bring on contractions and labour. If a large part of the placenta separates your baby may suffer from oxygen restriction and severe FOETAL DISTRESS.

If heavy bleeding continues natural clotting factors may be used up, causing further bleeding. This can become a life-threatening emergency and urgent action is essential.

trapped between the wall of the uterus and the placenta. Usually some blood flows into the vagina and some is retained.

Minor degrees of concealed abruption may not cause symptoms and have no effect on your baby.

Occasionally there is no visible bleeding but there is excruciating pain.

Risk factors

Most often, abruption occurs without an obvious cause. Some conditions are linked with a higher risk. They include:

* Severely high maternal BLOOD PRESSURE (a sign of pre-eclampsia).
* Thrombophilia in the mother, with excessive blood clotting (page 59).
* A diet that is deficient in vitamins, minerals and antioxidants and essential fatty acids, particularly before conception, because these deficiencies may be associated with poor implantation.
* Smoking or taking recreational DRUGS, particularly cocaine and crack cocaine.
* TWINS.
* An accident involving a severe blow to the abdomen.
* Rarely, the obstetric procedure 'external cephalic version', used to turn a breech baby, may trigger separation.

Action plan

Modern emergency maternity care has dramatically reduced the risks associated with placental abruption, and the sooner treatment begins the better the outlook.

Medical care

Your midwife or doctor will make a diagnosis after a clinical examination, an ultrasound scan and cardiotocograph (CTG) monitoring of your baby's heartbeat. Treatment depends on how much of the placenta has separated from your uterus, the amount of blood lost, your baby's wellbeing and the stage of pregnancy. Any other difficulties you are having (such as high blood pressure) will also be taken into account.

▨ MINOR OR MAJOR ABRUPTION

If the area of separation is small, your baby is not in distress and your condition is stable, you may be able to go home and rest. You will be offered close monitoring and scans for the remainder of pregnancy, in line with the procedures for a HIGH-RISK PREGNANCY. If there are signs of reduced placental blood flow and function your doctor will advise you when it is safest to deliver your baby early.

Major abruption

The diagnosis is usually obvious. Your doctor may give you an intravenous drip and take blood tests to check your blood count and clotting ability.

* If your baby shows no signs of foetal distress and your condition is stable, your doctor may advise induction of labour and a vaginal delivery if you have passed Week 36.
* Your uterus may not contract properly after delivery. As this raises the risk of heavy bleeding after birth, you will be given medication to stimulate contractions as you give birth to the placenta.
* If the area of separation is large, your baby is at high risk of foetal distress and you are at risk of heavy blood loss. Immediate delivery by CAESAREAN SECTION may be the best course of action.
* If you lose a lot of blood you may need a BLOOD TRANSFUSION and may require treatment for shock. If your blood is not clotting normally, the clotting factors will be replaced during the transfusion. This will reduce the risk of bleeding during and after delivery. Clotting factors are made in your liver and they return to normal in a day or two.
* PREMATURE BIRTH may save your baby's life. Depending on his wellbeing he may need care in a SPECIAL CARE BABY UNIT (SCBU).

Outlook

With prompt expert intervention, almost all mothers with severe placental abruption and more than 90 per cent of their babies survive. Foetal distress and premature birth present the greatest risk to babies. It is best to act quickly, as long delays between the onset of symptoms and hospital care are the most dangerous for mum and baby.

Very rarely, women have placental abruption in more than one pregnancy and this may be associated with an underlying medical problem such as high blood pressure, kidney disease or excessive blood clotting (thrombophilia). In this case, all subsequent pregnancies require close surveillance. If you are at increased risk, you will be advised to reduce heavy work and rest as much as possible. Both prior to conception and also while you are pregnant, it is important to eat well and take prenatal vitamins and minerals, and omega essential fatty acids.

Play

See also Emotions, explorative urge; playfulness.

All babies are born with a strong explorative urge and a need to play (page 217). This drives them to learn and develop in the most enjoyable and effective way.

Your baby is able to play in the womb, where she rolls and somersaults and explores her body and environment. After birth she will invite you to join her playful dance.

The best toys are what nature provides – your voice, the way you look, your smell and your touch, being outside in nature. There are a myriad of toys designed for young babies and you will soon get to know your child's preferences. After six months, many babies have their favourite cuddly transitional object and this is an important part of play and security (page 52).

Your baby is absorbing a huge amount of information and her pace is slower than yours. When she has had enough or does not feel like being stimulated, she will show you by breaking eye contact, appearing dreamy or distanced, perhaps by crying and maybe by falling asleep. Rest and sleep time allows her to integrate what she experiences, and is part of the learning process. She will feel safest and benefit most from play when the balance of stimulation and rest matches her rhythms.

Some parents feel under pressure to have a specific amount of time each day actively playing. But babies do not have any agenda. On some days your baby will not be in the mood for physical play, and will prefer to rest in your arms. On others, she may be extremely explorative. Following her lead helps her learn her preferences are important – a wonderful lesson that will help her trust and follow her instincts when she is older.

Pneumonia, baby

See also Coughs and colds, baby.

The pneumonias are a group of illnesses involving infection of the lung. Most are caused by a virus (between one and two in 300 babies), need no treatment and pass quickly. Much less common are bacterial pneumonias (two in 3,000), which are relatively serious and may be life-threatening if untreated. Severe pneumonia is a rare disease.

Viral infections involving the lower respiratory tract are very common, and are often, inappropriately, called viral pneumonia. Viral pneumonia is infectious and is occasionally followed by a secondary bacterial infection. Rarely, bacterial pneumonia may be present at birth, often called congenital pneumonia. This can be caused by GROUP B STREP, E. coli and CHLAMYDIA. Pneumonia can also be contracted from baby powder – some babies mistake it for a bottle and gasp a mouthful into their airways. Pneumonia from inhaling powder may be fatal.

Most pneumonias start after a cold when, instead of recovering, a baby gets worse and temperature rises. Newborns whose immune system is not mature are more susceptible, as are premature infants and children with physical disabilities who are always lying horizontally.

What happens

- Your baby's breathing will become faster – more than 50 breaths a minute – and he may grunt, will look unwell and will be lethargic.
- Your baby may have a fever, seem chilled or shiver.
- Your baby may have blue lips and nails if he is not getting enough oxygen.
- The space beneath the lower ribs may be drawn in as your baby breathes.
- Your baby may cough out blood-tinged sputum (mucus and saliva).
- Your baby may indicate pain on one side of the chest – this is the infected side.

✚ Red flag

If your baby shows any of the above symptoms you must get him seen by a doctor very urgently.

Action plan

- Your baby's chest may be checked through X-ray.
- Your baby will be given antibiotics, which usually bring a marked improvement in two to three days.
- Your baby may be admitted to hospital if difficulty with breathing interferes with feeding or he appears to be deprived of oxygen. In hospital he may be given intravenous antibiotic, fed via a tube and given oxygen.

Fortunately, modern antibiotics are extremely effective and complete recovery can be expected in nearly every case within seven to 14 days. Unless your baby has other problems, such as heart or lung disease, a further episode of pneumonia is rare.

Poo, baby

See also Colic; Constipation, baby; Diarrhoea, baby.

It's amazing how much time parents spend inspecting their baby's nappies. There are no rules as to what is normal, only guidelines. A baby's stools will change regularly as she develops from a newborn through her first year, depending on what she eats, and whether she is breast- or bottle-fed. You'll soon be an expert on what's normal for your own baby.

What colour?

The colour of your baby's motions will change in her first days and weeks.
- For the first three or four of days after the birth, your baby will pass sticky, green-black 'meconium', a substance that has built up in her intestines during pregnancy and is made up of bile, mucus, cells from the bowel wall and amniotic fluid. It is a good sign your baby's bowels are working normally.
- After a day or two, once feeding is established and the last of the meconium has passed through, the stools will turn a brown-green and be loose and grainy in texture, before becoming golden yellow and soft in consistency.
- Breastfed babies who are not fed solids tend to pass very liquid yellow stools. The smell is often sweet, like breast milk.
- Bottle-fed babies tend to pass pale yellow or yellowish-brown poo and remnants of the formula will leave it looking bulkier than a breastfed baby's, as formula is not as efficiently digested as breast milk. Formula-based poo also smells stronger (more like adult poo).
- Your baby's stools may regularly change in consistency and colour, too, going from soft and mustard-yellow in colour to yellow with green specks, and then back again the next day. This is completely normal.
- When your baby starts eating solids, the colour of the stools may vary according to what she eats. For example, carrots lead to orange stools, and broccoli to green stools, and her poo will become more solid. By the end of the first year, when she is finger painting, the colours may be quite alarming if she puts her paint-covered hands into her mouth!
- When she's eating solids, foods such as sweetcorn may pass through undigested.

How often?

The range is broad.
- A breastfed baby may poo at each feed, up to six or eight times a day or more ... or only once every three to seven days. There's no need to worry about the frequency as long as the stools are soft and easy to pass.
- After a number of weeks, your breastfed baby may establish a rhythm, pooing at certain times of the day. Naturally this will alter if she feeds more or less, or is unwell.
- Bottle-fed babies given formula milk normally need to pass a stool each day to stay comfortable and avoid constipation.

Poo that may be of concern

Diarrhoea

Symptoms include very runny stools and sometimes an increase in volume and frequency. Poo may spurt out of your baby's nappy. A breastfed baby is less likely to suffer from diarrhoea as breast milk contains natural pro-biotics that strengthen the 'good' gut bacteria, helping them combat the micro-organisms that cause diarrhoea (page 35). Breastfeeding reduces food intolerance which can cause diarrhoea.

Constipation

This is indicated by passing no stools for longer than a day if bottle-fed or on solids, or for more than three days if breastfed. Symptoms include a red face and straining on passing a stool, perhaps with crying, and hard stools. Streaks of blood in your baby's stools may occur if she's constipated, as straining can cause small tears in the skin around her anus. Do get this checked out by your health visitor or GP to eliminate an important cause, such as infection.

Green frothy poo

This may be a sign that your baby is taking in too much lactose (the natural sugar found in milk). This can happen if she feeds often but for short periods only if breastfeeding and misses the rich milk at the end of the feed to fill her up. Make sure she finishes feeding from one breast before offering the other. It may also be caused by overfeeding or underfeeding with a bottle, or is a sign that your baby has an infection of the digestive system. If the symptoms of green frothy stools last longer than 24 hours, consult your health visitor or GP to try to find the source of the problem, as it may be due to a lactose or other intolerance (page 14).

Pooing and emotions

Pooing is as natural and essential as breathing. Your baby may find it pleasurable or uncomfortable, or she may be indifferent. Her attitude to poo begins to develop early and the words and actions of the people caring for her may influence her feelings, particularly if pooing is talked about as being wrong/bad/disgusting. Some psychologists believe problems such as constipation can begin early if a baby feels chastised for normal bowel habits. Each baby is unique, however, and you cannot tell how your baby may react. It's best not to say she's naughty for doing what's natural. Babies cannot be naughty (page 47).

There is a physiological connection between the brain and the intestines and bowel, known as the brain–gut axis. What happens in the intestines can affect the way you feel emotionally, and the way you feel and think can affect digestion. For instance, anxiety (with an associated release of stress-hormones that act on the intestinal wall) may disrupt regular bowel habits. If your baby's

digestion is causing her discomfort you may decide to consider her feelings (page 206) as well as what she is eating and drinking.

Post maturity

See Labour and birth, mother, overdue (post maturity).

Post traumatic stress disorder (PTSD)

See also Labour and birth, mother, your unique reactions to birth.

Post traumatic stress disorder (PTSD) is a collection of emotional, psychological and physical symptoms that arise after a traumatic experience. The symptoms can be extremely disruptive to everyday life. In many people's minds, it is something that is linked with war, accidents and natural disasters. For some women (and a smaller number of men) the birth experience is very stressful and PTSD may arise after birth or following the loss of a baby. In a severe form, PTSD affects around 2 per cent of women in their first year after the birth. Many more women have a milder form.

After the trauma, feelings and physical symptoms can take months to surface and a long time to recede. Typically, the extent of PTSD reflects the degree of intervention, pain or shock, but there is not always a correlation. Your experience depends on your personality, regardless of what other people say you should be feeling. Even if your symptoms are mild, recognising that they may be trauma-related makes a difference to what you need after birth to help you enjoy life, your baby and future pregnancies.

Causes

Many experiences may feel stressful and traumatic. Your life before the birth is significant because when you are pregnant and mothering a baby you are more open. If you have experienced trauma in the past your deeply buried feelings may surface now. There is a positive side: pregnancy might be a catalyst for resolving personal issues.

Memories of past trauma. The birth may have reminded you of previous traumatic events. Many past events may be significant, especially childhood sexual abuse, assault or previous trauma in hospital or difficulty in childbirth.

Anxiety and depression. If you have an anxious personality or have been depressed you are more susceptible to PTSD.

Trauma during labour. Perhaps labour was traumatic or you felt shocked and hurt that people around you showed little respect, or you felt mishandled or violated. Some women are traumatised by exposure to blood or being in hospital. If there was intervention such feelings may be stronger.

Pain in labour. You might have experienced levels of pain that were beyond your personal threshold and were deeply shocking. Being in intense pain can sometimes make women dissociate from the birth, feeling as if it happened to someone else.

Fear in labour. Fear is a natural aspect of the birth process but if you experienced intense fear for your baby's wellbeing, or of damage or pain or even of death to yourself, you may have suffered emotional trauma.

Dashed expectations and lack of control. If you had strong expectations and birth did not meet your ideals you may feel angry and let down. This is more likely if you felt out of control because you were not consulted about any action, or did not feel heard, or felt intervention was unnecessary, or that more could have been done for you or your baby.

Feeling inadequately supported. What happens after birth is important. If you are not lovingly supported you may miss the chance to talk and to integrate the experience of birth, and tension and painful memories may intensify.

Domestic violence. Ongoing emotional, physical or sexual abuse (page 548) is a potent cause of PTSD.

Symptoms

If you have PTSD you may experience some of the symptoms below. The effect will vary according to your personality and the degree of trauma. The symptoms may come and go.

Among the most frequent symptoms of PTSD, it is usually possible to divide them into categories: psychological (especially hyperarousal), DEPRESSION (or numbing symptoms), fatiguability and flashbacks.

* Hyperarousal symptoms include feeling anxious, irritable, constantly on your guard, upset and angry. You may feel afraid and panicky and may suffer panic attacks.
* You may feel down or depressed. PTSD is distinguished from postnatal depression by its characteristic state of high-anxiety, high body tension and being on high-alert mentally and physically, whereas depression tends to sap the will. The two can exist together.
* You may feel detached and numb, and consciously or unconsciously avoid anything that reminds you of the trauma. Your baby is a strong reminder and you may feel little or no attraction to him, a lack of interest and little bonding.
* Exercise tolerance, even as much as walking up and down stairs, may be very limited, and you may tire easily. This is called fatiguability.
* You may be plagued by vivid memories, flashbacks, nightmares, and become distressed and anxious when something reminds you of what happened.
* You may feel guilty but powerless to change your mood or get excited about parenthood.
* You may have difficulty concentrating and sleeping.
* Pain and a range of physical symptoms may disrupt your life. Your symptoms may include multiple aches and headaches, digestive symptoms and palpitations.
* You may crave or turn to alcohol or DRUGS.

Possible effects of PTSD

Difficulty bonding. You may feel emotionally distant from your baby. You may have dissociated from the birth experience and stress may have reduced the flow of love hormones. If you and your baby were separated after birth or you still feel afraid or shocked, bonding may be more difficult. If you have quiet time together after the birth, the flow of love hormones often picks up again. Difficulties with bonding can usually be repaired with time and loving support (page 210).

Not feeling able to be a mum. Some women feel as if it wasn't them giving birth, or their baby is not their own and then feel like a failure or a bad mum. This may make it more difficult for you to relax with your baby and trust your instincts to mother.

Feeling excessively controlling, or out of control. You may feel a power struggle with your baby, for example, about when to sleep or feed, and how to stop your baby crying, and find baby care challenging. Such issues of control may be a continuation of the struggle you felt during birth and may be played out in other relationships in your life, including with your partner and your parents. Being excessively controlling or being unable to take control is usually based on fear.

Anxiety, depression and isolation. PTSD is a high-anxiety state, and depressive thoughts and feelings may affect your life in many ways. You may avoid spending time with other people.

Sex and next pregnancy. You may feel nervous about having sex again (page 475). This may contribute to relationship breakdown, particularly if you find it hard to tell your partner what you really feel. It's common to be afraid of having another baby, and having PTSD makes an elective CAESAREAN in a future birth more likely.

Loss of trust in other people and lack of confidence. You may find it difficult to trust medical professionals if their conduct is connected with your trauma.

Other possible effects. You may feel excessively anxious about your own health or your baby's health. Your vagina and pelvis may feel especially sensitive. You may find it difficult to cope with periods, and premenstrual stress may increase. This may be coupled with a fear of medical care and a reluctance to seek advice. Some women are terrified of any examination and preventable problems may go untreated.

Action plan

Minor degrees of PTSD are very common and worthy of attention. Some health professionals do not recognise PTSD and may focus on your anxiety or depression or only treat the physical symptoms. Some women are reluctant to ask for help. If you feel you have failed somehow – particularly if you feel guilty that you're not happy with your new baby – it may be very difficult for you to admit to how traumatised you feel.

Prevention

Trauma cannot always be prevented, but there are some measures that could help. Preparing realistically for active birth (page 349) can be very important. This includes being informed about labour and pain relief, planning who will be with you, and being open about what happens on the day. It is useful not to have rigid expectations. Women who are well prepared often feel more in control on the day. Meeting the people who will care for you may help. If you have experienced traumatic events in the past, it is helpful to tell your midwife to allow the team supporting you to be sensitive. It is best to build a network of friends who can care for you after birth.

Postnatal care

Acknowledging a potential problem is an important first step. A friend or health professional may notice it, or you may raise the issue. The second step is to actively care for yourself (page 121).

- With PTSD it will be hard to care for yourself on your own. People who are aware of how you feel can help you, for example with cooking and cleaning, spending time with your baby, accompanying you to doctor's appointments or lending a listening ear.
- An important part of recovery is for you to tell your story. You can use a friend or family member but often formal psychotherapy (below) is very useful.
- Your baby offers you an opportunity to heal and relax, and there are many benefits of skin-to-skin contact (page 517) to help the shock to settle as you bond. If you feel detached from your baby or you are afraid of parenting, your partner, friends and family may help. There is further advice on page 210.

Psychotherapy and EMDR

Most doctors recommend psychotherapy as a key part of support. Going over the events with someone you trust helps your brain integrate the experience without switching to panic or defence. Your therapist may help you recognise your personal strengths and help you release the pain and move forward. Some women forget details and need time to develop trust in themselves and in the therapist, and then to open up. It is often useful to book an appointment to debrief with your hospital. This is discussed in the section on receiving bad news (page 45).

There are numerous possible approaches to treatment (page 46). For PTSD the most effective are believed to be cognitive behavioural therapy and eye movement desensitisation and reprocessing (EMDR), which uses eye movements to help the brain process flashbacks.

Medication

The suitability of medication as part of your treatment will depend on your personal situation. Medication can be effective, usually with symptoms such as insomnia, anxiety, poor concentration and depression. Once medication eases symptoms it may become easier to focus on the underlying feelings. The medications discussed for treatment of anxiety or depression disorders on page 176 are also used for PTSD where appropriate.

Body therapies

You are a physical-emotional 'bodymind' (page 73) and so your physical body retains emotional trauma. In conjunction with emotional therapy, sensitive body work such as OSTEOPATHY, ACUPUNCTURE or REFLEXOLOGY may release tension and stress. Homeopathic remedies are usually tailored to the individual but you may find some of the suggestions on page 223 work for you.

There is also advice and support available through the Birth Trauma Association in the UK.

Posture

Eating well, exercising, YOGA and resting will tone your body and help your comfort. Like most people, you may need extra care to stay in balance and avoid – or reduce – strains and any soreness you feel with the added demands of pregnancy, birth and baby care.

Your posture affects your entire body. Good posture helps to improve muscle tone, strength and energy levels. It reduces strain, stiffness and pain. It also improves the circulation of blood and lymph fluids throughout your body. Moreover, good posture allows you to breathe fully and easily, thus to improve the supply of oxygen and release of carbon dioxide for both yourself and, when pregnant, for your baby.

Pregnancy is a wonderful time to develop good posture. You are naturally more aware of your body and physical sensations at this time. Moreover, the normal discomforts that affect most pregnant women at some point, including pelvic or lower back pain, breathlessness and heartburn, draw your attention to relieving and avoiding further strain.

After the birth, every system in your body is readjusting to its non-pregnant state. During this time, your spine, ligaments and muscles are vulnerable if strained. Attention to your posture will protect your body as you lift, carry and feed your baby. For dads, good posture is just as important, even though there are fewer bodily changes.

Once you learn and practise good postural habits, they come automatically and will improve your health for life. Practising regular YOGA or PILATES is a great way to enhance posture, although it's important to tailor any routine to suit you: for example, if you have pelvic pain, avoid postures that involve opening the legs wide.

Tips for good posture

Standing and walking

Stand tall with weight evenly distributed on both feet, your buttocks tucked in and back straight, navel drawn in towards your spine. Avoid standing for long periods of time. Vary between sitting and standing throughout the day and wear low-heeled shoes or trainers.

Sitting

* Sit well back in your chair so that your lower back is fully supported and straight. Let your pelvis release down and lengthen your spine. Relax your neck and shoulders.
* You may find it most comfortable to raise the level of your seat.
* Avoid very soft low chairs and couches, particularly if your spine is bowed.
* Ensure that you are sitting comfortably if your work involves sitting (for instance at a computer or till). You may need to alter the height of your chair and the position of your computer, till or other work tool so that your back is not hunched and your feet are flat on the ground or an alternative flat support. Make sure you take regular breaks to move around and stretch.

- Try to avoid unbalanced sitting positions, such as crossing your legs. When you cross your legs you tend to put more weight on one buttock bone and curve your spine.
- When feeding your baby, have enough cushions to support your back and arm(s) and your baby's weight.

Lying and getting up

- Whether lying on your back or on your side, you may be more comfortable with your knees bent, as this reduces back strain. A great pose for resting is to lie on the floor with your legs raised, calves supported on a chair (page 516).
- When getting out of bed, keep your knees bent, roll onto your side and push up into a sitting position using your arms, and swing your legs out over the side of the mattress. Use the same principle of rolling onto your side before getting up if you lie on the floor, sofa or other support, and when you move out of a lying position during YOGA or PILATES practice.
- Use a high quality mattress for sleeping and rest in bed with pillows under your knees or between your thighs. Specially shaped pillows help reduce back pain in late pregnancy and improve sleep.
- Take particular care when getting into and out of the bath and the car and be careful not to open your legs too wide – especially if you have pelvic pain (page 43).

Bending, lifting and carrying

- Squat down or kneel rather than bend when reaching into low cupboards, making beds, gardening and so on. Always keep your back straight.
- Avoid heavy lifting. When lifting moderately heavy loads, such as shopping, bend your knees and keep your back straight. Distribute the weight evenly by dividing your shopping between two bags and holding a bag in each hand. When lifting a single object, such as a box of groceries, bend your knees and not your back, bring the object close to your body, take the weight on your legs and do not twist your waist.
- When carrying your baby or toddler, change from holding on one side to the other frequently. To take the strain off your hips, arms and shoulders, it is easy to use a sling to support the bulk of your child's weight.
- Your posture when breastfeeding is really

important and attention to this may help you avoid discomfort and strain (page 84).
- When you carry a car seat, be aware of how you can best balance your body without straining it. It's preferable to take your baby out and carry her separately. If you lay her to rest on a flat surface, rather than in the curved chair, or alternatively continue to carry her, this is better for her back as well.

Treating strains and soreness

During pregnancy, birth and parenthood your body adapts and there will be new sources of discomfort (page 430). In addition, you have patterns of strain resulting from your entire life – even from your time in your mother's womb and your own birth – and some of these may present themselves now.

In general, the sooner a problem is addressed the less likely it is to build up. Some areas of strain may reduce as you attend to your posture, exercise, such as regularly walking, and rest. Others may be relieved most effectively with extra help, such as with a good MASSAGE, osteopathic treatment (page 424) or physiotherapy. Most people feel their emotional energy improves as bodily strain is reduced, so there is an overall improvement in wellbeing.

Pre-eclampsia

See Blood pressure, high and pre-eclampsia.

Pregnancy testing

Today's home-testing kits are extremely accurate. Within seven days of conception, placental cells secrete the hormone human chorionic gonadotrophin (HCG) into your bloodstream and urine. All pregnancy tests detect the presence or absence of HCG.

- Urine tests are able to detect pregnancy by the first day of a missed period. Depending on the type of kit you have bought, you will look for a spot, a line or a colour that confirms pregnancy.
- You may want your doctor to confirm the news; some surgeries are happy to do this and use a urine sample also.
- If you need early confirmation of your

pregnancy (after fertility treatment, for example), your doctor is likely to recommend a blood test, which is the most accurate method of detecting HCG but it will take one to two days to be processed by the laboratory.

Being sure about the result

Positive results have over 95 per cent accuracy. A negative result is more likely to be incorrect, particularly if you conceived late in your cycle and HCG levels are still low. If you are experiencing signs of pregnancy or feel strongly that you are pregnant, ask your doctor to do another test, preferably a blood test. You may be advised to wait another week before retesting. An egg may have been fertilised, but HCG levels are low.

If your tests continue to be negative but your period still doesn't come, ask your doctor to rule out other conditions that could cause delay. They may advise an ultrasound scan (page 33) as an important investigation. If you have an ECTOPIC PREGNANCY (a pregnancy that takes place outside the womb) you will probably have symptoms including a tender abdomen and spotting or bleeding.

Premature birth

See also Emotions; Special care baby unit (SCBU) and neonatal intensive care unit (NICU).

Premature birth is when your baby is born before the 37th week of pregnancy (up to and including day 259 of pregnancy). In the UK, 6 per cent of babies are born premature. Like many parents, you may be surprised if labour begins early. Even if you have time to prepare for the birth, coping with prematurity is still a challenge.

During the important last weeks of pregnancy your baby's organs mature. If birth is early, he will need to mature fully without the protection of the womb. The earlier that birth occurs, the greater this challenge becomes for your baby and for the medical team, and the risks to health also increase if some of his body systems are not working optimally.

It is good to know that babies born after Week 32 usually do very well. With earlier birth the risk of complications rises, although advanced neonatal care has greatly improved the outcome. Babies born between Weeks 26 and 28 have an 80

per cent chance of survival, with 70 per cent of survivors having no long-term physical problems.

Premature birth, expected or not, commonly makes parents anxious and can be frightening and upsetting. This is an entirely normal reaction that is the beginning of what may be a lengthy process of acceptance and adaptation by all the family. Being informed about what may lie ahead may help you prepare. Part of dealing with an early birth is gathering a support network and finding nursing and medical staff who you feel good with. When your baby is born it may take courage to let yourself fall in love with him, particularly if he is not well and you are afraid you may lose him.

Depending on how early your baby is born, it may take days, weeks or months of care by the neonatal team to ensure he develops and reaches his full potential. Babies who have severe INTRAUTERINE GROWTH RESTRICTION (IUGR) may be born early and then need extra care to recover from the combined effects of IUGR and prematurity.

What may cause premature birth?

The majority of premature births are not predictable, and for many the cause cannot be identified. There are, however, some pointers that may increase the possibility of prematurity. For more information on each of the following, turn to the appropriate entry.

- Infection in the VAGINA and CERVIX which can cause premature rupture of the membranes (page 392), the most common trigger for premature labour.
- Cervical incompetence of the valve of the cervix.
- A previous premature birth.
- A pregnancy with TWINS OR HIGHER MULTIPLES.
- Poor maternal nutrition causing a deficiency in minerals and vitamins.
- Smoking, alcohol and the use of DRUGS inappropriate for pregnancy.
- A complicated pregnancy that may warrant early delivery, such as placenta praevia (page 442), DIABETES, high BLOOD PRESSURE and severe IUGR.

What happens if you go into premature labour

If you believe you may be in premature labour, whatever the time of day or night, call the hospital. If you are in labour a vaginal examination will confirm your cervix has begun to dilate. You will probably have painful and regular contractions. Depending on your stage of pregnancy and your baby's wellbeing, your medical team may want to delay birth. If you need to give birth to your baby early for medical reasons, your doctor will arrange the necessary medical care.

After Week 34

If you go into labour after Week 34, your medical team will want to ensure there is no added risk of FOETAL DISTRESS AND ASPHYXIA and then you will be able to go ahead with an active vaginal birth. Babies born around Weeks 35–37 rarely have major problems, although establishing feeding and maintaining temperature may mean a longer hospital stay.

Before Week 34

If you go into labour before Week 34, your medical team may want to delay labour to allow time for you to receive corticosteroid (dexamethasone) injections to stimulate the development of your baby's lungs, thus reducing the risk of respiratory distress and BREATHING DIFFICULTIES at birth. To reduce your contractions you may be given intravenous tocolytic medication and you and your baby will be closely monitored. The medication usually delays labour for 24–48 hours, sometimes longer.

In labour

In labour, your baby's heartbeat will be monitored frequently because he is more susceptible to foetal distress, particularly if he also has IUGR. You may be anxious by unexpectedly being in labour and you will benefit from the support and calming techniques such as breathing, VISUALISATION and MASSAGE.

Your medical team may avoid a number of procedures. Because a premature baby's skull is prone to excess moulding or bruising, it is best not to break the waters to speed up slow progress (page 376), as they protect against excess pressure. You may also be advised to avoid pethidine for pain relief because a small baby may be very sensitive and the drug may depress breathing at birth. An epidural anaesthetic is better. Your birth team may advise delivery by CAESAREAN SECTION if your baby is in a position that could make vaginal birth difficult or potentially hazardous, or if he shows signs of

foetal distress or asphyxia because a less mature baby is less able to cope with stress caused by low oxygen supply.

First contact

If possible it is ideal for your baby to feel skin-to-skin contact with you soon after birth: how soon depends on your baby's needs for medical help. It may be possible for your baby to be treated in the birth room and for you to welcome and touch him. Kangaroo care is practised in many hospitals and this is discussed on page 518.

■ AFTER BIRTH

Babies born before Week 35 are generally cared for in a neonatal intensive care unit (page 497). If your baby is older and he requires extra support or observation, he may be cared for in a SPECIAL CARE BABY UNIT (SCBU).

How your premature baby copes after birth depends on how early birth is, the cause of his prematurity and his weight. If your baby is born between Weeks 33 and 37 and has no underlying abnormalities, there is an excellent chance he will adapt quickly to life outside the womb and, after a short spell in a special care baby unit (SCBU), will be fit and feeding confidently and can come home. If he is born earlier he will need more intensive care. Smaller premature babies may be very ill and need intensive support but with advances in care, neonatal death (page 420) is increasingly rare. It is usually related to very premature babies or those who are very ill at birth.

Being with your baby

However young or small your baby, he will benefit from your presence and loving touch. You may be able to stay with him and hold him, or your time together may be limited to a few hours a day and touching him through the sides of the incubator. It is preferable to spend as much time with your baby as your circumstances allow and you may be able to set up kangaroo care (page 518) allowing continuous skin-to-skin contact so that you and your baby can be in contact most of the day. Your hospital team will advise you, and kangaroo care may be possible even if your baby requires intravenous fluids. You can walk around or sit with him snugly against your chest, with the drip and fluids next to you. Kangaroo care helps premature babies recover and grow optimally, and reduces feelings of stress for them, their mums and their dads. It is a powerful bonding force as well as a great healer. If you carry your baby like this, frequent feeding is easy. The neonatal team can help you and your partner. Both of you may need to take extra time off work in the first few months. This early time together is very important and it is best if it is not rushed.

If your baby is in special care for a long period, the memory of looking into his eyes and touching his soft skin will stay with you when you are separated. You may want to have a photograph so you can see him when you are apart. As time passes, you will be able to lay your hands on him, gently massage his limbs and stroke his face.

Feeding and nourishing your baby

Premature babies have special nutritional needs and the younger your baby is, the more intense his need for calories, proteins, minerals, vitamins and fluids. Breast milk is the best fluid, containing antibodies as well as all the constituents for body and brain development, and will be suited to your baby's needs from birth. If you are in close contact your body will respond to your baby's changing needs, and when you are skin to skin you also help your baby stay at a comfortable temperature and feel safe. Your care team may recommend additional feeds designed for premature infants. Occasionally, special formula is given instead of breast milk.

If your baby is relatively large – over 1.5kg (3lb 5oz) – he may be able to breastfeed successfully. The sucking reflex is usually present after Week 29. If he is too small or young to suck he will need to be fed via a nasogastric tube passed down his nose and into his stomach until he is large enough to breastfeed. You will be helped to express (page 89) so your baby can be fed your breast milk in this way. If your baby is very young and his digestive tract is still immature, he will need an intravenous drip to provide glucose and essential amino acids and fatty acids. These are crucial for normal brain development. The exact constituents of your baby's feed will depend on his individual requirements.

Breastfeeding tips

Emotionally, many mothers feel better if they can breastfeed their babies, and they and their babies benefit from long periods of close body contact. If your baby is not able to suck from birth, you may need a high degree of motivation to keep your breast milk flowing through expressing. Many hospitals supply breast pumps and provide a private place for expressing or breastfeeding. Expressing may be more successful if you have your baby with you. When you begin to breastfeed, the advice on pages 81–91 may be helpful while you and your baby settle.

* Colostrum is the early milk and it is highly nutritious. It is very useful for your baby in the early days.
* Your milk will flow more if you are able to express every three hours, even at night. You can freeze milk for later use but it's unlikely that you'll produce an excess in the first weeks.
* When your baby is able to suck, your milk flow will adapt to his needs. If your baby has been taking a bottle, it may be possible to encourage him back on to your breast.
* Your baby is small and may need help as he learns to latch on and feed. It may take you and your baby a few days to settle into a comfortable feeding partnership, and for your breasts to respond to his suckling with a strong let-down reflex to provide the nourishing hind milk. There is no hurry and the neonatal staff will help. Feeding frequently is best for you and your baby.
* If your baby needs to be monitored, you may still be able to breastfeed while the nurses take measurements.
* In the early months, your baby will be weighed frequently to check he is getting adequate nourishment. Weight gain will be charted and your neonatal care specialist will let you know whether your baby needs more frequent breastfeeds and/or supplementary milk.

Health risks for premature babies

Babies born before Week 37 are more likely to have health problems. The risks rise for babies born before Week 32. While many premature babies do extremely well, it is useful to be aware of potential risks so you can be alert for signs and give your baby optimum care.

The list below may seem daunting. It may help to remember the risks are only potential –

it does not mean your baby will definitely have problems. He will be unique. Some babies are strong-spirited and get through very difficult stages with relative ease. Others seem upset and take longer to become independent. Close physical contact, which reduces stress and pain and encourages healing and growth, along with regular feeding and professional medical care, will offer your baby a great deal of support. The potential complications listed here are covered in full in this guide:

- HYPOGLYCAEMIA, drop in blood sugar, which is guarded against with appropriate feeding.
- HYPOTHERMIA, fall in temperature, which is usually prevented with the constant temperature of an incubator or through kangaroo care.
- BREATHING DIFFICULTIES if the lungs are immature. Ventilation assistance may be needed and a cortisone injection to boost the lungs prior to birth is often helpful. Having your baby against your chest supports regular breathing.
- Internal BLEEDING into the brain.
- Heart abnormalities (page 288) may occur in a tiny minority and exacerbate breathing difficulties.
- Infection is a risk because your baby's immune system is immature and some special care treatments may potentially introduce infection. Antibiotics are frequently needed.
- EYE AND VISION problems, such as impaired vision and retinopathy (page 479) may occur in rare cases.
- JAUNDICE may be caused by an immature liver and bruising at birth.

Taking your baby home

Your baby will probably be ready to come home when he is gaining weight, has a stable temperature in an open cot, can feed from a bottle or your breast without difficulty and has a mature and stable heart and is breathing well. There may be a room for you to stay with your baby before discharge.

Like most parents, you may feel a mixture of excitement and anxiety when it is time to take your baby home. The SCBU will have discharge guidelines and specific details relating to your baby. Before leaving, he may be given immunisations (page 536), screening

tests (for example, for vision and hearing) and you will be shown how to continue with any special care.

At home it may take time for all of you to adjust and for your baby to adopt a day–night routine after being in the brightly lit ward. The transition is often smoother if both parents have time to be at home. Carrying your baby with you through kangaroo care at home helps him feel secure and bond and relax with you.

■ LONG-TERM DEVELOPMENT

Your baby's age is calculated from the date of birth but this does not take into account that he may have missed up to three months of developmental time. This is very important during the first year but by the third or fourth year the differences disappear. Paediatricians correct for the effects of prematurity until the age of three years, when they conduct routine development tests. It is preferable for you to take things as they come and interact according to what your baby can do.

Your baby is likely to thrive with close contact and mental and physical stimulation. MASSAGE is something you can easily do at home, even while you hold your baby; and later, when your baby is strong enough, swimming and playful exercise or baby gymnastics (an extension of massage techniques) are useful. In the SCBU your baby will have spent a lot of time lying on his back, so being carried and having time on his tummy while you're with him can be very beneficial.

Requiring ventilation support after birth rarely leads to long-term breathing difficulties, although ASTHMA is a little more common. Babies who have been born early do, however, tend to have more than their fair share of coughs and colds, some no doubt due to increased susceptibility to infection.

Growth and development

Your baby's personal catch-up growth (see below) will depend on his genetic potential as well as his weight at birth, and his nutrition in the womb (page 323). If your baby was born weighing more than 1.5kg (3lb 5oz) he is likely to catch up with other children as he grows. However, if he weighs less at the time of birth than expected and there has been IUGR, he may remain smaller than other children of his age whose birth weight was not low.

Slow growth

If your baby is tiny and finds it hard to feed in the early days, he may lose weight and take up to 2–3 weeks to regain his birth weight. Being small also increases the risk that he may be unwell, and less able to tolerate intravenous nutrition, so that it may take longer to catch up. Babies in the uterus grow very rapidly during the last trimester and it is hard for a premature baby to keep up with this pace if he is ill. For most babies a phase of slow growth usually rights itself and weight gain begins to match the rate a baby usually gains in the uterus. Kangaroo care (page 518) has been proven to improve the rate of growth among premature babies.

Faster growth

When the faster growing phase begins, the body gives priority to development of the brain. Next, your baby will put on weight and lastly his length will increase. His body proportions differ from those of a full-term baby and this fast growth phase helps to reverse any nutritional defects as long as he is nourished with adequate minerals and vitamins. There are special milks and additives for meeting the increased nutritional needs of premature babies.

Catch-up growth

For your child to become the same size as his full-term peers, growth needs to be faster than usual. This is called catch-up growth. Some 85 per cent of premature babies have catch-up growth and then follow a normal growth chart by two years of age. Catch-up growth can continue until a child reaches normal size at adolescence. Most people born prematurely are not below average size in adulthood.

Some reasons a child may not catch up fully by two years of age include:

- Starting out very far below the growth chart with a long, long way to catch up.
- Ongoing problems that increase nutritional requirements or make it hard to obtain calories if metabolic rate is increased.
- Illness and a consequential reduction in feeding.

- A tendency to have a low appetite and need ongoing encouragement to feed.

Development in childhood

Your baby will be given follow-up assessments by a paediatric team to check for problems that occur more commonly among premature babies (page 456). The earlier any condition is detected, the sooner treatment can begin, and this greatly improves the outlook. For instance, if hearing is impaired and adequate support is given, potential delay to language development may be minimised.

As a group, babies born prematurely are known to have poorer concentration and many need extra support when they begin school; but each child is an individual. Most premature babies are referred to a 'developmental follow-up' clinic. Re-assessment occurs over the first five years as developmental difficulties may emerge slowly over time. You will probably be keen for your child to attend all the usual health checks and the extra tests. The clinic may be a valuable source of support for you and a place where you can meet other parents of premature babies.

Caring for you

It is important to take note of your needs, and do what you can to meet them, particularly if you feel pressurised or upset. The combined effect of baby care and stressful or uncomfortable emotions can be draining. If you were shocked or frightened by your baby's early birth it may take some time for your reaction to surface. The advice in the CARING FOR YOU and PARENTING entries might be useful as you consider how to allocate your time and care well for yourself. If you are stressed, feel down or very anxious, the section on EMOTIONS may give some useful pointers. Remember that other parents are often a great source of friendship, support and reassurance. In addition to local baby groups, a group specifically for parents of premature or unwell babies may offer a lot of positive support for you.

Puerperal psychosis

See Depression and anxiety, pre- and postnatal.

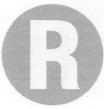

Rashes and spots, baby

See also Skin, baby.

During her first year, your baby may get a number of different rashes. Sometimes their cause is not obvious, and they fade almost as suddenly as they appear. Occasionally, a rash may be uncomfortablse, or it may indicate a medical condition, such as an infection, that requires treatment, or there may be a way to prevent the rash from occurring.

✚ Red flag

Call your doctor or seek medical advice immediately if your baby has a rash:

- that is associated with a fever of 38°C/100.4°F or higher,
- and fever after exposure to heat (heat stroke),
- that appears suddenly and does not fade or turn white when pressed beneath a glass – this may indicate a meningococcal rash (page 409),
- that does not disappear after three to four days or appears to be getting worse, or you suspect the rash is related to an infection such as chickenpox, measles or parvovirus,
- or your baby's body takes on a blue colour (page 482).

The following list may help you find a potential cause for a rash. You may use it as a guide and refer to the references in the following pages or to relevant entries but always contact your doctor if you are concerned.

Clusters of small red spots could be:

- mild erythema toxicum, a common and harmless newborn rash;
- CANDIDA or thrush, often in the folds of the skin, neck, armpits and nappy area, which is uncomfortable but usually simply treated (see page 117);
- heat rash, linked with being too hot, or with a fever or infection, which usually disappears when a baby cools down or a temperature is treated (for more see opposite);
- urticaria or 'nettle' rash, which is often a reaction to food or something touching the skin (page 460); or
- MENINGITIS (spots larger than 2mm in diameter that don't disappear when a glass is pressed on the skin), which requires urgent medical care (page 410).

Red spots with yellow centre could be:

- acne (separate spots), harmless, often related to hormones, and passes naturally; or
- erythema toxicum (red blotches, reddened skin), common and harmless newborn rash.

Rash over whole body could be:

- an allergic reaction to something (page 15), particularly if it's itchy;
- any virus especially CHICKENPOX, which is typically itchy and your baby may have a fever;

- very rarely MEASLES, where the rash is usually preceded by a fever and runny nose; or
- very rarely RUBELLA, where pink flat spots tend to begin on face and ears and spread to the trunk, and there may be a fever and some swelling.

Small white spots could be:
- milia, harmless, usually on the face, and disappears in several weeks; or
- candida (page 117), especially if on the tongue.

Red patches or scaly skin could be:
- the skin is adjusting to being in air, and harmless;
- cradle cap (page 163), particularly when on the head; may be in the nappy area or on the eye brows, and is harmless and rarely irritating; or
- eczema (page 204) is a less common cause.

Raised spots, maybe blistered or seeping fluid, could be:
- herpes (page 300), which is rare in babies.

Blue spots could be:
- normal pigmentation that tends to settle as a baby ages (Mongolian blue spots, overleaf).

Acne and milia

Around 20 per cent of babies develop neonatal acne, which looks just like adolescent acne, often spread across the nose and cheeks and across the shoulders. The spots may be red or have a small yellow head on them. Neonatal acne is due to blocked sebaceous glands in the skin and does not indicate a predisposition to develop acne as a teenager.

Milia literally means millet seed, as it looks like little white seeds. It often occurs on the face and may be present on large areas of the body and is harmless. It disappears within several weeks of birth.

Candida (thrush)

Candidiasis is a fungal infection that often begins as a nappy rash (page 418). The rash causes a red area, usually flat with sharper borders, and sometimes small pustules, usually in skin creases where there is warmth and moisture. The rash on the skin is often associated with oral thrush, with white spots in the mouth, or genital thrush. If your baby is affected by this you may be too. For more information, see page 117.

Cradle cap

Cradle cap is characterised by greasy, yellow or brown scaly patches of skin on the scalp. It is not irritating and although it may persist for months, in some babies it passes soon, or is easily treated (page 164).

Eczema (atopic dermatitis)

Eczema is an uncomfortable skin condition that often requires careful treatment, combined with attention to something in a baby's diet or environment that may be causing the reaction. Its characteristics and treatment options are discussed on pages 204–6.

Erythema toxicum

Erythema toxicum is a harmless rash seen in newborn babies and consisting of multiple red blotches with pale or yellowish bumps at the centre, which give a nettle-rash-like appearance. It occurs in 70 per cent of full-term babies. This rash usually peaks a day or two after birth and disappears within a week. It differs from acne in which the skin is pale and the bumps are separate from one another.

Heat rash (prickly heat)

Heat rash appears when your baby is too hot and her skin pores become clogged by sweat. Some babies develop this rash quickly from being over-dressed or overheated in an already warm atmosphere. It appears as clusters of little red spots and can occur anywhere on the body. It shows up most often in folds of the skin and on parts of the body where clothing fits snugly – on the neck, under the arms or near the edges of the nappy.
- The first thing to do is remove unnecessary clothes.
- Keep your baby in a cool environment and if she still appears hot, use a fan or sponge her gently with a flannel or cloth soaked in cool, but not cold, water.

* The rash will disappear within an hour unless your baby is still too hot.
* If it persists it is best to check your baby's temperature (page 239); treating an elevated temperature tends to result in the rash disappearing. Some viral illnesses are accompanied by a red rash and a fever.

Measles, mumps or rubella

If your baby has a fever or other symptoms accompanying a rash, it is always important to ask a doctor's advice. It is very rare for babies to have measles (page 406), mumps (page 417) or rubella (page 466) before the age of 12 months.

Meningococcal rash

The rash associated with MENINGITIS tends to consist of red spots that are more than 2mm across, spread rapidly and do not disappear when a clear glass is pressed to the skin. The rash will almost always coincide with other symptoms in your baby, such as signs of illness and irritability.

Mongolian blue spots

Mongolian blue spots on the lower back and buttocks are more common among babies of black, oriental or Asian families. They are often mistaken for bruises. In fact they are areas where the skin's pigment is blue or blue grey. They are harmless and tend to fade as a baby gets older.

Naevus (birthmark)

A naevus is a mark that is apparent at birth or appears within the first few weeks, and usually disappears within the first year (page 52). More rarely, a birthmark may need specialist dermatoccical care.

Nappy rash

Almost every baby has a rash in the nappy area at some point. The various possible causes, along with prevention suggestions and treatments, are discussed on pages 418–20.

Scaly rashes

After birth the skin is usually smooth although some babies have very dry skin that peels and flakes. This is most common in babies who are post mature by a few days. It goes away as the underlying skin becomes rehydrated and natural oils are replenished. Mildly scaly or dry skin usually responds well to an emollient (page 205), which is a cream that hydrates the skin, or use a natural oil such as almond oil. If the scales are brown and greasy, and on the scalp, this may be cradle cap (page 163).

In very rare circumstances the skin remains very scaly. This may be caused by a developmental anomaly called icthyosis (which means fish scales). Your doctor may offer a series of tests to establish a diagnosis.

Urticaria ('nettle' rash)

A red rash is common on the forehead, thighs and abdomen and may have raised areas. It is not eczema, and may wax and wane. It usually disappears by the age of three months and is typically caused by an ALLERGY to food or to substances touching the skin. The treatment is similar to the allergic type of eczema (page 205).

Homeopathy

The main remedies used for urticaria are listed here (homeopathy for the previous conditions is discussed in the relevant entry). You may give the most appropriate in 6c potency three times a day for three days and re-assess:

* *Apis* when the skin is inflamed, hot, red, itchy and looks shiny, is worse from heat of any kind and much better for cold applications.
* *Natrum Mur* for recurrent or on-going urticaria, usually at the joints, particularly the hands or ankles, that is white in appearance and perhaps linked with emotional stress.
* *Urtica Urens* if the rash is red, raised and blotchy and looks like nettle stings; feels itchy and prickly and is worse from heat and at night.
* *Rhus Tox* when the rash is very itchy, can form blisters, is concentrated on forearms or hands, makes your baby restless; and the itching is relieved by warm bathing.
* *Urtica Urens* tincture is good for soothing the

skin – 10 drops in a bath or a sponge wash with 10 drops tincture to 250ml (½ pint) water.
- Porridge oats in a pop sock in the bath can also alleviate itching.

Reflexes, baby

See Labour and birth, baby, checks following birth.

Reflexology

Reflexology involves touching and massaging the feet to stimulate health in the whole body. It is immensely relaxing and therapeutic and promotes general health and immunity.

Reflexology originated in Chinese ACUPUNCTURE and has links with Native American and Inca traditions. A reflexologist recognises 'qi' energy points on the sole of each foot that correspond to specific glands, organs and systems in your body. Through your feet, a reflexologist tunes in to your energy flow and what is happening in various parts of your body. They may sense energy blocks caused by illness, stress or injury, which are interfering with the normal activities of cells, organs, nerves and muscles. Treatment helps to improve your energy flow, vitality and health and can affect hormonal balance, sleep quality, mood, physical comfort and so on.

When a reflexologist takes your feet in their hands and applies pressure, the feeling of relaxation and tranquillity grows. When your body is deeply relaxed, circulation improves and energy flow is refreshed. This brings energy to cells, helps to balance essential hormones, assists elimination of toxins and helps to maintain equilibrium. Pressure frees up the flow of energy, and this may be temporarily uncomfortable as tension is released in the tissues. After treatment, most people feel relaxed and rejuvenated.

Reflux

See Vomiting, baby.

Relationships

Relationships are what life is about. We are genetically driven to care, nurture and love, and to play and explore together. Humans cannot learn or thrive in isolation. We need relationships to understand ourselves, and to learn how to understand others. When relationships feel good and we feel loved and accepted by someone else, we feel good about ourselves. We are also biologically driven to have fear, anger and separation anxiety to protect ourselves. If a relationship makes us feel uncomfortable our defence mechanisms emerge.

If you are in a couple the way you relate to one another will affect both of you and offers a model for your baby. He learns from what you do, from the looks you exchange, the way you touch and the tone of your voices, much more than from the words you say.

What we learn in our earliest relationships colours the way we approach relationships for life. In some couples, one partner is in a controlling role while the other is submissive or complacent. This, like many other possible scenarios, tends to be a repeat of what each person experienced in his/her family of origin (page 207). In your relationship, you and your partner will have some different values from your individual families of origin about parenting and about how a spouse 'should' behave. The roles are often not consciously chosen, and tend to be a repeat of your family, but you can change if the roles do not feel right for one or both of you and you are ready to move on.

The transition into parenthood may be the best opportunity you have ever had to be lovingly honest, clear the cobwebs and nourish a friendship that will in turn nourish you and your baby. If you have chosen to commit to one another for life, the investment of time and emotional energy to do this is obviously worthwhile.

ARGUMENTS AND CONFLICT

There will be times when you and your partner have different opinions, different needs and feel in conflict. This is natural – by nine months after the birth around a quarter of couples feel their relationship has improved. Another quarter say it is about the same. The remaining half say their relationship has gone downhill. There is a high chance you'll face rocky periods as part of the lifecycle of being together. Conflict may often be fruitful if it allows you to feel closer, and honestly expressing your anger, disappointment and upsets is part of being intimate.

Conflict and discomfort are an integral part of any relationship and they can be a stimulus for change. You both play a role in how this manifests in your partnership and your family environment. When there is conflict your baby will be aware of it. This may inspire you to deal with problems as they arise. How you deal with conflict will be an important and deep teaching for your baby, from birth onwards. Conflict may pass if you do not address it, but it is likely to surface again. You may need courage, patience and perhaps support to communicate and to reach compromises.

Action plan

Every relationship requires effort. The requirement tends to be greatest at critical times, and when your new baby joins you the dynamics of your relationship will change. A little effort will go a long way to help keep intimacy, trust, communication and mutual respect alive.

When you disagree, it's important to talk about it. But if you are arguing it is best not to do so in front of your baby. He needs to be protected from overt anger and violence. It will help to consider your emotions and feelings and your partner's – the information on page 208 may help. Sometimes, tension may arise when one of you is feeling depressed or anxious and it may be important to get appropriate support (page 176). SEX is also an issue for every couple. The simple act of having quality intimate time together may be like a magic ointment that puts an end to bickering and rekindles intimacy.

Many couples feel that with a baby days are taken up by chores, responsibilities and work. It can feel as if you move from one thing to the next and rarely connect with one another. If you remember only one piece of advice, it may be this: let yourselves be playful. Your baby, who is

playful, spontaneous and loving, can be a great teacher and a gift for your relationship.

Active listening

Not all communication comes through words: much is conveyed through body language and tone of voice. Active listening – really listening to others – allows you to hear their words and pick up on messages that aren't being said.

Active listening is a powerful way for you and your partner to talk and to hear one another. You could try it to kick-start communication if you are feeling distanced, and it is usually very helpful if you need to reach a compromise or a new solution. It is a good way for you to discover and accept your differences of opinion.

Disagreement may become agreement, or you may agree to disagree, without one of you being 'wrong'. Initially you may need to make a conscious effort to 'hear' what is said without projecting your own interpretations.

It may take a major shift in your usual approach to listen with no intention to fix. This often applies to men who are used to fixing. Doing nothing but listening may feel uncomfortably powerless. The conversation may bring up feelings of anger, fear or guilt that may be challenging for you. You might think it is easier not to listen in the first place but it is worth trying. Listening is often difficult for people who did not feel listened to as children.

Active listening can take as little as five minutes. You may be very surprised by the results.

* Create a quiet time with phones switched off. Look at a watch and time each other as each of you takes a turn to talk for three minutes, with no interruptions. When you have had three minutes take a short quiet break and then your partner speaks.
* Focus on what your partner is saying. Do not talk, reassure or ask questions – just listen.
* If you are distracted by thoughts, be aware of them, and let them go and listen again. If you become angry, acknowledge it to yourself and come back to actively listening. This is difficult if you think your partner is wrong and you are right. Your partner's view may be different from yours but it is valid. There is always more than one way to solve a problem.

- After speaking, do not discuss your thoughts for 24 hours until you have had time to process your feelings.
- If each of you has a turn to listen and be listened to you will feel what it's like not to have to defend your position. Many disagreements disappear when your values and differences are acknowledged.
- Next day, try active listening again. This is a good foundation when you begin a discussion. Try not to react immediately to what is said; rather, let it settle and come back to the subject later. Treat problem-solving as a joint effort and let go of believing that there is only one correct solution (yours).
- Where your conversation brings up several issues it is best to talk about each one individually.

Compromise will be easier in some areas than in others. Begin with the minor issues and approach larger problems when you feel comfortable with this way of conversing. Remember that some 'big' problems are made up of smaller points – agreement and compromise may be reached in stages.

If communication is breaking down, it may help to have someone with you as a mediator or supporter. If things feel deeply uncomfortable, upsetting and stuck, you may need to put in extra effort and gather lots of support for you and your baby as you try to avoid – or cope with – breakdown (see below).

■ BREAKDOWN AND SEPARATION

Almost all couples experience difficulties, and unfortunately breakdown is common after childbirth, and sometimes in pregnancy. Sometimes, other relationships break down: friendships, relationships with parents and in-laws, or sibling relationships.

Breakdown is not always final: it can provide the basis of a breakthrough when a new relationship is born from the ashes of the old. Relationships can be restored most easily when the breakdown is acknowledged and one of you sets things in motion to correct it.

On occasions, separation is the best option, not only for parents but also for their baby. While two parents living in harmony is the ideal

for a baby, if the parental relationship involves excessive anger, negativity and stress, and particularly if there is VIOLENCE OR ABUSE, it is preferable to live apart.

What happens

Every relationship is unique and it is not possible to be prescriptive about the causes of breakdown. In all cases, both partners contribute to the conflict. It is common, however, for new parents to have very little time together and for communication to be lacking or unclear. Unexpected differences and cultural expectations may become apparent. If there are complications in pregnancy or your baby is unwell or very demanding this can also put huge pressure on your relationship.

Action plan

If your relationship is ailing and breakdown seems possible there are three key things to consider:

- Are we caring for ourselves (page 121)?
- How can we communicate (page 462)?
- How can we be supported in the way we need?

You and your partner may benefit from the presence of a third party. A counsellor or therapist may be more objective and supportive than a friend or family member.

Feeling supported is important as you cope with your feelings and practical tasks. If either of you has postnatal depression (page 174) it is best to give yourselves time to recover before you separate. If you are in an abusive relationship (page 546) it is really important to communicate this to someone who is in a position to help you. Early separation may be essential.

If you decide to separate you will need loving support as you discuss childcare and access, finances and housing; and to ensure your baby is being loved and cared for well. Please give yourself time and space to relax and reflect on what is happening and to be with your baby. You will always be linked by your baby and separating while maintaining communication is best for your baby. You may each need personal emotional support (page 162) as you adapt to the new situation.

Respiratory distress syndrome

See Breathing difficulties, baby, rapid breathing and grunting.

Restless leg syndrome

With restless leg syndrome (RLS) your legs feel extremely uncomfortable while you're sitting or lying down. There may be cramping or tingling, and your legs may twitch and jerk involuntarily. It is reasonably common for the condition to appear for the first time in pregnancy (affecting up to 15 per cent of women) and then to disappear within a month after birth. While RLS lasts, it may be mildly annoying or absolutely maddening – particularly if it stops you from sleeping. The condition is not well understood but some measures can bring relief.

What happens

No one knows exactly what causes RLS. Some researchers suggest the condition may be genetic. It could be caused or worsened by an imbalance of the brain chemical dopamine, by iron deficiency, or by pregnancy hormones (and it is often worst in the last trimester). Stress tends to aggravate it. It usually gets worse in the afternoon or evening and at night.

Sensations include a feeling of crawling, creeping or tingling inside your foot, calf or upper leg. You might feel CRAMPING, burning or pain and have an overpowering urge to move your legs, or be unable to prevent your legs from moving of their own accord. Leg movements while you're sleeping are likely to keep your partner awake, and just as likely to stop you from having a good night's sleep. Hundreds of twitching or kicking movements may occur during each night.

Action plan

When your legs feel uncomfortable or begin to twitch, you'll probably feel like getting up and moving around. This can help the feeling go away, for a while. It is likely to return again, particularly when you sit or lie down to rest. You can try a number of other techniques, listed below. If nothing works for you, the priority is to nourish yourself with sufficient rest, good food, company and exercise, to help you cope until after the birth when the RLS is likely to reduce or disappear.

Self help

* Some simple stretches may help. If you have a YOGA, PILATES or exercise teacher, ask for advice and see what works for you. Even if relief is temporary, this may help you sleep and rest. Standing and facing a wall, with your forearms resting just above head level and one leg stretched back while the other knee is flexed is often effective.
* Good nutrition, including essential fatty acids (page 263) and plenty of water is important.
* If there is a link between your daily activities and/or what you eat, you may be able to alter the pattern. Try keeping a journal and monitor what you do to help you establish if there is a link.
* Soaking in a warm bath and massaging your legs might relax your muscles.
* Using a hot or cold compress, or alternating the two, might lessen the sensations.
* You may need to alter your daily routine so you can get sufficient sleep, such as having a lie-in or taking regular naps. It is thought that fatigue can worsen symptoms, so it's worth trying to get as much sleep as you need (page 495).
* Moderate exercise, maybe a walk or swim every day, might help, but don't exercise intensely too near to bedtime.
* If RLS is making you stressed you may benefit from counselling or psychotherapy to relieve your anxiety.
* VISUALISATION may help to relax your muscles.

Medical help

Talk to your GP. The syndrome cannot be confirmed with a lab test, but your symptoms will be obvious.
* If your symptoms are mild, an over-the-counter pain reliever may help and your doctor may

prescribe ibuprofen. You must be careful of the doses while you are pregnant (page 408).

* Sometimes, treating an underlying condition such as iron deficiency or peripheral neuropathy greatly relieves symptoms of RLS. Your doctor may recommend iron supplements.
* Although several kinds of drug treat RLS, none can be taken safely during pregnancy.

Homeopathy

Homeopathy may be useful. You may try one of the following remedies in 6c potency am and pm for two to three weeks and then re-assess the situation. If there is no improvement, please consult a homeopath.

* *Zincum Met* if you experience constant movement of the legs and jiggling of the feet with a sensation of formication (insects crawling on the skin) which may prevent sleep; and applying pressure to the area or rubbing helps.
* *Rhus Tox* if you have a constant desire to move your legs and feet in bed; moving brings some relief but this is temporary and symptoms soon return.

Retained placenta

See *Labour and birth, mother, bleeding following birth.*

Rhesus factor

See *Blood group and rhesus factor, mother.*

Rickets

Rickets is an abnormality of the bones in children, usually caused by dietary deficiency. Bone is constantly being broken down and built up. In rickets there is a lowered rate of bone production that can no longer make up for normal bone breakdown. This leads to a decrease in bone density. Rickets is now seen infrequently in a healthy and well-nourished population.

There are many different types of rickets based on a deficiency either of vitamin D, or of the basic building blocks of the bones – calcium and phosphorous. Vitamin D exists in three different forms and all can be made by the body, from the action of sunlight on the skin, and can be obtained from food. Formula milk contains added vitamin D.

PREMATURE babies may rarely develop neonatal rickets, which can cause fractures and impaired growth, and respiratory distress. It is diagnosed on X-ray and in blood tests. Vitamin D-deficiency rickets may appear in children unable to absorb the vitamin because of disorders of the bowel or the liver. Babies with severe kidney disease may also be affected.

In otherwise healthy full-term babies, rickets can appear because of exclusive BREASTFEEDING beyond 12 months that is associated with delayed weaning. The use of low-calcium foods and reduced exposure to sunlight may contribute to the increasing numbers of otherwise healthy children developing nutritional rickets.

Current recommendations that babies are given vitamin drops (page 559) are primarily intended to ensure babies get adequate vitamin D, as well as other nutrients. Rickets can be readily and effectively treated with vitamin D, calcium and phosphate supplements. Almost all babies are cured after treatment but in severe cases there may be some deformity of the leg bones with bow legs and knock knees (pages 80 and 330). Treating rickets needs specialist help, usually from a paediatrician and dietician.

Roseola infantum (sixth disease)

Roseola infantum (also known as sixth disease and exanthem subitum) is a viral illness caused by two common viruses, herpes virus types 6 and 7. It most commonly affects children between seven and 13 months old. The illness brings on a cold-like or respiratory illness that may be followed by a high FEVER lasting two to five days, but most commonly is a three-day illness. In 5–10 per cent of children the high temperature triggers a febrile convulsion. Your child may have a sore throat with swollen glands in the back of the neck. As the fever ends, a pink, raised rash appears on the trunk of the body. The pink-red spots blanch (turn white) when you touch them, and individual spots may have a lighter area or 'halo' around them. The rash usually spreads to the neck, face, arms and legs, and fades after one to three days. The rash can often appear when a baby seems otherwise well. The illness is called sixth disease as it is the sixth one in the series – mumps, measles, rubella, chickenpox, and Parvo B19 (also called fifth disease).

Your child will be infectious for five to 15 days following initial exposure to another infected child. The disease is spread through respiratory fluids and saliva, and is not particularly contagious (unlike chickenpox, for instance). Adults rarely become infected because they will have acquired immunity in childhood.

Action plan

* You can make your child more comfortable by treating her fever, keeping her cool and using infant paracetamol in appropriate doses (page 429). Antibiotics will not help.
* Encourage your baby to drink well and rest.
* Because the symptoms related to roseola may mimic other illnesses before the rash appears, your doctor may investigate other possible causes.
* HOMEOPATHY may ease your baby's symptoms and the first remedies you use may be to treat her fever (see pages 240–1). For best results, it would be advisable to consult with your homeopath.

Routine and structure

See Parenting, rhythm and routine.

Rubella (German measles)

Rubella – originally known as German measles – is usually a mild, self-limiting disease. Most adults in the developed world have been infected or vaccinated as children and are now immune. Routine vaccination is available for children (page 539). For the very small number of women who are infected in pregnancy, rubella carries serious implications because it may lead to foetal infection and developmental damage. This is known as congenital rubella syndrome.

What happens

Rubella infection brings on a rash of pink flat spots on the face and ears that spreads to the trunk. It is similar to the PARVOVIRUS rash, and may be accompanied by pain and swelling of the joints of the hands, feet and knees, a slight fever and swollen lymph nodes ('glands'). Symptoms begin two to three weeks after exposure and will pass in a few days. An infected person may infect others for around one week before symptoms begin, and for a few days after symptoms have passed. Rubella is spread by inhaling infected particles.

Action plan

All pregnant women are tested for rubella immunity: over 90 per cent are immune.

If you are not immune

* If your test is negative, you are 'rubella susceptible' and need to take care not to be in contact with any infected person. If you have been immunised but your antibody levels have fallen, you may still have partial immunity.
* You will be offered vaccination after birth but not while you are pregnant. However, if you inadvertently receive the vaccine while you are unaware of your pregnancy this does not imply that your baby is at risk: there have been no cases of CONGENITAL ABNORMALITIES associated with the vaccine.

Infection in pregnancy

* If you develop a rash, with or without symptoms of swelling or stiffness, visit your doctor.
* Rubella infection can be confirmed through a blood test that checks for a new infection (a high level of IgM antibodies). If your initial test is negative it can be repeated two weeks later to see whether antibodies develop.
* If rubella is confirmed within the first 12 weeks of pregnancy, you will be offered genetic counselling (page 267). Your baby is highly likely to be infected and congenital rubella brings an 80 per cent chance of congenital abnormalities that may range from cataracts and deafness to heart defects and learning difficulties. Planning for the future of your pregnancy will not be easy and you will need a

great deal of support from your family, friends and medical team. Termination will be an option.

- If you become infected between Weeks 13 and 17, your baby is at risk only of deafness. Infection after Week 17 carries no risk to your baby.
- When a pregnancy with infection is carried through to term, a baby can be tested for rubella infection. If your baby is born with congenital rubella she may have a low birth weight and remain contagious for many months.

Rubella in a baby

In the very unlikely event that your baby gets rubella from contact with the infection after birth, reduce her FEVER with appropriate doses of infant paracetamol. Your homeopath may also prescribe remedies.

Keep your baby away from any pregnant women or women planning to get pregnant. As adult infection is more common in men, it is a good precaution to warn all adults with whom you will be in contact. Recovery is usually complete, although there is a minimal risk of deafness.

Ruptured membranes

See Labour and birth, mother, spontaneous and premature rupture of membranes.

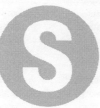

Sacral dimples

Sacral dimples are common, and occur in 2 per cent of babies. They appear as a small depression in the lower back, in the mid line just above the division between the buttocks. In almost all cases, this is a simple depression in the skin and causes no problems whatsoever.

Very unusually they may connect with the deeper parts of the spine. In this situation there is nearly always another finding, such as a tuft of hair in the dimple, or the dimple is situated higher up the back, or there is another associated lump. The higher the dimple is, the more likely it is to be associated with defects in deeper tissues.

A doctor will usually inspect the pit and see if it is possible to see the base of it. In addition, a quick examination of the reflexes of the legs, and a check of the flow of urine can quickly rule out any other abnormality.

Only if there is a suspicion by yourself or your doctor that there is any other cause for concern will further tests be discussed. An ultrasound scan of the dimple is often used to check that there are no other features that may need more complex investigations. In particular, the ultrasound looks to make sure the spinal cord has not been involved in the dimple.

Safety in pregnancy

During pregnancy most women are aware of potential hazards and avoid activities that carry risks. Recreational DRUGS, smoking and alcohol are covered separately and there is guidance on eating and weight.

Sport and exercise

Exercise is very good for you, but keep within safety limits (page 227), take care not to overheat, and make it fun. Exercising on a regular basis is better than widely spaced spurts. Always ask a professional teacher if you are unsure of safety.

In general, don't start a new exercise in pregnancy without guidance, and avoid climbing, horse riding, scuba diving, squash, step classes, water skiing, sky sports and anything that is fast or involves impact or sudden twists or turns.

If you're already a jogger, do no more than two miles a day. If you're not a jogger, don't start now. In mid- to late pregnancy fast walking is safer than jogging. If you are a competent skier it is safe in early pregnancy to cross-country ski below 2,000m (6,500ft). Downhill skiing and high-altitude skiing are not suitable.

Sex

Usually, making love is safe and cannot damage your baby. The safety issues are discussed on page 473. If you have had a history of MISCARRIAGE or BLEEDING during pregnancy, it is wise to abstain from sex for the first 14 weeks. In late pregnancy, sex is safe unless you have a history of PREMATURE BIRTH or your waters have broken.

There is no risk if you use condoms to prevent infection but spermicides are not needed. As long as you are comfortable, the following are safe: oral sex, anal penetration, masturbation, vibrators (but not deep penetration) and lubricators, including natural carrier oils (such as almond or grapeseed) and

KY jelly. Vaginal douches are not safe as they can upset the balance of the vaginal microflora. In later pregnancy, side-by-side and 'spoons' positions are gentle positions that do not put pressure on the abdomen.

Leisure and day-to-day activities

- Bleaching facial and body hair and electrolysis. Both are safe, though avoid the nipple area if you are BREASTFEEDING.
- Body piercing. Don't have a new piercing in pregnancy because of the additional risks that infection might cause. If you already have genital piercings, it is better to remove the rings during pregnancy, long before birth.
- Depilatories. It may be preferable to shave or wax during pregnancy. Your skin absorbs the chemicals used in depilatories.
- Electric blankets. Turn off an electric blanket before getting into bed to avoid overheating. It emits an electro-magnetic field, though levels are considered to be safe.
- Gardening. Best to avoid gardening in pregnancy to avoid the slight risk of contracting TOXOPLASMOSIS from the soil. If you choose to garden, wear gloves and avoid excessive bending and lifting heavy loads. Delegate jobs involving lifting and climbing.
- Hair colouring and perms. There is no conclusive evidence regarding the safety or otherwise of hair dyes. The chemicals in hair-colouring agents are absorbed through the scalp, not each hair shaft, so streaking or highlighting may be preferable to reduce any potential risk. Always wear plastic gloves when dyeing. Henna is a semi-permanent vegetable dye considered to be very safe. Perming may not work well in pregnancy, and the chemicals may not be safe. To achieve curls you could use the old system of twisting shafts of hair and securing them with rags or you could make numerous plaits, or you may use a heated appliance to curl or straighten your hair.
- Heating appliances. Gas and solid fuel heating carry the risk of carbon monoxide poisoning. Arrange inspection of any gas stoves, heaters, fireplaces or wood-burning stoves in your home and place a carbon monoxide detector nearby.
- House cleaning. Wear gloves and avoid products that have strong fumes and warning labels. Keep windows open for ventilation. Look into alternative products (such as vinegar for cleaning windows).
- Loud music. Your baby is cushioned within your uterus and will probably enjoy the music you listen and dance to. The combination of sound and your feel-good hormones is a powerful mix. There is no evidence to date that a baby's hearing can be damaged by exposure to music in pregnancy. If you are at a live gig, or at a party where the music is loud, the important thing is to stay within limits that are comfortable for you.
- MASSAGE. Check that the carrier and essential oils you use are safe in pregnancy.
- Painting and decorating. Avoid contact with oil-based paint, polyurethane floor finishes, spray paints, turpentine, white spirit and liquid paint removers. Water-based paints are a safer choice. Good ventilation is a must. Take care if you are removing or sanding old paint (pre-1970), which may contain lead, a toxic chemical, and avoid electrical work.
- Pets. If you have cats, use gloves when clearing out the litter tray because of the risk of toxoplasmosis infection. Better still, get someone else to do it.
- Saunas and Jacuzzis. Raising your core temperature significantly has the potential to cause birth defects, especially in the first trimester. Use for very short periods only.
- Tattoos. Existing tattoos are no problem. Avoid having new tattoos in pregnancy.

Chemicals and work hazards

A drug or chemical that is known to carry a high risk of causing birth defects is known as a teratogen. The link is a difficult one to ascertain, and although some chemicals and drugs have been proved dangerous, not every drug has been tested.

Moreover, the risk of harming a baby's development in the womb is often associated with a combination of environmental and some genetic factors. It is estimated that of the 2–3 per cent of babies born with birth defects, fewer than 10 per cent of cases can be linked with exposure to teratogens.

Most chemicals are present in extremely low doses and pose very little threat to you or your developing baby. The risk depends on the level and frequency of exposure, the stage of pregnancy and your genetic make-up. It inevitably rises if you are exposed to a dangerous chemical on a daily basis and do not take adequate precautions Take steps to avoid exposure to:

- dry cleaning chemicals – tetrachloroethylene and ethylene glycol ethers,
- insecticides,
- lead, such as old paint,
- mercury (most commonly found in fish such as shark – see page 260),
- aromatic hydrocarbons, phenols, xylene and vinyl chloride (used in laboratories, art work and ceramics),
- radiation (such as X-rays). It is preferable to avoid X-rays of your pelvis or abdomen. If an X-ray of any other area is recommended by your medical or dental specialist you should be given a lead apron to screen your abdomen (see page 570), and
- infections (for example, if you work in healthcare).

If your line of work involves exposure to chemicals that pose a special risk in pregnancy, your employer is obliged to tell you and allow you to move to a safer position. This also applies if your job involves physical demands that may endanger you or your baby.

Pharmaceutical drugs

In general it is best to avoid medication and to take medicines only as advised by your doctor. Safety issues and commonly used pain relief medication are discussed on page 407.

Sex

See also Relationships.

During pregnancy and in the months following, your sex life will change. Lots of things happen as you change shape, sensitivity and aroma, and both of you have new feelings and responsibilities as your relationship enters a new phase.

Many couples experience a continuation of an enjoyable and adventurous sex life once children enter their family, and for some people sex just gets better and better, with new positions and techniques in pregnancy and new thrills after birth when intimate moments

together may be more widely spaced, but more delicious. Usually if sex has been good before pregnancy/birth, it is good afterwards, even if there is a considerable break before full sex resumes.

It's also common for couples to experience a minor, or a huge, reduction in sex. While time or your mood may mean you have less penetrative sex, close physical contact can help to maintain your intimacy. It is preferable not to make love out of a sense of duty, and to be honest with one another if you feel upset, guilty or anxious. There are many alternative ways to be intimate and to feel loved (opposite).

Some common thoughts

She may think...

- 'I never had such good orgasms.' (Superb, lucky you.)
- 'I really feel my vagina and the sensitivity is amazing.' (Time to explore and have fun.)
- 'I just don't feel sexy.' (Stay with this, it's okay. You may feel more sexy tomorrow, next week, next month. Don't forget making time for intimacy can help to rekindle the sexual flame.)
- 'I love my body and enjoy being touched.' (A wonderful opportunity to delight in sensuous pleasure.)
- 'I'd love to have sex but he doesn't seem to fancy me anymore.' (Talk honestly – it's better to talk than to let resentment or guilt build up.)
- 'I don't feel his penis in my vagina like I used to, it's much less sensitive.' (Oral sex and stimulation of your vulva may be more arousing; pelvic floor exercises may help to keep your vaginal muscles toned.)
- 'I feel fat and unattractive.' (Body image is closely linked with libido; you may feel better from some loving support, some different clothes, exercise or a change in food – for more, see page 72.)
- 'I'm too distracted – I can't suddenly have sex while the baby sleeps for 20 minutes.' (Try not to put yourselves

under pressure. Some days you will feel more horny and spontaneous than others. Remember, though, that sex may be more important and rewarding than housework!)

- 'My vagina is sore and I need time to recover.' (Take your time.)
- 'I'm scared of pain, the birth hurt so much.' (Take your time, talk and be gentle when you start touching again.)
- 'I'd rather have oral sex.' (Talk about it – this may be great fun for you both.)

He may think...
- 'I'm afraid I will hurt or touch our baby in the womb.' (Your baby is protected.)
- 'Our lovemaking is better than ever.' (What a pleasure.)
- 'I love feeling her softness and warmth.' (Great.)
- 'I'm too anxious about the labour and birth.' (It is okay to feel anxious, you can talk about your fears together and this is part of intimacy.)
- 'I really miss it now that she's not interested.' (Disinterest is usually only for a short while.)
- 'She loves the baby more than she loves me.' (Mothering is a powerful drive yet it is usually only a matter of time before a baby-focused woman can expand her attention beyond her baby. You may need to accept that lovemaking will be less frequent now, but it may still be brilliant.)
- 'How can we get intimate with our baby in our bed?' (Try making time when your baby will not disturb you.)
- 'I have been patient during pregnancy, and think it's time for me.' (Talk, let your partner know how you feel, she may not appreciate your needs.)
- 'She acts like her mother – how can I possibly make love to my mother-in-law?' (It may help to create time for the two of you, while someone is with your baby, so you can relax once more as friends and lovers having fun together.)
- 'I love having sex in bed and our baby never wakes up.' (Lovely.)

■ BEING INTIMATE

Intimacy is feeling connected, listening and being listened to, trusting, loving and feeling loved and accepted. Some say intimacy is 'into-me-you-see'. In your adult partnership, sex is only one of the manifestations of intimacy.

Intimacy without sex

Being intimate without being sexual is the friendly aspect of a loving relationship. Spending quality time together is intimate. Many things may nourish you both, including touch, chatting, caring for each other and playing. After the birth, falling in love with your baby may distract you from your intimacy as a couple. This is a natural stage and some couples need to put in a little extra effort to nurture their relationship.

- Maybe cook a meal or watch a movie together. When you are with your baby a cuddle or kiss is lovely.
- Some couples enjoy bathing or taking a shower together. A gentle MASSAGE at the end of the day may feel great.
- Loving touch does not need to be sexual to communicate love and trust or to feel good.
- If you both lead busy lives, you could book time in your diaries and make a commitment to keep the appointment, even if you feel embarrassed at using a diary to meet one another. Even half an hour works well.
- Try active listening (page 462). It is powerful and intimate.
- When your baby is older and you are happy to leave her with a loving friend or relative, a night away is a chance to dine, sleep and wake together without interruption.
- When you are separated by work or other commitments, a sexy note, text message, email or gift can do wonders to keep the flame alive.

After birth, most new parents are at times tired, anxious or preoccupied. Don't be surprised if it takes a while to let go and get into the mood. Managing your time to create space for intimacy is a useful skill to build.

If talking and attempts at intimacy don't do it for you, seeking help, perhaps beginning with your GP or a counsellor, may reduce any long-term effect on your family relationships. If one or both of you feel low and lethargic, this may be a sign of blues or DEPRESSION. Taking good care of yourself (page 121) can go a long way towards keeping passion alive and raising your energy if you feel down.

Libido and arousal

Listening to music, watching a romantic film, going out for a meal together or preparing a dinner for two at home all have the potential to be sexually arousing (it can be very sensuous to feed each other or to play footsie and talk about intimate things in a restaurant). Have fun and enjoy, and remember you may need to make time, particularly after birth.

Penetrative sex will not always feel appropriate. Your bodies have many erogenous zones and you may really enjoy being gently touched or kissed on your cheeks, ear lobes, neck or belly. Mutual genital masturbation and oral sex may feel great and you may both find it fun to try new things – if your clitoris is more sensitive, many new possibilities may open up. Sex can be playful and when there's no pressure to perform it can be really energising. Freedom from contraception may feel good.

Your needs will not always be the same. One of you may want touch, masturbation or penetrative sex, whereas the other may want to chat and be listened to. You can powerfully transform a 'stuck' relationship by listening and exploring different, possibly novel, approaches that meet the needs of you both. Whenever possible, tell each other what you want – you are not telepathic and incorrect assumptions can lead to confusion and upset. Many couples enjoy the intimacy of talking together and often find it incredibly erotic to share their desires and fantasies. Equally, being honest about a low sex drive can help both partners let go of the pressure to perform, and relax together.

Mother

Every woman's reaction to pregnancy and motherhood is unique. When libido is high, many women enjoy regular sex with their partner and/or get a lot of pleasure from masturbation. Self-touching can enhance femininity and is a chance to privately explore and enjoy. Being comfortable with the touch and feel of your vagina and the way it responds

may be fun, and a foundation of confidence and familiarity may improve your confidence and reduce inhibitions during labour. The vagina's softness and strength and its incredible ability to expand, open for birth and heal are part of a woman's many strengths. After birth, familiarity with your vagina may be important to keep you in touch with your sexual side. Your partner might enjoy stimulating you with gentle masturbation; later you may return the gesture.

Father

Your libido is also likely to be variable. You may love the changes to your partner's body in pregnancy and enjoy it if she is more sensuous, loving, affectionate or relaxed than usual. If your sex drive is higher than your partner's, remember that her urges may not reflect her feelings about you, but are a result of her pregnancy or the way she feels after birth. Some men find relief with erotic material and/or masturbation. A minority of women find this upsetting, in which case it's useful to talk. Some couples share erotic material they both find arousing.

Once your baby is born, other issues may arise. Some men feel more deeply connected than ever to their partners, full of admiration, and have a powerful drive to be close. Intimacy often continues and increases before sex resumes. Some men are confused about their feelings and do not enjoy making love to a 'mother'. Being around mum and baby breastfeeding may dull libido; or feeling excluded and jealous of mother-baby intimacy may contribute to resentment, pent up energy and, for a minority of men, a temptation to seek pleasure from another woman. Being open and accepting may help you if there is a period of low sexual activity. It may take time, love and some honest listening (page 462) to integrate your life change and be creative about ways to continue to enjoy sex and intimacy in your relationship.

Impotence
Some men experience low libido or impotence. There are many possible reasons, and pregnancy or demands from family life are just some of these. Impotence is often linked with

pressure to perform. There are other factors including whether you are tired and physically fit. It may not be realistic to flick a switch and make it all better, although things usually improve over time, with honesty and intimacy. The problem may disappear when you both feel undisturbed and free of time restraints (for example, if you get a night away, or your baby begins to sleep for longer stretches). Sometimes it takes a commitment to dedicating time for sex or intimacy when there are so many chores that need to be done. You may feel more excited if you find time to make love earlier in the day, before you are both tired, or if you change the location (don't always do it in the bedroom). You could talk about your fantasies, explore new positions; or postpone penetrative sex and focus on oral stimulation. If you masturbate but do not enjoy sex with your partner, easing up on the masturbation may increase your sex drive when you are with her.

▓ IN PREGNANCY

As long as your pregnancy is progressing without any concerns, you can safely have sex throughout pregnancy. Many women experience a surge of sexual vitality and enjoy more exciting orgasms than ever before. Some women go off sex for part or all of pregnancy. Most women, like men, have fluctuating libido.

Some parents feel strange about having sex when the baby is so close in pregnancy. Sexual penetration cannot hurt your baby as she is protected by the amniotic fluid, and the mucous plug in your cervix ensures semen or bacteria do not pass into your uterus. You can continue to safely make love until onset of labour. When a mum enjoys sex her baby also experiences sensations of pleasure and love, in part through the receipt of love hormones that are released in her body. If, on the other hand, sex is forced or abusive in any way, feelings of stress and fear may be experienced by a baby.

Mum's body and mind

Pregnancy brings about a range of changes. Your vagina, clitoris, and your outer vaginal lips and the tissues inside can all become much more sensitive. This may be a good

thing – sexual stimulation can become more fun. You may get multiple or very powerful orgasms. Alternatively, you may be so sensitive that even light touch feels uncomfortable. If you don't feel like sexual stimulation, you may enjoy being intimate in other ways (page 471).

Pregnancy is a great opportunity to try new things and to respond to the changing sensitivity of your vagina and breasts.

* You may like experimenting with the way you touch one another and the positions you use to make love.
* You may prefer to lie side to side, to be on top, sitting up, or on hands and knees to avoid direct pressure on your uterus.
* Orgasms are good for you. Orgasms can feel great and help you to relax and sleep well, while giving a healthy glow to your skin and improving your body image.
* Orgasms can trigger uterine contractions but even very strong orgasms cannot trigger premature labour.
* Oral sex is fine – your partner may or may not enjoy the change in taste as your vaginal fluid alters.

Staying safe

* If you feel light-headed, avoid lying flat on your back.
* Sex cannot cause MISCARRIAGE. Only if you have a history of recurrent miscarriages or have had a threatened miscarriage is it a wise precaution to avoid sex during the first trimester.
* If you have an incompetent cervix (page 127), sex with orgasm can increase the risk of miscarriage. It is safest to wait until a cervical stitch is in place.
* Sex cannot cause premature labour.
* If you use vibrators or other sex toys ensure they are clean and do not go beyond your comfort zone.
* If your membranes have ruptured avoid sex as it may introduce potentially harmful bacteria into your womb.
* If you have any vaginal bleeding, avoid sex and seek advice (page 63).
* Rarely, the placenta is low down in the uterus (page 442). In this case, sex could lead to bleeding and should be avoided.

▧ POSTNATALLY

The vast majority of couples enjoy a full, satisfying and active sex life after the birth of their children. Some couples resume sex soon but most wait weeks and some wait for months. If you're too tired, not interested or too sore, take heart – you may need to wait but it doesn't mean your sex life is over.

After the birth, for your baby the most important feeling is to be safe and connected – the dyad of mum and baby is the natural way. When your baby is in deep sleep she will not be easily disturbed, and many parents do make love with their baby safely in bed next to them. In fact, co-sleeping can reinforce intimacy between mum and dad. It doesn't work for all parents, though. There are many alternatives and when your baby is sleeping you may enjoy going into another room.

As new parents you will be spending time getting to know and falling in love with your baby. This may be more intense for the woman, particularly when she is breastfeeding, and men can feel excluded. Some women feel guilty about this, even though a reluctance to make love is often purely physiological – breastfeeding and hormonal changes of low oestrogen often reduce libido and may increase vaginal tenderness.

There will be new demands on your time, and you may both be tired and will need to rest and sleep when you can. In the first few weeks, your body may need to recover and vaginal sutures or tears take time to heal. Most women prefer to wait until after bleeding and postnatal pain have passed. Men can also take a long time to believe that their touch won't hurt, and to get their own sex drive back.

Both of you may have postnatal blues (page 219), and changes in your body image may also take a toll on your sex life. The transition into parenthood may cause the lover to recede for some time. Patience and acceptance will encourage the lover to re-emerge, and sex may become more fulfilling when you do start again.

Some couples feel empowered by their experiences of pregnancy and birth and become more open and even daring about voicing their sexual preferences. If sexual intimacy means a lot to you it is worth creating time by cutting down on other commitments. For some couples,

particularly for the man, making love infrequently can be a major cause of upset. Staying intimate can reduce this (page 471).

Will sex feel different?

After a vaginal birth, muscle tone in the vagina may decrease and for a time this may reduce pleasurable friction during sex. You and your partner may feel less sensation than before. Pelvic floor exercises help to improve the muscle tone (page 438) and tend to increase sexual pleasure and the intensity of orgasm. Your partner can also help: try contracting your pelvic floor muscles around his fingers or penis – it's a wonderful way to get fit, enrol his help and achieve orgasm! Your partner will receive more stimulation from the clenching sensation.

If sex is painful it may be from the healing of your vagina after the birth or because the lining is thin from breastfeeding hormones (see page 543). Do discuss any pain at your postnatal examination with your doctor.

After childbirth, many women feel different – almost virginal – and the first time they make love again is like the beginning of a new and exciting sexual relationship.

If it hurts

Pain when you make love (dyspareunia) may be due to a number of reasons. The most common cause is increased tissue sensitivity caused by your hormones after birth. Sensitivity may also increase if you feel emotionally low, or are anxious about making love. Lubrication tends to decrease if you are nervous about sex.

If the pain is around your vaginal lips, this may be because the vaginal lining naturally thins after pregnancy and when breastfeeding. Other possible causes after birth include bruising, grazes or cuts that haven't fully healed and infection, such as thrush. Deep pain after birth may arise from your pelvic muscles and will settle or need osteopathic treatment (there is more on pelvic pain on page 43).

● If it hurts, stop.
● If pain worries you, let your midwife or doctor examine you.
● If there is any bleeding after birth, contact your doctor who may check and reassure you.

- If your tissues are sensitive rest assured that hormonal changes will pass. It is worth encouraging lots of lubrication – foreplay may work for you (and begin with talking rather than touching), or try natural oils (such as almond or grapeseed) or KY jelly. Avoid petroleum-based gels if using latex condoms as the gel can damage the latex.
- You may find some positions more comfortable than others, such as woman on top, entry from behind. Shallow thrusts can be more comfortable than deeper ones.
- Women who are not comfortable with penetrative sex often find oral sex is fulfilling on its own, or as foreplay before gentle intercourse.
- Masturbation may help you relax and discover what feels good. You can do this alone or with your partner.
- Create time to be with your partner and to discuss what you feel. This may be a chance to go through issues that have affected your sex life for some time and to boost your intimacy (page 471). Counselling, psychotherapy or sex therapy may sometimes be useful individually or as a couple.

Discomfort will gradually recede and intercourse itself will help stretch and heal your tissues. It can be a great way of strengthening your pelvic floor muscles. If pain continues for months it is important to consult your GP or gynaecologist for a personal check-up.

Safety

It is normal to bleed after birth (lochia) for roughly three to eight weeks. If sex triggers abnormal blood loss it is best to check with your doctor. Common causes of pain are discussed on page 430. Talk to your doctor if you are uncomfortable.

Sex and breastfeeding

The breastfeeding hormone prolactin suppresses ovulation and oestrogen production by your ovaries, and focuses you on your baby.
- Some women feel they need all their energy for mothering, and prefer to postpone sex until feeding has stopped. Others enjoy both.
- Your partner may be less – or more – turned on

by your large breasts and by watching you feed your baby.
- Your vagina may feel tender, as breastfeeding hormones thin the lining.
- Hormones may reduce lubrication. You can boost this with oral sex, gels or oils.
- Your breasts may leak milk when you are aroused and with orgasm (caused by the release of oxytocin) so keep a small towel handy.

▓ WHEN THERE HAS BEEN TRAUMA

For some women, childbirth can be a traumatic experience. If there has been any degree of POST TRAUMATIC STRESS DISORDER, sex is one area of life that may be affected. This also applies to women who have suffered sexual abuse, assault or rape in the past. The emotional scars may remain for years. Whatever the original trauma, if you have had feelings of violation, loss of dignity or fear, then anxiety about sex and/or discomfort during sex may continue.

You may be afraid of vaginal pain, of physical exposure or of losing control (in orgasm, for example). You may simply not feel sexy, as if that part of you has shut down, particularly if you feel depressed or low. Being afraid or being out of touch may reduce your libido, decrease vaginal lubrication and make you more sensitive to touch.

For some women, trauma was not physical but felt at an emotional level, often linked with early life. Your family's culture may have left you with the firm impression that sex is dirty, wrong or sinful. In this situation, having sex may be associated with guilt and shame, and these emotions may make you too tense to enjoy the experience. Feeling sexy, having sex or talking about it may cause you to feel ashamed.

Reclaiming and exploring your sexuality can take a lot of time and gentle care. Like any other woman you need to heal after birth and find time and space for intimacy in a busy family life. You may need considerable support to explore the emotional issues that are pertinent for you and to build trust in your body, and in your sexual partner. Some of the advice in the post traumatic stress disorder entry (page 448) may be useful for you and it may be appropriate for you to focus on intimacy and trust (page 471) before progressing to genital touching or penetrative sex.

Sexually transmitted diseases

See also Candida (thrush), mother; Chlamydia; Gonorrhoea; Hepatitis; Herpes; Human Immunodeficiency Virus (HIV), mother; Syphilis; Trichomoniasis.

A number of sexually transmitted diseases (STDs) carry risks to women and – in pregnancy or during childbirth – may present a risk of infection to a baby. Occasionally, infection can affect a baby's development and/or lead to illness. Not all STDs are routinely tested for in pregnancy. If you believe you may be at risk of infection, or may have been infected in the past with any single disease, or you have a suspect vaginal discharge (page 541) you may want to be tested for a wider range of illnesses that may be transmitted through sexual contact.

Shingles in pregnancy

See also Chickenpox.

Shingles occurs when the dormant varicella virus in your body is reactivated, often many years after an initial chickenpox infection (see page 128). If you get shingles, your baby is safe because you – and therefore your baby – already have antibodies to the virus.

What happens

When the chickenpox virus is contracted, it travels from the skin along the nerve paths to the roots of the nerves, where it lies dormant. When reactivated, the virus travels via the nerve paths to the skin, causing blisters to form along the way. It is often very painful. It isn't known what triggers reactivation but you cannot develop shingles through contact with someone infected with chickenpox or shingles.

Shingles is not infectious through airborne droplets like chickenpox. But it can cause chickenpox in non-immune people through direct contact with fluid from the blisters. Pregnant women who get shingles have a higher than normal risk of developing pneumonia.

Action plan

There is no specific treatment for shingles. You may need painkillers (page 408) if the discomfort is severe. A soothing calamine cream on the blisters may be very helpful. Fortunately the blisters crust over and the pain reduces in a few days. Homeopathy may be helpful to ease symptoms but it is not appropriate to self-prescribe, so you will need to consult your homeopath.

Shoulder dystocia

See Labour and birth, baby, shoulder dystocia.

Sickle cell disease and thalassaemia

See also Anaemia, mother.

Sickle cell disease and thalassaemia are genetic (inherited) conditions that affect the red blood cells. In these conditions, there is an abnormality in one of the two protein chains (alpha or beta) that make up the haemoglobin molecule. The severity of either condition depends on whether you inherit a faulty gene from one or both parents. If you have one faulty gene you may be a carrier and pass it on to your children but show no or only mild symptoms yourself. If you have both genes you will develop the full condition, which causes anaemia. Your baby may be affected, depending on his genetic inheritance. Both conditions occur most frequently in areas where malaria is, or used to be, a major killer. It is thought that the mild forms of these conditions may give some protection against the malaria parasite.

Sickle cell disease

Sickle cell disease is an abnormality in the protein forming the haemoglobin molecule. It is most common in people (or the ancestors of people) from Africa, Central America (especially Panama), South America, Caribbean nations, Mediterranean countries, India or Near Eastern countries. When the red blood cells of people with sickle cell disease are unable to get enough oxygen, the cells become longer and curved, like the blade of a sickle. Sickle cells can get stuck in small blood vessels, which inhibits circulation to some parts of the body. This can damage tissues and internal organs and cause pain, particularly if the blockage occurs in the arms, legs, chest or abdomen. Sickle cell disease exists as several milder forms that occur when the second gene is not a sickle gene. When there is a single gene for sickle cell and one normal gene, this results in a milder condition called sickle cell trait. If the second gene is another haemoglobin variant such as HbC, the disorder is called HbSC (sickle c disease). This is less severe than sickle cell disease, but more severe than sickle trait.

Thalassaemia

There are several types of thalassaemia. Beta thalassaemia involves the beta haemoglobin chain and is more common among people who live around the Mediterranean Sea, such as Greeks, Italians and North Africans, and in people living in parts of the Middle East, India and Pakistan. Alpha thalassaemia involves the alpha haemoglobin chain and is more usual among people from Southeast Asia. The more severe forms, called thalassaemia major, lead to anaemia and other symptoms and require treatment with regular blood transfusions.

What happens

A carrier has both normal and abnormal haemoglobin, while a person with the full condition only has abnormal haemoglobin and will be anaemic.

Your baby

If you are at risk, your blood will be tested using a technique called electrophoresis. If you are found to have any abnormal genes, your partner will also be tested. If you are both carriers, your child has a one in four chance of having the full-blown condition, a one in four chance of being completely free of the condition, and a two in four chance of being a carrier. That means that there is a three in four (75 per cent) chance that your baby will either have a mild form of the disorder or will be unaffected. Amniocentesis or

CVS (chorionic villous sampling) can determine the exact composition of your baby's haemoglobin.

Severe anaemia due to sickle cell disease in the mother may affect the function of the placenta and may cause INTRAUTERINE GROWTH RESTRICTION (IUGR). A baby who has inherited sickle cell disease or thalassaemia with resulting anaemia will need close paediatric care to prevent complications. It may take months for the sickle cell anaemia to become apparent. In areas where sickle cell or thalassaemia is common, newborn babies are routinely tested by taking a blood sample from the baby after birth, and if this raises concern the test is repeated at six months. This is now routine in the UK and is part of the heel prick blood spot testing.

Action plan

Mother

The treatment for anaemia due to sickle cell or thalassaemia is not the same as treatment for iron deficiency anaemia. There may be excess iron in the circulation and so it is dangerous to be given more iron. Women with sickle cell disease or thalassaemia are usually treated in specialist units because they and their babies require close monitoring. During labour and birth it is important to avoid any situation where the mother is shocked or remains under significant stress that may lead to shock, or has reduced oxygen in her blood, because this may trigger a sickle cell 'crisis' and increase the risk of damage to internal organs.

Baby

Sickle cell anaemia and thalassaemia do not generally affect a newborn baby. If a baby has inherited sickle cell disease, abnormal 'sickle' cells build up as mature haemoglobin replaces the foetal haemoglobin. By six months, this brings on symptoms such as paleness due to anaemia, fatigue, poor feeding and failure to thrive. Rarely, it may lead to a sickle cell crisis where body tissues and internal organs can be damaged through lack of oxygen.

When a baby is well he will need routine penicillin and some folic acid to support red cell regeneration. Treatment of sickle cell crisis requires admission to hospital and specialist

477

treatment, including correction of anaemia by blood transfusion and control of pain.

Thalassaemia usually follows a similar pattern, affecting the baby only once mature haemoglobin replaces foetal haemoglobin. The effect can be minimal, with a haemoglobin reduction to around 10 gm/dl at nine months (the usual level is 12 gm/dl). Very rarely, there is severe foetal anaemia requiring intrauterine transfusion, and blood transfusions may be needed for life. Transfusions every three to six weeks provide healthy red blood cells and allow children to enjoy life to the full. Affected children need ongoing specialist paediatric care. Unfortunately a drawback is a build-up of iron, which the body cannot get rid of naturally. After 10 or more years, this excess iron may cause complications such as poor growth and development, liver and heart disease and even death. To prevent these problems, children with thalassaemia major need regular treatment to remove excess iron from the body.

Sickle cell and thalassaemia cannot be cured by drugs, but may be cured by a bone marrow transplant.

SIDS

See Sudden infant death syndrome (SIDS) and sudden unexpected death in infancy (SUDI).

Sight problems and blindness, baby

See also Eye infection and swelling, baby; Growth and development, baby.

Fewer than one in 10,000 babies is blind. Although some parents notice a visual impairment early on, it is common for it to go unnoticed for up to three months, particularly when a baby can detect light and shadow. Until blindness is diagnosed, or at least investigated, some parents are disheartened by their babies' seeming lack of response. It is usually helpful for parents to know when a visual impairment is present, so they are less upset by reduced eye contact and can enjoy many other ways to be close and to bond. Eye contact is an important part of the parent-baby dance and a powerful

bonding force and when a baby has limited or no sight, touch is often the most effective connecting force between parents and their baby.

As neonatal care has improved, the commonest cause of blindness, retinopathy of prematurity (opposite), has all but disappeared in the west. There are still a few rare diseases that cause permanent and complete or partial sightedness in babies, including cataracts, cortical visual impairment, optic nerve hypoplasia, albinism, optic nerve atrophy and retinal diseases.

Action plan

If your child does not fix on or follow your face, or her eyes wander randomly, ask your health visitor or doctor to check her vision. She will be referred to a paediatrician, and then to a specialist in children's eyes for an accurate diagnosis. If her impairment is due to delayed visual maturation her vision is likely to improve as she gets older. Although all forms of blindness are rare, conditions such as delayed visual maturation, where a baby delays in fixing and following faces and objects, and ocular albinism, where the pigment in the retina responsible for vision is deficient, are the more common causes. They are difficult to diagnose and you will need highly expert advice.

If your baby is visually impaired, you and your family may need to dramatically adjust many aspects of your lifestyle, with increasing compensation for her lack of vision as she becomes mobile. She will use all her other senses to make up for the absence of effective vision. You can make things as easy as possible, encouraging her development and enjoying rich communication, with the help of specialised teachers and therapists that your local educational and health authority can provide. National organisations for the blind (the RNIB in the UK) provide information and support for families.

■ CATARACTS

A congenital cataract is an opacity (cloudiness) in the lens of the eye that is present at, or develops shortly after, birth. Very few babies (around three in 10,000) are affected, and around one fifth of these have a family history of cataracts. Sometimes infection during pregnancy is a cause. Congenital cataracts may affect one or both eyes.

They account for the largest proportion of partially sighted and blind registered children in the UK. New treatment methods and earlier diagnosis may well improve this, with better techniques for removal of cataracts and in some cases, placement of artificial lenses.

What happens

The lens lies behind the pupil and focuses rays of light into the retina to form an image. Ordinarily, the lens changes shape as it focuses on objects at different distances. It is made of fibres that are arranged in a pattern that allows light to pass straight through, like clear glass. When this arrangement is disturbed, the transparency is lost and an opacity, which is the cataract, results. The image your baby sees will then be blurred, or blocked out. This deprives her of the visual stimulation she needs to develop vision normally and if left untreated may result in permanent loss of vision.

The normal structure of the lens may be disrupted if abnormal breakdown products (metabolites) accumulate, with retention of water within the lens; or when normal development is interrupted because of a genetic error or an environmental agent (such as the rubella virus, now much less common, causing just one or two cataract cases per year in the UK).

A small cataract may barely interfere with normal vision, but often the cataract is more severe and leads to lazy eye (underdevelopment of the visual system in the affected eye). Without adequate stimulation central vision can be permanently impaired. There may still be some degree of peripheral vision and an ability to distinguish between light and dark.

Treatment

Early visual development depends on stimulation of the eyes, so diagnosis within the first few weeks of birth is important. The most effective treatment is to surgically remove the cataract. Following this, your baby may need optical correction with a contact lens and/or glasses. If surgery to one eye only is required, patching the healthier eye for several hours a day through early childhood helps her use the less healthy eye. Otherwise she would

unconsciously prefer the healthy eye and the other might never achieve normal vision.

The outcome depends on the type of cataract. Some congenital cataracts only slightly impair visual development and never require surgery. Others need surgery and although complication may lead to difficulties such as glaucoma, optic nerve damage and retinal detachment, even when bilateral cataracts have been treated vision may eventually become near normal.

▥ RETINOPATHY OF PREMATURITY

Retinopathy of prematurity (ROP), sometimes called retrolental fibroplasia, occurs in fewer then 1 per cent of premature babies. It used to be the most common cause of blindness in children, but is much rarer these days due to better understanding of what causes the condition and improvements in neonatal care. ROP is caused by an initial constriction of blood vessels in the retina followed by rapid growth. New vessels grow in the wrong places, and can cause disturbances of the blood drainage pattern. When the blood vessels leak, they cause scarring. These scars later shrink, and pull on the retina, sometimes detaching it.

The severity of ROP is indicated by its grade, a measurement of how the condition has progressed. Most children have grade I or grade II ROP and there is a good chance for complete recovery, with no specific treatment except, in some cases, the need to wear glasses.

Grade I. There is a demarcation line in the retina. This indicates that the peripheral retina is not receiving a completely normal blood flow.
Grade II. The line has progressed to a ridge.
Grade III. There are abnormal blood vessels in the eye resulting in scarring and fluid. There is some chance that the abnormal blood vessels and fluid may regress and your baby may still have good vision, correctable with glasses.
Grade IV. The retina has detached. Once this grade has been reached there is little chance of the eye getting better. Vision may be limited or completely impaired.

Diagnosis and treatment

If your baby has a PREMATURE BIRTH or a low birth weight and is at risk of ROP she will be given:

- An eye examination at birth looking for cataracts or developmental abnormalities.
- An eye examination at four to six weeks of age.
- Follow-up eye examinations at appropriate times, particularly for premature babies.

You may want to lower the brightness of lighting around your baby: studies are underway to determine if this may help prevent ROP.

If your baby is diagnosed with ROP it is best for her to begin treatment as soon as possible, preferably within 72 hours. Some babies benefit from cryotherapy, which uses freezing to stop further damage to the retina. Another treatment uses laser photocoagulation to create small burns, which produce scars that seal the borders of the retina and help to prevent detachment.

When a baby has had ROP, she is susceptible to: retinal detachment, cataracts, glaucoma, squint, and short sightedness. Some babies may develop vision loss or blindness in adolescence. It is important, therefore, to continue with regular eye examinations.

Single parenting

Families have many settings – mixed couples, same sex couples, primary carers and single parents. All have difficulties and advantages. If you have sole responsibility some things will be harder to cope with and some things will be easier. Today many children are at some stage cared for by one parent and nine out of 10 single parents are women.

A journey that begins in partnership, involves separation and then living as a single parent, is often long and difficult. At first the outlook may be bleak and pain and anxiety may be intense. In the long term you may feel happier, stronger and more confident. With a focus on your personal strengths, your support network and your baby, there will be possibilities that can improve your situation. The most helpful strategies are to listen to yourself and to your child, trust and respect your instincts and seek and accept the support that will help you do this. Ultimately, the relationship between you and your baby is the most important thing in both your lives, and this can thrive when you care well for yourself. The advice in the CARING FOR YOU section may offer useful suggestions.

Staying healthy and financially afloat, meeting your baby's needs and your own may be the greatest challenge you have ever met. It may be hard to keep up your enthusiasm but having to manage stimulates action and when the results are positive you will feel good.

If you have a network of extended family and/or close friends committed to caring for you and for your baby, you may feel more supported than some of your friends who are in a relationship where their partner is not supportive. The mix of independence and companionship that can come with single parenting can be exciting.

Pregnancy and birth without a partner

- Women who are single tend to have more anxieties about what might happen after the birth. Acknowledging your fears in advance may help you set practical arrangements in place and reduce your anxiety.
- You may ask someone to join you on antenatal visits, go shopping for baby equipment and get your house ready.
- If you are coping with a relationship breakdown or with the loss of your partner, support of loving friends is essential. Counselling could help you integrate your feelings, stay well and feel present for your baby.
- During labour, having a trusted friend with you can improve your experience. Alternatively, or in addition, you may hire a DOULA.
- It is particularly important to arrange practical help in the weeks after birth.
- When you are supported, you are better able to give your baby the attention and love he needs. Your community offers many resources.

Parenting

Every parent has ups and downs and there will be joys as well as challenges. Being the sole carer for your baby has many advantages. For example, your two-way bond may be extremely close and there is no one to question your decisions. If another person criticises what you're doing, or offers opinions, you may feel good that you know your baby best and are doing the best for him. Alternatively, you may become upset and paranoid. It is important to spend time with people who make you feel good and offer constructive support and advice – going to local groups may be part of this.

Your friends may not always be aware when you need help, particularly if you put on a strong front. If you are used to being independent you may not have had much practice in asking for help. But you and your baby will benefit from company, love, distraction, fresh ideas, practical help and time apart from one another. It is okay – and important – to ask if you need help, of whatever kind (see page 123).

Communication between parents

If you have recently separated, feelings of anger, abandonment and loss are played out between the two of you. Parents often blame one another for what has happened. Actively listening (page 462) is particularly valuable and may reduce the time you spend in conflict. You might benefit from professional mediation.

Some mums or dads do not stay in contact, whether through choice, death or traumatic separation. When the second parent is completely absent the balance may be redressed by strong relationships with others who take an active role in your child's life. Babies are quick to place trust in loving carers and are experts at striking up friendships, but they also notice if familiar people disappear from their lives. A positive step may be to enrol an aunt, uncle or godparent who can be present on a regular basis and offer a 'family' connection.

Around a third of lone parents experience violence in their relationship and are concerned about their child having contact with the other parent. If you are affected, please turn to the entry on VIOLENCE AND ABUSE.

How might your baby feel?

Your child has a full range of emotions (page 206) and his spontaneity and zest for life may spur you on. When he expresses distress or anger it may be very difficult for you. You may blame yourself and feel guilty. His feelings reflect many things and may not be related to the absence of his other parent; and even if they are, that's okay. He has no control over his emotions and will express them freely: he is behaving normally and his main need is to be listened to, held and acknowledged (page 208). You may both benefit from the company of others and your baby may enjoy a mixture of male and female energy from other adults and children.

Finances and work

In terms of statistics, single parents are worse off financially than pensioners and poverty is a huge challenge. Many single parents need to become experts at living economically, and many need to change their lifestyle, sometimes drastically. There are no rules about how to negotiate this complex area and each decision will be unique. It may help to re-assess your arrangements at regular intervals.

Stigma

Without realising it, some people (including some healthcare professionals) are judgmental, and the way they act may make you feel uncomfortable. This is more likely where the single parent is a man. It is hurtful when you know that you are doing your best if you get disapproval instead of praise; or if you feel strong and happy and other people are pitying you. Tapping into a network of other single parents may be a good way to celebrate with others who are parenting alone and to be supported if your self-esteem has dipped or you are facing practical difficulties.

Sinusitis, mother

See Coughs and colds, mother.

Skin, baby

See also Rashes and spots, baby.

Your newborn baby may show very red skin in parts of, or all over, her body. This is entirely normal, and is due to the high number of red blood cells in her circulation. As these are broken down the redness disappears and this may result in yellowing (JAUNDICE), which usually passes in seven to 10 days.

You may also notice spots or rashes. In fact seven out of every 10 babies have a neonatal spotty rash (known as erythema toxicum neonatorum, see page 459). A spotty newborn usually becomes clear-skinned within a few weeks, and the opposite is also true – a clear-skinned babe can develop spots soon after birth. Occasionally, a rash may be linked with an infection or illness, and it is always important to seek your doctor's advice if your baby develops a rash. Rashes and spots are covered in more detail on page 458.

Skin tags

Skin tags commonly occur in front of the ear, around the anus, and the hymen in little girls. They are harmless and do not require treatment.

▨ CARE

Your baby's skin needs no special care – a gentle wash with water is sufficient. You may take your baby into your bath (before you put any soap products in) or gently wipe her body with warm, wet cotton wool. It is best to avoid or use a minimum of natural soap. Pure oils (such as almond, olive or sunflower) nourish your baby's skin and can be simply rubbed in after a light wash (see page 404).

▨ COLOUR

- Red: normal in newborns, tends to settle in seven to 10 days.
- Yellow: sign of jaundice, very common and usually passes in 10 to 21 days.
- Blue with marbling: normal.
- Blue on fingers, toes and edges of face: normal (skin needs warming).
- Blue on the tongue and lips: abnormal, needs investigating (see blue skin, below).
- Coloured marks: birthmarks/naevi (page 52).

Blue skin

Acrocyanosis involves a change in blood flow that causes a blue colour change to the skin, particularly in the hands, feet and around the edges of the face. There is no swelling or any other changes. It is harmless and will go when the skin is warmed, and reduces by one month of age. It may be more noticeable in babies with DOWN'S SYNDROME. Central cyanosis is a blue colour to the lips and tongue caused by low oxygen levels in the blood that remains when a baby warms up. It may indicate a serious heart (page 289) or lung abnormality and requires investigation.

Marbled skin

A mottled or marbled appearance to the skin ('cutis marmorata') is typical in the first few months after birth. It occurs because the nerve supply to the small blood vessels (capillaries) in the skin is immature and some blood vessels dilate (widen), producing a red colour, while others contract, producing pale or blue skin. It's more noticeable when your baby is cold. In a rare form known as cutis marmorata telangiectatica congenita, the marbling is more pronounced. In this disorder, the marbling is more pronounced and permanent, and may be worse from crying or temperature change. It is usually outgrown in adolescence. (There is no connection with Raynaud's Disease, which is a disease of the small blood vessels of the hands and feet.)

Skin, mother

Your skin changes during pregnancy. It stretches, darkens and the sebaceous glands that produce natural moisturising oils and the sweat glands that control heat loss become more active. A number of women experience uncomfortable changes, ranging from dryness to excessive oiliness, as well as acne, itches and rashes. In most cases, these conditions settle after pregnancy. Some improve greatly with attention to nutrition, through MASSAGE and with the use of appropriate essential oils, and it is important to avoid too much sun.

Common changes are:
- *Melasma*, or darkening of the skin, affects 90 per cent of women. It may occur on breasts, abdomen, labia and inner thighs and as a central line running from the pubic area to the chest. If it occurs on the face it may look like a mask. This is called cloasma. Freckles or moles may darken. Tell your doctor if you are worried that darkening is excessive.
- *Acne* may arise because the sebaceous glands swell and become blocked by oily secretions, due to an increase in testosterone in pregnancy. It can also reflect diet, particularly too much saturated fat, not enough water, or excess wheat and sweets. Acne medications are not recommended in pregnancy. The best treatment is to keep your skin clean with water and a mild, natural cleanser, and attend to your diet.

- *Dry skin* may be a problem. The best treatment for this is to drink plenty of water and use a natural moisturiser (vitamin E cream is good). If you live or work in centrally heated or air-conditioned rooms, the atmosphere can be very dry. Taking omega-3 and -6 essential fatty acids often helps.
- *Stretch marks* affect as many as 80 per cent of pregnant women, mostly in the last trimester. They usually begin as reddish marks on the abdomen, thighs and breasts, and fade gradually after birth. Many people believe there is no method of prevention, because stretching begins beneath the surface, although avoiding excessive weight gain may help. Using the same principles as for dry skin may also help.
- *Skin tags* are tiny polyps that sometimes occur where skin rubs together or on clothing, such as under the arms, beneath the bra or on the neck. They are caused by excessive growth of the superficial layer of skin and disappear after pregnancy.
- *Spider naevi* are red, flat spots on the face, hands and chest caused by pregnancy hormones dilating small skin blood vessels. If you press on the centre of the spot with a pencil, it turns white until the pressure is removed. Spider naevi disappear after pregnancy.
- *Itching and irritation* are common – up to 20 per cent of pregnant women complain of a generalised itch, commonly beginning over the front of the abdomen. It may begin early but is usually most intense in the last 10 weeks. Usually itching without rash is of no concern. Rarely, it can be a symptom of CHOLESTASIS, particularly when the hands and feet are affected, and is worth investigating with a blood test. If you have a rash, your midwife or doctor can check it.

▓ RASHES IN PREGNANCY

If you are prone to dermatitis, acne, allergic reactions or one of the many conditions that affect skin, pregnancy is a time when they may flare up. Sometimes they improve. There are also a number of pregnancy-specific skin conditions and some women get a rash that is not specific to pregnancy for the first time.

PUPP (pruritic urticarial papules of pregnancy)

PUPP is the most common rash related to pregnancy. It can be severe and really itchy. It may begin on the abdomen and spread to the thighs, arms and buttocks with angry red raised spots or bumps, but does not spread to the face. The cause is not known and it may last for months but clears within weeks of birth. Rarely it begins at birth. It presents no risk to baby or mother but can be so irritating that it disrupts sleep and may occasionally prompt induction of labour at or near term because of exhaustion. The irritation may be soothed with aloe vera gel after washing, and by wearing snug-fitting cotton clothes. Some women need corticosteroid cream and, in severe cases, oral corticosteroids. HOMEOPATHY can also help.

Prurigo of pregnancy

This is more common in women who have a family predisposition to allergic dermatitis. The skin appears red, is extremely itchy and may form small red dots and nodules that weep. It usually begins in the second half of pregnancy, particularly in the last few weeks, on the limbs and abdomen, usually on stretch marks. It may become worse after birth but clears in one to three months. It does not present any risk and usually responds to antihistamines or prescribed homeopathic treatment.

Papular dermatitis of pregnancy

This is an extremely itchy rash consisting of red, raised spots that look like insect bites and are spread out, occurring all over the body. Some spots may scab over. The spots continue to appear until childbirth when they clear rapidly. Coticosteroid creams can provide relief.

Herpes gestationis

Herpes gestationis is a rare disease that is not related to the HERPES viral infection. It causes pustules that may resemble the blisters of herpes or chickenpox, on the abdomen, arms and legs, and occasionally on the palms of the hands or soles of the feet. It usually responds to corticosteroid treatment. In severe cases, it may lead to fever and need treatment in hospital. Herpes gestationis usually resolves in late pregnancy but may flare up after birth. Babies can be born with this rash, but it usually clears up within a few weeks without treatment.

Infections causing rashes

Fortunately, the majority of rashes are benign and can safely be ignored. Yet when a skin rash appears it is important to exclude infections that may harm your baby by requesting an examination and a blood test.

- Infections that cause rashes and may affect your baby in pregnancy include RUBELLA, TOXOPLASMOSIS, PARVOVIRUS and CYTOMEGALOVIRUS.
- A skin rash in the vaginal area may indicate herpes or CANDIDA.
- After birth, a rash on your nipples may indicate candida, and this can be passed to your baby.

SKIN DISEASES AND PREGNANCY

If you have psoriasis, eczema or a tendency to allergic skin rashes, your problem may improve during pregnancy. Atopic dermatitis, however, may worsen. Some pregnant women develop allergic rashes to food, plants, perfumes or soaps for the first time. If you are a long-term sufferer you will probably be familiar with your sensitivities but these may change in pregnancy. If you do not know what triggers the rash you may consult an allergist or dermatologist.

TREATMENT OF SKIN CONDITIONS

If you have a rash, excessively dry or oily skin, your condition may improve with the following action plan.

Medical care

- Ask your doctor to check the cause of the rash or itching in case it has implications for you or your baby in pregnancy. A clear diagnosis is important.
- If itching is uncomfortable and is interfering with sleep, your doctor may prescribe antihistamine pills.
- If a rash is severe and does not respond to nutritional changes and gentle remedies, it may respond to corticosteroids that are sometimes added to barrier skin creams. There is some absorption into the blood stream but your baby is highly unlikely to be affected if a mild cream is used. For an extreme rash corticosteroid tablets may be recommended by your doctor.

Diet and lifestyle

Focusing on nutrition may improve skin and connective tissue quality. The main elements are antioxidants, essential fatty acids, vitamins and minerals (page 263). Ensure you drink adequate water: six to eight glasses a day. Avoid fried and fatty food and have whole grains and vegetables to provide roughage.

- Try calamine lotion. You can also moisturise with a pure carrier oil (lanolin-free vitamin E or grapeseed, for instance) in a light MASSAGE or in the bath. Use tiny amounts of unscented soaps and bathe once a day.
- Wear loose, preferably cotton clothing and make sure you are not overheated. Use cotton bed linen and try a different washing detergent for your laundry.
- Avoid overheating and drying the air in your house through air-conditioning and central heating: humidifiers often help as does additional ventilation.

Aromatherapy and acupuncture

- Use neroli, tangerine or orange oil in a bath or add to a carrier oil for a light massage. If you have stretch marks, apply the oil three times a day. After Week 24 you may use lavender, frankincense and geranium in low dosage.
- ACUPUNCTURE can help reduce itching or dryness.

Homeopathy

For chronic skin conditions such as eczema it is always best to consult a qualified homeopath. For irritating itching one of the following remedies may bring some relief in 6c potency, morning and night for up to a week:

- *Dolichos* is a specific remedy for itching in pregnancy without visible eruptions when the more you scratch the worse the itch, worse at night and exacerbated by warmth.
- *Arsenicum* for a ticklish, crawling itch that burns after scratching, dry, rough skin that may bleed from excessive scratching, is usually worse at night and better from warmth, and makes you feel restless, anxious and chilly.
- *Sulphur* when your skin feels red, hot and dry and burns after scratching, your whole body feels hot, worse after contact with water, and in bed or after any exertion.

There are also external applications:

- *Calendula* is soothing, used in tincture form by adding 10 drops to a bath or in a prepared cream applied twice a day.
- *Graphites* cream if the skin becomes excessively dry or cracks.
- *Urtica Urens* cream where the itching burns after scratching.
- It is possible to have combination creams made up by the homeopathic pharmacies.

For stretch marks, try *Calc Fluor* 6x (tissue salt) as it helps promote skin elasticity.

Skin-to-skin contact

See *Touch, skin-to-skin contact*.

Slapped cheek disease

See *Parvovirus (slapped cheek disease)*.

Sleep, baby

ADVICE

Sleep is a time for rest, and a time when your baby processes everything he has experienced. It is essential for his physical, emotional and intellectual development. Babies' sleeping habits are one of the most common sources of anxiety for parents, and TIREDNESS is one of the major problems new parents have to learn to cope with – and also aim to minimise.

There is no definitive sleeping pattern since each baby is an individual. Your baby knows when he needs to sleep and has a sleep cycle before birth. Most babies continue this cycle after birth – initially without a day–night rhythm – and adapt gradually. Guiding your baby takes months and it is useful to remember that he also takes months to mature physically to reach a stage when he is able to sleep soundly (and go without food) through the night.

If sleep becomes a problem, often a baby is not sleeping in any way 'abnormally' but the parents' expectations do not match reality. Broken nights are normal, but when parents do not have a chance to rest, either during the day or at night, or

a baby seldom sleeps for long stretches everyone gets tired. Many parents are surprised how much guidance some babies need. For some families, sleep is the most important and stressful issue they face in the first year after birth.

What happens

The different stages of sleep range from deep, dreamless sleep to light, dream (REM) sleep. Once in deep sleep your baby is unlikely to be stirred by noises, lights or movements. After anything from five to 45 minutes he'll surface to light sleep, and may twitch and smile as he dreams. If he's not distracted and still needs to rest, he may fall back into deep sleep. Your own cycle and the time you can spend in deep sleep are longer, usually 90 minutes.

Your baby may open his eyes during REM sleep and appear awake. This is a common reason for parents to say that their baby doesn't sleep well but it is completely normal. If you pick your baby up during this 'eyes open but asleep' state, he will probably become fractious and irritable. If he is left, he may fall back into deep sleep. His sleep pattern might be disturbed by physical sensations, dreams, the need for contact and reassurance, hunger, anxieties and many more issues. His rhythm will change as he grows and in response to what is happening in his life. As he gets older, your baby sleeps for fewer hours in each 24-hour period.

The following sleep entries give guidelines on the very broad range of 'normal' sleeping patterns in the first year, and suggestions that may help your whole family sleep well.

Your influence and expectations

It may be useful to consider your expectations. If they are not appropriate for your child you may feel you are struggling. Yet by simply altering your expectations a problematic situation may be transformed as you accept normality. Parents' expectations often reflect their childhood experiences. Some people think, '*I hated being told when to sleep, so I won't do that to my son*' ... '*Babies need to have 12 hours' sleep a night and that's the way I was brought up*' ... '*I slept through the night by six weeks and something is wrong because my baby isn't ...*'

Sometimes parents unconsciously make it difficult for their baby to sleep. Some people enjoy being with their babies so much, especially the feeling of touch, that they wake their baby too frequently. Most commonly, if parents desperately want their baby to go to sleep their babies may feel their anxiety, making the situation worse. Letting go of anxiety is often the key.

Postnatal depression

It is thought that DEPRESSION and sleeping problems are often closely linked, with tiredness and sleep deprivation contributing to, or exacerbating, depression, and adult depression sometimes contributing to a baby's unsettled sleeping. If you suspect a link, ask for extra help so you can catch up on your sleep. This may begin to alter the pattern.

Action plan

The ideal is to offer infant-led care. This means observing your baby's rhythms, and helping him to sleep soundly. Give yourselves time to settle into family life before aiming for a formal structure. Different patterns of infant care do influence sleep and behaviour, especially in the first month after birth. In societies where co-sleeping, close contact and breastfeeding are more common there is less disturbance in sleep. If you are loving and responsive, your baby will feel secure and you will have guided him well.

Boundaries

Your baby will feel safe and sleep more soundly when he is guided and supported in an age-appropriate way. The boundaries (page 432) you set (such as whether you co-sleep, when and where your baby naps in the day and so on) also need to take account of other family needs. Being loving and consistent requires a commitment to listening to your baby and to your own needs, and to assess and alter your boundaries as your baby grows and his needs change. You and your partner may need to talk about areas where you agree and where you differ.

Homeopathy

In addition to assessing your baby's daytime routine and ensuring that he is getting enough calories from milk and solids during the day, you may want to try one of the following remedies. Sleep, however, is a sensitive area and

depends on many factors including your baby's character, so it is best to consult a qualified homeopath who can consider your unique case.

If your baby is unable to fall asleep easily, you may give the most appropriate remedy (30c potency) in the evening and again on first waking. Try this for three to four nights and then re-assess. If he goes to sleep and then wakes for reasons other than hunger, you may give the most appropriate remedy at the first waking time and if necessary repeat the remedy again if he wakes subsequently. Try this for three to four days and then re-assess. If none of the suggested remedies fits the symptom picture for your baby, visit your homeopath.

- *Aconite* if your baby wakes around midnight seeming scared or anxious or wakes with a fright. During sleep he may be restless and jumpy. *Aconite* is often given to a newborn after a difficult labour.
- *Chamomilla* if your baby wakes frequently between midnight and 2am, seems over-sensitive to everything and is difficult to please, wails pitifully, is irritable and on edge, seems desperately tired but cannot sleep; there is relief from being carried around, but he wakes instantly if you try to put him down.
- *Coffea* for sleeplessness due to over-excitement, for example, if your baby seems hyped up but not miserable, and does not want to miss out on anything, he is hyper-sensitive to noise and in a very alert state. (If you are breastfeeding and drinking a lot of coffee, this may be a good remedy used in conjunction with cutting down your caffeine intake.)
- *Phosphorous* if your baby is easy-going during the day but out of sorts during the evening, is tired but can't let go to fall asleep, or falls asleep and wakes soon after seeming troubled, wants company and likes to be stroked back to sleep. These babies often develop strong imaginations as they grow older and have vivid dreams and nightmares at night. They tend to be very scared of the dark.
- *Pulsatilla* if your baby fears separation, is clingy, dislikes the dark and is restless at night, waking frequently, wanting reassurance and physical contact rather than a feed.
- *Stramoniom* for twitchy babies who have had a difficult labour (either very prolonged or extremely rapid), wake frequently at night in a panic and are jumpy and unsettled.

Safety and positions

Very few babies come to harm in their sleep and you may feel very relaxed that your baby will call out for you if he becomes uncomfortable or too hot or cold. Most parents, though, do have some concerns about the risk of sudden infant death syndrome (SIDS, page 503) and will want to be sure they are doing everything they can to avoid known risk factors.

There are many steps you can take to maximise your baby's safety. The advice below applies if your baby sleeps in a Moses basket or cot. If you sleep together, the safety tips on co-sleeping (below) apply to sharing an adult bed.

- It is safest for your baby to sleep in your room for at least the first six months.
- The current advice is to lay your baby on his back to sleep. This is because research shows there is less risk of SIDS in this position than when lying on the front. Remember that tummy time is vital for normal spine development and it is important to encourage your baby to play on his tummy when he is awake.
- All babies learn to roll when they get older, so your baby may end up on his tummy. By this stage he is able to roll back again if he needs to – he will find his own comfortable position.
- It can be dangerous if your baby's head gets covered in his sleep. Place him with his feet at the foot of the cot, with the bedclothes no higher than his shoulders – in this position he is less likely to wriggle under the covers.
- A baby sleeping suit is a popular alternative to sheets and blankets – if you use one, ensure your baby is not overdressed beneath the suit. Use a lightweight suit without a hood and ensure the neck is the right size so your baby cannot slip inside.
- Do not use a duvet or pillows in your baby's bed. Avoid electric blankets and hot water bottles, and collections of soft toys. Use sheets and blankets.
- Do not put your baby's cot next to a radiator or in direct sunlight.
- The Foundation for the Study of Infant Deaths recommends an optimal room temperature for your sleeping baby of 16–20°C (61–68°F). You may want to use a room thermometer to check.
- Ensure your baby is not overheated. Check his body by looking for sweating or feel his abdomen (not hands or feet, which can be cold when his core temperature is hot). If he is too hot, remove one or more layers of blankets.
- If your baby has a temperature, he needs fewer blankets, not more.
- In a cot, check the gaps between the bars are less than 6.5cm (2½in), and the space between the cot sides and the mattress is no more than 4cm (1½in).
- Do not smoke – or let anyone else smoke – around your baby, day or night.

Sleep, baby
Co-sleeping

For a small baby, sleeping with a loving adult is deeply calming. Among the mammal kingdom, humans are unusual in that they regularly sleep away from their parents, even as newborns. Yet in common with other mammals, human babies have an intense need to be with their mums, and mothers may become very distressed by separation (page 220). A lioness may fiercely protest if she is separated from her newborn cub; a human mother may be very vocal or alternatively may not be outwardly expressive, but inside feel sad and confused. Co-sleeping is one way that humans can feel connected, and protected, from birth. Parents who co-sleep with their babies invariably say they love it. Over 50 per cent of parents of two- to three-year-olds allow a child to sleep in their bed for at least part of the night. In many families, parents and children enjoy sleeping together regularly or from time to time for years. This is true in the west and in many cultures world-wide.

It may be useful for you and your partner to talk about your preferences in advance of birth. If you don't agree, you will have time to explore the options. Your ideas about how and where a baby 'should' sleep may reflect the opinions of your parents and it may take courage to try something different.

Whatever you choose, it is worth remaining flexible. You may plan to have your baby in a nursery but after the birth feel that the natural thing is for you to sleep together. Alternatively you may plan to sleep with your baby but discover that he – and you – sleep better when he is not in your bed. The safest place for a baby to be for the first six months is in his parent's room.

Safety

* Co-sleeping may be safer for a baby than sleeping separately. This is providing you do not smoke and are not under the influence of drugs or alcohol, and avoid the risk of overheating. Your body is acutely tuned into your baby's body signals. Your own body is able to warm up or cool down to create the optimal temperature environment for your baby. You will not roll over and squash your baby.
* You can extend the size by placing an extra bed on the side of your existing bed to accommodate your baby and still ensure a good sleep for all of you.
* Take care not to over-dress your baby or use excessive covering, or overheat the bedroom. Avoid heavy duvets – use sheets and blankets instead. If he gets cold, he will let you know.
* If you have consumed alcohol or taken any drugs that dull your sensory awareness (these may be prescription drugs or recreational) you may put your baby at risk of dangerous smothering or overheating. Do not share a bed in these circumstances.
* Sleeping on a sofa with your baby is never appropriate – you need a large bed to be safe.
* If your baby is ill with a FEVER keep one side of your bed uncovered and cool. This may help keep his temperature down.
* If your baby rolls over you may worry that he'll fall out of bed. A low bed and a spare mattress on the floor minimise the risk of injury. You may choose to sleep on a futon or mattresses on the floor for a while (this makes it easier to extend your bed if you wish to). Ensure your baby cannot slip between the bed and the wall.

Potential advantages of co-sleeping

Baby

* Your baby has minimal separation from mum and dad.
* Being close and smelling and feeling you is lovely for your baby.
* This feels safe, and it is the most natural place to be.
* Your baby knows that mum and/or dad will respond promptly if he calls out.
* Breastfeeding is easy: your baby can learn to feed when he wants yet barely wake you.
* It's easy to fall asleep after a feed.
* Your baby gets all the benefits of skin-to-skin

touch through the night, great for growth and wellbeing (page 517).

Mum and dad

* Many parents say there is little that is as delicious as having the presence of their baby in bed.
* Breastfeeding is easy, with minimal disruption for mum.
* It's easier to sleep deeply in between feeds.
* Closeness minimises separation anxiety (page 220).
* It may be a precious opportunity for dad to be with baby if he is at work most days.

Potential disadvantages of co-sleeping

Baby

* Some babies like to be swaddled and sleep best in their own space, preferably a basket beside the parents' bed.
* Rarely, your baby may be woken by you.
* If your baby is windy or has colicky pains he may need to be rocked and winded after a feed, but it is easy to get out of bed.

Mum and dad

* You both need to sleep. If sharing your bed makes it difficult, work out what suits you best. You may begin the night together and then move to separate beds. On some nights, one of you may sleep with your baby. You may decide to encourage your baby to sleep on his own.
* Your baby may become dependent on you in order to fall asleep. When you wish to help him to fall asleep alone, he may need gentle guidance. You might settle him in your room and join him in bed later.
* Your personal space and intimacy are important and if this is missing because your baby is in bed with you, begin by creating time to be together.
* Many couples make love with their baby sleeping in bed, or in a cot nearby. As a newborn, your baby may already be used to you making love, having experienced it during pregnancy. If sharing your bed is hindering sex, there are daytime opportunities to make love, or do so without your baby in your bed and then welcome him in later.
* Often dad is the one who sleeps in a separate room. This may work well for you all, but

sometimes a dad feels left out. It's worth talking if it happens.

- If one of you has to work the next day, you may use ear plugs or a mask or use another room. You can talk about your boundaries concerning sleep, and when it is appropriate to encourage your baby out of your bed/room.

Baby leaving your bed

When you consider it is time for your baby to leave your bed, it is preferable to do so gradually by creating a safe, secure space for him. Initially this may be a bed or cot in your bedroom, and sleep begins there. If you wish to use another room then create a warm environment and begin by putting your baby to sleep there during the day and gradually begin to do this at night. If your baby objects and you sense he is not ready, simply wait and try later.

When you do make the separation the priority is to listen to your baby, and to let him know what is happening – respecting his needs as well as your own as you set up a new and loving boundary around sleep.

Sleep, baby
Controlled crying

The technique known as 'controlled crying' has been advocated as part of a 'sleep training programme'. In short it involves leaving your baby to cry when it is (in your view) time for sleeping. Many people feel this method is harsh and controlling and will not try it: some parents who try it become upset. There is a balance between the pain of leaving your baby to cry and the projected pay-off of having more sleep at night. Sometimes days or weeks of painful attempts do not produce the desired results – this is not a guaranteed route to peaceful sleeping and some babies respond far better to the security of knowing mum or dad is near at hand.

If you want to try controlled crying, remember to listen to your gut feelings. Separation anxiety is a core emotion for you and for your baby (page 220) and can make you both feel very uncomfortable. Yet this technique may feel appropriate for you and offer your baby and

family comfortable boundaries. If you find a happy balance and can be there for your baby and help him discover it's safe to go to sleep, and you and your partner end up getting more sleep, you have done a good job.

Action plan

Some sleep-training practitioners advocate controlled crying from an early age, even from birth. This is not appropriate – your baby needs time to settle after birth and the most comforting place for him is with you or another adult. As a newborn he needs to fall asleep according to his personal bio-rhythms. Before practising 'controlled crying' think about how your baby feels. If your baby is already fearful or anxious, or seems unwell, do not begin. It is better for him and for you to wait until he seems settled and you feel you understand his range of cries.

If you are ready, you can try leaving your baby in his own room:

- Before leaving your baby in any room, give him time, over a number of days or weeks, to get used to that room and sleeping there.
- Stick to your normal evening pattern, such as bath, massage, feed, then settle your baby safely and comfortably.
- You may want to tell a story or sing before you leave the room. If he falls asleep while you do this, then there's no need to leave him to cry.
- If your baby cries, allow a few minutes for him to fall asleep. You may choose to look and if he's okay, withdraw and give it another few minutes.
- You may need to go in and reassure him. Let him see your face, maybe whisper gently. If he is in a rocking crib, gentle motion may be very soothing. A gentle touch may help.
- Try not to disturb him too much – don't pick him up unless he's very agitated. Don't turn the light on or take him into a brightly lit room.
- You may need to gently reassure him several times before sleep finally comes.
- If your baby wakes and is upset in the night, or finds it difficult to settle after a night-time feed, you may choose to bring him into bed with you where you and he can both drop off to sleep easily. You may find co-sleeping (page 487) is less disruptive for the whole family but this depends on your unique circumstances.

Some babies fall asleep alone after a few nights of controlled crying. Others get more worked up and do not respond. If you feel clear about your aims and you are gentle with your baby and with yourself, and you remain consistent, you both may gradually adapt. Go with your gut instinct – it is not a 'failure' if you pick your baby up. Some parents try controlled crying until they 'know' emotionally it's not for them or their baby.

Controlled crying and being there
It is possible to try 'controlled crying' without leaving your baby. Some parents, particularly those who co-sleep, may choose to lie with their baby while she cries, remaining reassuring and offering soothing comfort. If this is a break from the norm of falling asleep at the breast it may take your baby a few nights to get used to it, gradually crying less each night.

Sleep, baby
Newborn (0–4 weeks)

What's usual?

* It is usual for a newborn baby to sleep between 16 and 19 hours in every 24-hour period.
* Your baby is likely to wake every two to three hours to eat, and may often sleep for less than an hour. Depending on your baby, this may apply equally at night and during the day.
* In the early days, hunger may be the most common reason for your baby to wake up, and because his appetite changes according to his needs, his sleeping pattern may change, too.
* It is normal for newborn babies to fall asleep at the breast. Your breast is a comforting place for your baby to be.
* Your baby may fall asleep in the car. If he is in a car seat take him out when you have finished your journey and lie him flat; this is important for optimal spine development. Many parents find it is most convenient to leave their baby asleep in the car seat when the drive is finished, but regularly sleeping with a slouched and unsupported back is not good for a baby's physical development and should be avoided. This applies throughout childhood.
* In each 24-hour period your baby may have at least one long snooze lasting from two to five

hours. This is often after 10pm. He will also have at least one period when he is particularly alert – this is often early evening or first thing in the morning.
* It is unusual for babies to sleep for more than four or five hours at a time, although some do sleep for longer, maybe for up to eight or 10 hours. This is all right, provided your baby is gaining weight as expected and seems well.
* Many babies fall asleep as and when they need to. But there will be times when your baby finds it difficult to drop off and will need your help to calm down. Signs of tiredness include crying, yawning and drooping eyelids.

What you can do

* Be with your baby.
* This is the babe in arms period and if your baby is held and warm and fed, and feels safe, he continues the pattern of sleep, dreaming and wakeful exploration that he had in the womb. This is most likely to be smooth when mother and baby are together.
* Your baby's body naturally responds to light and dark and to feelings of fullness and hunger with genetic and physiological changes. These contribute to his sleep pattern and he is able to self-regulate effectively if all his needs are met – including his need to be with you. He may appear to notice the difference between night and day – and sleep more at night – within one week, or not until he is four or more weeks old.
* Your baby is likely to sleep more soundly, and disturb you less, if you sleep together in the same bed or in the same room (see page 487).
* Some parents wish to establish a bath and bedtime habit in an attempt to lengthen the first sleep period of the night. The first long sleep is often after 10pm. Other parents refrain from structured routine in this early period and wait a little longer before introducing a bath and so on at the end of the day. Your baby will indicate when he feels relaxed and together you are likely to settle into a rhythm that suits you both.

Causes for concern

Hungry babies tend to wake frequently. This may be misinterpreted as a 'sleep problem' when it is perfectly natural, and just what the baby needs. Watch out for excessive sleeping with associated feeding difficulties. Although these may be two unrelated problems, there is a chance they are linked in some way. The key is to monitor your baby's weight gain, and to ask your health visitor for advice. Some babies, especially those who bottle-feed, will sleep up to six or even eight hours. Some are more sleepy than others in the first weeks after birth. As long as your baby is thriving, this is not a problem. However, if your baby is small it is realistic to expect him to wake more often to feed, and going for longer than five hours is not usual. In that case you may need to wake him for feeds (page 86).

✚ Red flag

If your baby is underweight, PREMATURE, is not gaining weight adequately or is unwell, allow yourself to be led by his feeding requirements and place less emphasis on the timing of sleep. You will be offered advice by the specialists caring for him.

Sleep, baby
4–12 weeks

It is not possible to be prescriptive about how a baby *should* sleep at any particular age. Some time between the age of four weeks and 12 weeks, however, your baby will have grown sufficiently to sleep for more extended periods. This may reflect the fact that he is feeding for longer. If you are breastfeeding, your body will recognise his pattern, delivering milk that has sufficient calories and protein to keep him going for longer.

What's usual?

- It's usual for babies to continue to wake frequently for feeding.
- It's usual for babies to cry when they wake, although if your baby is sleeping in your arms, against your body or in bed with you, he may be much calmer, particularly if your breast is easily available.
- It's usual for the length of sleep at night to increase and for a baby at this stage to spend longer periods of time awake during the day.

- It's usual for a baby to sleep for four to six hours at a stretch at night, and within this time to surface several times from deep sleep into dream or semi-waking state.
- It's usual for a sleep pattern to feel 'settled' for a day or two, maybe even a week, and then alter. Your baby may sleep more during a growth spurt, and will also be easily disturbed by uncomfortable feelings including digestion, pain, anxiety or feelings of isolation, illness and reactions to medical care (such as VACCINATIONS).

What you can do

- Be there for your baby.
- Giving your baby solid food is not a recipe for improved sleep: it may have the opposite effect as your baby isn't ready.
- Even 'topping up' with extra formula milk is not a good idea, though you may hear it recommended. If your baby's growth is on track it is not in his interests to be overfed. A breastfed baby can never be overfed.
- If your baby falls asleep only at your breast, by 12 weeks you may feel it's time to help him reduce the dependence. Try to keep him awake for a full feed then gently take him away from your breast and rock him to sleep in your arms.

There are popular techniques that may encourage your baby to sleep longer at night. For example:

- Babies respond well when the adults around them help them feel safe and relaxed, and a calm atmosphere before bed is often very valuable. The gentle touch of water and hands and the soothing lilt of your voice in a dimly lit room, undistracted by multiple activities, sights, sounds and so on, may help your baby to release physical, mental and emotional tension. A habit of bath time and possibly a MASSAGE then a quiet feed around the same time each night may work well for your baby.
- Take care not to disturb your baby when he's in light sleep.
- Keep your baby's room dark or very dimly lit.
- It may be helpful to ensure your baby takes full feeds in the day (for example, by squeezing the palm of his hand, stroking his cheek or taking his socks off if he dozes early in a feed).
- Play and conversation when he's awake offer an important balance to sleep. Remember that your baby is unique and his needs alter from day to day – too much stimulation (for

example, overwhelmed with new experiences, people, places and feelings) can over-activate his nervous system, making it difficult for him to sleep soundly; too little may leave him with excess energy so that it's hard to relax.

Causes for concern

If you are concerned, the reasons are likely to be similar to those in the first month (page 490). If your baby is happy and gaining weight there is no concern. If your baby seems to be settling into a pattern but it doesn't last, this is normal. Your baby is changing so much each day and his sleep will reflect this.

Sleep, baby
3-6 months

Around the third month, your baby may naturally begin to sleep for longer at night. Ideally he will wake only when he is hungry and you may be able to predict when this will be and ensure you sleep between these times. But he may also wake because he is uncomfortable, wants to be with you or has had a dream.

During the day, you can expect your baby to have fewer short dozes and instead sleep for one, two or three longer periods. It is easier for your baby to fall into this rhythm if there is a typical structure to the day and he feels comfortable and safe. Babies who are constantly on the move from one location to the next, or whose usual rhythm is disrupted (for example, on holiday) often have difficulty sleeping.

Helping your baby sleep at night

Most babies need help to get used to sleeping longer at night. Do what feels comfortable for you. There is no single right way but there is usually a comfortable way where a baby can be helped to sleep better and the whole family, consequently, is more rested. Most babies respond to repeated patterns of activity and rest and having a familiar bedtime may help your baby feel settled. Some of the tips below may be useful now and you might also want to use some of the tips suggested for babies aged over six months (opposite).

Bedtime

Performing a similar set of actions before bed each night that relax your baby allows him to unwind and also gives your baby a sign of what is coming (bedtime). When the habits become familiar (maybe in as little as three days) your baby will recognise them and feel safe. You might want to bathe, massage, feed and dress him, tell stories or sing – anything that is pleasurable and soothing for him.

* Between three and six months is a good period to introduce a bedtime routine. At this age your baby responds well to cues, and is less capable of overcoming the need to sleep than he will be after six months. Bedtime habits established early on may stick for years.
* If you want your baby to go to sleep at 8pm each night but he is usually alert until a 10 o'clock feed, start by making this feed earlier by 15 minutes every other day. You can calm him beforehand with cuddles or a gentle massage.
* Feed him where he will be sleeping. Reduce noise in the house (such as the television, music, other children, chatter), ensure he has a clean nappy and is comfortable, and settle him in your usual way.

Night time

* It is normal for a baby to surface from sleep briefly 10 times at night and he may grumble or briefly open his eyes then go back to sleep.
* Your baby is likely to surface with wide open eyes or a cry when he needs a feed. If he wakes before you expect him to and cries himself back to sleep he will wake again soon, even more hungry. It is best to give him comfort and a feed if he is hungry.
* Some parents gently wake their baby for a feed before they go to sleep around 11pm or midnight in the hope of reducing hunger later in the night. Sometimes this works, and a baby then sleeps for six or seven hours. Some babies cannot rouse themselves to take a full feed, and still wake in the middle of the night.
* If things are going well, remember it's important to remain flexible: if your baby is upset and crying when he 'should' be asleep, he needs you. He is not able to regulate his feelings. If his cries are unanswered he may stop crying out of despair rather than satisfaction. This 'protest-despair' experience is very stressful (page 168).

Daytime sleeping

If, by 14 weeks, your baby wakes more than once between the hours of midnight and 6am and doesn't go back to sleep easily, helping him regulate his sleep during the day may help him sleep better at night.

* If your baby sleeps for two or three hours twice a day, shortening one nap could help him sleep longer at night. As he surfaces from deep sleep gently wake him, perhaps offering the comfort of a feed. See how he reacts.
* If your baby sleeps from 2 to 5pm keep him awake afterwards until bedtime – a feed, a play, a massage and bath and another feed may set him up for a good sleep.
* If he naps between noon and 3pm, let him have a rest around 5pm for about 30 minutes if he's tired, and then work towards bedtime in your usual way.
* If your baby falls asleep outside nap times it's because he needs to – you can alter the rest of the day's structure accordingly. It may be time to review your expectations in response to his new needs. He will have sleepy days and wakeful days and as he grows he'll need less sleep during the day.

Daytime play and feeding

* What your baby does when awake contributes to how he sleeps. Keep daytime active and interesting, with some quiet non-sleeping time.
* Try to keep the last 30–60 minutes before 'bed time' quiet so he doesn't go to bed while his mind is racing.
* Satisfy his thirst and hunger – regular feeds help stabilise energy levels and lead to calmer sleep.
* If your baby is energetic and will not sleep during the day, create two periods of at least 20 minutes, one in the morning and one in the afternoon, when things are quieter than usual. Tidy away toys, put on some relaxing music, give him a massage or take him for a walk. He needs this time to relax, otherwise his body may hold excess energy as tension, making it difficult to relax and sleep.

Comfort objects

Many babies need 'crutches' to help them fall asleep. So do many adults! Some parents worry that their baby needs a particular thing at night but it is entirely normal, as it helps him feel secure. Your baby's reliance on any 'crutches' is one of many boundary issues you will face – at three months it may be fine for him to fall asleep at your breast, and at six months you may not want this to happen regularly. It is best to find a favourite support item that suits both of you.

The advice for helping him sleep without you (page 489) may be useful, and you may encourage him to have a number of comfort objects. Many babies develop a strong attachment to a blanket or teddy, or an item of mum's clothing, or a dummy (page 194). These are all security objects (page 52) and attachment to them is a natural and healthy part of a child's progression towards independence. Giving a baby a dummy at bedtime may help quiet him (page 194), although he may cry later when it falls out of his mouth and he can't get back to sleep by himself. Many babies love to be rocked. Sometimes it is fine to rock, for example, during afternoon naps, and sometimes it is not, for example, in bed with you at night.

Your baby's attachment to a comfort object may not be a problem for you. If so, you will be relaxed and let him separate from it in his own time. If it is causing him to sleep poorly, you may try to replace it with something else (such as a blanket instead of a dummy), and encourage a gentle withdrawal, starting when he naps during the day. Unless there is a persistent problem, though, it is fine for him to be attached to a comfort object – and this will pass in time even without your encouragement.

Sleep, baby
6 months plus

At six months and onwards, babies have a natural tendency to sleep less during the day and more at night. They are also keenly exploring their environment and will be better at fighting tiredness when they think there are other more interesting things to do. This may bring new difficulties.

Between six and nine months of age, an ideal sleeping pattern is 12 hours at night and three hours during the day – divided into two or three naps. While every baby has different tendencies, this total of 15 hours suits most babies well. The exact timings of naps and bedtimes will depend on your lifestyle and your baby.

Even by nine months or later, though, only a minority of parents enjoy uninterrupted nights on a regular basis. You may want to encourage your baby to sleep for longer, and you will no doubt be offered many tips by family and friends. With consistency and persistence, and a willingness to be flexible and try more than one approach to see what works for you, you may all have a full night's sleep regularly. Mums and dads who resolve a night-waking problem often experience positive changes to their energy and feel as if someone has handed them and their family a new lease of life.

If your baby wants to stay awake

The more your baby can move and communicate, the more interesting life becomes and the more boring seclusion and sleep may seem. Some babies make a fuss if they are put in bed when they'd rather be active, even when they are tired. You cannot control how upset or angry your baby gets but he will find it easier to fall asleep if he is not highly agitated.

When you notice your baby is getting tired or you want to begin calming him, let him know. '*I am going to take you to bath/bed/etc. in a few minutes, okay? Let's play for a little bit more before we go.*' Your baby will by now understand a lot of words and his body picks up your intention: advance notice is easier to integrate than sudden change. He is likely to settle more easily if he also has 10–30 minutes of calming down time. You may do this with a bath, a massage, some singing, story telling or a feed. You may also try homeopathy remedies (page 486).

Fear of being alone

Around the age of six to nine months, all babies experience separation anxiety (page 220) with intensity. At this age your baby begins to understand that he is separate from you. If your baby begins to sleep less soundly this may be playing a part.

You cannot tell how long your baby's fear of separation will last until it has passed. You can, though, tell him that you know how he feels. It will probably help to make more time to be with him at moments of separation, including bedtime. This comes as a surprise to many parents who have looked forward to having more time to themselves. You can help your

baby pass through this transition without lasting anxiety by following the tips below.

If your baby won't settle to sleep

Most parents discover that with love, consistency, patience and perseverance their baby wakes less at night and goes to bed with greater ease. Some of the suggestions here may be useful for you. Some will not apply if you are co-sleeping (page 487).

* On the way to bed, follow a similar relaxing set of actions. This may incorporate a bath, massage, and saying good night to other people, or to toys or pictures.
* Spend time holding your baby and focusing on him before you lay him down to rest. A familiar blanket or an item of your clothing may be comforting for him.
* When you put your baby in bed, stroke his head or back, give him a kiss and say good night. You can stay sitting next to him and keep eye contact, letting him know you are there.
* If you leave before he falls asleep, let him know you are going and will be close by.
* If he cries, go to him and let him see you. You may want to touch him and could say, '*I hear you are upset. It is time for sleeping now, I think you're finding it difficult. It's okay.*' If you are committed to sleeping separately, unless he is very distressed it is helpful to resist the urge to pick him up, but remain with him and be reassuring. He needs your help to learn that it is safe to sleep in his own space.
* It is up to you to gauge whether it is comfortable for your baby and for you if he cries for a few minutes without you. Some babies cry for a very short period, as if from frustration and to release a last bit of pent up energy, then fall asleep quickly. Others cry vigorously, find it difficult to calm down without help and prefer to sleep with mum and/or dad. Your baby may show both reactions depending on his feelings from day to day.
* If you leave while your baby is crying, watch the clock and go back to him in three to five minutes. He may fall asleep in this time or he may still be awake and need to see, feel and hear you.
* You might need to go in three or four or more times to settle him. Letting him cry but leaving him alone is part of a controlled crying method that you might want to try. This is explored in more detail on page 489.

Coping with night waking

If your baby wakes occasionally, this may be due to illness, discomfort, overheating or cold, vivid dreams, hunger, or – if you're not at home – an unfamiliar environment. It is likely he will go back to his usual sleep pattern when the disruption is past. If you have recently weaned him, he may be woken by digestion feelings. If he has eaten sugary foods during the day (including fruit juices, pop, sweets, cakes and biscuits) or has a food intolerance, this can stop him sleeping.

If your baby regularly wakes at least once a night, and/or has difficulty falling asleep, he'll need your help. The first step is to tackle any possible cause during the day.

- You may need to wake your baby gently from daytime naps to reduce overall daytime sleep.
- You may need to review daytime feeding times to ensure your baby is getting sufficient calories during the day and reduce hunger at night.
- If your baby is sleeping at night in a cot, either in your room or on his own, you can help him become familiar with it by staying with him as he falls asleep in it for at least one nap during the day.
- Altering pre-bedtime habits may help your baby relax and wind down.
- If daytime is not stimulating or your baby is missing time with mum and/or dad, one of the reasons for waking may be a need for contact. Creating more time to be together during the day may help.

Early mornings

Many babies wake up, joyous and excitable, long before mum and dad want to leave bed. The average wake-up time is 6–7am, with a variation of one to two hours either side.

You may be content to snuggle with your baby and feed him, then doze off together. If you want things to change, you may be able to make a difference, but remember your baby has powerful sleep–wake rhythms and some babies are early wakers. You may try reducing the length and/or number of daytime naps; encouraging him to eat sufficient calories (page 558); and ensuring he gets plenty of physical play and fresh air daily.

You can also make the room darker. Hang thicker curtains or use an extra piece of dark cloth. If there is no light when your baby wakes he may drift back to sleep. You could introduce a clock or light with a timer-switch that gives a sign for morning. Set it to come on at his usual time of waking (say, 6.20am) for two or three days and draw his attention to it. Say: 'Look, the light is on and it's time to get up.' Then set it to come on five or 10 minutes later for the next two days and gradually move the intervals. Your baby may associate the light or noise with waking up and this may help him to sleep for longer in the morning.

Sleep, mother

See also Tiredness, mother.

Getting enough sleep is a basic human need. Many people believe it's essential to have a full eight hours a night but research suggests that five to six hours of restful sleep are sufficient. The best guide is how you feel: quality of sleep is most important.

Your body is flexible and your hormones and nervous energy alter in pregnancy and after birth so you can thrive on shorter stretches. Going into a state of deep relaxation for 10–15 minutes can sometimes be as revitalising as three hours of light sleep.

Sleep is one of the major issues for parents after birth. There are no medals for putting up with too little sleep, however, and it is important to get what you need in whatever way suits your baby and family. You know how being tired affects you. It may make you irritable and can be a factor in anxiety and DEPRESSION. If your tendency is to value action and 'busy-ness' you might find it hard to take time to rest. It really is okay to prioritise sleep so that you can enjoy your life and your family. Once your baby is born, it is normal to be tired and you may become an expert at cat-napping.

Action plan

Sleeping comfortably

- A useful starter is to let go of unrealistic expectations. If you are ready for a broken night, good sleep will be a bonus. It is normal to be tired when you have a baby.

- A supportive comfortable mattress and a well-ventilated room make a huge difference to quality of rest.
- In pregnancy, when sleeping on your side, you can use a pillow under your bump or between your legs. If you have HEARTBURN, try sleeping with your back and head raised on a bank of pillows.
- If the need to pee is waking you, try drinking less after 6pm.
- If you are having vivid or troubling dreams, keeping a dream diary may help you let go of any tension that remains with you.
- There are homeopathic remedies to aid restful sleep (below).
- A slow-burning snack before bed may prevent restlessness from a sugar low in the middle of the night. It is very helpful to avoid alcohol and caffeine or a big high protein meal before sleep.
- Restless legs occur in 15 per cent of pregnancies, mainly in the last six weeks. Tips for easing the disruption are discussed on page 464.
- Try having a bath or shower, followed by a VISUALISATION before bed.
- You may want to sleep separately sometimes, or discover that sleeping together as a family is the most restful option (page 487).
- If your baby's breathing keeps you awake, try using ear plugs or turn down the baby monitor if you are in separate rooms. You will wake when she cries.
- HYPNOTHERAPY is often helpful and you may learn techniques or use a recording to help you sleep and rest.

Daytime tips
- A balance of EXERCISE and rest is optimal.
- YOGA improves the quality of rest and sleep.
- Being peaceful through meditation, visualisation or deep breathing exercises may help. Even five minutes can make a huge difference.
- Eating at regular intervals, avoiding sugar highs and lows, reducing caffeine, and getting sufficient vitamins and minerals will help keep your energy from dipping.
- Get sleep during the day when your baby sleeps. Turn off the phones and pin a note on the door to minimise disturbance.
- Remember to use your network of support. There may be people in your family or community who can stay with your baby while you take a rest.

Winding down at night
MASSAGE can be wonderfully relaxing and energising. Try the essential oils lemon, grapefruit and jasmine combined with a carrier oil for massage or in a bath (page 35). Lemongrass and melissa can lift your energy after birth. To relax before sleep, try lavender (after Week 24) or some tangerine oil, perhaps in a warm bath or for a gentle face massage.

Homeopathy
The following remedies in 30c potency may help. If you have trouble falling asleep, you may take the most indicated remedy and repeat half an hour later if you are still awake. If you have no problem falling asleep, but find that you wake in the middle of the night, then take the most indicated remedy, and if you are still awake, repeat half an hour later. You may try this for three to four nights. If there is no change, you shouldd consult a homeopath.

- *Aconite* for sleeplessness with acute anxiety, with restlessness, nightmares or disturbing dreams; an inability to feel comfortable with much tossing and turning; waking around midnight in a complete panic.
- *Kali Carb* for sleeplessness, often in the third trimester, from an over-active mind and particularly waking between 2am and 4am; often accompanied by backache and night sweats.
- *Coffea* if you are over-excited, nervous, restless and cannot quieten your mind from racing thoughts.
- *Nux Vomica* if you are a light sleeper and any sound disturbs your sleep; you may wake at around 5am or 6am and are unable to continue sleeping; you may feel snappy, irritable and highly strung.

▨ RELAXATION

The advice on POSTURE gives suggestions that will reduce tension and imbalance. You may also wish to try one or both of the following simple exercises to relax. Do not do these if you feel faint.
- Lie on the floor with your head supported on a book to take the pressure off your neck. Place your calves on a low chair or couch until the lower half of your spine is completely flat on the floor. Your thighs should be at right angles to your back, and your calves parallel to the floor. Performing this relaxing posture for 5–20 minutes two or three times a day diminishes backache and headache

and can be deeply energising. Stop if you feel faint or short of breath.

- 'Legs up the wall' is another good method of relaxing and releasing the pressure on your back. Curl in a foetal position, on your side, with your buttocks as close to a wall as possible. Turn gently onto your back, with your legs upright and flat against the wall. Try to get your buttocks as close to the wall as possible and gently let your legs slide open into a comfortable 'V' shape – it needn't be wide, and it must be comfortable. Hold for a few minutes while concentrating on your breathing. Stop if you feel faint.

▓ INSOMNIA

If tiredness or insomnia become a problem, the following additional suggestions may be useful.

- Bear in mind that there may be an underlying medical condition that is causing – or contributing to – your sleep problem. Seek medical help and if a problem is identified, once treatment begins you may notice a considerable improvement.
- If anxiety, stress or depression are affecting your sleeping, you may need support (page 176).
- If your legs twitch or jerk when you lie down to rest, you may be affected by restless leg syndrome. Please see page 464 for advice.
- It is preferable to avoid taking medication, but it may sometimes help. Any sleeping pills or medication need to be prescribed by your doctor. It is important to ensure they know about any other medication you are taking, such as medicines for anxiety and depression.
- Herbal medications can be powerful and it is always best to consult a herbalist before taking any in pregnancy or while BREASTFEEDING.

Smell

See Growth and development, baby, smell.

Smoking

See Drugs, smoking.

Special care baby unit (SCBU) and neonatal intensive care unit (NICU)

See also Premature birth.

About 10 per cent of all babies delivered in the UK each year are admitted to a special care baby unit (SCBU). The majority are born at term and have minor problems. A small number are ill, often premature, and require intensive care. Babies born before Week 35 are generally cared for in a neonatal intensive care unit (NICU). Most babies admitted to the NICU also have low birth weight (less than 2.5kg/5.5lb) and/or a medical condition that requires special care. TWINS, triplets and other multiples are often admitted to the NICU. Babies with medical conditions such as heart problems, infections or birth defects are also cared for in the NICU and there may be an intermediate or continuing care area for babies who are not as sick but do need specialised nursing care.

Larger district hospitals usually have a NICU and can care for the majority of premature babies. Very immature babies, usually under 26 weeks' gestation (development in the womb), may require tertiary – or level three – care with the most sophisticated facilities and highly trained neonatal specialists. If your baby needs to be transferred, he will travel in a portable incubator accompanied by one of the NICU staff.

How you may feel

The emotions of parents whose babies need special care vary widely. While you may feel relieved that the care is available, you may also be frightened and upset. Some parents feel ashamed that their baby is so small and fragile or that they have somehow failed. This loss of self-esteem may be even more pronounced if other members of the family are upset, angry or accuse the mother or father of doing something wrong. You may feel guilty and resort to a string of 'if only's ...' 'If only I had noticed a discharge, if only I did not smoke, if only I had not moved to a new house, if only I had the perfect diet.' This is a very common reaction.

You and your partner will both need support as you go through what is likely to be an emotional and testing period. If your baby becomes very unwell, feeling supported will be even more valuable.

You may believe that you will soon awaken from a bad dream. As the weeks pass the truth dawns and this may be when you and your partner feel low. It is also a time when support diminishes as family and friends become involved in their own lives. You will then need to care for yourselves and one another, and to rely more heavily on your medical team and counsellors.

What happens

Inside the unit

A NICU is usually brightly lit and filled with equipment. There is generally a lot of activity with babies, doctors, nurses and parents all present in the same room.

Babies in the NICU usually wear only a nappy – and sometimes caps to prevent heat loss from their heads. Your baby may have a variety of high-tech attachments. These can be off-putting at first. They may include tubes for feeding, suction to clear the lungs and lines to monitor heart rate, breathing, oxygen and temperature. A 'long' intravenous line may be inserted to allow intravenous nutrition and blood sampling. Phototherapy lights help in the treatment of JAUNDICE.

Depending on your baby's wellbeing he may be with you, held close and skin to skin in 'kangaroo care' for most of the time, or for brief intervals. This is proven to promote growth and health in premature babies and is discussed on page 518.

The medical team

Premature babies need a supportive environment to help them continue to mature and develop as they would in their mother's womb. The role of the team is to provide the best possible environment for your baby. Your baby may be subjected to tests, procedures, noises and lights very different from the warm, dark environment of the womb, and the team will do what they can to provide comfort.

Care involves many aspects: from meeting comfort needs and helping your baby feel secure and develop normal sleep patterns, to decreasing stimulation from noise, lights or procedures and following your baby's individual rhythms so that care can be given when he is awake and least stressed. There have been many advances in

special care, not just in technology and medicine, but also in meeting the emotional and developmental needs of babies. Changes are bringing many benefits, including shorter hospital stays, fewer complications, improved weight gain, better feeding, and enhanced parent/infant bonding.

You may sometimes be confused by conflicting or scientific comments made in good faith by the staff. The best remedy for this is to ask questions – even if you worry that they may be seen as trivial – and ask for regular updates and make notes. You will soon get the hang of SCBU jargon. Feeling supported in difficult circumstances is further explored on page 176. The hospital may provide reading material or a video on neonatal care. Neonatal teams are usually very caring and encouraging when parents wish to be more involved. They will help you to change nappies, and wash and feed your baby while they gently act as supervisors. As your baby's medical needs diminish your mothering role will increase.

Stating your preferences

Your input is very important and you will do your best if you feel comfortable. When you are upset or unsure, try to talk to someone on the unit. It may seem difficult to question or criticise those on whom your baby's life depends, but if you are not happy about some aspect of the care, and you express your concern tactfully, you will fulfil your obligation to your baby. The unit may offer an independent counsellor or parent representative who can help you offer your views to the staff. Most parents get on well with a number of the staff and have an ongoing relationship with some members after discharge.

Your relationship with your baby

Parenting a premature or sick baby is a very stressful experience. Yet relationships and love develop over time and there will be plenty to make up for early separation and concern. Being with your baby, accepting him for who he is, offering love and encouragement, gentle touch and eye contact are all powerful ways to begin bonding while your baby is in hospital.

It may be difficult to allow yourself to fall in love with a tiny baby who requires intensive medical help and who may not survive. In the short term you may find it easier to remain objective and rational. Once you are home, it may be easier to go into your feelings, which could range from shock and fear to anger and guilt. Research suggests that emotional expression helps parents to fully accept the reality and move forward, and to bond with their babies. If you feel supported by your partner, friends, family and the neonatal team then you will have more emotional strength and reserves to be there for your baby.

Being separated

If you are separated from your baby, a picture is helpful. If separation is prolonged and you are in a different hospital your partner may be able to visit and spend time with your baby and then come back and describe everything to you.

Fathers

Fathers are very important but never more so than after a premature birth. As a dad you offer emotional and practical support to the mother and may take on a managerial role while attending to practical details. In the early days you may spend a lot of time visiting your baby. If you cannot get to the unit until after the senior staff have gone home and you wish to discuss things, it will be helpful to arrange to meet them. Some men are devoted and very caring but neglect their own needs. Your strong feelings may or may not be similar to your partner's, and you also need support and gentle encouragement to acknowledge and process your feelings.

Siblings

Your older children may feel very confused. They were expecting a baby and were probably not expecting you to be away for any length of time. It is well worthwhile spending time telling them what happened, however old they are. They will get an idea from the tone of your voice just how you feel. Explain that the new baby needs your attention, a special room and nurses to help him and you do love and adore them. The NICU may let your children visit. Then the nurses can explain to them about all the wires and tubes. It may be possible for an older child to touch their tiny sibling. You may have a present waiting for your older child when they come to visit and something for them to give their brother or sister.

A long hospital stay

Hospitals differ in their policy regarding when babies are able to go home. A baby who is very healthy but small will be discharged at a lower birth weight than a baby who is unwell. Usually babies who have been born prematurely need to weigh over 2,000g (4.4lb) before they can go home, unless receiving 'kangaroo care' (page 518).

Waiting to go home

There are many things that you can do to reduce the waiting time or make it more acceptable.

* Prepare your home for your baby and stock up on clothes and nappies that are the right size. You may place provisional orders to be delivered when your baby returns home. Getting ready in this way is a very optimistic sign.
* Organising your time around your work and commitments to other children is part of a long stay in hospital. You and your partner will need to plan to spend time with your baby individually and as a couple. You may find that in the hustle and bustle of daily life your relationship does not get the attention it deserves. A night out or a quiet evening with a video at home is one way you may try to maintain intimacy (page 471).
* You may both want to spend as much time as possible with your baby, perhaps even moving in to the hospital, and may be welcome to put toys or pictures close to your baby. Try to MASSAGE, 'kangaroo' and stimulate your baby as much as possible.
* If you have decided to breastfeed then you'll need to pump or express milk frequently to maintain your milk supply (page 455).

Coming home

Most pre-term infants, even those with very complicated problems, will go home. The transition may lead to a withdrawal state and anxiety for you and your baby. You will mirror one another: your baby will reflect your mood and anxiety in his behaviour, feeding pattern, cry and overall development, and you will be affected by your baby's mood and rhythms.

Once home, it is important for your baby to be held and carried in a sling with warmth and body contact to make up for the isolation of the incubator. Different babies vary in their response to high-tech treatment. Some take it in their stride, while others show signs of strain by being irritable and CRYING a lot. Massage and cranial OSTEOPATHY combined with lots of contact are a great help. Sharing a bed (page 487) can also be a lovely way to get to know your baby, for him to feel comfortable, and for your family to bond.

Spina bifida and neural-tube defects

Neural-tube defects are serious congenital abnormalities in which the development of the brain and spinal cord is incomplete. The neural tube forms very early on in the life of the foetus and then develops into the brain, spinal cord and vertebral column. If it fails to form properly during the first four weeks of foetal development, this results in varying degrees of permanent damage. The reasons for incorrect formation are not clear. Around one in 1,000 babies are affected by neural-tube defects.

Spina bifida is the most common of the neural-tube defects and also the most frequent disabling birth defect. The other two neural-tube defects are anencephaly and encephalocoele. Anencephaly results in an incomplete skull and underdeveloped brain, and a baby will not survive after birth. Encephalocoele is a hole in the skull through which brain tissue protrudes.

What happens

In spina bifida, the spinal cord is not protected in the bony spinal column. Spina bifida occulta is the mildest form, where one or more vertebrae are malformed but are covered in skin. It affects roughly 5 per cent of people. Most are unaware of it and it causes no problems. In more serious forms, the membranes around the spinal cord or even the cord itself are exposed. This is a meningocoele.

With spina bifida and a meningocoele, there may be nerve damage with either loss of motor power (paralysis) or sensation (numbness). The effect is related to the number of vertebrae involved and the level of the spinal defect and may include bladder and bowel dysfunction, muscle paralysis and orthopaedic problems including spinal curvatures, hip dislocation or club feet (page 143). Some children born with spina bifida

walk without assistance; others need braces and some require a wheelchair.

About 80 per cent with severe defects develop hydrocephalus (page 281), where the cerebral spinal fluid builds up, causing pressure within the brain and an enlarged head, and there may also be learning difficulties. A small number have difficulty feeding and swallowing. Hydrocephalus may occur without spina bifida.

Action plan

Prevention
Folic acid supplements have reduced the incidence of neural tube defects considerably. All women who may become pregnant are urged to take 400mcg of folic acid every day, even if pregnancy is not planned, and to continue to take it in pregnancy. Many breads, flours and breakfast cereals are now being fortified with folic acid. If you have had a previous pregnancy with a neural-tube defect or have spina bifida yourself, you need a higher dose of folic acid (usually 800mcg). It is best to consult your doctor about your personal requirements. Nutritionists believe other vitamins and minerals are also important for normal development and a well-formulated multivitamin and mineral supplement is preferable to folic acid alone. Do not take extra folic acid by taking more multivitamins, though, because some vitamins could be harmful to your baby when taken in excess (page 264).

Antenatal diagnosis and care
Antenatal ultrasound scanning is increasingly accurate in detecting neural-tube defects. Severe defects may show at the 12-week scan. Smaller defects are visible on later scans. The defects are not detected with amniocentesis and CVS. If your baby shows signs of a neural-tube defect, you will need the advice of your obstetrician, paediatrician or genetic counsellor, and considerable support. The medical team will discuss the potential effect on your baby's future and options for surgical treatment. You may elect a termination of pregnancy. Foetal surgery at around Week 25 is still experimental. The long-term benefits are not known and there are risks.

After birth
Babies with spina bifida require extensive health evaluation and treatment. The treatments range

from surgery to ongoing care in a stimulating and loving environment. Babies with open spina bifida usually have surgery within 24–48 hours of birth to repair the skin defect. This reduces the damage, although it frequently cannot prevent some permanent disability. A baby may require multiple operations. Treatment for hydrocephalus, if needed, involves inserting a valve and tube (shunt) into the skull to drain off excess fluid (page 282).

In severe forms of spina bifida, there will be some paralysis below the level of the open spinal cord, and your child may need walking aids, or achieve independent mobility by using a wheelchair. The older child may have problems with bowel and bladder control but modern techniques can usually ensure continence is well managed. This is important both for social reasons and to keep kidneys healthy.

Some children with spina bifida may take longer than average to achieve a sitting balance. Giving your baby adequate support will help him use his hands freely to play. It is also helpful to stimulate your baby by making him aware of the parts of his body that have less feeling, and letting him know when you are going to do things, such as nappy changing, as lower areas of the body are less sensitive to touch. Ask your health visitor about support available in your area, such as a portage scheme (a pre-school home advisory service).

Most children born with spina bifida live well into adulthood and are able to join in normal life. More and more young people with spina bifida are growing up and having families of their own. If hydrocephalus is not present at birth, intelligence is often normal but some children with spina bifida do experience learning problems. The majority of children with spina bifida and hydrocephalus go to mainstream schools, often with extra assistance in the classroom. ASBAH (Association for Spina Bifida and Hydrocephalus) in the UK is a useful resource.

Spiritual life

Some people who have not previously thought of themselves as spiritual may experience a new sense of their own spirit in pregnancy, as if it is awakened by the new life within. Many feel their existing spirituality deepening as pregnancy progresses, and with the experience of meeting their new baby. If your spiritual life is important to you, nourishing this is a central part of caring for yourself and welcoming your baby.

If your life as a parent reduces the time you have 'for you' you may need to be creative to ensure you continue to nourish your spirit. You might ask others to care for your baby while you spend private time in prayer or meditation; you might go to a place of worship or contemplation with your baby.

Aside from dedicated spiritual practice, there are endless opportunities to honour and nourish your spirit, and your baby's, each day. You may feel this as you look into each other's eyes, as your baby smiles or cries, and as you rest together in bed. Your baby will often rest in a state of consciousness that is meditative and peaceful, both when he is awake and when he is drifting into or out of deep sleep. When you are relaxed together you tend to mirror one another, and he may take you with him into a calm and spiritual place.

Squinting

See Eye crossing and squinting, baby.

Sticky eye

See Eye infection and swelling, baby.

Stillbirth

Death of a baby in the womb after Week 24 is called stillbirth. It is a devastating loss, yet it is rare. In the UK fewer than one in 200 (0.5 per cent) babies is stillborn between 24 and 42 weeks. This is a rate that has fluctuated very little in the last 10 years, but has fallen dramatically since the 1950s. Over the previous 50 years, stillbirths declined by over 75 per cent, from around one in 50 in 1950. This dramatic fall is largely due to better attention to nutrition, monitoring in pregnancy, improved diagnosis and treatment of maternal conditions, and drug avoidance.

Sometimes loss can be anticipated. However, 50 per cent of stillbirths happen without warning. Most deaths occur before labour. The loss can be extremely difficult to accept, and the process of coming to terms with the reality may be long. The cause of stillbirth is not always known. Where a cause is found it is most commonly due to developmental problems linked with CONGENITAL ABNORMALITIES (in about 15 per cent), and these are often detected by an ultrasound scan in the second trimester. The chance of a stillbirth is increased in high-risk pregnancies, accounting for about 5 per cent of stillbirths, particularly when there is severe INTRAUTERINE GROWTH RESTRICTION (IUGR).

Even though the population of pregnant women in general is at low risk, individuals may be at higher risk. For example, mothers whose country of birth is outside the UK have 30 per cent higher rates of stillbirth, and multiple births have higher rates. In the UK, about 3 per cent of all births are multiple (TWINS or higher) but account for 11 per cent of stillbirths. Stillbirth rates are higher among babies born before their due date, and lower birth-weight babies.

What happens

The first sign of death is usually an absence of foetal movements. A healthy baby can be expected to move at least 10 times a day either as a single run of 10 kicks or spaced out. During labour the absence of the baby's heartbeat is the diagnostic sign.

Action plan

If you notice a change in your baby's kicking pattern and have felt fewer than 10 movements in 24 hours, contact your midwife or doctor. You will be assessed with an electronic monitor to listen to your baby's heartbeat, which can be confirmed using an ultrasound scan. In most instances decreased movement turns out to be insignificant but it can be an indication of a problem. In rare cases heartbeat is absent and the baby is no longer alive.

If you are told this tragic news, your emotions may range from total shock and numbness to extreme anger or tearful hysteria. Your midwife will be there with you and a doctor will confirm the diagnosis. Most hospitals now have counselling facilities and you may value the support as you decide what to do. As long as your health is not in danger, you can take a day

or two to come to terms with what has happened before you make a decision about whether to induce labour, or to wait for it to come on spontaneously. You may wish to have your baby by CAESAREAN SECTION but a section carries more risks to you, so you will probably be advised to give birth vaginally. Many parents who have experienced a stillbirth feel that the process of giving birth, although extremely difficult, is an important part of grieving.

Most couples choose to have labour induced in hospital. If you prefer to wait, but if labour has not begun after seven days, induction is recommended because there is a small risk of bleeding from a clotting abnormality that can develop after this time.

Labour

Induction of labour is often handled with careful sensitivity and it is helpful to know in advance what level of support you are likely to receive and what pain relief is available. Another couple who have had a similar experience in your hospital may be able to give you valuable advice, and you may ask to talk to the people who will be caring for you. You may choose to have a close friend or family member with you or present nearby.

Early induction of labour may be a slow process because your cervix may not be ripe. Induction (page 374) begins by inserting into your vagina a gel containing prostaglandin that helps to ripen the cervix. This may be followed by an intravenous oxytocin infusion. Labour may be very long and very painful. With the knowledge that your baby will not be alive, your energy may be low and you will need lots of support from your medical team and birth partner. Some women choose to avoid pain relief altogether. Others ask for an epidural.

Stillbirth in labour

If foetal distress and perinatal asphyxia occur (that is, severe lack of oxygen affecting a baby just before, during and after birth), in most instances a baby is delivered safely (page 249). If asphyxia leads to a stillbirth, it comes as a greater shock. You and your partner have to greet and say goodbye to your baby at a time when your hormones and hopes are geared to welcoming. This is confusing as well as upsetting. Asphyxia prior to labour or in labour accounts for under 2 per cent of stillbirths.

After the birth
Most hospitals have bereavement rooms where the parents can remain with their baby after the birth. This time together is an excruciatingly painful yet constructive part of the grieving process. Grief, healing and recovery, plus the practicalities involved when a baby is lost, are covered from page 399.

Stomach pain

See Abdominal pain.

Strep B (GBS)

See Group B Streptococcus.

Stress

See Emotions, stress.

Styes

See Eye infection and swelling, baby.

Sudden infant death syndrome (SIDS) and sudden unexpected death in infancy (SUDI)

See also Loss of a baby; Sleep, baby, advice.

The tragedy of a baby dying suddenly and unexpectedly always presents questions about what might have been the cause. All sudden deaths in infancy are investigated, and about 25–30 per cent will be found to have an underlying cause, usually some form of overwhelming infection or undiagnosed CONGENITAL ABNORMALITY (present before birth). These are classified as SUDI (sudden unexpected death in infancy). Extremely rarely, the cause linked with SUDI may be suspected to be a non-accidental death, in which case a child protection enquiry with police investigation and possible prosecution may occur (page 133). In the remaining 75 per cent of cases no cause is found, and these are certified as SIDS (sudden infant death syndrome), formerly described as cot death. Not all instances of SIDS happen at night or in bed, which is one reason why the term cot death has been replaced. There appears to be no suffering in most cases, and death occurs very rapidly, usually during sleep.

SIDS is the leading incidence of death in infants over one month of age. The next most common occurrence is linked with causes related to congenital abnormalities. The UK rate of SIDS is around one in 1,600. This is three times fewer than 10 years ago, when it was approximately one in 500. In part, this is due to better understanding of the risk factors and how to reduce them by paying more attention to the health of mothers in pregnancy and new approaches to the care of babies after birth. The peak age-related risk period for SIDS is around two to four months. The majority of deaths occur during the winter months (October to April in the Northern Hemisphere).

Risk factors
Researchers believe that SIDS probably has more than one cause, although the final events leading to death appear to be similar in most cases. Recent factors identified as increasing the risk are co-sleeping (in the same bed) if either parent is a smoker or regularly drinks excess alcohol. Co-sleeping without these additional factors is thought to be protective for breastfed babies, and some statistics suggest that co-sleeping with regard for safety may reduce the risk of death by roughly 20 per cent.

The risk reduction as a result of exclusive BREASTFEEDING is also about 20 per cent, and if the two factors are combined the advice is to breastfeed and co-sleep – but only if you do not smoke or drink.

SIDS is about 10 times more common among PREMATURE babies (affecting 1 per cent), among TWINS AND HIGHER MULTIPLES, babies who had severely restricted growth in the womb (page 322), and among boys.

Action plan

In the unlikely and traumatic event of unexpected death, you will find your baby not breathing and lifeless. You and your partner will need a great deal of loving support from your friends and family in the short and long term. There is information on pages 399–403 about practical issues and possible emotions connected with the loss of a baby.

After a sudden death, the responsible authorities, namely health, social and police, will thoroughly investigate. A coroner is responsible for the investigation and a team approach helps to ensure that parents feel well supported. In this way, important information is communicated to the family, and explanations – whenever available – are given.

The investigation is usually done in a very sensitive and caring manner, even though parents and other family members may feel there is an intrusion at a time of grief and vulnerability. Although parents may feel they are under investigation, this is unavoidable if all possible causes of the traumatic event are to be looked into. Usually there will be a home visit, by a paediatrician and a specially trained police officer, and at this visit clothing and bed clothes may be removed for forensic examination.

The coroner may wish to arrange X-rays and post-mortem tests. Your GP, midwife or health visitor might be an important member of your supportive team. After the investigation has been completed, it is likely you will meet the paediatrician and other members of the investigation team, and the findings will be discussed with you, particularly any relevant factors that may help avoid such a tragedy happening again.

If parents feel that they are not being treated with sensitivity, either during an investigation or with follow-up support, they have a right to complain to the team leaders. Such complaints are uncommon and reviews of the team approach since the turn of the 21st century are proving to be especially valuable in identifying the causes of tragic loss, and offering the necessary support.

In the UK, there is a support programme for families expecting another baby following a tragic loss, called the Care of the Next Infant (CONI) project. Your health visitor and other members of your healthcare team may be involved in this.

For a detailed look at ways to grieve and move forward in this time of distress, turn to page 399.

Surgery, homeopathic support

If you or your baby requires surgery you will find details of the procedure and recovery advice under the relevant entry. For support before the operation and to assist healing and recovery, you may wish to use homeopathic remedies. It is always advisable to consult your homeopath prior to surgery, who may suggest giving the following remedies:

* *Aconite* is very useful for fear. One dose (30c) can be used just before surgery to calm yourself and/or your baby.
* *Arnica, Hypericum* and *Calendula* can then be taken together – usually given three times daily for up to five days. Each one supports post-operative healing in a different way.
* *Arnica* (30c) for shock and trauma, and to help reduce inflammation and bruising following surgery.
* *Hypericum* (30c) – the arnica of the nerves – for surgery involving nerve tissue with or without stitching, particularly to feet, hands, eyes, head or teeth.
* *Calendula* (30c) speeds up post-operative healing of wounds and scars.

Depending on the procedure you have undergone, the following may also be useful:
* *Phosphorous* (30c) if a general anaesthetic is used. This is usually given two hourly for up to three doses after surgery.
* *Staphysagria* (30c) heals lacerations and helps with the trauma of an invasive procedure, for instance if a catheter is used. If your baby seems jumpy, you may give this, in addition to the top three remedies, twice a day for up to two days.

Swelling (oedema), mother

See also Bloating and flatulence.

During pregnancy there is an increase in the amount of water in your body. This may cause some swelling (oedema), usually in the lower legs and ankles, wrists and fingers. You might also feel bloated with swelling around your abdomen. The swelling occurs when the extra fluid in your circulation seeps out of the cells and into the tissues. Although it is common and is usually harmless in pregnancy, swelling may be an indication of pre-eclampsia (page 68), particularly if your face is swollen. If your legs are swollen, press the skin over your shin bone. If there is a white, pitted mark that lasts for over 30 seconds, this is oedema.

What happens

Swelling is more common if you are carrying TWINS, are overweight or gain excessive weight or if your family has a tendency to retain fluid. Some women experience massive swelling during normal pregnancy and it settles completely after the birth. It is more likely in hot weather and when you have been standing for a long time. Swelling usually reaches its height at the end of the day and diminishes as you lie in bed at night. The swelling is likely to increase towards term as your baby grows.

Swelling may be associated with varicose veins (page 544). If you feel bloated in your abdominal area this may be connected to wind and flatulence.

After the birth, excess body fluid is naturally excreted in the urine and during this time your legs may swell excessively for two or three days.

+ Red flag

Occasionally swelling may be due to an underlying cause that needs treatment.
* It may be a symptom of pre-eclampsia, particularly if your face becomes puffy. Other signs include high BLOOD PRESSURE, protein in your urine, headaches or ABDOMINAL PAIN.
* A very rare cause of oedema is kidney disease: regular urine testing for protein assesses this.
* If you have notable swelling of one calf, particularly with pain that does not improve with bed rest, this may indicate a deep vein thrombosis (page 545) with a blood clot in the calf vein and you must contact your doctor immediately. Other possible symptoms of DVT include breathlessness.

Action plan

Visit your midwife or doctor if you notice a sudden increase in swelling or facial puffiness because it is important to exclude pre-eclampsia, or if you suspect DVT. Otherwise, there are a number of things you can do to help yourself.

Exercise, yoga and diet
* Exercising improves circulation and redistributes retained fluids – walking is very effective. There are YOGA postures geared towards encouraging circulation in the legs, feet, hands and abdomen; a teacher can advise you.
* As part of a good diet (page 253) exclude added salt and include 1.5–2 litres (6–8 glasses) of water a day (not tea, coffee or fruit juice) to help your kidneys eliminate excess fluid. Some nutritionists advise cutting down wheat and dairy products to decrease fluid retention. Ideally, have a personal assessment.
* Essential fatty acids and fish oils (page 263) may help with oedema.
* Herbs and vegetables known to assist kidney function include celery, dandelion (also available as a tonic in health food shops), nettles and cleavers. Fennel is good for reducing bloating and can be used to add flavour to most dishes, but should not be taken in tonic or concentrated form in pregnancy.

Posture
* When you rest, lie on your left side as often as possible: this enhances kidney function. Try to do this several times a day for 20–30 minutes at a time, as well as at night.
* If your legs are particularly bloated, rest with them raised whenever you can.
* If swelling is marked in your legs you might find support tights comfortable, particularly if you have varicose veins. Make sure they fit properly in late pregnancy.

Homeopathy
You may take the most appropriate remedy in 30c potency three times a day for up to three days and then re-assess.
* *Apis* for oedema in your ankles, feet, hands and fingers when you cannot tolerate heat in any form, your fingers and toes may swell quite severely and you feel stinging or burning in the affected area, worse from

3–5pm and better with cool applications, cool bathing and cool air.

- *Natrum Mur* if there is a feeling of heaviness with swelling that may also be in the legs, you feel restless and want to keep moving the swollen area, you feel worse from heat, but better from rubbing the area and after perspiring.
- *Arsenicum* for oedema in the hands and feet with tingling and burning. Feet may feel a bit numb and swollen, there is restlessness and a desire to move the feet constantly or walk around. You may feel better from keeping warm.

Aromatherapy

Sandalwood, patchouli and, from Week 24, lavender and a low dose of geranium can be helpful in a bath or diluted with a carrier oil and used for MASSAGE.

Symphysis pubis dysfunction

See Back and pelvic pain.

Syphilis

Syphilis is a SEXUALLY TRANSMITTED DISEASE (STD) caused by the bacterium *Treponema pallidum*. Although uncommon, it is highly contagious and tends to occur in epidemics – sometimes large outbreaks – especially among those with multiple sexual partners who do not practise safe sex. Fortunately, syphilis can be treated during pregnancy to reduce the potential risks to mother and baby.

If you are infected in pregnancy and you do not receive treatment, there is a risk of your baby having congenital (present at birth) syphilis. The potential risks can be prevented in up to 75 per cent of women with syphilis in pregnancy when appropriate antibiotic treatment is given. Occasionally, babies of infected mothers may have congenital syphilis infection but no outward signs, and the infection can be successfully treated using antibiotics at birth. Very few babies show any physical signs of syphilis infection, but in rare cases there may be FITS, developmental delay, skin and mouth sores, infected bones, ANAEMIA, JAUNDICE, or a small head (microcephaly). There is also a chance that syphilis may be a cause of stillbirth.

What happens

The primary stage of syphilis infection is usually marked by the appearance of sores (called chancres), which are similar to HERPES sores and last three to six weeks. These sores can sometimes go unnoticed, especially if occurring internally, such as in the vagina or anus. If antibiotics are not administered, the infection progresses to the secondary stage within months, marked by a non-itchy rash, fever, swollen lymph nodes (glands), weight loss and tiredness. Without treatment, the infection progresses in years to the tertiary stage with damage to organs, including the brain and the nerves.

Action plan

Standard blood analyses of pregnant women in the UK test for syphilis. If your test appears positive, you may be offered a second test to verify the result. A single dose of penicillin is enough to treat an infection contracted within the previous year but for long-term infection you will need a course of antibiotic injections. If you are allergic to penicillin, other antibiotics can be used. A low level of antibodies will stay in your blood for years after treatment. There are no over-the-counter treatments. It is sensible to be tested for other infections including CHLAMYDIA, GONORRHOEA and HIV. At birth, a sample of your baby's cord blood may be sent to confirm there is no infection and she may be given follow-up blood tests at one and six months. If infected, she can be successfully treated with antibiotics.

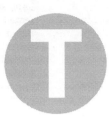

Taste

See Growth and development, baby, taste.

Tay-Sachs disease

See also Antenatal tests.

Tay-Sachs disease is an inherited condition that leads to blindness, seizures, dementia and early death. The first signs usually appear after six months, and the condition then steadily worsens. Tay-Sachs is one of a group of chemical (metabolic) disorders caused by a deficiency in an enzyme that controls the way lipids (fats) are processed by the body, particularly in the brain and the nervous system. Each disease in this group is characterised by a different enzyme deficiency. The deficiencies have major effects on health and development. Tay-Sachs is more common in certain populations, particularly Ashkenazi Jewish families, but can occur in other racial groups.

Tay-Sachs is caused by a recessive gene. This means that if a child inherits the gene from only one parent he will be a carrier and may pass it on when he grows up but will not develop the disease himself. Whether or not one or both parents are carriers can be detected through a blood test taken before or during pregnancy. If both parents are carriers of the gene there is a one in four chance their baby will be affected and a one in two chance he will be a carrier. An amniocentesis or CVS is usually advised to check whether the baby is affected. If the result is positive the parents have the choice of termination of pregnancy.

Unfortunately, there is no treatment for Tay-Sachs, and the effect of the disease is usually very severe. Even with dedicated care, children with Tay-Sachs disease do not usually live beyond the age of four. Advances in treatment mean that stem cell or gene transplants may become an option in the future.

Tears

See Labour and birth, mother, episiotomy and tears.

Teeth and gums, mother

Many women experience oral and dental problems during and after pregnancy. The most common is gum inflammation, or gingivitis. VOMITING from morning sickness may encourage erosion and loss of enamel, but holes occur as a result of poor dental hygiene, not as a result of pregnancy. Mouth ulcers tend to become less common in pregnancy.

◼ GINGIVITIS

Gingivitis causes very red gums that are often swollen, shiny and tender and bleed when brushed or when hard foods are chewed. There may also be bad breath and/or a bad taste in your mouth. Symptoms often begin early, reaching a peak by the eighth month. Hormones and increased blood flow can cause swelling but the main cause of gum disease is the bacteria in dental plaque that settle at the gum line between teeth and gums. Bacteria are likely to build up if you consume high-sugar snacks and drinks and neglect oral hygiene. If your gums are soft because of gingivitis, you may also notice your teeth moving slightly. This usually returns to normal in the postnatal period, provided you brush effectively.

Action plan

It is as important as ever to look after your dental health when you are pregnant, with attention both to oral hygiene and what you eat.

Diet
Sugars are easily fermented and can combine with harmful bacteria in the mouth and the sticky layer of plaque on the teeth. The combination results in the production of acids, which dissolve the minerals in the enamel and dentine of teeth.

- If you eat a sugary snack between meals, always rinse your mouth with water or brush your teeth afterwards. If you feel the need to eat between meals, nibble on raw vegetables or fruits that encourage saliva flow, which helps to balance acid levels in the mouth.
- Avoid sugary drinks, particularly carbonated colas, as well as sweets including minty 'breath fresheners'.
- Avoid smoking, which can cause gum disease.

Dental care
- Continue to care for your teeth by brushing morning and night and regularly flossing. Your dentist can advise on toothbrushes and flossing techniques.
- If you vomit, rinse with a dilute neutral fluoride solution to refresh your mouth and help to re-mineralise the softened tooth tissue. If you brush your teeth afterwards, use a soft toothbrush but don't brush every time you are sick because too much brushing can erode enamel and dentine.
- Visit your dentist twice in pregnancy (be sure to tell your dentist that you are pregnant) and regularly after birth so early signs of gingivitis can be spotted. Your dentist (perhaps with a dental hygienist) may remove plaque to guard against cavities and gum disease.
- If you have cavities, it is safe to have them treated while you are pregnant. The care is generally free to women in the UK during pregnancy. Avoid X-rays if possible, although they are safe provided your abdomen is screened with a lead apron to protect your baby.

It is safe to have a local anaesthetic. The amounts that enter your bloodstream will not affect your baby. Filling material presents no risks to you or your baby.

- If you have pain or infection, ensure that any medications you are given are safe for pregnancy.
- In the third trimester, turn slightly on your side in the dentist's chair so the pressure of your uterus is directed away from the large blood vessels that run along the back of your abdomen.
- If you discover after the birth that you have gingivitis, a programme of three-monthly cleaning and plaque removal combined with a healthy diet and good brushing and flossing can help your gums return to normal.

Homeopathy
The following remedies may help gingivitis. You may try the most indicated remedy three times a day for three days and re-assess.

- *Mercurius* when gums feel soft and spongy; sore to the touch and when eating, and can bleed easily when brushing teeth; there is increased salivation and an unpleasant metallic taste in the mouth.
- *Natrum Mur* when teeth are sensitive to both hot and cold; gums are inflamed and sore and lips feel dry and cracked.
- *Phosphorous* for sore gums that bleed easily and teeth that feel loose or numb.
- *Kreosotum* for inflamed, red – sometimes bluish – gums that bleed on touch; teeth feel painful with increased salivation and a bitter taste in the mouth.
- *Hypercal tincture* used as a mouthwash may help. Ten drops in 250ml (½ pint) boiled, cooled water, rinsed in the mouth three times a day. Do not swallow; merely rinse your mouth.

Teeth, baby

CARE

Even before your baby's teeth push through, they are vulnerable to decay. This is evident if the newly erupted teeth have white, yellow or brown spots that won't brush off.

- Limit – or preferably avoid – sweets and sweet drinks.
- Avoid giving a bottle of juice.

- A bottle of juice or milk given at night may be even more harmful because the liquid pools in the mouth and provides an environment for bacteria to grow.
- Choose sugar-free medicines, as those that contain sugar can encourage decay.
- If your baby enjoys drinking from a cup, perhaps from six months, you could encourage her to let go of the bottle by around 12 months because sucking on a bottle is more likely to encourage tooth decay. (Not all parents or health professionals agree with this approach, however, as some babies benefit enormously from the soothing effect of sucking.)

Once the first teeth appear, you can clean them with a wet cloth, a moistened cotton wool bud or very soft baby toothbrush. Do not use toothpaste – the early days are to get your baby used to a dental care routine with a 'brush' morning and night (the evening clean is most important). Introduce baby toothpaste gradually, in small amounts. The cleaning is essential because whatever your baby eats and drinks, bacterial plaque will continually form on her teeth and needs to be removed.

Fluoride supplementation is recommended from six months onwards in areas where there is not enough fluoride in the water. You can contact your local water board for details about your own tap water and you may want to discuss it with your doctor or dentist – too much fluoride can also be harmful.

▥ INJURY

Injuries to teeth are common and fall into three basic categories:
- A minor fracture is when a small chip breaks off a tooth, is not serious and can wait for dental attention. A larger break needs to be looked at as soon as possible. If a nerve root is exposed it may be very painful.
- A tooth that is loose or pushed out of position (luxation) requires immediate dental care. What may appear to be a loose tooth could possibly be a fracture. An X-ray can assess the true extent of the injury. Loosened teeth need to be stabilised while the socket tightens.
- If a tooth is knocked out, you may be able to save it if you rinse it clean with water and place it back within 30 minutes. This is very

difficult with a young child and the most important thing is to make your way to the dentist. The reason for re-implanting the tooth is in part cosmetic, as the early loss of a tooth may be quite noticeable. However, the presence of the milk tooth, even if not alive, does help guide the permanent tooth into the correct position as it is growing.

Teeth that turn dark after damage are dead because the blood and nerve supply has been severed. Baby teeth that turn grey are usually left alone unless they become infected, in which case a dentist may remove the tooth to prevent the infection from damaging the permanent tooth bud that lies beneath.

Teething

Very few babies are born with any teeth. It is usually two to three months before teething begins and longer before the first tooth appears. Your baby may not complain, although usually teething causes some distress – and sometimes a lot of pain. Teething symptoms commonly include general grumpiness and CRYING, sore ears, dribbling, red cheeks and red gums, waking in the night and fussiness over feeding, and sometimes a NAPPY RASH and even a FEVER. While teething, your baby may coincidentally develop a common illness, such as a cold or cough, so if you are concerned, visit your doctor.

What happens

The gum may appear red and swollen as each tooth emerges. Sometimes your baby may show signs of teething and then calm down without a tooth appearing. This is quite normal. Often the first teeth to appear cause the greatest irritation. Molars may erupt with considerable pain. Baby teeth will all be replaced by adult teeth from the age of six or seven onwards. Your baby's first teeth are likely to appear in the following order, although variation is quite normal.
- From six to 10 months – lower central incisors (front teeth).
- From eight to 13 months – upper central incisors, lateral incisors (either side of the front teeth).
- From 10 to 16 months – lower lateral incisors.
- From 13 to 19 months – first upper and lower molars.

* From 16 to 23 months – upper and lower canines (cuspids).
* From 25 to 33 months – second upper and lower molars.

Action plan

The following remedies may work on occasion, but not necessarily every time.
* Cooled or frozen rubber teething rings can give relief.
* Try rubbing ice on sore gums.
* Teething gel or granules available in chemists may help.
* If your baby is eating finger foods, chewing on a piece of apple, raw carrot, dried fruit or a crust of toast may give some relief.

Homeopathy for teething

For acute teething when your baby is upset by the pain, you may use an appropriate remedy, 30c potency, every two hours for the first six hours and then repeat three times a day for three days – then re-assess. If there is no improvement, consult a qualified homeopath.
* *Chamomilla* is the No.1 remedy if the gums are inflamed, your baby is clearly in pain, is sensitive, irritable, wants something and then refuses it, cannot be pacified, has one flushed cheek and one pale, may be colicky and have watery, greenish stools and is better for being carried and having something in his mouth.
* *Belladonna* for teething accompanied by a fever and distress with symptoms that occur suddenly and intensely, a flushed face, red gums, hot mouth, perhaps ear pain (usually on the right), a hot head and cold feet, worse for sudden movement and bright light.
* *Arnica* for gum inflammation and pain. It may be given in addition to another remedy.
* *Pulsatilla* if teething is accompanied by ear problems, congestion and yellowish mucus with snuffling, crying, clinginess and showing improvement with fresh air.
* *Calc Phos* if the teeth are appearing late, and there may be digestive problems, particularly with wind or diarrhoea. This can be given with another teething remedy in a low (6x) potency six times morning and night for up to two weeks.

While teething, your baby could benefit enormously from constitutional treatment. The immunity gained from you in the womb starts to wane from around six months, while her own immune system begins to strengthen in response to her environment. If her system is stressed by teething she may be more susceptible to other ailments.

Testicles, baby

▓ SWOLLEN (HYDROCOELES)

A hydrocoele is a collection of fluid around the testicle in the scrotum. It affects about 20 per cent of all newborn boys. The swelling is painless and the fluid is usually absorbed.

What happens

Fluid from the baby's abdomen passes through the neck of a balloon-like structure that runs along the spermatic cord and around the testicle. Normally the balloon neck is sealed before birth. If it fails to close, fluid continues to seep through and causes scrotal swelling. If the hydrocoele has a large enough opening, an inguinal HERNIA may also occur. Hydrocoeles are more common among PREMATURE babies.

Action plan

A hydrocoele is normally absorbed within a few months. If not, it usually disappears by the end of the first year. If the swelling grows or does not get smaller with time, an inguinal HERNIA may also be present. Your doctor can do a simple check for this by shining a torch light behind the scrotum. If the beam of light is not visible, a hernia is present. If the scrotum illuminates, then the hydrocoele alone is present. An ultrasound scan confirms the diagnosis. Hydrocoeles only require repair if swelling is still present after two years, which is the case for one in 1,000 boys affected at birth.

▓ TESTICULAR TORSION

Torsion means 'twisting'. Torsion of the testicle is caused by a CONGENITAL ABNORMALITY of the covering of the testicle. This allows the testicle to twist within its sac. It is mainly a problem in boys over seven years old. This twisting can cut off the blood supply to the testis, bringing sudden pain and swelling of the scrotum. It is a surgical emergency.

Torsion of the testis can occur before birth, when it is called neonatal torsion. It is extremely rare and when this happens the testicle needs to be removed surgically. The other testicle will be examined by the surgeon to make sure it will not twist. In boys who are born with only one testicle, the cause is most likely to have been a neonatal torsion, occurring before birth, with the damaged testicle being absorbed.

If torsion of the testicle after birth is suspected, it is important to have exploratory surgery as soon as possible. If the twisting is remedied within six hours of the torsion occurring, there is a 90 per cent chance that the testicle can be salvaged. After this time, the chances that the testicle will survive reduce dramatically and the testicle may need to be removed.

▨ UNDESCENDED (CRYPTORCHIDISM) AND RETRACTILE

A boy's testicles form inside his abdomen. Around Week 36 they descend through the inguinal canal and into the scrotum. One testicle (testis) is normally higher than the other. When a testicle does not move down, it is described as undescended, a condition known as cryptorchidism. Some one in 125 boys has some form of undescended testis and in 15 per cent of these cases both testicles are involved. Premature babies are more likely to be born with cryptorchidism. Most testicles descend spontaneously within nine months of birth.

What happens

Testicles absent from the scrotum may:
* remain in the abdomen (14 per cent),
* remain in the inguinal canal in the groin on the way to the scrotum (85 per cent),
* be completely absent (1 per cent), or
* have disappeared due to the very rare neonatal testicular torsion (opposite).

In boys born with undescended testicles, 50 per cent descend by six weeks after birth, 66 per cent by three months and 75 per cent by nine months of age, all without intervention. After nine months of age it is very rare for the testicle to descend without medical treatment, however,

and so referral to a specialist paediatric surgeon is recommended. If a testicle remains within the abdomen, the higher temperature of the body may inhibit the normal production of sperm and affect future fertility. An undescended testicle is also frequently associated with inguinal hernia, and is more vulnerable to injury.

Retractile testicle

If an undescended testicle is suspected your doctor will first check for a retractile testicle. In cold weather, a testicle that has moved into the scrotum may temporarily get pulled back up into the inguinal canal by the cremaster muscle. This condition requires no treatment because retraction is a normal reflex pattern in response to a cold temperature. It will descend again when the outside temperature is warmer, perhaps when your baby is in a warm bath.

Action plan

All boys have their testicles checked during their neonatal examination and again at six weeks. Premature babies are examined closely when they reach their expected date of delivery, and again every three months.

If one or both of your baby's testicles remain undescended, your baby may be given an ultrasound scan to check the location. You may be advised to wait for a year to see if they descend of their own accord. Be observant for swelling in the groin, which may indicate an inguinal hernia: this needs prompt investigation and treatment.

If there is no descent by the end of the first year, surgery by a paediatric urologist can bring it into the scrotum. The procedure causes little discomfort and most children feel well and resume normal activity within a few hours. Current surgical practice allows some operations to be done by laparoscopic procedures ('keyhole' surgery). If your baby is referred for surgery, do ask the surgeon exactly what procedure will be used.

In extremely rare cases where the testicles are absent, you will be given advice by a paediatric urologist and your baby may be offered hormonal tests and treatments and a sex chromosome analysis. Rarely, absent testes may be part of AMBIGUOUS GENITALIA.

Future testicular health

Boys born with an undescended testicle appear to have an increased risk of infertility. And although testicular tumours are very rare, there is a greater chance of developing testicular cancer if there has been a history of an undescended testicle, even if subsequently brought down into the scrotum. The risks reduce with earlier surgical correction. When your child gets older, let him know that he had an operation to bring his testicle down and that he needs to examine his testicles regularly for lumps or swellings.

Thalassaemia

See Sickle cell disease and thalassaemia.

Thermometers/
taking temperatures

See Fever, baby.

Thrombocytopaenia

See Bleeding and blood-clotting disorders, baby.

Thrush

See Candida (thrush), baby; Candida (thrush), mother.

Thumb sucking

See also Dummies.

Your baby sucks his fists and may suck his thumb or fingers in the womb. Some babies do this so vigorously they are born with sucking blisters on the lips and fingers. Sucking is a reflex action in the first three months of life, and is a natural instinct. After birth half of all babies do suck their thumb or fingers. The habit may persist for years.

What happens

Babies usually suck because it feels nice, physically and emotionally. Sucking is essential to the normal development of the palate and the muscles of the tongue. When your baby sucks his thumb he also presses on his mouth in some way – often the pressure is on the roof of the mouth. Some babies do this as a way of 'balancing' their system: the pressure in the mouth helps to push up their head and has effects throughout the bony system of the jaw and skull. It may be an important way for your baby to ease an imbalance. Another benefit may be to ease a head or ear ache. Once the initial need (to introduce balance, or reduce pain) has passed, the habit of sucking may remain.

Sucking for comfort does not mean your baby is unhappy. There may be occasions, however, when persistent sucking is there to 'fill an emotional hole' if your baby or child feels neglected or upset. It may begin when a sibling arrives, with a house move or something else that disrupts his world, or if he feels unsafe. Again, the habit may persist, either because the emotional insecurity persists, or because a physical habit remains even though feelings of insecurity have passed.

Action plan

Sucking the thumb is not a concern or wrong. It is best to avoid corrective measures, especially in young babies.

If you are concerned about dental development, the best course of action is to visit a specialist paediatric orthodontist if the thumb sucking continues into toddler years or is still present at school entry to discuss precisely what is happening in your baby's mouth and the potential effect of the sucking.

Thyroid function

The thyroid gland in the neck produces thyroid hormones that regulate energy levels and hence control the activity of cells throughout the body. Thyroid hormones also cross the placenta to the baby and so are crucial in early foetal development. Thyroid function is easy to measure with a simple blood test. Rarely, a thyroid disorder in a mother may result in abnormal thyroid function in a baby (opposite). The foetal thyroid begins to function at 12 weeks. Thyroid hormones contain iodine and if there is a deficiency of this mineral in the diet, the gland may enlarge, causing a swelling in the neck. This is called a goitre. Deficiency is rare in Europe because iodine is usually added to salt.

Thyroid, baby

See also Thyroid function.

▨ OVERACTIVITY

An overactive thyroid (hyperthyroidism) in an unborn baby can cause fast heart rates, poor growth and other problems such as swollen throat. The condition is usually caused by maternal thyroid disease, especially Graves' disease, an autoimmune disorder in which the immune system produces antibodies that stimulate excess thyroid hormone production (overleaf). In this condition, the antibodies that make the mother's thyroid overactive pass into the foetal circulation. Untreated maternal hyperthyroidism in pregnancy can lead to hyperthyroidism in an unborn baby. Even if a mother has had her thyroid disease treated, especially by surgical removal and is on thyroid replacement treatment, her baby can still have an overactive thyroid, as the mother's antibodies are still present.

These days this type of complication is rare if the mother's thyroid problem is under the care of a specialist.

Action plan

Thyroid antibodies can be measured in the mother's blood during pregnancy to predict neonatal thyroid overactivity. An ultrasound scan of the thyroid will detect an enlargement.

In general, when a mother has (or has been treated for) hyperthyroidism, a baby's thyroid function will be checked weekly for the first two weeks as symptoms may be delayed for seven to 10 days after birth.

In the rare case that a baby is affected, she may appear small and very active, and may have other typical symptoms such as swelling around the neck – called a goitre – and irritable mood, including difficulty sleeping. If severe, thyroid overactivity may cause failure to thrive, JAUNDICE and a variety of other symptoms including heart failure. The diagnosis depends on the doctor linking the problem with the mother's thyroid problem. An affected baby needs intensive

medications to reduce her thyroid activity. After treatment, the thyroid will return to normal levels of activity, and treatment can be stopped. This may take several months.

▨ UNDERACTIVITY

When your baby has a heel prick test (page 338) in the first week after birth (days six to eight) one of the conditions she will be tested for is congenital hypothyroidism. The disorder results in an underactive thyroid gland so levels of the thyroid hormone, thyroxine, are low. Thyroid hormone is essential for brain and body development and screening is vital because very early treatment of the disorder results in normal development.

Around one in 4,000 Caucasian babies and one in 30,000 non-Caucasian babies is affected in North America and Europe. Among these, some have temporary congenital hypothyroidism, which gives similar early symptoms to the life-long deficiency and requires the same treatment, but only for a few months. This temporary type of hypothyroidism is confined to preterm infants. After the age of two or three years, medication can be reduced to ascertain whether the condition is permanent and, if it is, replacement of the thyroid hormone is then needed for life. Rarely, the thyroid gland is absent.

What happens

In most cases there is no specific reason why the thyroid gland did not develop normally, although occasionally the disorder may be inherited.

Babies with congenital hypothyroidism often appear normal at birth, usually because they have a small amount of functioning thyroid to get them going in the first few weeks, or thyroxine reaches them via the placenta. Some have symptoms such as:

- reluctance to feed,
- jaundice that does not clear,
- a puffy face with a flattened bridge of the nose and occasionally a swollen tongue,
- low muscle tone,
- persistent CONSTIPATION,
- umbilical HERNIA, and
- failure to gain weight.

The long-term effects include impaired learning skills and delayed physical development.

513

If the standard heel prick test shows normal thyroid function, you will probably not be informed. With a positive test result another confirmatory test is usually performed, and your baby may be given an ultrasound scan that examines the state of the thyroid gland.

Action plan

Treatment involves replacement of the missing thyroid hormone in pill form. It is extremely important that these pills be taken because thyroxine is essential for all the body functions and for brain development. Your paediatrician will prescribe a dosage that suits your baby's weight and current thyroid function. The pill can be crushed, then administered in a small amount of water or formula or breast milk. Thyroxine should not be mixed with soya milk formula as this product interferes with its absorption.

With very early replacement of adequate thyroid hormone, every week is important and with follow-up and care the outlook for your baby is excellent. The main problem is remembering to give the treatment every single day – without fail!

Thyroid, mother

See also Thyroid function.

▓ OVERACTIVITY

Around one in 500 pregnant women have an overactive thyroid (thyrotoxicosis/hyperthyroidism). This is most commonly caused by an autoimmune disorder called Graves' disease where the mother's immune system produces antibodies that stimulate thyroid hormone production. A diagnosis is usually made before pregnancy. Signs include swelling in the neck that may be accompanied by swollen, bulging eyes, insomnia, palpitations, feeling anxious and weight loss.

Action plan

- Treatment is with carbimazole tablets that decrease excess thyroid output. It is preferable to begin treatment before conception as this improves fertility and reduces the risk of MISCARRIAGE.

- Sometimes excessive activity is reduced by injecting radioactive iodine, which is taken up by the thyroid. The radiation then destroys the cells. Although a very effective treatment, it should never be given during pregnancy because the baby's thyroid gland could be damaged. Radiation treatment is used only if drug treatment is not successful.
- In pregnant women, propylthiouracil is the safest drug. However, because it can affect the baby's thyroid gland, rarely causing underactivity, it is very important to be monitored closely with blood tests for thyroid function in the mother so the dose can be adjusted.
- Some of the symptoms caused by too much thyroid hormone, such as tremor or palpitations, can be improved by beta-blockers. These are useful to control symptoms rapidly and to enable the dose of propylthiouracil to be reduced.
- Rarely, overactivity in the mother's thyroid can stimulate antibodies that cross the placenta and cause overactivity in the foetal thyroid gland (page 512). This can be checked by measuring levels of TSH receptor antibodies in the mother's blood and measuring the size of the foetal thyroid on ultrasound scan after 32 weeks.

▓ PROBLEMS AFTER PREGNANCY

Within a few months of birth, one in 20 women develop inflammation of the thyroid gland, a condition called postpartum thyroiditis, caused by the production of autoimmune antibodies during pregnancy. The condition is painless and causes little gland enlargement. Thyroid hormone output may rise, causing overactivity that may last weeks or months. Thyroid hormone levels usually return to normal but the problem may be followed by a fall in hormone levels, and underactivity. The symptoms are sometimes missed and mistakenly attributed to lack of sleep, nervousness or postnatal depression.

- Beta-blockers may help if there is overactivity resulting in symptoms such as tremor or palpitations.
- Thyroxin can be used to treat underactivity until normal function returns.
- The condition usually passes within four months but may recur after subsequent pregnancies. Some women develop a permanently underactive thyroid gland.

■ UNDERACTIVITY

About one in 300 women of childbearing age develop an underactive thyroid gland (hypothyroidism). However, this problem often remains undetected because there may be no obvious physical symptoms. An underactive thyroid can cause weight gain, tiredness and depression and may cause infertility and recurrent miscarriage, if untreated. Children born to mothers with severe untreated hypothyroidism during pregnancy score lower on IQ tests than those on thyroid replacement.

The underactivity is usually caused by the development of antibodies against the thyroid gland in a condition called autoimmune thyroiditis (Hashimoto's disease). An overactive thyroid gland may, over time or with surgical or radioactive thyroid treatment, become underactive.

Action plan

If you have been treated for hypothyroidism, the medication dose may be increased during pregnancy according to your needs, determined by thyroid blood tests carried out every two to three months. There are no side effects as long as the proper dose is given. After birth, you will return to the pre-pregnancy dose and your thyroid function will be checked after two months. It is safe and essential to continue taking the medication when BREASTFEEDING.

Time

See Parenting, time and space.

Tiredness, mother

See also Sleep, mother.

The extra demands of pregnancy and altered sleep patterns may make you tired. Once your baby is born and your nights are disrupted it is normal to feel tired. The key then is to increase the quality of your sleep and rest periods, and be patient, because sleep will improve when your baby is older and sleeps for longer. Occasionally, an underlying medical condition, persistent

discomfort or anxiety, leads to low energy, fatigue or insomnia.

What happens

Physical and medical causes

* Hormones alter the metabolism of your body so your sleep patterns will alter in pregnancy.
* In late pregnancy when your uterus is large, you may have difficulty getting comfortable in bed and you may have to pass urine frequently.
* Physically carrying your baby before and after birth may make you tired. If you are fit and well nourished your energy will be higher.
* Symptoms such as nausea and VOMITING, HEARTBURN or chest problems and back or pelvic pain (page 43) may sap your strength. After birth, and maybe before, ANAEMIA or thyroid underactivity (above) reduce energy.
* If labour has been long, tiring and/or traumatic and you have pain it may take days or weeks to feel you have your strength back.

Daily life

* A diet deficient in vitamins and minerals can contribute to low energy, particularly if you consume lots of sugary foods and caffeine that give initial highs followed by lows (page 261). Sugar lows can contribute to nightmares.
* Too little EXERCISE and relaxation may cause insomnia (page 497).
* Your EMOTIONS may be draining. You may feel your energy dip if you are anxious or confused or if there is conflict in any of your relationships.
* If you are feeling low or depressed this will contribute to listlessness and fatigue. Anxiety is a key issue in reducing sleep time. Anxiety and DEPRESSION often co-exist. You may get into a vicious cycle where you become anxious about not sleeping and this may worsen insomnia. Vivid dreams may also make sleep less restful.

Action plan

There are many possible ways to boost and balance your energy. Caring for yourself is always important (page 121), and it helps to accept that life has changed. You will probably find that reducing the number of tasks you set yourself to do each day will help you use your energy well. When you are tired, it is sometimes useful to move about and exercise (page 226) or get some fresh air – sometimes what you need is to rest. Getting a balance will help you feel good. You have cycles and your circulation, brain waves and nervous energy periodically slow down. This is roughly every 90 minutes but alters depending on what's happening in your life. Your baby displays his own rhythms and shows you how it is possible to totally let go. If you are very busy, even five minutes of relaxation makes a difference. Here are some tips to help you unwind:

- Sitting with your back well supported or lying flat on a rug or mat on the floor when your body is fully supported is restful.
- You could use yoga and breathing to deepen relaxation of all your muscles.
- Music or a relaxation tape, possibly after a bath, may be very soothing.
- A very restful technique is to lie flat on your back on the floor, with your calves resting on a chair, at right angles to your thighs. If this makes you breathless in late pregnancy, do not use this posture. You can do this after birth with your baby resting on your chest.
- If you find it impossible to relax, you may need to release emotional tension, perhaps with guidance from a psychotherapist or with ACUPUNCTURE, OSTEOPATHY, REFLEXOLOGY or massage.

If you are constantly tired, and particularly if you're having difficulty sleeping at night, some of the suggestions for addressing insomnia on page 497 may be helpful.

Homeopathy

If you need an energy pick up, you may select from the following remedies. You may take the remedy in 30c potency three times a day for five to seven days, and then re-assess.

- *Kali Phos* if you feel overloaded and stressed, irritable, weak and forgetful and perhaps have backache.
- *Phosphoric Acid* if you feel absolutely exhausted and overwhelmed, want to be alone, when even talking involves too much effort and you crave refreshing drinks and fruit.
- *Gelsemium* when you feel physically and emotionally weak, and drowsy with muscular

weakness, particularly after being ill with a virus.
- *Sepia* when you feel shattered on all levels, moody, snappy and irritable, although indifferent emotionally to those closest to you, despite the fatigue, and vigorous exercise makes you feel better.

Tongue tie

The tongue is connected to the floor of the mouth by a band of tissue called the frenulum. When babies are born, the frenulum extends towards the tip of the tongue. As baby and tongue grow, the frenulum retreats, allowing further extension of the tongue out of the mouth.

Tongue tie (ankyloglossia) occurs when the tongue is anchored firmly to the base of the mouth. Because the frenulum tends to naturally retreat after birth, this seldom causes a problem. In a small number of babies it may interfere with feeding, or the anchoring may persist, in which case it is helpful to cut the frenulum.

What happens

If your baby has tongue tie, he may not experience any difficulties, and the anchoring may gradually loosen. Tongue tie may, however, make it difficult for him to latch on well, and he may compress your nipple (instead of the areola around it), which will be uncomfortable for you, and does not encourage plentiful milk flow. If the sucking position continues, your baby may not get sufficient milk and there is a risk of nipple trauma and MASTITIS for you. Some babies with tongue tie also find it difficult to bottle-feed.

Action plan

Tongue tie may be obvious, and a midwife or paediatrician may spot it soon after your baby's birth. Alternatively, you may become concerned because your baby has difficulty feeding. Tongue tie is an unusual cause of feeding difficulties (page 83), but if it is the root cause, it can be easily treated. A quick procedure to cut the frenulum may be recommended. This must always be done by a surgeon experienced in the procedure for the best results and lowest risk to the baby.

- A trained health professional will wrap your baby in a towel, divide the tongue-tie with sterile scissors and bring him back to you quickly so that you can feed him. The procedure takes roughly one minute.
- If this is done before your baby is eight months old, it is done without a general anaesthetic. Most doctors believe the procedure is relatively pain free. Some babies sleep through the cutting. Sometimes a baby cries, but usually for under a minute. Holding your baby closely and feeding him straight afterwards is a good way to soothe him. There are other tips for relieving pain on page 408.
- After cutting, a few drops of blood are normal. The bleeding will stop quickly, except in unusual circumstances where a baby has a blood clotting abnormality (page 56). A white patch may develop under your baby's tongue, and take 24–48 hours to heal.

If your baby has tongue tie but is not having any difficulty feeding, your doctor may take a wait-and-see approach. As your baby grows his tongue may separate from the floor of his mouth, so there are no long-term problems. If the tongue tie does not improve, your baby may have difficulty with eating solid food. When children start dating as teenagers, tongue tie may become an issue. Surgical correction can be done in older children or teenagers, when it is carried out under anaesthetic.

Torticollis (wry neck)

See Wry neck.

Touch, skin-to-skin contact

Being held against your skin is the natural habitat for your newborn baby. It offers warmth, security and love, and reduces feelings of separation and discomfort. Most hospitals now follow 'best practice', which involves handing a newborn baby to her mother as soon as possible after birth so they can rest together skin to skin.

It is universally recognised that a baby's health and wellbeing, and the bond between mother and baby, are enhanced by close contact. Being close is a basic need for your baby and for you. Most parents say it is exquisite to feel their baby snuggled on their chest.

The first hour after birth is an important period but touch is always important. Touch is part of BREASTFEEDING, and you may want to hold or rest with your baby at other times. In many families the pleasure of being close continues for years, through cuddles, sleeping in the same bed (page 487), bathing and swimming together, and MASSAGE. The benefits are always there.

■ BENEFITS FROM BIRTH

Immediately after birth your baby is vulnerable. She needs to feel warm and protected. Keep your baby with you unless advised otherwise for medical reasons. If medical care is needed, come together as soon as you can. Being touched and held after birth provides warmth and security and is an apt replacement for the feeling of being in the womb. This is a lovely way to enter the world and feel welcomed while experiencing first new contact with mum, and many new sounds, sights and smells. A baby who is separated from her mum may become very stressed, and the stress hormones (page 310) can reduce temperature, increase heartbeat, interfere with regular breathing and hinder feeding, as well as other effects.

Skin-to-skin touch has been proven to:
- Regulate breathing rhythm, improve oxygen intake, and reduce periods of irregular breathing or apnoea (page 102).
- Regulate body temperature (your body temperature can rise or fall by a whole degree or more to warm or cool your baby optimally).
- Regulate heartbeat.
- Reduce anxiety (it may lower stress hormone levels as much as tenfold).
- Reduce pain.
- Boost circulation of love hormones (see page 307), helping you and baby feel good.
- Reduce CRYING.
- Improve bonding between mother and baby.
- Improve bonding between father and baby.
- Assist successful breastfeeding.
- Improve mother's mood and wellbeing, reducing the risk of DEPRESSION.

Skin-to-skin contact can greatly improve growth, development and health and is increasingly recommended for PREMATURE babies. Kangaroo care (below) is an extension of this approach and ensures babies are in touch with mum (or dad) for as long as possible.

In bed

At night, if you sleep together (page 487) you and your baby will continue to feel the benefits of being close. It is very easy to put a nappy on your baby and then for her to be skin to skin with you or your partner in bed.

With massage

You may know how delicious it is to MASSAGE and be massaged. Alternatively, having a baby may be your first opportunity to experience this. There is guidance on massage on page 404.

■ KANGAROO CARE

You may wish to spend many hours in skin-to-skin contact with your baby. In the early days you may lie together in bed. If you want to keep your baby with you when you are dressed you can kangaroo. Kangaroo care is a practice that originated in Colombia in the late 1970s and has been adopted worldwide because of the advantages for premature babies. It is also good for full-term babies. Kangaroo care means securing your baby skin to skin against your chest. Babies that 'kangaroo' appear more relaxed and content. Kangaroo care also helps parents feel close to their baby, and gives them confidence in their ability to meet their baby's needs. Mothers who 'kangaroo' show improved breast milk production.

You may want to try it. You could use a boob tube, as long as this feels secure, with a wrap around cardigan or shirt on top of this; or there are purpose made wraps. Your baby needs to be held securely between your breasts, her tummy against your chest and her arms spread out. Her head will rest to one side and you can ensure her nose is clear so it is easy for her to breathe. The wrap or boob tube needs to cover her back and hold her safely. To ensure you are doing it right, so your baby is safe and you do not feel strain, it is best to talk to a professional – a neonatal nurse or your health visitor may help you – and there are tips on the internet.

Kangaroo care can continue for as long as you both enjoy it. Carrying your baby in a papoose or sling, with clothes on, is a good second best because your baby can still smell you, feel your heartbeat and movements, hear your voice and breathing, and know she is safe.

For babies needing special care

If your baby requires special care and is well enough to be held kangaroo style, your own body is capable of naturally providing a more supportive environment than an incubator. It is possible to hold your baby when you sit, stand, rest, sleep or walk, even if she is on a fluid drip. If your baby's need for care means she must be in an incubator all the time, being touched by you offers many benefits, and is an important way to help her feel loved and for the bond between you to develop.

Toxoplasmosis

Toxoplasmosis is an infection caused by the microscopic parasite *Toxoplasma gondii*. It is most likely that you acquired the infection in childhood and are now immune. Very few women are not immune and only one in 500 has the infection in pregnancy. In these rare situations infection may lead to serious health complications for a baby. A small number of babies are born with toxoplasmosis (congenital toxoplasmosis). The impact varies widely, and over half of the babies infected have no symptoms. Another third have a mild form of the disease. Roughly 10 per cent of infected babies have a severe form, which may cause blindness, mental retardation or even death. It is important to follow strict hygiene measures during pregnancy to eliminate any risk.

What happens

Infection may not cause symptoms in adults. In some people it causes flu-like symptoms including sore throat, aching muscles, swollen lymph nodes (glands) and tiredness. The infective parasite is found in many animals, but cats are the only animals to pass the infective forms through their faeces, and kittens are more likely to carry the parasites than are older cats. If you have lived with cats before becoming pregnant, you may have contracted toxoplasmosis and developed immunity. Grass-eating animals acquire toxoplasmosis by ingesting soil where infected cat faeces have been present, and the parasite forms cysts in the muscles. These can then be passed on to humans in meat products that have not been well-cooked. The parasite may also be passed on to humans from handling infected soil, and through eating unwashed fruit and vegetables that have been in contact with infected soil.

Infection in pregnancy

Women who are first exposed to the parasite more than three months before becoming pregnant will not infect their babies. If you become infected in the first three months of pregnancy, there is a risk of around 45 per cent that your baby will be infected. The infection is likely to be mild but there is a small chance of MISCARRIAGE or stillbirth, and a higher chance (around 30 per cent) of damage to your baby's eyes and/or brain. If you are infected in the last three months, your baby is much less likely to contract the disease. Signs of the disease may not be present at birth, but may appear later.

Action plan

Even though the risks are low it is essential to take precautions to prevent toxoplasmosis.

Precautions

Cats often use gardens and sandboxes as litter boxes, and can pass the Toxoplasma parasite in their faeces. If possible, delegate jobs such as gardening or cleaning out cat litter trays to someone else during the time you are most at risk. Otherwise, follow these precautions:
- Wear gloves when gardening or doing any task that involves handling soil.
- Wear latex gloves when touching raw meat.
- Wash your hands well if you touch raw meat, after gardening and before preparing or eating food.
- Thoroughly wash salads, fruit and vegetables and ensure all meat products are well cooked.
- If you have cats or are in contact with cats, feed them dry or canned cat food.
- Avoid handling stray cats or kittens.
- If you have a litter box, wear gloves and clean the litter box every day to get rid of any parasites before they become infectious. Wash

your hands well afterwards. Alternatively, someone else can do this.

Diagnosis

You may want to consider having a blood test for Toxoplasma. This is not routine in the UK, so you need to request it. This may be a wise precaution, especially if you have contact with cats or garden regularly. A specific test can detect antibodies. IgM antibodies are produced in large numbers during the initial infection. IgG antibodies appear later to confer longer-lasting immunity. Therefore the presence of IgG antibodies denotes an old infection and no risk to your baby, whereas IgM denotes a new infection with the associated risks. As time passes, levels of IgM diminish and levels of IgG rise. Blood samples may be repeated in two to four weeks to assess any change in antibody levels. This allows accurate dating of the initial infection and your doctor can predict the risk to your baby in this pregnancy.

If your doctor predicts a high likelihood that your baby is affected, you may be referred to a specialist centre for ultrasound scanning and possibly foetal blood sampling. Drug treatments in pregnancy may reduce the effects of the disease but they are not completely effective in treating an unborn infected baby, and do have side effects. If your baby is diagnosed with the infection you will be offered advice and counselling as you consider the options for treatment and future implications.

Transfusion

See Blood transfusion, mother.

Travel in pregnancy

Many women travel in pregnancy without problems. While you are pregnant the main things to consider are: your comfort, your baby's health and the stage of your pregnancy. Against this you'll also need to consider any particular healthcare you require. If you are on holiday, taking time off may be so relaxing that many unpleasant symptoms disappear. Remember, though, that your energy is needed to nurture your body and your growing baby, so don't overdo it.

When to call a doctor

If you are away from home and you experience any symptoms that concern you, consult a doctor immediately. These include BLEEDING, abdominal cramps, contractions, ruptured membranes, excessive leg swelling or headaches.

When is the best time to travel?

The best time to travel is probably around the middle three months of your pregnancy (second trimester) when you are likely to begin to feel more lively and there is usually less need of medical care.

* *First trimester.* Whether travelling by car, train or aeroplane, you may experience difficulties such as nausea, perhaps with VOMITING, and fatigue. Travel wristbands based on ACUPUNCTURE can alleviate nausea, and plenty of rest and relaxation is the first step to take if you have TIREDNESS and low energy.
* *Second trimester.* This is the best time to make a long journey. The risk of MISCARRIAGE greatly reduces after Week 12 and the risk of premature labour remains low unless you have a past history.
* *Third trimester.* You may choose to stay at home or within easy reach of your surgery or hospital. From Week 32 your antenatal appointments will become more closely spaced. You may not be able to fly from Week 34 and insurance companies may not provide cover.

When travel is not recommended

It is always best to consult your doctor if you are travelling far from medical facilities. Your doctor will be able to assess the risks, recommend precautions and advise you of any reasons to avoid travel. You may be advised against travel if you:

* Have a history of recurrent miscarriage (this risk reduces after Week 12).
* Have cervical incompetence – see page 127 (do not travel until the stitch is safely in).
* Have a history of premature labour or premature rupture of membranes (page 391). (Travel is inadvisable after Week 27.)

* Have placenta praevia (page 442) or a baby with INTRAUTERINE GROWTH RESTRICTION (IUGR).
* Are carrying more than one baby.
* Have pre-eclampsia (page 68) or DIABETES, unless it is well controlled, or another health condition that requires frequent medication or observation.
* Have severe ANAEMIA and plan to fly (your baby may receive less oxygen than she needs).

Where it's not advisable to go

* High altitudes – above 2,000m (6,500ft).
* Areas with ongoing outbreaks of life-threatening food- or insect-borne infections, especially where chloroquine-resistant Plasmodium falciparum malaria is endemic.
* Areas where live-virus vaccines are recommended (opposite).
* Areas that are excessively hot, unless you are able to acclimatise gradually and you increase your fluid and salt intake accordingly.

What to take with you

* Your medical notes.
* Your doctor's phone number.
* Plenty of healthy snacks and fresh water to drink, to keep up your energy levels on the journey.
* An extra cushion for comfort, particularly after Week 20.
* Light, loose-fitting clothes (you may feel warmer than usual) and comfortable shoes that allow your feet to expand if you are flying or stay seated for long periods.
* Support stockings if you have any swelling or prominent veins in your legs. They are recommended for everyone to prevent deep vein thrombosis (page 545) and swelling during flying or long car journeys.

Your travel medical kit

Some additions to your everyday first-aid kit might include:

* Pregnancy multivitamins and minerals, especially folic acid tablets.
* Oral rehydration powder, in case of DIARRHOEA.
* Anti-fungal cream and pessaries to treat vaginal CANDIDA.
* Antibiotics that are safe for pregnancy in the event of diarrhoea or a chest infection. Ask your doctor for a prescription.
* Insect repellent that is preferably free of DEET (diethyltoluamide) or contains only a low percentage (10–35 per cent). The chemical is

absorbed by your skin and may, in theory, affect your baby. You can spray it on clothing rather than directly on your skin. There are a number of herbal repellents available, but these too need to be cleared for safe use in pregnancy. A mosquito net is useful (and may be essential, depending on the area) at night.

* Sunscreen with a high sun-protection factor.
* In the third trimester, you may want to take urine dipsticks so you can check for protein to rule out pre-eclampsia.
* A HOMEOPATHY travel kit advised by your homeopath.

Travelling by car
When you travel by car, always wear a seatbelt. As your abdomen grows, fix the lap section of the belt across your pelvis beneath – not over – your abdomen, with the other strap passing over one shoulder, between your breasts and around the side of your bump. If there are air bags fitted, move your seat back as far as is comfortable when you are in the passenger seat. In the event of an accident, be examined urgently. Use support stockings for long trips.

Travelling by plane
Commercial air travel poses no special risks to a healthy pregnant woman or her baby. Each airline has its own policy, so it is best to check when booking. You may need to carry documentation stating your expected date of delivery. Domestic travel may be permitted until Week 36, while international travel is commonly not allowed beyond Weeks 32–34. Flying does not bring on labour but there are practical difficulties involved if a woman goes into labour on a plane.

Air pressure and oxygen: It is not safe in pregnancy to fly in an unpressurised cabin, but on commercial planes the cabin pressures are safe. The amount of oxygen in the atmosphere is lower than on land but your baby experiences an even smaller drop than you do. The effect is insignificant unless you have anaemia. If you take a small unpressurised aircraft on a short flight of under one hour it is safe.

Metal detectors and radiation: Security checks, which may involve a magnetic field, do not present any risk. Cosmic radiation is known to increase at altitude and the effect is related to the time in the air. Exposure is unlikely to pose any risk to your developing baby if you fly just once or twice.

Keeping hydrated: The main risk associated with air travel is dehydration, because of low humidity. Drink plenty of water at regular intervals – 1 litre (2 pints) for every two to three hours' flying – and eat healthy snacks to maintain your energy levels.

Movement: Walking around, up and down the aisle, every two hours or so will help keep your circulation moving, reduce swelling, stiffness and cramp, and reduce the risk of deep vein thrombosis. If there's room, stretch your arms and tense and relax the muscles in your legs for a few minutes.

Where to sit: You may be able to book a seat with more leg room.

Preventing deep vein thrombosis: You are advised to wear support tights for any flight longer than four hours, drink water and avoid alcohol, and move around the cabin every two to three hours. Consider taking a low-dose aspirin (75mg) before the flight to thin the blood (page 409).

Vaccinations for international destinations
If you plan to travel to an area where immunisation is advised, you will need to consult your doctor, perhaps in conjunction with a travel health clinic or centre for tropical diseases. Some vaccines use a live, attenuated (weakened) virus and/or bacterium and there is a theoretical risk that a mother could become infected and pass the infection to her baby, and this could carry a risk of developmental damage. Thus live vaccines are best avoided, especially during the first trimester while your baby's organs are developing. It is also best to avoid them in the three months prior to conception.

While you are away
* Find out the address and contact numbers of local doctors.
* Do not drink water unless you know it is safe. Choose filtered and boiled or bottled water (check the seal is intact). In pregnancy, using an iodine purification system is not recommended. Avoid ice and ice-based drinks.
* Eat only food that has been well cooked and is served piping hot to the table. Avoid: cold or lukewarm food that has been exposed to air,

salads if local water quality is dubious and unpasteurised milk.

- If you suffer from diarrhoea, guard against dehydration by drinking adequate clean water with medically prepared rehydration solution. Well boiled, cooled water should be safe. Rice milk is an effective substitute. You can take a stool sample to a health clinic or hospital for analysis.

- If you travel to a country where malaria is endemic, aim to keep risks to a minimum. Try not to go out of doors between dusk and dawn, especially if you are near a river or swamp. When you do go out, wear long sleeves, trousers and socks and a hat. Sleep under a mosquito net and use measures such as insect repellent and mosquito coils. Discuss malarial prophylactics with your doctor.

- There are many insect-borne diseases that may harm you and your unborn baby. Not all occur in tropical countries. West nile virus, for example, is endemic to large parts of the USA and Canada. Always check the disease status of any country you are planning to visit well in advance of travel. Travel health clinics and many airline websites have regularly updated travel health information.

Travel with your baby

See also Travel in pregnancy.

If you travel with your baby you may have many enjoyable times. There may also be times when you feel stressed and tired – travelling with a baby can be demanding. It's worth planning ahead and adapting where necessary so that your travelling time, as well as the time you spend in your chosen destination, is as relaxing as possible. If possible, travel with your partner, or a friend or relative.

For advice on specific destinations it is important to consult your doctor about any potential hazards and health risks, bearing in mind that while some are well-known (such as Malaria in India) there are others that fewer people are aware of (such as west nile fever in North America). It's also essential to talk to the travel company/hotel operator about family-friendly facilities. Going to places unsuitable for babies, and/or where everyone else is single and adult, tends to be doubly stressful.

Within sensible limits, most travel is possible with a young baby, from car trips and train journeys to transatlantic flights and some adventure holidays. There are a number of specialist holiday companies for families. Insurance is important. Check the policy closely, paying careful attention to medical cover both for you and for your baby.

■ CAR SEATS

Always use an approved car seat for your baby, but never put it in a seat where there is an airbag. Make sure the straps fit snugly so that neither your baby nor the seat can move more than two finger widths. When he is very small, if he slips down in the seat, place a rolled up cloth between his nappy and the strap that passes through his legs.

■ TRAVELLING ABROAD

It is best to avoid travel to areas where malaria and other illnesses are a risk as infections can present very significant dangers to babies. If you do choose to travel to a region where malaria prophylaxis and vaccinations are needed, appropriate up-to-date and expert advice must be sought prior to departure. If you are BREASTFEEDING, your own medication will not pass to your baby in the milk. He needs his own protection. When you arrive at your destination, or prior to arrival, it is useful to gather contacts for medical advice and facilities, should you need them. While you are away, be as meticulous about hygiene as you would be in pregnancy.

When to call a doctor

Some babies adjust to travelling easily. Some find it unsettling. While you may take this into account if your baby doesn't appear his normal self, it's worth getting prompt medical attention if you are at all concerned. This applies particularly if you are in a country where there are contagious diseases and you are not familiar with the symptoms.

Your medical kit

A medical kit is an essential piece of travelling equipment. In addition to general FIRST-AID remedies, you may want to pack the following:

* Barrier cream – your baby may become hot or slightly dehydrated, both of which may lead to nappy rash.
* High-protection sun block formulated for babies.
* Insect repellent specially formulated for babies – plus mosquito netting impregnated with permethrine if you are in a mosquito environment.
* Oral rehydration powders in case you or your baby gets DIARRHOEA.
* HOMEOPATHIC remedies recommended by your homeopath.

Travelling by plane

It is inadvisable to take your baby on a plane before he is two weeks old if born at term, or two weeks after his due date if premature. Ideally, your baby should be at least two to three months old before he flies. By then, his immune system will be stronger and better able to resist infection, you'll have settled into a routine, and by this time you may both be comfortable with breast- or bottle-feeding.

The biggest concern about flying with a baby is exposing him to the re-circulated air in the aircraft, which may contain viruses and irritants. Airlines do not allow any baby younger than one week to fly unless you have a doctor's note.

* When flying, dress your baby in loose, comfortable clothing. Reduced air pressure in the cabin makes air in the bowel expand and can cause abdominal, colicky pain.
* When crossing time zones, keep one watch set to your home time so you can keep to your baby's schedule.
* Feed your baby during take off and landing. Sucking and swallowing help to equalise ear pressure and reduce ear pain. If he is not hungry, offer a bottle of water or diluted juice. Let him breastfeed or drink from a bottle whenever he wants. Babies become dehydrated in the dry cabin air more quickly than adults.
* Many airlines provide cribs and can fix them securely.
* After a flight, watch for signs of ear pain. This is caused by changes in cabin air pressure. If your baby is uncomfortable he may cry or scream within half an hour of landing, become restless and irritable, particularly if he is lying down, or be unable to sleep. Some babies shake

their heads. Pain usually passes by the following morning.

Trichomoniasis

Trichomoniasis is an infection caused by a single-celled parasite, *Trichomonas vaginalis*. It is transmitted through sexual contact and inhabits the vagina and urethra (the tube through which urine passes out of the body). It is often present without symptoms, but can cause a thin, frothy and yellow-green discharge, with an unpleasant fishy smell. The discharge makes the skin around the vagina sore and inflamed and there may be itching and pain on passing urine. Trichomoniasis can spread to cause inflammation of the bladder – cystitis (page 170).

A very small number of women are infected in pregnancy, sometimes with other SEXUALLY TRANSMITTED DISEASES. Rarely, trichomoniasis may be responsible for pneumonia in a newborn (page 446) who becomes infected during delivery. An infected baby may develop a FEVER, and in girls there may be a vaginal discharge. It may be a contributory cause of prematurity.

Action plan

A smear or vaginal swab test can diagnose the infection and treatment is needed for both sexual partners. Treatment is usually with the medicine oral metronizadole. It is safe in late pregnancy and during BREASTFEEDING, and babies can be treated similarly. Once treated, trichomoniasis will not recur unless there is re-infection from another person.

You may use a homeopathic remedy described for vaginal discharge, page 542.

Tuberculosis

Although still rare, tuberculosis (TB) is on the increase and is more common in the UK today than it was 20 years ago. Babies are more vulnerable than healthy adults and, in the rare event of childhood infection, face a greater risk of complications including MENINGITIS. A vaccine exists, involving a weakened strain of TB, called Bacillus Calmette Guérin (BCG). Children are not offered routine vaccination unless they live in an area with a high prevalence of TB. Treatment is important if your child is infected. Treatment can also be given to you if you become infected during pregnancy.

What happens

Tuberculosis is a bacterial infection (*Mycobacterium tuberculosis*) passed on by droplets in the air, usually when an infected person coughs. Adults are generally much more likely to spread the disease than children, whose mucous secretions usually contain very few bacteria and whose cough isn't strong enough to produce airborne droplets. The disease is quickly destroyed when exposed to fresh air and sunlight and is not easily contracted except by repeat infection, and so is more common among poorer communities. The most vulnerable adults are the elderly, people with compromised immune systems (such as HIV infection, chemotherapy patients), and malnourished people living in overcrowded, poor quality housing among others who are infected.

There is a slight risk of infection by another form, bovine TB (*Mycobacterium bovis*), which can occur in dairy cattle. It is passed on through consuming unpasteurised infected dairy products, especially milk. All milk sold through shops is routinely heat-treated to eliminate this risk, but avoid milk and milk products from other sources unless you know they are safe.

The most common symptoms are a persistent fever, coughing and night sweats, although an infected infant may also be relatively well, with minimal symptoms, or just appear tired with some weight loss.

+ Red flag

If your baby has been in contact with someone with TB and has a lasting fever or a cough that doesn't respond to medicine, or perspires excessively while she sleeps, alert your paediatrician immediately. A clear diagnosis and treatment are vital.

Action plan

* A tuberculin skin test involves injecting an extract of *Mycobacterium* into your baby's forearm. Your doctor will check the area after two days. If a small, firm bump appears, or if the skin becomes swollen, itchy and red, this shows a TB infection is or was present. The infection may have been present before your child developed active TB.
* Your child will need a chest X-ray to determine whether the disease has infected the chest. If the X-ray suggests an infection, your paediatrician will culture your baby's cough secretions or the contents of her stomach to determine specific treatment because different TB strains require different antibiotics.
* If your baby is infected but has not developed the disease, she'll be given medication (isoniazid) every day for six to nine months to prevent active TB. If your baby has active TB she'll probably be given three or four medications for about six months, with regular checkups. Though your baby is likely to feel better after a few weeks of medication, it's vital that she completes the entire course. If she doesn't, the disease may return in a drug-resistant form.

TB in pregnancy

* Treating TB is a highly specialised area. You will need advice from a specialist in the field as some of the drugs used cannot be given to pregnant or BREASTFEEDING women.
* It is possible but extremely rare for a baby to contract TB from her infected mother in pregnancy. It would only occur if the mother had bacteraemia (bacteria in the blood), which does not occur if the mother receives prompt treatment.
* Breastfeeding while on treatment is safe. Vitamin B6 (pyridoxine) supplements are often given to a baby to counteract a deficiency in the mother caused by drug treatment.
* If TB in the mother is diagnosed only after birth, she needs to be kept separate from her baby until she is confirmed as non-contagious, or until her baby has been vaccinated against TB. The vaccination can be given at birth.

TB immunisation for children

If you live in a community where TB is prevalent, your baby may be offered immunisation. It is best to discuss the pros and cons with your GP or health visitor.

Twins and higher multiples

Today, with routine scans, it is extremely rare for the diagnosis of twins to be missed. Discovering twins may be a delight for you, or it may be a shock, even after fertility treatment. You may feel anxious about how you will give birth and cope with two babies, and at the same time look forward to double rewards. There are support groups for parents of twins and you could make contact during pregnancy and perhaps spend time with a family who has twins. This might help you to prepare. If you have triplets or more, you may receive extra help from local social services.

There is no doubt that twins, particularly if they are identical, have a deep bond. They grow together in the womb and communicate with one another non-verbally on a level that few people can access. Sometimes twins are late in using verbal language because of this, and they often rely heavily on one another for emotional support. Ultrasound scans show twins in the womb touching through the membranes that divide them.

What happens

Identical or monozygotic twins
These develop from a single fertilised egg that divides into separate embryos. The babies are the same sex, the same genetic make-up and very similar physically. Identical twins do not run in families, and occur randomly in three to five in 1,000 pregnancies. They share a single placenta, although each has his own amniotic membrane and sac and umbilical cord. Two-thirds of identical twins share a chorion, the second and the outer membrane (monochorionic). The other third each have their own chorion.
Monochorionic twins need to be monitored particularly closely during pregnancy as they are at a higher risk of developing complications because one of the twins may have a lower blood flow and grow less well if there is twin-to-twin transfusion (page 528).

Non-identical or dizygotic twins
These result from the fertilisation of two eggs, each by a separate sperm, and are no more alike than any other siblings. They each have separate membranes, placenta and umbilical cord. Non-

identical twins occur in five to seven in 1,000 pregnancies. The tendency to release two eggs at ovulation is inherited, rises with fertility treatment and is more common over the age of 35 years.

Siamese or conjoined twins
These are very rare with only 12 cases in the UK in the last 50 years.

Potential complications
Symptoms of pregnancy, such as nausea and VOMITING, are often more severe with twins, and your uterus will be 'large for dates'. You will feel heavier in the later stages than if you were carrying only one baby. Throughout pregnancy you will be more closely monitored.

Half of all twin pregnancies result in healthy full-term babies, usually at about Week 37, with no complications. The other 50 per cent of twin births are PREMATURE (before Week 37), and these babies usually require a period of time in a SPECIAL CARE BABY UNIT.

* The most significant potential complication is premature birth, often due to excess amniotic fluid, particularly with monochorionic twins. After birth, premature twins are more prone to the problems of immaturity than a premature singleton.
* INTRAUTERINE GROWTH RESTRICTION (IUGR) is common. It is usually mild but there may be a dramatic difference in size and one baby may be up to 1kg (2lb 3oz) smaller than the other. Severe IUGR may necessitate an early birth.
* Twin-to-twin transfusion only occurs in some monozygotic (identical) twins, where one twin receives less blood and lower nutrition, and may show IUGR and even ANAEMIA during pregnancy.
* There is an increased risk of placenta praevia (page 442), where the placenta is low and may cover the cervix, necessitating delivery by CAESAREAN SECTION.
* The incidence of foetal loss is higher in twin pregnancies, particularly with identical twins. An early ultrasound scan under six weeks may reveal two amniotic sacs but one of the embryos has been absorbed. An obvious MISCARRIAGE may occur. In a tiny minority, one baby may stop growing after 12 weeks and the foetus that would have miscarried will shrink and will be born after the living twin. Very

rarely, particularly with identical twins, one foetus does not receive sufficient placental blood flow and may be stillborn (page 502). The impact from the LOSS OF A BABY is significant and difficult because there is joy that one baby is alive and sadness for the other.

- Pre-eclampsia (page 68) is more common, particularly with identical twins.
- You may be uncomfortable from pressure on your back and internal organs: you may have pain in the back or pelvis, or swelling (oedema) in your legs, INDIGESTION and HEARTBURN and BREATHLESSNESS.
- The incidence of iron-deficiency ANAEMIA, urinary tract infections, PILES and varicose veins (page 544) is higher than with a single baby.

▨ CARE IN PREGNANCY

Antenatal care is important for you as well as for your babies, and you will probably be offered more frequent check-ups with your midwife and obstetrician or a foetal medicine specialist. Caring for yourself is important, too (page 121), because there are higher demands on your body than with a singleton pregnancy.

Medical care
Close monitoring ensures your BLOOD PRESSURE, digestion and back and pelvis are not causing concern, and checks your babies. You may be offered ultrasound scans at four-week intervals, or more frequently if your doctor is concerned about one of your babies.

Later in pregnancy their foetal heart patterns (using cardiotocograph or CTG) may also be monitored. If there is any suggestion of IUGR, monitoring will intensify and you may be advised to stop working relatively early in pregnancy.

Nutrition, weight and exercise
A balanced diet (page 253) is very important. It is not necessary to eat twice as much, however, nor is it safe to take double the dose of vitamin and mineral supplements recommended for pregnancy.

You can expect to gain more weight than in a singleton pregnancy – 15.9–20.5kg (35–45lb) is the average weight gain (page 564) – so watch your diet and avoid calories that will add further

weight. You may need to eat smaller amounts more frequently, as your stomach will be under pressure from your growing uterus. With the extra weight and the energy required to nourish your babies, you'll need to rest regularly and choose gentle yet effective EXERCISE – such as walking, swimming and YOGA.

Planning ahead
It's a good idea to look into the financial and practical implications of paid help if you won't be getting assistance from your family. Parents of twins do need help. And because twins are more commonly born early, prepare from Week 28. You'll need two of everything.

▨ LABOUR AND BIRTH

Some twins are born vaginally, yet because of an increased risk of complications during labour, most twins in the UK are born by CAESAREAN SECTION. The method of delivery will be your choice, but if your doctor anticipates any problems or if you go into labour before Week 37, a caesarean may be the safest option. Sometimes the first twin may be delivered vaginally but because of awkward positioning the second may need to be delivered by caesarean. It is usual to give birth in a high-dependency unit so extra medical help is at hand.

In an ACTIVE BIRTH (see LABOUR AND BIRTH, MOTHER), the cervix usually dilates more rapidly and labour is a little shorter. If you are comfortable being upright, the flow of blood to the placenta will be maximised. The birth team will monitor the wellbeing of your babies with extra vigilance. It is common practice to ensure an anaesthetist and a paediatrician are available.

The main difficulty with twin births is the delivery of the second twin. The most common presentation is for both twins to be head down but often the second is breech (page 342). Your doctor will check your babies' positions with ultrasound before or during labour, and after the first twin is born, your second baby's position is re-checked. If the head is down, the membranes around the amniotic sac may be ruptured to encourage birth and if contractions do not begin within 10 minutes, you may be given oxytocin to stimulate your uterus. If the second twin changes position and is breech or lying transversely (page 345), a caesarean section will be advised. Triplets are usually delivered by caesarean.

During a vaginal birth, the delivery of the placenta is usually managed actively, which means you will be given an injection of oxytocin to encourage delivery (page 391). This is to reduce excessive BLEEDING, which is more likely because of the large surface area of the placentas.

▓ LIVING WITH TWINS

After the birth, you will quickly focus on caring for your babies. There is a long-established belief that only women who cope well with babies have twins, so rest assured you will probably be fine.

Feeding your babies

If everything goes well with the birth, you will have both babies with you soon afterwards and you can establish BREASTFEEDING as soon as possible.

- Because newborns eat often, you may be feeding almost constantly, and provided your nipples do not become painful, this is good because the more your babies feed, the more milk you will produce. When you are used to it, both babies can feed at the same time provided you are comfortable and they are well supported on pillows. You may favour the rugby hold position (page 85). If you find it hard to hold and feed two babies at once you may cradle one and rest the other on a pillow, and swap for the next feed. Dad may be there to hold one baby while you feed the other.
- If one or either of your breasts is red or lumpy, change your feeding position and alternate your babies: one may suck more strongly.
- If you are planning to bottle-feed, your babies you will need to be very well organised.
- Some mothers find that alternating bottle-feeding and breastfeeding for each baby helps avoid exhaustion and anxiety.
- However you feed, it helps to feed both babies at the same time or you will be feeding virtually non-stop. When one wakes for a feed, wake the other – night and day. With luck you will all fall into a reasonably predictable pattern, although you may find your babies have very different sleeping rhythms.

Feeding takes up a lot of time and, as with every other aspect of baby care, you need to be very well organised and have adaptable babies if you are going to get sufficient rest in the first few months after birth. Use the help that you've arranged during pregnancy and rest as often as you possibly can. If your mind is buzzing and you find it hard to relax, try VISUALISATION or yoga-based breathing exercises to help you switch off. You will need to maintain a high fluid intake and nourish yourself well. This will be easier if there is someone who can cook and clean for you, at least in the early days.

Your emotions

Parents say that having twins is double the trouble but also double the joy. There may be knock-on effects to your relationship so it helps to create some undisturbed time with your partner regularly. You will need lots of extra support to make this a reality (see page 122). You'll also benefit from space to yourself.

From the beginning most twins learn to accept that mum cannot be in two places at one time, and most mums learn how to switch off and ignore some crying. It may be easy going, or you may find that one twin (or both) complains. Although you may feel pressurised and caught up in the whirl of getting through each day, it is important to make time to be with each of your babies separately, and you will develop a unique relationship with each one. They will have different personalities and different needs: one may be dominant, one placid, one big and hungry, the other slight and quiet.

As you get to know each baby better, you will be able to meet their needs and when their needs are met they are likely to be less demanding (page 120). If crying becomes a problem you may try ear plugs – you can still comfort and be with your babies, just with lower volume. As the weeks pass, your babies will amuse one another and you will have more time for other things. This aspect of life with twins is one that many mothers of single babies envy, and it gets better as twins grow and play together.

You may feel confused or guilty if your feelings are not the same for both your babies, particularly if one is in special care and the other is not. It may be helpful to talk to a supportive friend or professional, and also to create time to be with both babies. If you feel ambivalent towards one it may be worth putting extra energy into getting to know his unique ways and just being together. You may want to contact other parents and health professionals through groups such as TAMBA, the Twins and Multiple Births Association, in the UK. If you are finding daily life very difficult, or troubling feelings towards one or both of your babies are intense, some of the advice in the EMOTIONS entry may be useful.

Twin-to-twin transfusion syndrome

See also Anaemia.

Twin-to-twin transfusion syndrome (TTTS) is a disease of identical (monozygotic) twins caused by abnormal connecting blood vessels in a shared placenta. In TTTS, blood from the 'donor' twin is transfused through the placenta into the 'recipient' twin. TTTS is believed to affect as many as one in 1,000 pregnancies. If left untreated, TTTS has a mortality rate of over 80 per cent and can cause severe disability in survivors.

What happens

The recipient twin is often larger and the increased blood volume can result in heart failure. This twin may have too much amniotic fluid and may develop swelling in the body tissues called HYDROPS. The donor twin is often smaller and may become anaemic and the small amount of amniotic fluid volume may interfere with chest and muscle development.

TTTS may cause symptoms in the mother, such as premature contractions, abdominal growth and pressure, and breathlessness, more pronounced than in other twin pregnancies.

Diagnosis

In early pregnancy, a scan will show whether the twins share one placenta (monochorionic twins). If so, regular ultrasound scans will be performed by a foetal medicine specialist trained to detect TTTS. The condition may become evident by four to five months.

Action plan

Treatment is available at specialist regional centres. The principle is to reduce the number of blood vessels communicating between the twins to decrease the blood passing between the babies. This is done by very experienced specialists using scans and laser equipment. Delivery by elective caesarean section is usually considered the safest option to reduce further risk posed by a normal vaginal delivery to one or both twins.

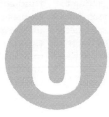

Ultrasound

See Antenatal tests.

Umbilical cord

See also Hernia; Labour and birth, baby, being born; cord compression and prolapse.

In pregnancy, the umbilical cord has been your baby's lifeline, delivering oxygen and nutrition and removing waste products. It may even have been sampled during the pregnancy or used for blood transfusions.

▨ CARE AFTER BIRTH

At delivery, many hospitals allow the placental blood to pass through the cord, so that about 60–80ml of blood re-enter and remain in your baby. This appears to be important in giving baby a store of red cells that can be broken down to release iron for future cell production and growth. Even in a newborn needing medical care, there are often 60 seconds available for blood to flow before the cord is cut and clamped (page 334).

Sometimes the umbilical cord is used for special procedures if there are health concerns. The umbilical cord arteries or vein can be sampled to check the wellbeing of your baby after birth. Catheters can be inserted to allow samples to be taken and drugs and fluids to be administered.

The shape of your baby's umbilicus (belly button) does not depend on how the cord is cut.

The cord stump

Your baby's umbilical cord stump will separate around seven to 10 days after birth. The cord separates simply by 'bacterial action' at the base. After separation there is a pink raw area. This usually develops a skin covering over a few days, and heals, leaving a belly button. Approaches to care differ: you may choose to leave the area alone, or to gently clean it once a day with cotton wool soaked in cooled, pre-boiled water, or to use a weak tea tree solution.

The best homeopathic care is to add Hypercal tincture to your baby's bath water (10 drops per bath). This acts as an antiseptic solution as well. If healing is slow, you can give your baby Calendula 30c, morning and evening, for five days.

Occasionally healing is slow, and a raw area is left which can ooze and appears sore. This is called an umbilical granuloma and sometimes needs treating (overleaf).

▨ INFECTION (OMPHALITIS)

In rare cases the stump may get infected: if so, it will become inflamed, the surrounding skin looks very red, and there may be pus or discharge and a foul smell. Your baby may have a fever. It is important to tell your midwife or doctor because although this type of infection can clear up quickly it may spread to deeper structures.

Action plan

The best way to prevent infection is to leave the area well alone and expose it to air whenever possible. Allowed to dry in air, the cord rapidly withers and separates. Bacteria on the skin are essential to allow the cord to soften and separate. You can minimise infection by folding the top of nappies down to keep the stump clear of urine. It is safe to clean the area in a bath or with cotton wool dipped in boiled, cooled water. If the umbilical cord fails to separate by 10–15 days, visit your GP.

Medical care

In most cases, no treatment other than keeping the cord dry and clean by gently wiping with moist cotton wool is required. Your doctor or midwife may advise you to use a special alcohol solution or an antibiotic powder or ointment. These usually clear up the infection, although they can delay healing and separation. Your doctor or midwife will keep an eye on your baby in case of infection spreading.

Homeopathy

You may add 10 drops of *Hypercal* tincture to your baby's bath and/or bathe the area with cotton wool soaked in a dilution of 10 drops of *Hypercal* tincture to 250ml (½ pint) of boiled, cooled water. There are a number of anti-sepsis remedies that can be given, but it is best to consult your homeopath.

Umbilical discharge not connected to infection

If your baby has an umbilical granuloma (below) this causes a discharge and may need treatment. Very, very rarely (in one in 10,000 babies) the cord continues to ooze a clear fluid despite apparent healing. This represents a persistent connection of the bladder with the umbilicus, called a patent urachus. The connection needs to be closed through surgery.

■ SINGLE ARTERY

Ordinarily, the umbilical cord contains three blood vessels – two arteries and one vein. In up to one in 100 babies, however, only one umbilical artery is present. The condition is more common among TWINS and where the umbilical cord attaches to the edge of the placenta, rather than in the middle. It may be detected on antenatal ultrasound scans, but often is not known until the placenta and cord are examined after birth. A foetus can thrive with a single artery and if no other abnormalities are seen during antenatal scans,

this should not cause any problems for you or your baby. Very occasionally, there may be restricted growth (page 324).

A single artery may occasionally be associated with other CONGENITAL ABNORMALITIES, so you may be advised to have a further or more detailed ultrasound scan before birth. If another physical abnormality or a marker for a serious chromosomal abnormality is found, you may wish to go ahead with an amniocentesis (page 21). It is wise in late pregnancy to ensure that your baby's growth rate is normal. Your baby will be given a detailed clinical examination after birth. If the antenatal tests suggest the need, your baby's kidneys or heart may be closely checked with ultrasound scan after birth.

■ UMBILICAL GRANULOMA AND OTHER LUMPS

An umbilical granuloma is a small area of raw scar tissue that has not been covered by skin after the umbilical cord has separated. This small piece of pink, fleshy tissue contains no nerves and so your baby will not feel anything if it is touched. It may produce a discharge and can bleed. Umbilical granulomas occur in roughly one in 20 babies within six months of birth and most disappear in a few months. Some need to be cauterised by a doctor or health visitor, using silver nitrate. Occasionally surgery is needed.

Pyogenic granuloma occurs in roughly one in 1,000 babies older than six months if normal skin growth over a wound is not efficient. This usually disappears within a few weeks but may need minor surgery.

Umbilical cord, blood banking and stem cells

Cord blood is the baby's blood that remains in the UMBILICAL CORD and the placenta after the birth. It is a rich source of stem cells, the immature cells from which nearly all other cells in the body can develop. Recently discovered 'cord-blood-derived embryonic-like stem cells' are not quite as primitive as embryonic stem cells, which can give rise to any tissue type of the body. However, cord-blood-derived embryonic-like stem cells are more versatile than 'adult stem cells' such as those found in bone marrow (which may be used to repair damaged tissue during life). There is a greater potential for cord-blood-derived cells to be manipulated in a laboratory to function as a variety of different cells. Cord blood is currently used to treat leukaemia, sickle cell disease, thalassaemia, some immune disorders and enzyme deficiencies. Scientists claim that in the future cord-blood-derived embryonic-like stem cells could be used to treat an even wider range of diseases including Alzheimer's, Parkinson's, diabetes and many others.

A cord-blood stem cell transplant uses cord-blood-derived stem cells to replace diseased cells and, for example, rebuild the person's blood or immune system. To be a success, the new cells must match the person's cells as closely as possible. Thousands of successful cord-blood stem cell transplants have been performed to date. Cord blood transplants have a higher success rate than bone marrow cell transplants and cord blood can be frozen for years before use.

Cord blood banking is the process of collecting blood from a baby's umbilical cord immediately after delivery. It is frozen for long-term cryogenic (freezing) storage in a private or state-run bank. There is a fee for private storage. The state-run NHS Cord Blood Bank (NHS-CBB) was established in 1996 with the aim of resolving the issue of the ethnic imbalance of donors represented on the British Bone Marrow Registry, by collecting stem cells from a far wider donor pool. The NHS-CBB collects cord blood following delivery of the placenta at a stage where it is considered a waste product, and this is usually done at the request of the family. The NHS Cord Blood Bank will provide stem cells to anyone in need. There is also an initiative to divide cord blood: some will be stored in state banks and the rest held privately for the sole use of the donor person.

The cells may later be used by the donor (they are a perfect genetic match), or by someone in the donor's family (a close genetic match), or in an unrelated individual (if the match is close enough). The risk that a person may need their own stem cells at a later date is very low indeed.

If it is your request cord blood is collected carefully after the placenta has been born. Sterile precautions ensure that the cells remain viable. Your midwife needs to attend to you and your baby so another person collects the sample. Cord blood can only be collected when there are sufficient cells left after the placenta is born and there is time and people available to collect the sample. If your baby is PREMATURE or low birth weight it is better to delay clamping the cord to provide the maximum number of blood cells for your baby in order to reduce ANAEMIA later. This is discussed on page 334.

The cord blood is then sent to the laboratory where the stem cells are separated from the other blood cells and frozen for storage. Not all hospitals allow collection by private banks. There are still some uncertainties about responsibility if the cells thaw out in the event that, for example, the storage facility develops a technical fault.

Underactive thyroid

See Thyroid, baby; Thyroid, mother.

Underweight, baby

See Weight, baby, failure to thrive (low weight gain).

Underweight, mother

See Weight, mother, underweight.

Urinary tract infection, baby

A urinary tract (kidney and bladder) infection is not always easy to detect. Infections are more common in baby girls, affecting one in 20, because their urethra is shorter than a boy's urethra.

What happens

If your baby is unwell, with FEVER, irritability or DIARRHOEA, is refusing feeds or has poor weight gain and her urine smells strong, this may indicate a urinary tract infection. An infection can be very painful.

Normal urine is sterile and is free of bacteria, viruses and fungi. An infection occurs when micro-organisms, usually bacteria from the colon, cling to the opening of the urethra, the tube that carries urine from the bladder to the outside of the body, and travel into the bladder where they begin to multiply. There is an increased risk of infection when there is an abnormality of the urinary system, and this may be diagnosed on ultrasound scans in pregnancy (below).

Action plan

For most babies, simple remedies such as ensuring adequate fluid intake help to prevent infections. Your baby needs increased fluids to help flush out the kidneys. Always wipe your baby girl from front to back to reduce the chance of bacteria travelling from the bowel to the bladder.

If you are concerned, a urine test can detect infection.

* A urinary infection may be treated with antibiotics, possibly for an extended period if the infection recurs.
* You may wish to give infant paracetamol (page 429) to relieve pain.
* When a urine infection is confirmed, a specialist will investigate the underlying cause. The tests mainly look for obstruction and reflux (below).

▩ URINARY OBSTRUCTION, HYDRONEPHROSIS AND REFLUX

A very small number of babies have an obstruction to the flow of urine or a reflux (backflow) of urine from the bladder to the kidneys that increases the tendency to infection. If the urine flow along the ureter, the tube between the kidney and the bladder, is obstructed or flows backwards, it leads to a condition called hydronephrosis where the ureters and the kidney become swollen and filled with urine. This may be visible on an ultrasound scan during pregnancy (in about 2 per cent of babies) or after birth, or the problem may become apparent with a urine infection in the first few months. Hydronephrosis may lead to long-term kidney damage that treatment

may prevent, so all babies with urinary infections are referred for specialist assessment to see if the reflux or back flow is a cause of the infection.

What happens

Possible causes are:

* *Urinary reflux* (vesico-ureteric reflux) involves urine flow in the reverse direction from the bladder back up the dilated (enlarged) ureter towards the kidney, leading to pressure on the kidney and an increased risk of infection.
* *Ureteric obstruction* is usually harmless. Some obstructions are found during antenatal ultrasound in mid-pregnancy or after Week 32. The condition arises from a narrowing of the ureter, where two different parts of the ureter have joined, one part growing down from the kidney, and the other part growing up from the bladder.
* Very rarely posterior urethral valves occur (only ever seen in boys). These narrow and block the urethra so that the bladder distends and the kidneys dilate with severe hydronephrosis on both sides. This damages the developing kidney. The distension is visible on an antenatal ultrasound scan at or before Week 20.
* The majority of babies found to have enlarged or dilated ureters have normal kidneys.

Action plan

Some foetal medicine specialists insert a catheter to drain the urine during pregnancy by means of amniocentesis and this relieves the effects of pressure. This may not, however, prevent damage to the kidneys. If hydronephrosis is suspected, after birth your baby may be given a low dose of antibiotics to reduce the risk of infections that could cause scarring to the kidneys. In many babies, the condition seen in pregnancy may clear up with no treatment, and the preventive antibiotic treatment is stopped.

* After birth the tests include ultrasound scan to check for two normal kidneys and to observe the size of the ureter and the bladder wall thickness and their ability to empty.
* In some centres a micturating cystourethrogram is carried out by passing a

catheter tube into the bladder via the urethra, injecting a dye and taking X-ray pictures to see if the urine refluxes. It involves a number of X-rays or the more up-to-date equivalent using ultrasound imaging. In some centres the availability of specialist ultrasound may avoid the need for a catheter test.

- Other tests involve injecting slightly radioactive materials (radioisotopes) into a vein and using a gamma camera to see the function of the kidneys and observe reflux or narrowing of the ureter.

Urinary obstruction and reflux generally improve by the age of three years, after which antibiotics are stopped because the risk of new scarring is minimal. Your baby will be followed up and surgery may occasionally be needed. If any form of reflux or other kidney abnormality is confirmed after the birth the preventive antibiotics are usually continued until a baby is at least one year old, and sometimes longer. You may wish to use homeopathic remedies to reduce possible side effects of the antibiotics (page 35).

If you have had one baby with hydronephrosis there is around a 30 per cent chance that a subsequent baby may be affected. Even if scans are normal before birth, it is advisable for your baby to have an ultrasound scan after birth.

Urinary tract infection, mother

See Cystitis and urinary tract infections, mother.

Urine, baby

Your baby will pass urine many times every day. She has no control over this. Plenty of urine, making a lot of wet nappies, is a sign of health and shows that your baby is getting plenty to drink. Less urine than usual may be a sign of dehydration, and it is important to avoid this. Ideally, urine is a light straw colour or almost colourless and has little smell. Dark or stronger smelling urine may indicate mild dehydration. An extra breastfeed or a drink of water may

help. If there are other reasons to think your baby may be unwell, or she has dry lips or is listless, seek advice. Dehydration is covered in detail on page 181.

Disposable nappies can absorb a lot of wee without feeling wet, so the best way to judge whether your baby is urinating frequently is by the weight of her nappy. If you are very concerned put a small cotton wool ball in the nappy. Check it every hour or so and when you notice it is wet it will quickly tell you she is passing urine.

Baby urine is very clean and has little smell when fresh. But if it remains in the nappy for a while, bacteria will produce ammonia from chemicals in the urine, and this may irritate your baby's skin. It is important to change her nappy regularly and wash her skin with water. Olive oil helps to protect her.

You may occasionally notice a light pink, orange or even red stain in your baby's nappy. This is caused by crystals made by a reaction between urates in the urine (which are normal) and chemicals in the fibres of the nappy. The crystals can appear when your baby is totally healthy, but are more likely if she has not drunk enough, making her urine more concentrated. It is more common in boys, as their urine tends to settle in the same place in the nappy.

If there is a red or brown stain that looks at all like blood, or your baby seems unwell and is not feeding normally, she may have a urinary tract infection, which is more common in girls (page 531), and you need to visit her doctor. Small amounts of blood in a baby girl's urine in the first two weeks are usually hormonal (page 62).

Small yellow or brown 'crystals' on the inner surface of a disposable nappy are the water-absorbing crystals. These leak out of the inside of the nappy if the nappy is torn and are harmless unless eaten.

Urine, blood and stones, mother

It is routine to have your urine checked for blood at each antenatal visit (page 32). Rarely, urine may contain blood or stones.

▓ HAEMATURIA (BLOOD IN THE URINE)

A number of different conditions can lead to haematuria. These include:

- *Cystitis*, where infection causes inflammation of the bladder wall, resulting in small amounts of blood being found in the urine. The urine can be 'cultured' in the laboratory – that is placed on a growing medium in a dish – to allow any bacteria present to multiply. The infection can then be identified. It is usually treated with antibiotics and increasing fluid intake. Drinking cranberry juice is also known to reduce bacterial growth (page 171).
- *Kidney stones* that become lodged in the ureter (the tube that connects each kidney with the bladder) may irritate the lining and cause bleeding (see below).
- *Microscopic haematuria* (minute particles of blood in urine) may occur if the glomerular membrane in the kidney, where urine is filtered from blood, becomes more porous. This may be due to a benign (non-damaging) condition of no significance or, very rarely, a more serious kidney problem. If an ultrasound scan reveals nothing abnormal and no protein is found in the urine, further tests can be completed after the birth.
- *False haematuria* readings may occur if blood from vaginal BLEEDING is collected inadvertently as part of a urine specimen.
- *Polyp or tumour* in the bladder or kidney is a very rare cause of haematuria in pregnancy. If large it will appear on ultrasound scan.

▓ STONES (CALCULI)

Kidney stones occur when there is an over-concentration of a particular substance such as calcium or oxalate in the urine. This may be due to a diet rich in certain substances or because the body produces too much. They are more likely if the urine is very concentrated, for instance when a person does not drink enough fluid. Most stones are the size of a grain of sand, but some may be much bigger and affect the flow of urine from the kidneys.

Many people have kidney stones but do not realise it, although the problem may cause repeated pain or urinary tract infections. It is usually only when a stone moves from the kidney down the ureter that symptoms occur.

These usually involve blood in the urine and pain in the back and down into the groin. In pregnancy, the pain may be mistaken for common pregnancy-related muscular pain.

An ultrasound scan will reveal the stone – X-rays cannot be used in pregnancy to investigate abdominal problems because of the risk to the baby. The majority of kidney stones pass by themselves. Removal of persistent stones is usually deferred until after birth because the pregnant uterus makes it difficult to perform the removal. If a stone is causing pain, treatment in pregnancy will involve pain relief, as directed by your doctor. Always drink plenty of fluids, especially in hot weather. If you are prone to calcium stones, reduce the amount of dairy products in your diet. Reducing spinach, chocolate, rhubarb and nuts can prevent oxalate stones.

Uterus, abnormal shape

The uterus develops in a girl foetus from two halves that fuse together. A cavity then forms. Typically, a uterus is pear-shaped and contains a regular cavity that connects the cervix below to the fallopian tubes above. There are possible variations from this pattern. Usually these do not cause problems but for a small number of women who are affected, special attention during pregnancy and when giving birth may be necessary.

What happens

The most common abnormality is an indentation (a septum) in the cavity at the top of the uterus. This is a septate uterus and usually causes no symptoms or complications. The next most common abnormality is a heart-shaped or bicornuate uterus. Here there is one cervix but the septum is more pronounced and the cavity is heart-shaped. These variants are quite common and 3 per cent of women are affected, with no genetic tendency. If only one side of the uterus forms, it may be associated with abnormal development of the kidney on the absent side. Very rarely, there is a complete double system with a double uterus and cervix and sometimes the vagina is also duplicated.

Most women with uterine variations do not have problems. Difficulties are more likely if the uterus is heart-shaped and are related to the degree of abnormality. If the heart shape is severe there is an increased risk of incompetence of the cervix and MISCARRIAGE, or breech presentation, or PREMATURE BIRTH. Very rarely there may be restricted foetal growth (page 322). After the birth there is more likelihood the placenta may be retained.

Action plan

* If you are aware that you have a bicornuate uterus, tell your doctor before conception, particularly if you have had previous miscarriages, a breech baby or a retained placenta. Investigations may include ultrasound scans with 3-D imaging and rarely laparoscopy (using a fibre-optic camera to look at your uterus). Treatment before pregnancy may include reducing the septum with minimally invasive vaginal surgery, although this is necessary only for a minority of women for whom it is a cause of recurrent miscarriage. If you have a bicornuate uterus, you will be seen frequently during pregnancy.

* You may be offered ultrasound scans to check your cervix for incompetence (page 127) by measuring the length and the canal diameter. Scans can also check your baby's growth and position and to see where the placenta has implanted. If the placenta is in the top of the uterus a retained placenta is more likely.

* If the canal of your cervix is dilated (widened), a stitch is inserted between Week 12 and 15 to prevent a miscarriage and reduce the chance of premature birth.

* A CAESAREAN SECTION is only necessary if your baby is in breech position (page 342).

* Labour may be very painful and/or progress slowly because the two sides of the uterus may not synchronise well.

* After a vaginal birth you may be offered oxytocin to speed up the birth of the placenta and prevent excessive bleeding.

* A double system is very rare, and when this occurs specialist advice is essential.

Vaccinations in pregnancy

See Influenza (flu), mother; Travel in pregnancy.

Vaccinations, baby

The Department of Health in the UK strongly recommends vaccination (also known as immunisation or 'jabs'). The programme usually begins when a baby is eight weeks old (page 538).

Some vaccines are given together. This is because they often enhance the way each one works and give a better result. If you spread out vaccinations you may not be doing your baby a favour – in fact she may develop a doctor phobia or needle phobia and there may be additional emotional effects. The recommendation to vaccinate a baby at two, three and four months is made because there are fewer reported side effects at those times.

Vaccination controversies

There are differing opinions regarding mainstream vaccinations. The anti-immunisation groups point to the risks of side effects as one of the strongest reasons not to immunise. Those who support immunisation believe the risks of side effects are far smaller than the risk of serious injury arising from an actual infection by a disease. Current estimates suggest one in three million babies will suffer a serious life-long reaction to immunisation. As many as 10 per cent will have a minor reaction.

If you are unsure about what steps to take, read as much as you can about the subject, talk to others, and consider the views of both sides, then weigh the risk of side effects against the risk of your child developing serious complications and the impact this could have on your child and family. Being well informed is important.

There is scientific evidence to support or reject the concerns of parents and, indeed, health professionals. Over the last 30 years the evidence of harm caused by any vaccine given in the UK has been subject to enquiry from the Vaccine Damage Tribunal. Since April 2000, the tribunal has heard 1,164 cases, and made payments in only 21 (so the true frequency of vaccine damage payments is very low). In this time many millions of vaccinations have been given.

The only alternative way to immunise your child against a disease is for your child to get that illness and develop her own antibody protection.

Homeopathy

Homeopathy cannot provide vaccination but does offer remedies that can strengthen the immune system or increase resistance to disease. Many parents choose homeopathic remedies to use together with standard vaccinations to reduce the risk of side effects.

Thiomersal in vaccines

Thiomersal contains ethyl mercury. In the past, very low doses were used in some vaccines to prevent contamination by bacteria and fungi. There is no thiomersal, and never has been, in any MMR, Hib, oral polio, meningitis C conjugate or BCG vaccines used in the UK. DTP vaccines contained thiomersal until September 2004, since when the thiomersal-free five-component vaccine has been used. The apparent rise in the incidence of autism in recent years has not been matched by any change in childhood exposure to thiomersal from vaccines in the UK. There is no evidence that autism is related to vaccinations.

Antibiotics in vaccines

Antibiotics are present in some vaccines as a precaution against bacterial contamination during manufacture. Because antibiotics can cause severe allergic reactions in a small number of children, some parents are concerned. Penicillins and cephalosporins, the antibiotics most likely to cause severe allergic reactions, are not used in vaccines. Only the antibiotic neomycin is contained in detectable quantities, and has so far never been clearly found to cause severe allergic reactions. The possibility that the trace quantities of antibiotics contained in vaccines cause severe allergic reactions remains theoretical.

▧ CHILDHOOD VACCINATION PROGRAMME

Childhood vaccination protects children against infectious diseases by stimulating the immune system to produce protective antibodies. In this way a child's immune system is prepared in advance against possible serious infection. Childhood vaccination does this by injecting the disease-causing organism, either in fragments of the bacterial cell wall, or in a dead or live-but-weakened form of a virus, into the child's body. This activates the immune system so that it can more easily deal with the naturally occurring form of the disease, should a child be infected with it. The protection offered by vaccination or immunisation is generally life-long, but some particular infections require boosters in order to ensure life-long protection, for example hepatitis B and tetanus vaccines.

The standard childhood vaccination programme is constantly being reviewed and you will need to take the advice of your GP, health visitor or paediatrician as you consider vaccinations for your baby. If your child is receiving medication of any kind (including over-the-counter and complementary remedies) you must ensure your GP is aware of this before vaccination.

Diseases that standard vaccines protect against

Haemophilus influenzae Type b (Hib)

This bacterial infection may cause illnesses including Haemophilus MENINGITIS, pneumonia, blood poisoning and ear infection.

Tetanus

Also known as 'lockjaw', this is a rare disease that can cause muscle paralysis and breathing difficulties, and may be fatal if untreated. It is caused by a nerve toxin produced by a bacterium (*Clostridium tetani*) commonly found in soil and especially in gardens treated with horse or cow manure. It can be caught from a wound, such as a prick, cut or burn, which leaves the skin open to infection.

Meningococcus Type C

This bacterium causes a type of meningitis that can have potentially serious effects. Meningococcus also exists as Types A, B and C. Type B is less common than Type C and causes a similar disease. There is no effective vaccine against Type B at present. Type A causes epidemics of meningitis in the tropics, and there is an effective vaccine but this is not given routinely in the UK.

Diphtheria

Although now very rare in the UK, this is a serious disease, which can damage the heart and nervous system and can be fatal.

Pertussis (whooping cough)

This is a very tiring and potentially serious illness for a child, especially under the age of one year (page 568). In the UK, nine babies die from this illness every year – 90 per cent of them too young to have been immunised. Many catch the disease from non-immunised siblings. This risk is being reduced by giving the first doses at two, three and four months and the next between three and four years.

Polio

This is a virus that attacks the nerve cells that control the muscles. It can cause paralysis in the limbs and/or the chest muscles, and can be life threatening. Because of a world-wide vaccination programme, it no longer exists other than as the strain used for vaccination in Europe, North America and most parts of the world. The aim is to eradicate it completely world wide. It is now given as a killed virus as part of a single combined-vaccine injection.

Pneumococcal vaccination

Prevnar is the trade name of a newly licensed pneumococcal conjugate vaccine that has been shown to protect against potentially serious infections with the bacterium Pneumococcus. It is effective in preventing meningitis, infection of the bloodstream, pneumonia, and infection of the middle ear caused by this organism.

Some mild local reactions are associated with giving this vaccine but they are not serious and are self-limiting. It is given with the other usual childhood immunisations.

The programme outlined here was standard in 2007.

At birth
- Hepatitis B may be given where a baby is at risk (page 294) and repeated at one month and six months. It is given within hours of birth, as this is a high-risk period where infection from a mother with the virus may occur.
- BCG (bacillus Calmette-Guérin – a weakened strain of tuberculosis) may be an option in the first eight weeks, depending on the risk of tuberculosis where you live, and whether you are planning to travel to regions with high risk of tuberculosis.

Two months
- Since 2004 children in the UK have been given a five-in-one vaccine. The vaccine is called DTaP/IPV/Hib and stands for diphtheria (D), tetanus (T),

acellular pertussis (aP – whooping cough), inactivated polio (IPV) and haemophilus influenzae type b (Hib). It is given in a single injection in the upper forearm or thigh. None of the vaccinations is live.
- Pneumococcal infection as Prevnar (Pneumococcal conjugate vaccine, PCV) – one injection.

Three months
- Five-in-one vaccine (as above) – one injection.
- Meningitis C (meningococcal group C or MenC) – one injection.
- The influenza vaccine is recommended for 'at risk' babies (such as those who have heart disease or another major illness) and can be given from three months to six months of age, but usually at six months, as maternal antibodies may protect to this age.

Four months
- Five-in-one vaccine (as above) – one injection.
- Meningitis C (as above) – one injection.
- Pneumococcal infection (as above) – one injection.

Around 12 months
- Hib/MenC (Haemophilus influenza type b/meningitis C) – one injection.

Around 13 months old
- MMR (measles, mumps and rubella) – one injection. The primary dose can be given at any age over 13 months but can be safely given from six months if there is a local outbreak of measles.
- Pneumococcal infection (PCV) – one injection.

Three years and four months to five years old
- Four-in-one injection: dTaP/IPV (diphtheria, tetanus, pertussis and polio) – one injection.
- MMR (secondary dose) – one injection.

Chickenpox vaccine

The chickenpox vaccine (against the varicella virus) is licensed for use in the UK but is not part of routine childhood vaccinations. It is a live virus vaccine to be avoided in HIV positive children. There is concern that if the chickenpox vaccine were to be added to standard childhood vaccinations there would be a greater number of cases of shingles in adults. However, the vaccine is a routine part of the schedule of immunisation across the USA, Canada, and several European countries.

Reasons for avoiding vaccination

* Don't vaccinate your child if she has a FEVER on the day the vaccine is due to be given.
* After a cold, your baby may have a runny nose and cough for a few weeks. As long as she has no fever on the day of vaccination it is unnecessary to delay giving any of the routine immunisations.
* Avoid vaccination if your baby has a severe congenital (present from birth) medical problem affecting her development and nervous system, particularly if an accurate diagnosis has not yet been made.
* If your baby has had FITS or seizures before the age of two months, it is best to delay vaccinations until the cause is identified.

Some parents are anxious about the safety of vaccination for other reasons. The advice from the Department of Health is to go ahead with vaccination even if:

* Your child has had the illness which the vaccine is designed to prevent (prior infection does not necessarily provide long-lasting immunity).
* Your child has had a mild reaction to a previous dose of the vaccine.
* Your child has an egg ALLERGY (overleaf). Your doctor will advise. The risk of reaction is so low as to be negligible and there is no evidence to support the avoidance of vaccination in any egg-allergic child.

Controversies regarding safety of vaccinations are discussed on page 536.

▓ MMR (MEASLES, MUMPS, RUBELLA)

The MMR vaccine is recommended as routine in the UK. It has caused more controversy than other vaccines and many parents wish to consider their choice carefully.

The vaccine is said to be 95 per cent effective at protecting a child against MEASLES, MUMPS and RUBELLA, any one of which carries a risk of potentially serious consequences. The MMR vaccine is a live-attenuated vaccine. This means it's a live virus that's been weakened so it won't cause the disease in your child, but as the virus replicates in the cells of her body this will cause her to produce an immune response. This should protect her if she comes into contact with an infected person.

In the USA, Canada and much of Europe the triple vaccine is combined with the varicella (chickenpox) vaccine in the 'MMRV' vaccine.

Timing the vaccine

Measles and mumps are both very rare conditions under the age of one year. The first MMR dose is therefore recommended between 12 and 15 months of age, with a secondary dose given between the ages of four and six years.

If your baby is exposed to the infection before immunisation

If your baby has been exposed to the measles virus and hasn't yet been immunised, it's important to talk to her doctor, as vaccination as soon as possible after the exposure to the measles-infected contact may be advised to help prevent your baby developing the infection. This is often recommended when there is contact in a nursery to help prevent epidemics. The same recommendation applies for contact with mumps and rubella infections, although the risks of infection causing complications are lower.

* If it's been six days or less since your baby was exposed, your doctor may suggest an immunoglobulin injection (page 406). This is not a vaccine, but provides the specific antibodies that mop up the measles virus directly to help prevent the illness. This is not necessary for mumps and rubella.
* If your baby is six months or older and it's within 72 hours of exposure, your doctor may also recommend that she receives one dose of the MMR vaccine. She will still need to receive the two routine doses of the vaccine at 12–15 months and at pre-school entry.

Safety concerns: autism and Crohn's disease

Since MMR was introduced in the UK there have been concerns among some parents about a possible link between the vaccine and a rise in autism (page 39), and between MMR and a later development of Crohn's disease (page 320). Extensive independent research from around the world has not confirmed any evidence of these links, and there is a need for detailed research to understand the causes of autistic spectrum disorders.

In the USA, MMR has been given for more than 25 years and around 200 million doses have been used. Autism and Crohn's disease have not been linked with MMR there. In Finland, where children have been given two doses of MMR since 1982, reactions reported after MMR were followed up. There were no confirmed reports of permanent damage due to the vaccine. A special study in Finland also did not confirm a link between MMR and autism and Crohn's disease.

Safety concerns: egg and antibiotic allergy

The MMR vaccine can safely be given to children who are allergic to eggs. It is prepared using chick cells to grow the virus, but contains no egg protein. Rarely, an allergic reaction is triggered by the child being sensitive to the small amount of antibiotic present in the vaccine, not to egg protein. If your baby has an allergy, the doctor can make special arrangements for the immunisation to be given safely in a setting where any extra help which may be needed is immediately available.

Giving separate measles, mumps and rubella vaccinations

Giving the vaccines separately may be possible by private arrangement but may not be safer in terms of complications. It prolongs the period of time during which your baby is susceptible to the three diseases – mumps, measles and rubella – and the number of additional injections could potentially distress your baby.

■ POSSIBLE REACTIONS

Although most children have no reaction to vaccination, all children are different. Some may have a rare reaction and, much more rarely, an allergic or other severe reaction.

Mild reactions

* Sometimes redness and swelling may develop where the injection was given within six to eight hours. This will slowly disappear and is not a cause for concern.
* Sometimes a small lump develops where the injection was given. This lump can last for several weeks and then disappears.
* A baby may be miserable within 48 hours of vaccination. Some babies become irritable and show signs of a headache, sometimes with a high temperature. Doziness, crying, irritability or a raised temperature of 38.5°C or more, taken with a digital thermometer in the rectum (page 239), can last for up to 24 hours. If it goes on beyond 24 hours you should consult your doctor, although the cause may often be a coincidental illness, and not due to the vaccination.
* A mild rash, perhaps with a mild fever and swollen glands, may occur within five to 12 days of measles immunisation.
* You may ask a homeopath to prescribe remedies for your baby before and after vaccination. These may help to reduce anxiety and discomfort and minimise reactions. The chosen remedy will depend on your child's unique constitution, age and history of illness and vaccination to date. Your homeopath may also prescribe something for you if you are anxious about the procedure.
* A dose of infant paracetamol suspension (page 429) as directed by your health visitor or doctor will help reduce discomfort for your baby and will help bring down her temperature if it rises.
* The BCG vaccination is a small amount of a live but weakened strain of bacterium given to protect against TUBERCULOSIS where children may be at risk. It is injected under the skin. This causes a local reaction at the site of the injection with a small pus-filled blister. This then bursts and needs to be kept clean until it heals, a process that takes up to 12 weeks.

Uncommon reactions

* Very rarely, children can have allergic reactions straight after vaccination. For this reason, you will be asked to stay in the health clinic for up to 15 minutes after the injection has been given. The usual signs of a serious allergic reaction are a rash that covers the face and body, a swollen mouth and throat, breathing difficulties and shock. If your child does react and is treated quickly, usually with an injection

of adrenaline and antihistamine medicine, recovery will be complete. People giving immunisations are trained and their surgeries equipped to deal with these allergic reactions.

Severe reaction

A severe reaction is very rare indeed and risks of long-term damage directly caused by the vaccine are small.

- If your baby reacts to the vaccine in a severe way, specifically with prolonged screaming and crying for 48 hours, which starts within 24 hours of vaccination, or a fit (seizure) within 24 hours, inform your doctor. The doctor may prefer not to give the product again. However, it is now difficult to obtain alternative vaccines, so your child may miss out on receiving the full protective course. It is important to seek expert advice before making your decision.
- Having a fit is no more common after vaccination than at any other time for young babies but it is important to talk to your doctor, nurse or health visitor if this happens. In the unlikely event that your baby had already had a fit this would be taken into account as part of her medical history but would not automatically rule out vaccination.

There is a small chance of reacting to the five-in-one vaccine (page 538) with any form of reaction, and the risk of a reaction rises after four months of age. Delaying immunisations beyond four months of age seems to be associated with a higher number of reactions, both major and minor, presumably because the infant immune

(page 538)

+ Red flag

Let your doctor or nurse know if you have any concerns over your child's developmental progress or if your baby:
- Has a high fever.
- Is showing worrying signs of distress.
- Has had a bad reaction to any other immunisation.
- Has had or is having treatment for cancer.
- Is HIV positive.
- Cries for over 24 hours after the immunisation.

---

system is more mature, and can respond with a larger reaction. The protection resulting from immunisation before four months of age is as good as that resulting from giving the immunisations after six months of age, but with a lower risk of reactions, and parents may need to take this into account when making decisions about the timing of vaccinations.

Vaginal discharge and infection

The vagina constantly produces a film of mucus to keep the tissue moist and maintain the correct pH (acid-alkali balance). A thin and milky, mild-smelling vaginal secretion is normal because 'good' bacteria live in a healthy vagina and protect against harmful microbes. In pregnancy, your cervix secretes an increased amount of cervical mucus and discharge may increase. If you feel discomfort or itchiness, or develop a discharge that is yellowish, greenish or foul smelling, you may have an infection. In addition to discomfort, some infections carry a risk of harming a developing baby so it is important to inform your doctor or midwife. In pregnancy, vaginal infections often recur and may not resolve completely until after the birth.

What happens

Every woman will notice an increase in vaginal mucus in pregnancy. This is perfectly normal. If the mucus increases and is accompanied by other symptoms, such as unusual discharge or irritation it may be a sign of the following:
- *Bacterial infections.* These include VAGINOSIS, CHLAMYDIA, GONORRHEA and SYPHILIS and can be treated and cured in pregnancy to clear symptoms and protect an unborn baby. GROUP B STREP (GBS) poses a risk to your baby so you may wish to be treated in labour.
- *Fungal infections,* such as CANDIDA *albicans* (thrush). These can be treated.
- *Viral infection.* Genital HERPES or HIV cannot be cured, but can be managed to ease symptoms. Special measures can be taken to greatly reduce the risk to a baby.
- Sometimes irritation and itching may be a skin rash, often related to an ALLERGY.

- Occasionally a discharge of clear urine-coloured fluid signifies rupture of the membranes. This is amniotic fluid leaking.

Action plan

Always get any abnormal discharge from the vulval area checked. If you think you are leaking more urine than usual (incontinence), your midwife will need to exclude a leak of amniotic fluid (page 23), which may be potentially dangerous for your baby.

If you have symptoms, arrange to be examined. A vaginal swab is used to take a sample of the discharge that can be cultured in a laboratory. Different swabs are needed to test for bacterial, viral and chlamydia infections and your doctor will recommend the most appropriate. Group B Strep (GBS) may also be detected using a rectal swab. Routine antenatal testing for vaginal infection differs from hospital to hospital.

Sometimes a test is negative when there is an infection. If symptoms continue it is worth being tested again. If you test positive for a vaginal infection that may be sexually transmitted, it is sensible to ask to be tested for other SEXUALLY TRANSMITTED DISEASES and HIV and for HEPATITIS B and C. Testing involves a vaginal swab or a blood test. Your partner should be tested as well.

If your discharge is heavy:

- Try wearing a panty liner. Change it regularly to keep the area fresh and clean. Do not use tampons, which could introduce bacteria and lead to infection.
- You may feel better if you wear loose-fitting clothes and cotton underwear.
- It could help to avoid perfumed toiletries as they can cause irritation and make matters worse.
- Do not douche, especially during pregnancy. There is a danger of altering the normal vaginal bacteria and making an infection more likely.
- If you have a proven infection, consult your doctor for treatment. Each type of infection warrants individual treatment, outlined in the relevant entries in this A–Z.

Homeopathy

Following your specific symptoms, you may try one of the following in 30c potency, four times a day for two days. If your symptoms are improving, continue with the same remedy for another two days and re-assess. If there is no change whatsoever in two days, re-assess and you could try another remedy. If your symptoms are worse please consult your doctor or homeopath. When you bathe, adding 10–15 drops of *Calendula* tincture in the bath may ease itching and burning.

- *Kreosotum* for a burning profuse, foul-smelling discharge (it may smell like rye bread) that stings, is milky or yellow in colour, itches and irritates and can be accompanied by pains in the lower back and general weakness.
- *Nitric Acid* for a pinkish or greenish stringy, smelly discharge that itches, irritates and burns, comes with splinter-like pains and feels worse in the evenings. *Nitric Acid* is often used for chronic vaginosis.
- *Pulsatilla* for thick milky or creamy-yellow bland discharge, accompanied by itching but not much irritation and burning compared to the other remedies. You may feel weepy and need consoling.
- *Mercurius* for thick, lumpy, discharge, foul-smelling, itchy and burning and you feel chilly and sweaty.
- *Sepia* for a white or yellow discharge that can sting. You may have dragging pains or a heaviness in your abdomen, vaginal itchiness, irritation or dryness. Your moods may be changeable and symptoms are worse during the day.

Vaginal pain

See also Sex, pain.

During pregnancy, your labia may soften and become fuller and more sensitive. This usually causes tenderness rather than pain. Your clitoris may also enlarge and become more sensitive to direct touch or tight underwear. This may be pleasurable, or a source of discomfort. Sometimes pain in pregnancy arises from the joint at the front of the pelvis: this is known as dysfunction of symphysis pubis (page 43).

After a vaginal birth, it is very common to feel discomfort in the vagina and around the anus and perineum (the area of tissue between the anus and vagina). This may last for several days or for weeks, and tends to be worse after delivery involving medical instruments and when there have been stitches. If you have a graze and/or stitches after birth, your vagina will sting when you urinate until the tissues have healed. There is advice for reducing discomfort after stitches on page 371. Breastfeeding keeps oestrogen levels low, which affects the lining of your vagina, keeping it thin. You may feel more sensitive or perhaps uncomfortable during sexual stimulation.

Vaginal pain may also relate to one of the following, dealt with elsewhere in this book, and may require a doctor's advice and treatment.

- *Infection*. Discomfort with stinging or itching and perhaps a discharge or odour (see page 541). Pregnancy makes you more susceptible to thrush (page 117).
- *Dysfunction of symphysis pubis* (DSP). This may underlie pain around your vaginal and pubic area (page 43).
- *Cystitis*. Bladder infection can be very painful, usually with stinging or burning on passing urine (page 170).
- *Varicose veins*. These are a rare cause of sensitivity (overleaf).
- *Vaginal prolapse*. This is not common. It causes pain and/or a feeling of the inner vaginal walls coming down (page 317).
- *Piles and anal fissures*. These may cause pain in your anus, which may radiate through your perineum and vagina, particularly when you need to pass a stool (page 440).
- *Birth injury*. If you have had stitches or a deep tear or episiotomy the area may remain painful for many months. Initially the pain may be related to infection in the area but later on it may be from scar tissue.

Vaginosis

See also Vaginal discharge and infection.

Bacterial vaginosis, also known as gardnerella vaginitis, is one of the most common causes of vaginal discharge. It is called non-specific vaginitis and can be present without symptoms. It may be transmitted through sexual contact but this is not an exclusive route. Men also carry the infection but do not show symptoms. The infection cannot be spread by sharing clothes or in swimming pools. Nor can it be spread from a pregnant woman to her unborn baby, but it has been linked to premature rupture of the membranes (page 392) and PREMATURE BIRTH, so early treatment is worthwhile.

What happens

Vaginosis bacteria often live in the vagina in small numbers without presenting any problems. The bacteria favour conditions that are not too acid and their numbers increase if the environment becomes more alkaline, as in pregnancy, perhaps giving a vaginal discharge with an unpleasant fishy odour. The smell may be strongest after sex but there is unlikely to be any itching.

Action plan

A vaginal swab can be tested for organisms.

- Treatment is with antibiotics in tablets or as an antiseptic vaginal gel. The usual choice is metronidazole for use once the first trimester has passed. If treatment eradicates the infection, it may reduce the risks of premature birth.
- If you have had a premature birth in a previous pregnancy, you may consider asking for a test, as infection may have been a factor.
- Probiotic yoghurt or pills may help to replace the lactobacilli in your bowel and vagina, thus preventing the gardnerella bacteria from thriving (for details of how to take this, see page 35).
- Nutrition can build up your immunity to this and other common infections.
- If you would like to use HOMEOPATHY, please refer to the remedies listed for vaginal discharge.

Veins, mother

The veins in your body undergo many changes during pregnancy. Blood volume increases, pregnancy hormones relax and dilate (widen) the vein walls and the veins expand, particularly in your pelvis, labia, thighs and legs. This can lead to potential problems, ranging from harmless visible veins to a rare but potentially life-threatening condition – deep vein thrombosis (opposite).

■ PROMINENT AND VARICOSE VEINS

When veins swell because of increased blood flow, they become prominent, visible as blue lines beneath the skin and perhaps slightly raised. They are common on the abdomen and breasts. Sometimes, as a vein expands, the valves in the wall stretch and lose their ability to stop the backflow of blood. As a result, the vein becomes varicose. These are most common in the legs, thighs and labia and also appear near the anus. Probably 30 per cent of women get them. Varicose veins often run in families (due to an inherited tendency to thin connective tissue), are more likely if you are carrying TWINS, are overweight, or stand for long periods (for example, at work).

Varicose veins often throb, particularly at the end of the day, and may be associated with swelling, often in the lower legs. Varicose veins present no risk to a baby and usually improve after pregnancy. Labial veins always disappear completely after birth but varicose leg veins may not resolve completely if the extent of stretching means that the valves are no longer strong enough to prevent a build-up of pressure. You might find the problem increases in subsequent pregnancies.

Action plan

Medical care

Surgical removal of varicosities is not recommended during pregnancy because of the high blood flow in the veins at this time. It is best to wait for three to six months after birth, by which time the veins may shrink. You may prefer to wait until you've completed your family because each pregnancy puts additional strain on your venous system.

+ Red flag

If you have pain in the veins that does not disappear when you rest or if they are red and sore, further investigation is needed to exclude phlebitis (inflammation) or deep vein thrombosis (opposite).

Lifestyle, diet and exercise

- Good-quality elastic support tights are essential to minimise pressure on your veins. If the veins are severely affected, use the tights whenever you are out of bed. Support is very important after delivery (a high-risk time), particularly during and after CAESAREAN SECTION, to prevent a deep vein thrombosis, and will help your veins return to their normal state.
- Avoid clothing that restricts blood flow. This includes tight trousers and socks with elastic tops.
- Reducing the pressure on your legs may prevent or decrease the extent of varicose veins. Try to put your legs up above the level of your uterus for an hour or two during the day and raise the foot of your bed by about 15cm (6in) at night.
- If you are taking a long flight, use support tights, drink water and walk around regularly and take a single low-dose aspirin (75mg) before the flight.
- Take care to avoid gaining excessive weight. A diet rich in vitamins and minerals and antioxidants reduces the risk of thrombosis.
- EXERCISE often by walking or swimming to maintain circulation and prevent thrombosis.

Aromatherapy and massage

A cold compress (page 36) can offer relief, as can gentle MASSAGE. Use gentle upward massage strokes and never massage directly over a varicose vein. Try lemon essential oil mixed with a carrier oil (page 35). After Week 24 you can use geranium in a low dose.

Homeopathy

The suggested remedies below may be taken in 6c potency, three times a day for up to one week before re-assessing. If there is no change after one week, your homeopathic practitioner may advise an alternative remedy. If pain is severe and persists, seek medical advice.

- *Hamamelis* (No. 1 remedy) for varicose veins where there is soreness, congestion, heaviness of legs and thighs, a constricted, stinging feeling in the veins, worse from pressure and movement and better at night, perhaps with a history of poor circulation. If there are few guiding symptoms, this would be the remedy of first resort.
- *Sepia* for purple varicosities on the vulva and legs with a feeling of heaviness, when the whole system feels sluggish (perhaps with

constipation or piles) but better for fast movement and warmth.

- *Pulsatilla* for poor circulation with cold hands and feet, bluish, swollen veins that are tender and sting. There may be changeable symptoms, turbulent emotions, and a tendency to be worse sitting or standing and better for gentle exercise, fresh air and pressure on the affected area.
- *Fluoric Acid* for chronic varicose veins that are knotted and sensitive with a burning sensation, better for walking fast and from bathing in cool water.
- *Carbo Veg* if you feel chilly, particularly your hands and feet, yet veins are burning and itching and your skin appears mottled. Useful for varicose veins on the vulva, groin and legs, especially if pain eases in fresh air and you feel better elevating your legs.
- *Lachesis* for hard, ropy, purple, distended veins, usually on the left leg, with pulsating pains exacerbated by heat and worse after sleep.

SPIDER VEINS

Sometimes blood vessels become visible as red spots that are spider shaped and may be up to 3mm in diameter. These consist of capillary blood vessels that have been dilated by the hormones. They disappear if you touch them lightly, then reappear when you release the pressure. They are harmless and will become invisible when pregnancy is over.

THROMBOSIS AND PULMONARY EMBOLISM

From the moment you conceive, your blood-clotting system is very active. It coagulates (clots) most easily in the first week after you have given birth. This has the advantage that it prevents excessive BLEEDING at birth but it also increases the risk of you developing a blood clot, or venous thrombosis. This is a rare but potentially serious problem that usually occurs in the pelvic or leg veins.

The risk associated with thrombosis is that if the clot or embolus is dislodged it may travel to and block the pulmonary veins in the lungs, causing a pulmonary embolism. This rare event can be life threatening as it reduces the amount of oxygen the blood receives. Early diagnosis and treatment of thrombosis prevents serious, even life-threatening complications.

What happens

When a superficial (surface) leg vein becomes inflamed (phlebitis) it feels hot, red and tender and the leg may swell, usually only around the swollen vein. With care this will not necessarily progress to thrombosis.

In more dangerous, deep vein thrombosis the usual symptoms are pain and swelling of the calf or the thigh. The pain of a deep vein thrombosis is not relieved by bed rest or by elevating the leg. In 50 per cent of thromboses, though, there is neither swelling nor pain, particularly if the clot is in one of the pelvic veins. 'Silent' thromboses are more dangerous because they are not treated early. If the clot travels to the lungs to give a pulmonary embolus, symptoms may vary from minimal breathlessness to severe chest pain, shock and collapse.

A number of factors increase the risk:
- A blood disorder leading to abnormal blood clotting (page 58).
- Prolonged bed rest before or after the birth, also following operative surgery, including caesarean section.
- A previous episode of deep vein thrombosis or pulmonary embolism.
- Existing large varicose veins or inflammation in the veins.
- Being overweight and/or being a smoker.
- A family history of pulmonary embolism or deep vein thrombosis.

✚ Red flag

Call your doctor immediately if:

- You have a swollen vein or leg with pain that does not improve with bed rest.
- You have even mild symptoms associated with pulmonary embolus, such as breathlessness. Severe chest pain or shock needs urgent medical attention.

Action plan

Prevention
- If you have had a previous thrombosis or embolism or thrombophilia, you may be given

anticoagulants (blood-thinning drugs such as aspirin or heparin) as a precautionary measure.

- If you have a caesarean section you can reduce the risk of thrombosis by using elastic stockings and becoming mobile within hours of surgery. Many hospitals give heparin injections to thin the blood while you are in hospital.

- Superficial phlebitis (inflammation) carries a low risk of embolism provided there is no underlying deep vein thrombosis and the swelling is treated with anti-inflammatory tablets and cream. You must wear support tights and it is important to remain mobile to reduce the risk of the clot extending into deep veins. Anticoagulants may rarely be needed.

Diagnosis and treatment

- A deep vein thrombosis is confirmed by ultrasound scan of your leg veins and can be treated with anticoagulants. Heparin is the drug of first choice because it does not cross the placenta. It is administered by injection under the abdominal skin once or twice a day. However, if heparin is used for more than a few months, it may cause OSTEOPOROSIS. After pregnancy it can be gradually replaced with warfarin to keep the blood thin. The doses must be carefully monitored to prevent over-thinning and internal bleeding. Depending on clot size, treatment may continue for a few months. Aspirin may be prescribed in careful doses in conjunction with heparin in pregnancy.

- During pregnancy, the diagnosis of a pulmonary embolism can be confirmed on CT scan (a computer-aided X-ray image) but the usual ventilation/perfusion scan uses radioactive isotopes and is not used because of radiation risk to the baby.

- A pulmonary embolism is an emergency. It is treated with heparin to thin the blood and prevent further clot formation. If the embolus is large, additional intravenous medication may be administered to break down the clot and improve blood flow to the lungs. Rarely, if these measures do not help a mesh is inserted into the large chest vein to trap blood clots before they reach the lungs. It is removed a few weeks later when the clot has dissolved.

- In the first week after birth, ensure you are mobile and receiving anticoagulants if these are needed.

- If you have a thrombosis or embolus you may require anticoagulant treatment during any subsequent pregnancy as a precaution. Your blood can be tested after birth to diagnose an increased clotting tendency (thrombophilia).

Violence and abuse, baby

See Child protection and abuse.

Violence and abuse, mother

See also Child protection and abuse.

It is a sad fact that battering and abuse against women is most common during pregnancy. Around 10 per cent of women suffer physical, emotional or sexual abuse, most often in their own homes. Physical abuse is a more common cause of antenatal complications than vehicle accidents or falls. Abuse may begin before conception but it sometimes starts during or after pregnancy.

When there is abuse towards a mother, this is a strong indicator that a baby or child may be abused in the future by the perpetrator (page 131). Appropriate measures taken in pregnancy can help to protect a mother and reduce the risks for her baby in pregnancy and beyond.

If you are or have been a victim of violence you may find it difficult to share the truth, even with friends. During pregnancy, however, you have access to a wide network of medical, practical and psychological support. This may be your first chance to confide in people who listen and help you bring about change. You are now responsible for two people – your baby and yourself. Although separation is sometimes the only way to put an end to aggression, some families do survive intact.

What happens

Abuse may involve physical, psychological or sexual violation, often between intimate partners. In pregnancy, physical abuse is often directed towards the abdomen or the breasts. Psychological and emotional abuse includes verbal harassment and threats, intimidation and destruction of possessions, and forced isolation. Sexual assault may include rape and mutilation of the breasts and genitals. Sometimes the effect of violence may hinder a baby's growth (page 132), cause PREMATURE BIRTH or LOSS OF A BABY. Abuse shatters many lives and it can take years to pick up the pieces.

Abuse is a form of control and dominance. It often involves a man being violent to his partner, although abuse may be present in other relationships (including a parent-child relationship, even when the child is a pregnant adult and mother to be). Some people have a personality trait that inclines them towards violence, and some repeat the aggressive treatment they received as children. During pregnancy, men with a tendency to aggression or jealousy may feel threatened by their unborn child. An abusive man becomes a 'different person' when he is violent.

An abuser often blames his victim and over time a woman may believe she is at fault. Some battered women deny the truth: they are afraid of how their attacker will punish them if they seek help, or they feel ashamed, embarrassed or guilty. Despite the pain of staying in an abusive relationship, women often develop ways to hide the truth; there may be a drive to protect themselves, their relationship and/or their partner. Sometimes being abused feels preferable to being alone.

Some effects of abuse in pregnancy

Abused women are prone to a number of emotional and physical ills but doctors or midwives may not sense a problem during routine antenatal care. Women who are being abused or have suffered abuse in the past are more likely to have pain such as headache, back or pelvic pain, DIARRHOEA with irritable bowel syndrome, unrelenting TIREDNESS or significant anxiety and DEPRESSION. There is also a greater dependence on alcohol and addictive DRUGS. Some women delay or miss antenatal visits for fear that signs of abuse will be noticed or for fear of intimate questions, physical touch and examinations. Illnesses, drug or alcohol use and avoidance of routine checks may leave a woman feeling isolated and more fearful, and may carry profound implications for the development of her child.

Your baby in pregnancy

Your baby is well protected from physical injury in the womb. He is, however, sensitive to touch and will feel the impact if you are struck with force. He hears well by Week 15, and can sense the sounds and your reaction when someone shouts at you and you become tense or afraid. He picks up hormonal messages in the fluids he receives through the umbilical cord and may develop a stress-reaction when levels of stress hormones in your body are high. If there is ongoing violence, your baby will be exposed to stress throughout pregnancy.

Your baby is an individual with a unique set of genes and a unique temperament, and many factors, including nutrition and the love he receives, affect his physical and emotional wellbeing. If he experiences a lot of physical or emotional abuse directed towards you this is likely to affect him. It may be that stress arising from domestic violence results in a small and stressed newborn who adapts poorly to life outside the womb. But he may be very resilient and your love could help him thrive. The possible effects are discussed on page 132. The long-term impact will also be influenced by the environment your baby experiences after birth – the way your baby is held, loved and cared for is hugely important.

Labour and birth

One result of being abused may be a high state of anxiety. Labour and birth are influenced by many things, including your body and state of mind, and your baby's size, resilience, health and position. In labour, fear can restrict the flow of helpful birthing hormones, hinder progress, increase sensitivity to pain, and raise the likelihood that intervention will be needed. You may find it hard to say what you need – particularly if a person who has been abusing you is present. Birth may feel traumatic, and this brings a greater risk of POST TRAUMATIC STRESS DISORDER. Alternatively, birth may present a wonderful opportunity to celebrate and the arrival of your baby may be a catalyst for a new start.

After birth

After the birth abuse is usually a continuation of an earlier pattern. Occasionally it may begin as a reaction to the huge life change. A man might feel envious of the new baby and upset that he has been displaced. If your parents have been abusive to you this may continue as they try to control how you mother your baby. If you are being abused, parenting will inevitably become more challenging. Your baby is also at risk.

In relationships where there is domestic violence, children witness about three-quarters of the abusive incidents. About half the children in such families have themselves been badly hit or beaten. Toddlers often become anxious, complain of tummy-aches, find it difficult to sleep, have temper tantrums and start to behave as if they are much younger than they are. A small number of abused women abuse their own children, perhaps because aggression is the only means of control they know.

Action plan

The first step is to seek support so that others can offer you practical help and be there for you emotionally. If you have asked for help before but received a reaction of disbelief or denial it is worth trying a second time, or exploring a different option. There are dedicated help lines and your antenatal care team may include sympathetic people you have not previously known.

Being at the receiving end of aggression may leave you feeling small, at fault, wrong and submissive – qualities that might make it hard to recognise the extent of the abuse and to ask for support. It takes a lot of courage and loving support from one or more people who acknowledge and value your feelings to speak up and take action. When you have a baby your motivation to change may be many times stronger.

A priority may be to seek alternative accommodation, or you may be okay where you are and benefit instead from someone to come and stay with you or visit regularly to help with domestic chores and share a cup of tea and a chat. It is important to talk about what has happened and to discuss options for the future, including the birth and your plans when your baby has been born. A therapist (page 162) may offer non-judgemental listening and advice. Part of support is help with appreciating that you do not have to go through this alone, you are not at fault, and change is possible. You might ask your GP or midwife for a recommendation, enquire about a local or national support group or group therapy. Any counselling will be treated in the strictest confidence.

Your baby is aware of your moods. He will know if you love and accept him, even though you may be hurting or afraid, and you can tell him this, even before birth: talking honestly and positively to your baby alters your own stress hormones and calms you (page 310).

Pregnancy and birth

Letting your medical team know what you are going through is important because it will help them to care for you. It may be possible to have more time at an appointment and to have a companion or chaperone with you. During labour, doctors and midwives may find it easier to support you with understanding and tact. Planning to have epidural anaesthesia may be important to reduce discomfort and fear.

Whether you choose to tell your medical team or not, it will be helpful for you to ask someone you trust to be with you during labour and birth. When you are cared for by people you trust your labour is more likely to go smoothly (page 347).

After the birth

If your life situation has not changed in pregnancy, it is important to make changes once your baby is born. Many women who are abused feel isolated and helpless, and appreciate help in identifying options for change. Some show symptoms of post traumatic stress disorder (page 449). Counselling or a local or national support group may help. Your health visitor and GP may be at the centre of your supportive network. They may help you arrange practical support, put you in touch with individuals and organisations, including legal professionals if necessary, and give advice if you are experiencing other physical or emotional symptoms (such as ongoing pain and depression).

You may need extra support as you care for your baby and build a loving bond (page 210). If you are still at risk of violence, a social worker may be involved as a matter of protecting you and your child (page 133). Abuse may be one of the factors causing post traumatic stress disorder.

Your baby

If you feel cut off from, or abusive towards, your baby, or you know or suspect your abuser is hurting your baby, it is important to confide in someone. The priority is for your baby to be safely cared for while you receive help and support. It may be enough to ask a friend or relative to take over childcare while you take time out; or you may need to look for a longer-term solution (page 133). It may be reassuring to know that many women feel angry with their babies. It is when the urge cannot be controlled that it is time to reach out. This is preferable to staying in a situation in which you may both be hurt. It takes a lot of courage to admit to feeling overwhelmed and concerned about your baby and to ask for what you need in order to enjoy a safe and loving relationship.

One of your baby's key requirements is to feel safe, loved and accepted. With positive and loving experiences, your baby may be happy, explorative and healthy and bring intense joy to your life. It will be a challenge, however, to offer safety and appropriate attention if you feel under threat or if you are highly anxious or depressed. In order to care well for your baby, you will need to care for yourself and seek support, as suggested above. It may be useful to know that if your baby felt stressed in pregnancy he may continue to be irritable or anxious after birth, but this does not necessarily continue. Loving care and contact with you can help him feel settled and relaxed. Suggestions for helping your child feel safe are given on page 208.

Staying in an abusive relationship

If you remain in an unsafe home it is a good idea to have to hand a telephone number of someone who can help and/or a police number, plus identity documents, keys, money and a suitcase with essential items. Social workers or health visitors can help you make a plan. On the bright side, in some relationships when abuse is addressed and both partners receive help, behaviour patterns do change and family life may become loving and rewarding.

Homeopathy

It is best to visit your homeopath for a specific remedy, and to do so regularly if you are receiving therapy, because a number of different emotions may surface. Many people find remedies for depression, grief and anger (page 176) helpful. *Staphysagria* is one of the main remedies for long-term abuse when suppressed anger builds into deep resentment that is suppressed or simmers beneath a facade of pleasantness before exploding.

Vision difficulties

See Sight problems and blindness, baby.

Visualisation and self-hypnosis

Taking time to relax through visualisation recharges your batteries and expands your mind. It may help you through labour and birth: labour can be visualised and experienced as segments of contractions that can be managed easily. In some cases, previous traumatic memories can be worked through using visualisation as one of the tools. You can perform a visualisation at any time, for example when you're feeding your baby or having a bath, or you can make it more formal in an undisturbed setting.

After birth it is vital for you to have lots of good quality rest. Visualisation enables you to slip into deep relaxation where you can take your mind away to a safe place that you have chosen to visualise. This is your private sanctuary, your well-deserved space of peace. In this place you choose to feel safe and nurtured, and allow all your rhythms to wind down and your body to regenerate. You can go there by closing your eyes and saying to yourself, 'I am going to my safe place now.' Over time this will become a trigger for relaxation.

It is useful to take several short visualisation breaks during the day. Ten minutes is equivalent to at least 30 minutes of sleep. If you have been woken up at night you may find it easier to drift back to sleep by doing a relaxing visualisation.

Before you start a visualisation, get comfortable and warm. Breathe deeply and relax from your head and shoulders down your back, into your pelvis and to your toes. You may enjoy focusing on an imaginary spot ahead of you until your eyelids become heavy and close as you relax. Watch thoughts arise and intrude on your visualisation, let them fall and then re-focus.

The visualisations here are for you to play with and use whenever you wish – their power will surprise you.

Visualisation: for new energy

- Imagine yourself on a warm summer day walking through a meadow. You can hear the sound of a river. You lie on soft, green grass and look up at leaves moving in the breeze ...
- Let yourself relax and watch wisps of cloud moving across the blue sky ...
- Feel your body sinking into the softness of the grass and hear the sound of birds and wind-rustled leaves ...
- Feel yourself lying still as you become one with nature ...
- You are in harmony.

Visualisation: for gentle birth

You can practise this or a similar visualisation in pregnancy as you prepare your mind for the day of birth. On the day it will then be easier to slip into this state and you may find it very relaxing and encouraging.

- Deeply relax all the muscles in your body – from the tips of your toes to the top of your head. Look into your womb and make contact with your baby.
- Every thought and feeling you experience is shared by your baby. Allow yourself to think positive thoughts about your coming birth experience. Remember that you and your baby are working in close co-operation to create a wonderful birthing experience.
- Now focus on the birthing part of your body.
- Take your inner eyes into the deepest part of your abdomen, and locate your pelvic circle of bones, which provides the frame on which the muscles of your abdomen, lower back and thighs are attached. Just as the muscles in your body have the ability to move, know that the bones in your pelvis also have an inherent ability to expand at the joints and ligaments.
- Between now and the birth powerfully visualise that the inner diameters of your pelvic space are becoming wider and wider every day. As your baby grows, ask the head to gravitate down into the lowest part of your uterus so the top of your baby's head is in close contact with the inner opening of the cervix, the neck of your womb. Mentally prepare the birthing space so that by Week 36 your baby's head can easily find the optimum position for birth.
- Flex your own head so your chin is tucked onto your breastbone. Mentally transmit that image to your baby and ask her to adopt this position. Also ask you baby to face towards your spine slightly to the right or to the left so that the smallest diameter of her head sinks into your pelvic birthing space.
- From Week 36, as your baby's head grows comfortably within your pelvis, encourage mutual moulding between your pelvis and her head so that birthing becomes gentle for both of you.
- Encourage your baby to feel calm and nurtured so the placenta produces generous quantities of all the hormones to prepare your birthing spaces for a gentle open-release at birth.

▩ HYPNOSIS

When you spend time doing a visualisation you often slip into a state of self-hypnosis. 'Hypnos' in Greek actually means sleep, but hypnosis is closer to an altered state of mental awareness when the brain waves flow as 'alpha' waves (as they do in meditation). This is a natural state of mind and the human brain drifts in and out of hypnosis spontaneously. Consciously encouraging it may be useful to create relaxation as it helps muscles and blood vessel walls relax, increasing circulation, stabilising blood pressure and slowing heart rate. It can help you feel energised and confident.

Entering hypnosis is easy if you know how. To be guided into hypnosis you can talk silently to yourself or ask someone to talk to you in a flowing and gentle rhythm, as if there is no punctuation and no break between sentences. You can learn this method if there is a class near you or from a DVD.

Vitamin K dependent bleeding

See Bleeding, baby, vitamin K dependent bleeding.

Vitamins

See Food and eating, mother; Weaning, baby.

Vomiting and nausea, mother

Nausea with vomiting occurs in 70 per cent of pregnancies, typically starting by Week 4 or 6, peaking by Weeks 8 or 12 and resolving spontaneously by Week 16. It can occur at any time of day or night, although it may be more intense in the morning, hence the term 'morning sickness'. Some women feel queasy at intervals during the day and some vomit once or several times, daily, for weeks. Around one in five women still feel sick in late pregnancy. Nausea and vomiting are usually not a cause for concern. Severe vomiting that leads to weight loss and dehydration is called hyperemesis (page 553). Nausea tends to be worse in a first pregnancy and in women who have a poor diet, and/or are carrying TWINS.

What happens

The exact connection between vomiting and pregnancy is not well understood. The nerve centre for nausea is situated in the brain and it is unclear how the hormonal changes of pregnancy affect the brain's cells.

* Later in pregnancy, nausea may occur as your enlarging uterus presses on your stomach.
* Nausea can be brought on by muscle tension, particularly in the diaphragm or upper abdomen, and this may be aggravated by poor POSTURE, anxiety and TIREDNESS. A vicious circle often begins with nausea giving rise to fatigue, and fatigue bringing increased muscle tension, a tendency to slouch rather than sit upright, perhaps excessive eating of sweet foods, and increased nausea.
* If you have an underlying tendency to nausea, for instance travel sickness, you may be more susceptible.
* Nausea may reflect anxiety about your personal and family circumstances or ambivalence at becoming a mother. These and other feelings linked with anxiety are explored on page 174.

Implications for you and your baby

The majority of women function well despite nausea, even though it can be tiring and upsetting. Physically, there are no long-term health problems related to nausea, although if you eat an excess of bread, sugary foods and juices to reduce the feeling you may gain excessive weight. Occasionally an underlying emotional or stressful issue is brought to light by persistent and severe vomiting. This may put a strain on your family relationships or lead to DEPRESSION. Some women feel so upset they consider terminating the pregnancy. The passing of sickness is usually accompanied by a joyful high.

Your developing baby obtains adequate nutrients from reserves of vitamins, minerals, proteins and fatty acids that have been stored in your body before conception. Even if you have intense vomiting in early pregnancy that settles, your baby is likely to continue to grow normally. Babies born after severe vomiting and hyperemesis treatment may weigh roughly 200g (7oz) less than average but their development is normal.

Action plan

If you are well nourished before you become pregnant, you are less likely to suffer from nausea, and if it does occur your energy levels will be higher. To cure nausea or vomiting, try homeopathy or acupuncture first (overleaf) – these are safest. To alleviate nausea, a good resource is a balanced diet.

Rinse your mouth with a gentle fluoride rinse each time you vomit. This will freshen your mouth and protect your teeth from stomach acid. Use a very soft toothbrush twice a day – not immediately after you vomit because stomach acids may soften the enamel and excessive brushing could cause erosion.

Food and eating

* Where you can, avoid the sight and smell of anything that makes you nauseous. If a home or workplace smell is a problem, try burning an aromatic essential oil.
* Try to eat small quantities of complex carbohydrate every three to four hours to avoid sugar lows (page 261) and to neutralise your stomach acid.
* If you eat lots of refined bread, sugary food and drinks because they make you feel better, take care that you don't gain excess weight, although this may be less important for a few weeks than keeping yourself going. Nuts and seeds are usually well tolerated.

- Have a snack before sleep or if you wake at night and before getting up in the morning. Carry snacks around with you so you don't find yourself without food in the late afternoon, often a queasy, low-energy time. A complex carbohydrate is best, such as an oat biscuit or rice cake.
- Even if you cannot tolerate food, it is important to keep drinking – dehydration will make you exhausted and weak and, if severe, may lead to hyperemesis (opposite). Drink small amounts every hour or two, rather than large quantities, to avoid bloating. Focus on water and a variety of herbal teas: ginger, mild mint or hot water with a slice of lemon. Ginger tea is often effective. Fruit or vegetable juices or soups contain essential electrolytes and minerals as well as liquid.
- For vitamin and mineral supplements, you may prefer a tonic to a tablet or try crushing pills to a powder and sprinkling on your food.

Lifestyle
- Managing stress may reduce nausea. If you have been feeling nervous about your baby, an ultrasound scan may help to allay your anxiety.
- VISUALISATIONS or meditations may ease stress symptoms.
- Slow, restful YOGA postures and breathing techniques (page 105) may help to release muscle tension.
- When you feel nauseous, allow yourself 15–20 minutes to relax.

Homeopathy
You may match your symptoms to one of the symptom pictures below and take the appropriate remedy in 30c potency four times a day for up to three days and then re-assess.
- *Sepia* for constant nausea, empty feeling in the stomach, a desire to eat but the thought or smell makes things worse, you are better for eating little and often, feel very tired, irritable and upset, worse first thing in the morning and between 3pm and 5pm.
- *Ipecac* if you have no relief from vomiting or eating and feel worse from any motion; you are pale and prostrate with nausea, and you are salivating, suffer empty retching and have no thirst.
- *Arsenicum* for persistent nausea and vomiting that leads to exhaustion, faintness, restlessness and chilliness, when you are anxious about your

health and your baby's health and there is relief from sips of hot drinks and company.
- *Nux Vomica* if you feel relieved from vomiting, although this may require lots of empty retching and gagging, you feel overstressed and over-stretched, irritable, constipated and crave an uninterrupted sleep.

Acupuncture
Acupuncture can be very effective.
- The point Pericardium 6 is the usual focus, and in full treatment this would be combined with other acupuncture points according to your needs. Pericardium 6 is two finger-widths above where your wrist and your palm meet, in line with your middle finger. Massage this point with your thumb in an anti-clockwise direction, with moderate pressure, for two minutes on each wrist, two or three times a day.
- Acupressure travel sickness wristbands are available from chemists, with instructions for locating the acupuncture point – press the buttons to increase stimulation.

Aromatherapy
Massage with essential oils can be powerful in breaking a cycle of vomiting and helps to replace tension with calm. You could add a few drops of essential oil to a warm bath and have a good soak. Ginger is good, or try lavender after Week 24.

Medical care
If you are vomiting and have INDIGESTION or HEARTBURN, you may be prescribed medication to reduce acid production. Anti-nausea medication may be essential if the vomiting is causing you to feel weak or dehydrated or shows the characteristics of hyperemesis (opposite). The medication acts on your brain to reduce vomiting. None of the anti-nausea medications are licensed for use in pregnancy because of the possible side effect on a developing baby, but if vomiting is severe your doctor may consider treatment essential.

Dopamine antagonist drugs (such as metoclopramide and prochlorperazine) have been used for decades and to date there is no association with any harmful effects for developing babies, although some women do feel drowsy. Suppositories are beneficial if you vomit excessively. Your doctor will tailor medication to your needs.

On very rare occasions an inner ear infection may cause vomiting and can be treated. This is usually accompanied by dizziness.

■ HYPEREMESIS

Hyperemesis is a condition characterised by excessive vomiting with dehydration and the loss of more than 5 per cent of pre-pregnancy body weight. Fortunately it is very uncommon (affecting only three in 1,000 women) and usually responds to hospital treatment involving intravenous fluid therapy to replace water, plus electrolytes and sugar, and anti-nausea medication.

A tiny proportion of women require prolonged treatment and support, particularly those carrying twins. Excessive vomiting may lead to inflammation of the oesophagus and even bleeding from the inflamed area. It may be necessary to treat the acidity with antacids or drugs to reduce acid production.

H2 blockers and proton pump inhibitors are usually very effective but these are prescription-only medications and it is important that your doctor knows you are pregnant. Replace vitamins and minerals as part of the treatment programme. In a tiny number of women with very severe hyperemesis that is resistant to medication, corticosteroids are effective.

Vomiting, baby

For the first few months, all babies bring up a small amount of milk after some, most or all of their feeds, often with a burp but no sign of any force. This is possetting – not vomiting. It is completely normal, particularly in the first 12 weeks after birth, and rarely causes distress. Providing your baby is thriving and gaining weight it is not a cause for concern. When your baby possets, he brings up two to three spoonfuls of liquid. Vomiting, which is different, involves bringing up a large amount of stomach contents through the mouth and sometimes the nose. All babies vomit at some time. On occasions this is a sign of an underlying problem such as an infection that will respond to treatment.

When vomiting is not a cause for concern
Occasional vomiting is seldom linked to a serious health concern. A single occurrence may simply

be a sign that your baby is a little unwell or overfilled with milk, and is usually self-limiting.

✚ Red flag

When vomiting may be serious

- Repeated vomiting that occurs suddenly, particularly if linked with DIARRHOEA and/or a high temperature, may be a sign of infection that requires treatment.
- Usually the main concern is that repeated vomiting may cause dehydration (page 181), which if severe needs hospital treatment.
- In a small number of cases, ongoing vomiting (particularly if 'projectile' or forceful) is a sign of a disorder in the digestive system such as pyloric stenosis (overleaf).
- Vomiting may be a symptom of concussion following a head injury.
- Green or bright yellow staining of the vomit indicates that your baby is bringing up bile as well as his food/milk, and needs to be investigated by your doctor to exclude a bowel obstruction.

What happens

When a baby vomits, contractions of the stomach force food contents up the oesophagus (food tube) and out of the mouth and sometimes nose. The milk or food is often partially digested and may look curdled, and because it contains stomach acid it may make your baby uncomfortable, a feeling like heartburn. If your baby inhales vomit, he may cough and gag, become breathless and panic until the vomiting or retching has stopped and his airway is clear.

Vomiting is seldom dangerous – it is the resulting dehydration (if vomiting is repeated) that can present a problem. A normal healthy baby will not choke on vomit. Even when asleep, your baby has well-developed reflexes that will prevent him from inhaling vomit.

Possible causes of early vomiting

By far the commonest reason for vomiting is being fed too much. The excess food/milk may come up with effortless reflux or possetting, or with a burp.

Reflux

At the level of the stomach, a valve in the oesophagus relaxes to let food into the stomach, and closes to prevent food mixed with stomach acid from refluxing back up into the mouth. If food does come back, even part of the way, this is called reflux or gastro-oesophageal reflux.

All babies reflux: this is normal and is part of the process causing possetting. If reflux causes pain from the acid content of the food, your baby may appear unsettled after feeding or reluctant to feed. Reflux may also cause him to vomit. The reflux is likely to pass as your baby grows older, and typically improves when your baby spends more time upright (in your arms, or sitting and later standing and walking) and with the introduction of solid food (although it is not helpful to introduce solid food before he is sufficiently mature, i.e. not before six months of age, see page 557).

There are many simple treatments.

* Babies are placed on their back to sleep to reduce SUDDEN INFANT DEATH. This practice has increased the incidence of reflux. When your baby is awake it is best to be upright in a sling or in your arms; hold your baby upright during and after a feed. Car seats also encourage reflux.
* Try giving him less milk at each feed, and feed more often.
* If he is over six months and eating solids, increasing the solids in his diet may be effective.
* If you are BOTTLE-FEEDING do not add cereal or thickener to the milk, or use more formula powder than instructed. This could dangerously increase sodium content and may contribute to dehydration. Occasionally, a specialised thickened milk feed, such as Enfamil, may be prescribed.
* Occasionally a prescribed antacid, such as Gaviscon Infant, brings relief.
* A very few babies with reflux have failure to thrive (page 559), and this is probably the only group for whom medical treatment with antacid drugs, rather than just Gaviscon Infant, or anti-reflux drugs, or rarely surgery is needed.
* Sometimes reflux is a symptom of milk ALLERGY OR INTOLERANCE. If this is diagnosed, follow specialist recommendations regarding an alternative formula milk.

Disorders of the digestive system

Early vomiting rarely occurs because of a disorder of the digestive system. However, occasionally projectile vomiting may be due to the following:

Intestinal atresia/intestinal malrotation

Forceful vomiting after each feed with bright yellow or green vomit may be due to bowel obstruction. This needs to be checked urgently by your paediatrician. An X-ray or ultrasound scan can establish the cause. The obstruction may be due to intestinal atresia (absence of a normal opening) or the bowel may be twisted (intestinal malrotation). These rare conditions also lead to CONSTIPATION.

Pyloric stenosis

If your baby projectile vomits with progressive intensity and frequency after every feed, this may indicate pyloric stenosis, another rare intestinal condition. The symptoms of pyloric stenosis usually begin from the third week but may not start until as late as the twelfth week. It is more common in boys and is caused by an excessive thickening of the pylorus muscle that obstructs the stomach and stops it from emptying into the small bowel. Your baby may be upset from the vomiting, and from being continually hungry. Weight loss can occur quickly. It is important to get an accurate diagnosis and, if necessary, treatment with a relatively simple operation where the thickened pylorus muscle is opened. Once the operation is complete, feeding generally returns to normal, growth resumes and your baby's weight is likely to quickly catch up with his peers. If he seems nervous about feeding he may need gentle reassurance as he gets used to feeding without vomiting, pain and being hungry.

Overfeeding

Occasional projectile vomiting is not a sure sign of pyloric stenosis. Many babies initially thought to have this condition are actually being overfed.

Possible causes of later vomiting

Infection

Infection is a common cause of vomiting after 12 weeks, and occasionally before this. When the infection has passed, perhaps with the aid of antibiotic treatment if the cause is bacterial, the vomiting will clear up of its own accord.

Very occasionally viral infection causes vomiting before 12 weeks.

* About 90 per cent of vomiting after the twelfth week is caused by viruses, predominantly rotavirus.
* If your baby has a cold or cough this may trigger vomiting. It is likely to happen at night while your baby is not upright and mucus is more difficult to expel.
* Vomiting may be a symptom of a throat or ear infection. It may also be a sign of a urinary tract infection.
* More serious infections that may lead to vomiting include MENINGITIS.
* A bacterial infection causing vomiting is likely to cause abdominal pain and bloody stools. When accompanied by diarrhoea, vomiting is often a sign of a bowel infection such as gastroenteritis or food poisoning (page 181).

Vomiting with blood

* If you can see blood in the vomit, this is not necessarily a cause for concern. If you have cracked nipples your baby will take in blood as he breastfeeds. It is safe to continue feeding and the blood will do no harm.
* Less commonly, blood in vomit may be a symptom of a bleeding or blood clotting disorder (page 62) and needs urgent attention.
* Very rarely, bloody diarrhoea with vomiting indicates haemolytic uraemic syndrome, a disease usually triggered by the Escherichia coli bacterium. Treatment requires hospital admission, and specialist care. For other causes of bloody stools, see page 61.

Action plan

Visiting your doctor

You need to visit your doctor if:

* There are signs of dehydration – dry lips but wet inside the mouth, troubled but not excessively fretful, and tiring easily.
* Your baby is under six months and has been vomiting for more than 12 hours.
* Your baby is over six months and has been vomiting for more than 24 hours.
* Your baby has other symptoms that are of concern, such as ear pain, diarrhoea or FEVER.

+ Red flag

You **urgently** need to call your doctor and you may need to take immediate FIRST AID measures (page 3) if:

* There is blood in the vomit unless you have cracked nipples.
* The vomit is bright yellow or bright green – bilious vomiting that could indicate a bowel obstruction.
* Your baby's abdomen appears to be more swollen or has unusually prominent veins.
* Your baby seems to have abdominal pain for more than two hours, lasting longer than a usual attack of COLIC.
* Your baby has signs of moderate to severe dehydration – mottled or pale skin, listlessness, dry lips and mouth, absence of urine.
* Your baby cannot keep any fluid down.
* Your baby has a high fever above 38.5°C (100.8°F).
* Your baby has had an abdominal injury or a knock to the head.
* Your baby is having a FIT (convulsion).
* Your baby is receiving medicines for seizures or a heart condition and cannot keep these down.
* Your baby may have ingested a poison (plant, medicine, chemical).
* Your baby appears to be choking.

Treating your baby at home

The key is to prevent dehydration by giving your baby fluids. It is important to introduce the fluids gradually and in small amounts. If you are BREASTFEEDING, let your baby suck for a short time every five minutes. If not, offer your baby water or a rehydration solution (page 182) one hour after the last vomiting attack. Begin with a sip or teaspoonful every 15 minutes.

There is no best position to prevent inhalation unless your baby is unconscious. If so, turn him on his side, and allow secretions to drain from the mouth.

Medical care

- You can use infant paracetamol (page 429) to reduce a fever. If he cannot keep this down and the fever persists, your doctor may prescribe paracetamol suppositories.
- When your child is vomiting repeatedly, stop any medicines he is taking, unless they are critical (such as anti-convulsant drugs or drugs for a heart condition). If more than one dose is missed, call your doctor.
- Do not give anti-nausea medication or medicines to stop vomiting. These are only necessary if the vomiting is severe, in which case they are best given in hospital.

Homeopathy

For mild cases you may give the most indicated remedy in the 30c potency, three times per day for one day and re-assess. Continue with the same remedy if your baby is improving or change the remedy to a more indicated one and re-assess again 24 hours later. If vomiting is severe it is crucial to see your doctor.

- *Aethusa* for vomiting that occurs soon after feeding; usually curdled milk, that can be quite violent and your baby becomes sleepy afterwards.
- *Arsenicum* for vomiting with diarrhoea, your baby is restless and anxious and clearly uncomfortable, he is very thirsty, but as soon as he drinks everything comes up again.
- *Phosphorous* for vomiting that occurs once the contents warm the stomach. Your baby will seem cheerful, thirsty and want to be cuddled.
- *Silica* for a baby who vomits breast milk that smells sour – especially for babies who are not thriving, feel better for warmth and being wrapped up.

There are also remedies for reflux: these are best given with personal prescription from your homeopath.

Treatment in hospital

If you take your baby to hospital the doctors will ask you how frequently he is vomiting, when it began, whether it contains blood, if urine is being passed. Your baby's temperature will be taken and you will be asked about his recent feeding patterns and any contact he might have had with infection. Your baby will be examined and tested for dehydration and infections.

Most babies are offered a feed of clear fluid of about 0–90ml (1–3oz). If this is not vomited up within 30–60 minutes it is repeated. If your baby keeps the fluid down and appears well, he may be allowed home. Continue with usual feeds and supplement with extra oral fluids. Use oral rehydration solution (ORS) or Dioralyte in the amounts recommended on the package (page 182).

If your baby does not keep the initial feed down, then fluid may be given through a vein or through a tube into the stomach. Often this is sufficient to stop the vomiting, and fluids by mouth can then be restarted. If this is tolerated, your baby will be observed for a few hours, receive regular oral fluids and if these are kept down he may be discharged. Most babies recover within 48 hours on this treatment. Some babies have treatment for longer, usually to treat viral or bacterial infections or other causes of vomiting.

Von Willdebrand's disease

See Bleeding and blood-clotting disorders, baby.

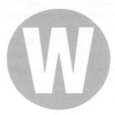

Water birth

See Labour and birth, mother, active birth in water.

Weaning, baby

In the UK, opinions regarding the best time to start a baby on solid food have changed dramatically over the last 50 years. Across the world, too, there are different philosophies. The UK's Scientific Advisory Committee on Nutrition (SACN) currently recommends exclusive BREASTFEEDING for six months from birth to give optimal nutrition for your baby. By six months of age, your baby's digestive system will have matured sufficiently to begin eating solids. It is vital to continue breastfeeding your baby, or alternatively give formula milk, until 12 months, and sometimes beyond, in preference to unmodified cow's milk.

Within these guidelines, each individual baby should be cared for according to her unique needs. It is recognised that, in the UK and across much of Europe and the USA, parents introduce foods earlier than six months for many personal, social and economic reasons. If you are unable to follow the SACN recommendations, or choose not to, seek the support of your health visitor or other advisor to ensure you provide the best nutrition for your baby.

Weaning before six months

Giving your baby solid foods before his neuro-muscular co-ordination, intestines and kidneys are sufficiently mature can increase the risk of infections and development of allergic illnesses

such as eczema and ASTHMA. It may also bring on colicky symptoms (page 144), worsen existing colic, lead to CONSTIPATION or (less commonly) DIARRHOEA.

If your baby is not growing as expected for her age (page 559) it is not appropriate to give solids before six months. A thorough medical examination is important and your doctor will make recommendations according to your baby's needs.

If you give your baby solids before six months in the hope of getting a longer sleep at night, think again. Her body may not be ready for it. She will sense your frustration and may overeat and put on unnecessary weight. She may even become anxious and begin an unhappy relationship with food. There are other ways to help her sleep (page 492).

Introducing solids, from six months

- Respond gently to your baby's signals. Offer food when she's alert and content and let her set the pace and gradually get used to eating.
- Offer something smooth with a gentle flavour, cooled to room temperature. Hold her on your lap and give her food with your finger.
- Later, you can introduce a soft plastic spoon. It is best to sterilise all the spoons and bowls that she uses.
- Begin with baby rice mixed with your baby's usual milk. Give one spoonful a day, at lunchtime, after an initial drink. If she has difficulty digesting she is likely to feel settled by bed time.
- If your baby seems happy after four to seven days of having one spoonful a day, introduce another, and build up gradually.

* Introduce puréed pear and soft puréed vegetables.
* You can gradually increase texture as your baby gets used to eating, and when she is teething or has teeth she may enjoy chewing on solid pieces, such as cucumber or apple.
* Although most babies love sweet food, they are not so partial to it as toddlers seem to be. Give your baby a variety of vegetables and savoury dishes, with fruit purées as a second choice, and avoid sweets, sweetened yoghurts, doughnuts, cakes, ice-creams and so on. Use organic where possible, and wash all fruit and veg well.
* Always end the day with a milk feed.

Take advice from a health visitor or a specialist baby book as you broaden the range of foods you give. Guidelines are based on what's known about babies' digestive systems, but they are only guidelines. Your baby will have her own reactions, likes and dislikes.

What your baby needs

Your baby requires around half the number of calories you need each day and can get sufficient from her milk and from healthy meals that include fat. Vegetable fats are preferable and you may give yoghurts, hard cheese, and so on that have a valuable fat content. If you make milk-based meals (such as cheese sauces) choose full-fat milk, as the calorie content of skimmed or low-fat milk is insufficient.

Breast milk and formula milk, in combination with a well-rounded diet of fish, vegetables, beans and pulses, offer appropriate quantities of vitamins and minerals and protein (for more on sources, see page 263). Fibre is also essential and comes from many sources including vegetable skins. Vitamin supplements are also nationally recommended (opposite).

Foods to avoid

* Current advice is to delay giving cow's milk or powdered skimmed milk mixed with water until 12 months; but it is okay to give processed dairy products such as baby milk, yoghurt, hard cheeses – from six months.
* Don't give soft or blue cheeses such as Brie or Stilton because of the risk of LISTERIA.
* From six months it is okay to give gluten-containing products (including bread), but keep the amounts low. Exceptions may be made if there is a history of gluten allergies in your family, in which case the advice is to avoid gluten until the end of the first year.
* Avoid granary and high-fibre bread and wheat bran, which are too difficult for your baby to digest.
* Avoid egg whites until 12 months.
* Avoid nuts and nut products until the age of three.
* Adding salt or sugar to baby foods is also unnecessary and can be a cause of excess weight gain and high BLOOD PRESSURE in later life.
* Don't give your baby excessively sugary foods, fruit juices, colas and cordials, crisps, biscuits and so on. If you give your baby rusks, check the ingredients because some are high in sugar.
* Don't give products containing unpasteurised honey to your baby, or indeed eat them yourself, as the unpasteurised honey may contain botulinus spores that can cause a serious illness. It is safe to give your baby pasteurised honey, because the heat of pasteurisation destroys the botulinus.

Meal times

Balancing your baby's diet is important and can make a difference to her moods and sleeping pattern. Once weaning is established, it is best to give solid food every three to four hours. A three-meals-a-day rhythm may be more readily established if your baby is BOTTLE-FEEDING; if she is breastfeeding it is normal for her to snack from your breast at intervals as well as having three meals a day. She may do this for 18 months or more.

Playing and exploring

Your baby may love selecting from a range, perhaps slices of banana, cooked carrot, avocado, pear. Don't limit meals to purée mixes, or worry whether she eats all that's on the plate, as her appetite will change from day to day. And enjoy: messy meals are the norm and your baby's urge to explore (page 211) is not naughty!

Gagging and choking

Many babies are sensitive to lumps in their food and may gag and cough. For most babies this soon passes but if the stage persists try going back to purées and give finger foods, such as bread or apple. A very small number of babies remain sensitive and need the help of a speech therapist. This occurs more often in children who have been born prematurely or have had other difficulties in the newborn period. Sensitivities to lumpy foods are more common among babies for whom milk feeding or the experience of eating solid food has been challenging.

Milk requirements

From 6 months
Solids are a supplement to milk feeds but they do not replace milk feeds. By six months the recommended milk intake is five breast feeds or five bottles of 250ml (7–8fl oz), giving a total milk intake of around 1,125ml (32fl oz) plus small amounts of solid food.

7–9 months
Your seven- to nine-month-old baby needs to consume at least 600ml (21fl oz) of milk a day. You may give some of this as part of his cooked meals (for example, 30–60ml [1–2fl oz] in a cheese or creamy vegetable or pasta sauce) but most will come from your breast or a bottle. Between six and nine months most babies have three or four milk feeds a day, usually at breakfast, mid-afternoon and bedtime, and an optional extra mid-morning.

If your baby goes through a growth spurt or goes off his food when he is teething or feels unwell, let him feed from your breast as often as he likes, or if you are bottle-feeding, increase the amount until he is keen to eat solids again.

The final milk feed before bed is the most leisurely. If he's still hungry after a large bottle or after feeding at both breasts, look back over what he has eaten during the day: you may need to increase the size of his meals.

Vitamins

Infant vitamin drops are currently recommended from six months for breastfed babies, and from 12 months for bottle-fed babies, until the age of five. This is primarily because of the increasing risk of rickets due to vitamin D deficiency (page 465) and to ensure each child has adequate vitamin stores throughout childhood. Children who have a good appetite and eat a wide variety of foods, including fruit and vegetables, probably receive adequate vitamins in their diet, but are still advised to take vitamins until they are five.

The most common supplement is ABIDEC, a liquid preparation. This contains peanut oil. If your baby is known to be allergic to peanuts it is safest to avoid this preparation. However, despite many years of study, no direct link with allergic reactions or with later development of peanut allergy has been apparent. There are other products available in the UK. Later, you may give a proprietary vitamin capsule or chewable vitamins. The most recently developed products, including ABIDEC, now contain omega fish oils.

Webbed toes

Webbed toes are much more common than multiple toes but often go unnoticed by parents because webbing can occur to varying degrees. This is very commonly found running through generations of families and even in whole communities. Webbing occurs when the skin fails to separate between two toes during foetal development. The toes can be surgically separated for cosmetic appearances or if the webbing interferes with normal toe movement needed for walking.

Weight, baby

See also Intrauterine growth restriction (IUGR).

▓ FAILURE TO THRIVE (LOW WEIGHT GAIN)

Of all the challenges facing parents, the issue of growth, especially weight gain, causes the greatest amount of concern and conflicting advice. Failure to thrive is not specifically defined in medical terms. It is a growth disorder of infants and children due to nutritional and/or emotional deprivation and resulting in loss of weight or poor weight gain. It is often linked to delayed physical, emotional and social development. Children who fail to thrive don't receive or are unable to take in or retain adequate nutrition to gain weight. The condition is more common in PREMATURE babies and it may be linked to medical problems.

Most babies who are investigated do not show failure to thrive: 98 per cent do not have a significant growth problem. The first few months are a common time for parents to worry that their babies may not be growing adequately and parents' concerns are taken seriously.

What happens

If you fill in the growth chart (page 274) in your baby's record book regularly, you will notice a gradual upward trend. At times, your baby's weight gain may level off, there may be obvious growth spurts and she may sometimes lose a little weight. This variation is normal. In true 'failure to thrive' (affecting just 2 per cent of babies) weight gain is lower than expected, or the growth chart drops down two or more percentile curves over time. If this happens, you and your doctor will probably want to investigate and treat the cause.

The first month

A healthy baby may lose up to 12 per cent of her body weight, and some breastfed babies up to 17 per cent, in the first week after birth at full term. This is because she draws on fat and glycogen stores for energy while feeding is established. The loss is normal, but it can be reduced with lots of skin-to-skin contact (page 517). After this weight gain is progressive. A baby born prematurely or weighing less than 2.5kg (5lb 8oz) may not lose as much weight initially, and many small babies gain weight rapidly to catch up.

Breastfed babies often gain weight more slowly than bottle-fed babies in the first two weeks. By far the most frequent cause is feeding difficulties. This problem is more common among women who leave hospital before feeding has been established. Typically, when a mum receives guidance and support to address feeding difficulties this helps a baby obtain the calories she needs.

About 10 per cent of newborns need additional help because of weight loss in the early weeks. Because of difficulties with feeding, a baby may become more jaundiced, and appear to lose weight due to inadequate fluid intake, resulting in dehydration. In this case it is important to ensure that there is no underlying medical cause, such as a urine infection.

Up to six months, and beyond

The average baby born at full term doubles her birth weight by six months and triples it at one year. A premature baby attains her birth weight at about 10 days after birth, and then her weight increases as normal, providing she is able to tolerate her feeds. Babies born small due to INTRAUTERINE GROWTH RESTRICTION (IUGR), rather than from prematurity alone, often lose no weight after birth, and are hungry feeders.

When a baby grows more slowly than expected, she may become apathetic and irritable, and may not reach milestones such as sitting up, walking and experimenting with language at the usual age. Being poorly nourished may also affect mental development, and may increase susceptibility to illness and infection.

What causes failure to thrive?

The cause of failure to thrive may be broadly sorted into three categories:
* A baby is eating but not being given enough milk or food.
* A baby has a medical problem that interferes with food intake or digestion, leading to malabsorption.
* A baby's requirements are higher than normal due to illness or infection.

Your doctor may be able to pinpoint a specific cause. If eating is painful for your baby, she may be fractious when you feed her, and the challenge of consuming food may affect calorie intake.

Possible causes
* BREASTFEEDING difficulties are a common cause. They include poor position (page 83), low milk flow (page 94) and difficulty sucking (page 99), which is more usual among premature babies or babies with a cleft lip or palate.
* When your baby begins to eat solids there may be a temporary levelling off or slowing of weight gain as her body adjusts.
* Occasionally an ALLERGY OR INTOLERANCE affects weight gain and, for a small number of babies, intolerance to milk affects weight gain before solids are introduced.
* Digestive difficulties resulting from conditions such as gastro-oesophageal reflux (page 554),

DIARRHOEA or VOMITING may affect consumption and absorption.

- It is possible that your approach to feeding may be the cause, perhaps feeding too infrequently in the initial months, or giving your baby too few calories when she is eating solids. This may be due to misinformation, or to a fear that your child may gain too much weight. A low-fat adult diet is not suitable for a child. Your baby needs a high-calorie intake (page 558) and still needs milk when eating solids.
- Illness with an infection, which forces rapid use of nutrients, sometimes brings about failure to thrive. Other rarer medical causes may be involved.
- CONGENITAL ABNORMALITIES such as CYSTIC FIBROSIS, liver disease, metabolic disorders and coeliac disease that limit the body's ability to absorb nutrients may affect growth.
- A small number of children fail to thrive as a result of neglect. They are not fed enough, or not touched lovingly or held often enough. Being held and having skin-to-skin contact promotes the body's manufacture of growth hormones.

Genetics

Genetics may play a part. If you are slim, your baby may inherit the same trait. Genetically determined small children often grow in a similar pattern to their parents. Small but normal need not be a cause of concern. If your baby is growing along her own line on the growth chart, this is not a sign of failure to thrive. If your baby's small size reflects intrauterine growth restriction there may be related issues (page 323) that require attention. Some genetic conditions and chromosomal disorders, such as DOWN'S SYNDROME, do carry a greater tendency towards failure to thrive.

Action plan

Diagnosing the cause

It is important to know why your baby is failing to thrive. Your doctor may examine your baby and arrange blood count, urine analysis, and blood chemical and electrolyte tests to get useful information. If a disease or disorder is suspected the doctor may perform tests to identify or exclude the suspected condition.

Your doctor, perhaps with the help of a dietician or breastfeeding counsellor, will ask you what your baby eats and how she behaves when she eats. He or she may recommend that you keep a food diary in order to calculate your baby's calorie intake. You may be asked about your own diet and lifestyle if you are breastfeeding.

Treatment

In most cases, treatment is straightforward: increase calorie intake. If your baby receives and absorbs additional calories, her weight may increase within a week and she may be more settled. It may take longer before your baby reaches the normal range for her age. The advice, encouragement and practical help you receive will be important. Your midwife, health visitor or lactation consultant may make a real difference if you wish to continue breastfeeding to offer your baby the benefits of your milk. You and your baby may be supported by a nutritionist, and perhaps by an occupational or speech therapist if your baby has difficulty sucking or swallowing, or a milk intolerance. Occasionally, a family therapist may be involved if there appear to be bonding difficulties or relationship issues. Depending on the cause, a specific child specialist may be part of your baby's care team. If the reason for slow growth is thought to be related to your baby's family environment, a social worker or psychologist may provide support.

Touch and time together

While your attention is on breast- or bottle-feeding or the foods you give your baby, it is important to remember that she needs touch in order to grow. Spending time together, preferably skin to skin, can boost growth and can improve your milk supply and your baby's digestion. This applies even if your baby needs tube feeding (overleaf) or in the unlikely event that she requires special care.

Breastfeeding

During the newborn period, successful breastfeeding usually leads to an increase in weight. You may need guidance if you are experiencing positioning difficulties or pain, and support if you feel anxious, because anxiety may affect your milk supply. It may be useful to look at your own eating routine and to spend more time with your baby. The calorie content of your breast milk adjusts to meet her needs when you feed frequently and are in touch with one another.

Supplementing breastfeeding with formula
Occasionally, it is appropriate to introduce supplementary feeds. If you are bottle-feeding, you may be advised to alter the type of formula milk. Rarely, a doctor may prescribe a high-density milk formula.

Treating vomiting or diarrhoea
If your baby is regularly vomiting or has diarrhoea, identifying and treating the cause (pages 553 and 181) is likely to help.

Increasing calorie intake for your weaned baby
If your baby is weaned, adjusting her diet may be a simple case of ensuring she has calorie-rich foods (page 558). Your doctor may recommend specific foods.

Allergy
If your baby shows an allergy or intolerance, you may need to alter your diet, if you are breastfeeding, or try different formulae before her weight stabilises. It is always important to consult a specialist.

Tube feeding
In very extreme instances, a baby may need to be tube fed, particularly if she is ill. This can be done at home and parents are shown how to put the tube in place. About half the caloric needs can be delivered through a continuous drip of liquid milk or supplemented liquid milk at night while day-time eating remains as normal. Once weight increases the tube can be removed.

Treatment in hospital
If a weight problem continues, a baby may need to be admitted to hospital where she can be fed and monitored continuously, and may stay until weight gain is adequate. The hospital team will attempt to identify any underlying medical causes for the slow growth. These teams are highly supportive of babies and parents. Typically, a baby with poor weight gain is admitted to a children's ward. Babies who have been home for any length of time are not usually readmitted to a SPECIAL CARE BABY UNIT.

Family meal times
If your baby does not eat readily or becomes upset at meal times, you may become frustrated. It is common for parents in this position to feel at fault or inadequate, even though the cause of eating difficulties is often out of their control. It is helpful to observe your reactions at meal times. If you become tense or angry, this may increase the stress your baby feels and magnify the problem. If meal times become a war zone, a pattern of frustration may continue for many years. Things may become easier with support from your GP, health visitor, nutritional therapist or another health professional, so that meal times can become more enjoyable, even if your baby has specific dietary needs.

■ OVERWEIGHT AND OBESITY

See also Weight, mother.

Obesity is now recognised as a global epidemic, and being overweight in childhood may be a significant risk factor for being overweight, obese or having eating difficulties (page 200) in later life. Eating habits start before birth and in infancy.

In the UK, 10–20 per cent of children are obese by the age of six, although figures suggest there may be a slight improvement by 2010, among boys more than in girls.

Obese children are twice as likely as normal-weight children to become obese adults. Being overweight can lead to enormous social consequences, such as teasing and exclusion, low confidence and poor educational achievement. The health risks include premature heart disease and high BLOOD PRESSURE, onset of DIABETES, early onset arthritis, and aggravation of ASTHMA.

In pregnancy, your health and your diet are important to set your baby's tastes, and after birth you play a crucial role in your baby's eating patterns. It is now well established that bottle-fed babies are more prone to obesity in later years, because a bottle-fed baby can be overfed. Breastfed babies cannot be overfed and although breastfed babies tend to gain weight initially more rapidly than bottle-fed babies (page 275), prolonged breastfeeding is not a factor contributing to obesity. What your baby eats and drinks when she is weaned is very significant.

What happens

A tiny fraction of children develop obesity because of a specific genetic disease. This is known as endogenous obesity. However, by far the most common cause is excessive calorie intake and reduced energy use. This is 'exogenous obesity' and is almost exclusively linked with family and cultural habits around food and exercise.

Your baby, like you, has fat cells (adipocytes). These increase in number when calorie intake increases. The process begins in the womb and continues through to adolescence. If your baby develops a higher than normal number of fat cells in the critical period between conception and her first birthday, the risk of gaining excess weight increases. Developing excess fat cells through childhood and adolescence is similarly significant. An overweight problem that develops in later life may have its roots in the early years.

Everybody needs to consume calories for energy, but many overweight children are not physically active and do not use the energy provided by food – instead, it is stored as fat. Many babies spend more time sitting and lying than their parents did. Prams, car seats, baby chairs and other convenient objects actually deny them the chance to move and exercise as much as they naturally need to.

Action plan

Prevention is possible and powerful. If you can help your baby build a good foundation in pregnancy and the first years of life, you may help her avoid obesity for life. If your baby's weight chart places her in the upper zone, your health visitor may talk to you about eating patterns and suggest preventive measures as part of daily life.

Your habits and values

You may be surprised how useful it is to look at your own eating habits and the attitudes you have towards food, body image and weight. Emotional and cultural issues will come into play. The way you were fed as a baby is likely to affect the way you feel about feeding your own baby. It is common, for instance, to use food to distract from physical pain, or to suppress uncomfortable emotions and feelings or even avoid difficult conversations. Adults often knowingly or unconsciously use food in a similar way to placate a crying baby or toddler. There are other significant family views, such as believing a baby needs to look chubby to be healthy, or a mum deserves to indulge in rich foods and sweets in pregnancy. Some families have an opposite view that any sign of excess body fat is unhealthy.

You and your partner may decide to look at your own values and family backgrounds and discuss what the effect could be for your baby. The advice on page 567 about what to do if you eat when you are not hungry may be useful.

Eating in pregnancy

Weight gain is normal in pregnancy (overleaf). If you or your midwife believes you are gaining excessively it is time to check whether you are consuming too many calories, and consider ways to slow the gain. It is never appropriate to lose weight in pregnancy, but there are many ways to keep your gain optimal. This is looked at in detail on page 565.

* If you consume sweets or sweet drinks, you and your baby will experience a sugar high followed by an energy slump – this is the 'sugar trap' (page 262). This pattern may become habitual for your baby, and could be reinforced if you give her sweet foods and juices when you wean her. A balanced diet supplemented by appropriate vitamins and minerals may help you to avoid sweet snacks in pregnancy and think ahead to weaning foods that are healthy and low in sugar.
* If you have diabetes, you will need to monitor your blood sugar levels closely during pregnancy because poorly controlled diabetes can be associated with above-average growth in a baby.
* If you have an eating disorder (page 200), dealing with this problem before the birth may help you enjoy parenting and feel less anxious.

After birth

* Breastfed babies cannot overeat. You and your baby are in harmony and your body produces milk to meet her needs, altering its calorific and fluid content constantly.

- Overfeeding is more common among bottle-fed babies but if you monitor the spacing and size of your baby's feeds this is easily avoidable (page 76).
- If you are worried that your baby seems overweight, the first thing to do is ask your health visitor or doctor to weigh her and check her height. She may appear chubby yet still be within a completely acceptable margin of weight gain.
- Try not to compare your baby to other babies, but follow the advice of your health visitor. Every baby is an individual.
- If you are breastfeeding (page 81), continue to eat nutritious, well-spaced meals so that your baby gets a healthy balance of nutrients and calories without regular high-sugar feeds.
- Never give your baby juice in a bottle. Juice is a potent cause of weight gain and tooth decay.
- When you wean your baby, avoid giving calorie-concentrated foods such as sweets, crisps, biscuits and cakes. Ask your health visitor for advice if you are concerned that your baby eats too much or always seems hungry.
- Encourage your baby to play regularly, even when she isn't walking. As she moves her arms and legs, pushes herself up and supports her weight, this helps her develop and use the energy she consumes in her milk or food. You may use MASSAGE and gentle physical play to help her enjoy feeling physical. Reduce the time your baby spends in a baby car seat and use a sling to carry her. EXERCISE is a crucial aspect of balanced health.
- As your child becomes increasingly independent and eats more solids after the first year, remember that snacks between meals, particularly if they are sweet or loaded with fats, are a potent cause of excess calorie intake.

Weight, mother

See also Eating difficulties, mother.

▄ GAIN IN PREGNANCY

There are guidelines for recommended gain because too much, or too little, may mean that conditions are not optimal for your baby's development or for your health. Your care team will keep an eye on your gain at antenatal checks.

Your weight reflects not only what and how much you eat but also how you feel emotionally and your lifestyle. Every woman's body changes in a different way, and it is more helpful to be aware of your personal progress than to compare your weight gain to that of other women. You may delight in your new shape and your growing belly. Alternatively you may feel uncomfortable, perhaps embarrassed. Some weight gain is healthy and essential in pregnancy.

What happens

Ideally, weight gain begins after the first missed period and continues until the birth – precisely how much you gain depends on your physiology, your baby and your eating habits. More significant than the gain during pregnancy, however, is your weight before conception. If you are underweight (page 567) or poorly nourished, this can be harmful.

How your body gains weight in pregnancy (approximately)

Breasts:	450g–1.3kg (1–2lb 13oz)
Placenta:	675g (1lb 8 oz)
Amniotic fluid:	900g (2lb)
Uterus:	900g–1.6kg (2–3lb 8oz)
Maternal fluid/ blood:	2.9kg (6lb 6½oz)
Baby at term:	3.1–3.8kg (6lb 12oz–8lb 6oz)
Maternal fat stores:	3.6–4.5kg (8–10lb)
Total:	12.5–15.8kg (27lb 10oz–34lb 9oz)

Body mass index and recommended gain

It was once thought that weight gain should be limited to no more than 6.8kg (15lb). Current recommendations are based on pre-pregnancy body mass index (BMI). BMI is a formula based on weight-to-height ratio endorsed by the American College of Obstetricians and is used in the UK. BMI is preferable to only measuring weight, because it also takes height into account. Taking your weight in kg and dividing it by the square of your height in metres gives your BMI. BMI charts are available in most clinics.

Weight gain in each trimester

There are guidelines for weight gain in each trimester (three-month period). Please remember

Weight at conception	BMI	Gain recommended
Underweight	Below 19.8	12.7–18.2kg (28–40lb)
Normal weight	19.8–26	11.4–16.0kg (25–35lb)
Overweight	26–29	6.8–9.1kg (15–20lb)
Obese	30–40	6.8kg (15lb)

Pregnant with twins: Target weight gain 15.9–20.5kg (35–45 lb).

The optimal weight gain for a woman who is 1.6m (5ft 2in) or smaller is the lower end of these recommended ranges.

these are only guidelines, and each woman gains weight differently, so do not be too rigid.

In the first trimester (Weeks 1–13): an ideal weight gain is 1.4–1.8kg (3–4lb).

In the second trimester (Weeks 14–26): an ideal gain is 225–450g (½–1lb) per week. This amounts to a total of 3–6kg (6½–13lb). It is often the easiest time to eat well.

In the third trimester (Weeks 27–birth): a similar gain should continue until the end of the eighth month. In the final month, weight gain may slow down, so the gain for the whole trimester is 3–4.5kg (6½–10lb).

Action plan

It is best to keep weight gain as steady as possible – your baby requires nutrition from day to day. Your midwife or a nutritional therapist may help you assess whether your diet provides sufficient calories and nutrients. Your doctor or midwife will help you to keep on track. There is practical advice in the section on eating (pages 253–65).

If you have a goal, choose a target gain that does not put unnecessary pressure on you. Weigh yourself no more than once per week. If you recognise you are out of your target range, it is important to discuss the situation. If you are concerned your weight gain (high or low) may affect your baby, you may ask for an additional ultrasound assessment of your baby to ensure his development is on course.

If there is another issue, such as stress, anxiety or depression, lifestyle steps may help. For instance, stress can often be managed with a few adjustments to the way you plan your time. If you have an eating disorder, pregnancy

is a good time to address it. You may do this through your midwife or with confidential counselling (page 162).

▇ LOSS AFTER BIRTH

Weight loss does not happen the instant your baby is born. Your body takes time to release the fluid you have accumulated and also needs to retain some extra fat stores for BREASTFEEDING. Within six weeks, most women lose around two-thirds of the weight gained in pregnancy, and many women look four to six months pregnant for some months. The rate of reduction varies enormously, however, and depends on how you feel emotionally and physically after birth, whether you breastfeed and what you eat. The weight gained in pregnancy usually falls away within three to nine months of birth.

Not losing enough weight

Whatever your body shape or your tendency to gain or lose weight, it's more important to attend to nutrition than to the figures on the scales. Yet it will be obvious if you are losing weight slowly, or indeed if you are continuing to gain. If so, it is worth seeking advice, reducing your calorie intake and exercising regularly. While you are breastfeeding, the same intake as pregnancy (page 256), is fine – on some days you may feel you need a little less, and on others a little more.

Some women say it's hard to eat nutritiously because they have little time to prepare food. There may be a number of people in your immediate family or in your group of friends who would be very happy to cook some meals for you and help you build your skills for cooking and preparing nutritious snacks. Continue with the pregnancy vitamin and mineral supplements.

It is important to attend to your weight at this time because some women find that a cycle of progressive weight gain begins in pregnancy and spirals after each baby.

Losing too much weight

While you're breastfeeding, a sharp fall in weight could affect your milk supply, and if you're undernourished this will make it harder to enjoy your baby and your life.

If you are losing weight normally and you feel well in yourself and your baby is thriving, there is no cause for concern. If your loss is rapid or excessive and especially if you are feeling unusually weak or tired, consider your calorie intake and whether you are getting sufficient nutrients. Consult your GP or midwife and request a thyroid function test. Rarely, thyroid overactivity can lead to tiredness and weight loss (page 514). Taking supplements (page 264) may improve your digestion and absorption, while exercise or YOGA might boost your appetite.

■ OVERWEIGHT AND OBESITY

Being overweight and, especially, obese can carry considerable health risks and often has a very negative effect on self-esteem. The risks increase as your weight rises.

Obesity is defined as weighing more than 20 per cent above expected for your age, height and body build – that's an excess of approximately 2.5 stone (15.8kg or 35 pounds) or a BMI (page 564) of 30–40. Obesity is far more common than being underweight.

Pregnancy is a common time for the problem of being overweight to begin. If you develop a habit of eating excessively and if the weight gain continues after birth, you may have begun a long-term struggle. For some women, the weight gain comes after birth: adjusting to a new lifestyle that includes sufficient EXERCISE and time to buy and cook nutritious food can be gradual.

What happens

Being overweight is a reflection of the way you eat, exercise and work, your relationships and, underpinning all of these, your self-esteem.

- Excess weight results from eating more calories than your body burns. The main causes are sugar, fat and insufficient exercise.
- Eating large quantities or high-calorie sugary foods may be part of a life-long habit. Alternatively, cravings (page 255) may start in pregnancy. You may use food for comfort or to relieve boredom.
- There may be a gene that controls weight and metabolism and predisposes to excess weight. This is being researched.
- Obesity can result from dieting (page 256): the vast majority of dieters regain all the weight they initially lose, plus roughly 5kg (10lb) extra.
- You may become overweight if you have been bulimic and are controlling your purges but not your food intake.
- Some people are obese because of biological problems such as malfunctioning thyroid gland and it is worthwhile having a blood test. Sometimes physical disabilities limit exercise and physical activity.
- Occasionally excess gain in pregnancy may be a sign of gestational DIABETES. This is a form of diabetes that first appears in pregnancy. It usually resolves after the birth but may indicate an underlying risk for diabetes that returns later on.

+ Red flag

Uncommonly, a rapid gain of more than 1kg (2lb) per week in pregnancy could signify the onset of pre-eclampsia (page 68) and requires urgent attention.

Increased risks associated with high weight

If your weight is significantly high, extra medical care may be necessary because you are at greater risk of gestational diabetes, high BLOOD PRESSURE, carrying a LARGE BABY and having difficulties in labour (although maternal gain and a baby's size do not always correlate). You are more susceptible to complications with anaesthesia and CAESAREAN SECTION. Your doctor may find it difficult to feel your uterus and need more scans to monitor your baby.

Extra fatty tissue can cause breathing problems, and the abdominal pressure may lead to INDIGESTION AND HEARTBURN and put extra stress on your knee joints. Excess weight can be a potent contributor to DEPRESSION.

Action plan

When weight gain is due to consuming excessive calories, the simple solution is to alter what you eat. The benefit begins as soon as you cut down, and it's best to begin before you get too far into pregnancy. The advice in the section on foods to eat, calories, dieting and emotions may help you meet the challenge of changing your habits (pages 253–65).

Creating a nutrition-friendly environment

Everyone has their own eating habits. You may feel hungry each time you pass the cupboard where the biscuits are stored. You might reach for a sweet whenever you watch television, or stock up on nibbles when you go for a long drive. Simple awareness may bring change without the need for major resolutions. Something as straightforward as not stocking high-sugar, high-fat 'treats' but keeping a store of healthy alternatives (such as fruit and nuts) may make a big difference.

If you want to eat but aren't really hungry

With a good basic nutritional foundation, and little or no 'treats' in the house, you may notice you reach less and less frequently for excess food. Exercise and eating every three to four hours (page 262) will also help. If you eat to satisfy emotional hunger, what are you hungry for? Many people use food as a substitute for love; sometimes it may be a punishment. If you need help to be objective, counselling (page 162) may be the key.

Do not diet

Dieting (page 256) is never appropriate in pregnancy, so please don't aim to lose weight if you begin pregnancy already overweight. Take a measurement of your body mass index at the beginning of pregnancy, and ask your midwife or nutritional advisor to calculate a recommended gain for you. Through pregnancy and after birth, if you care for yourself with nutritious eating and exercise, you are on the right track. Setting a target weight to reach nine months after birth is often realistic.

Medical care

If you begin pregnancy already overweight or gain excessively during pregnancy your health risks rise. A slight excess gain is minimally risky, particularly if you are well nourished with adequate vitamins and minerals.

▇ UNDERWEIGHT

Being slightly underweight is rarely a health issue, particularly if your diet contains sufficient vitamins and minerals to encourage your baby to thrive. Being significantly underweight before conception, however, means that you have fewer nutritional reserves on which your baby can draw. For your baby, your weight and nutritional status when you conceive is more important than weight gain in pregnancy. Even so, losing weight in pregnancy is not a good sign and you and your baby may be deprived of nutrients.

What happens

Being under average weight is usually a reflection of a diet low in minerals, vitamins and essential fats, and/or calories. For some women, it reflects an allergy or intolerance that inhibits absorption of food. It may be linked with lifestyle habits that demand more energy than you get from food – such as excessive exercise or high stress levels. Occasionally, low weight is due to thyroid overactivity. In a severe form, being underweight may be a sign of anorexia and/or bulimia (page 200). Rarely, low weight gain is linked with maternal illness or severe bowel disorders like colitis or Crohn's disease connected with malabsorption.

If you are significantly underweight before conceiving, you could find it hard to accept the weight gain of pregnancy. Some women react to this by eating small amounts so although they grow with pregnancy, after birth they remain underweight. If you are not receiving sufficient nutrients, including calories, you may feel tired and emotional and particularly touchy around food. This applies to men as well as women.

Low gain in pregnancy

A slow gain in the first trimester is common and is rarely a cause for concern. Fortunately, nature protects babies of mothers who feel too sick to eat well during the first three months. A baby does not need many calories at this stage and the reserve of vitamins, minerals, essential fatty acids and proteins built up by the mother before pregnancy will be sufficient. Not gaining or even losing weight in the early weeks isn't likely to cause problems, nor is it related to your baby's rate of growth.

An overall low gain, however, that is less than 6kg (13.2lb) during pregnancy, is likely to concern your care team. This is because low gain can reflect poor nutrition and if your nutrition is inadequate this increases the risk that your baby may be PREMATURE or underweight (see INTRAUTERINE GROWTH RESTRICTION, IUGR). IUGR for a non-nutritional reason may cause low maternal gain. There is not always a correlation between a baby's weight and mum's weight, however. Some women gain at the lowest end of the scale, even though their babies grow at or above the average weight.

Action plan

The first step may be to attend to the practical details of buying food, cooking and eating. Many women appreciate encouragement and company, and it might be helpful to ask a friend or relative who loves cooking to spend time with you and share some tips.

If your calorific intake is low, try eating extra meals each day. You may need five or six small meals rather than three. Boost your intake with food that is nutritious: a handful of nuts with each meal, an extra glass of milk or cheese or yoghurt, an avocado, for example. You will need to experiment to see what feels right for you and professional nutritional advice may give excellent guidance. Vitamin and mineral supplements are important to ensure your baby has sufficient nutrients to develop and grow.

Most women find that long-term change also involves a willingness to consider their feelings towards food (page 258). If you have a more severe problem such as vomiting (bulimia) or anorexia (page 200) it is crucial to seek professional help.

Wheezing, baby

See Asthma and wheezing, baby.

Whooping cough

See also Coughs and colds, baby.

Whooping cough (pertussis) is a serious infection, caused by the bacterium *Bordetella pertussis*. It is associated with severe bouts of distressing coughing and wheezing, and can be life-threatening, particularly in babies aged under six months. A baby below six months may not cough at all, but may have episodes of apnoea, when breathing stops for a few seconds (page 102). Whooping cough can persist for months and is exhausting for the whole family. Vaccination against whooping cough is routinely offered to all babies in the UK. Around nine non-immunised babies die from pertussis every year in England.

What happens

Whooping cough often follows what seems to be a minor cold. It brings on episodes of coughing in runs (paroxysms) lasting up to five minutes, with a characteristic whooping sound on breathing in. Your baby will go red in the face and if coughing is severe, oxygen levels may fall and he may faint. Fainting stops the coughing and allows the body to recover.

Whooping cough has been called the 100-day cough because it often lasts this long before slowly easing. If your baby catches a cold in the year after the initial illness, the cough is likely to return, not from re-infection (the baby has produced antibodies to pertussis) but because his airways are sensitive (irritable).

Action plan

Even with antibiotic treatment, the cough may remain, although the risk of infecting other people can be reduced. Often by the time a diagnosis is made the baby's body has already produced antibodies and the bacteria have been eliminated. If so, the use of antibiotics will make no difference to the coughing, which is a reflex caused by the fact that airways are now inflamed and sensitive.

While your baby has the cough, follow the general advice for colds and coughs (page 157). If the coughing causes your baby to retch and vomit, when the coughing fit has passed, offer another feed. HOMEOPATHY may be helpful but it is essential to see a qualified homeopath.

Wry neck (torticollis)

Wry neck, or torticollis, is a twisting in the neck caused by muscle tightness or tearing and affects roughly 2 per cent of babies. There may be a small lump in the baby's neck and she may hold her head towards the injured side. The cause is unknown. Your baby may have had her head tilted to one side during pregnancy, which reduced blood supply to the muscle, restricting its growth and causing it to tighten. It may then be damaged as the muscle is stretched during birth. The resulting tissue causes the lump and further shortens the muscle.

Though a baby with wry neck may look uncomfortable, it is probably not painful. The muscle can be lengthened and strengthened and gently encouraged to turn away from the injured side with physiotherapy. OSTEOPATHY is also very effective.

Swelling disappears in four to six weeks and normal neck movement is usually established by six months. Because the head lies to one side, head shape may be temporarily affected, resulting in plagiocephaly or 'flattened head' (page 281), but this will right itself once your baby is sitting up.

Giving your baby tummy time is a great opportunity to allow the natural forces of gravity to help the muscles stretch. And by gently turning her head to the side she does not favour, the effects of gravity will gently stretch the muscle. The physiotherapist or osteopath will suggest movements and stretches for you to do with your baby.

Your baby's neck muscles will recover when confident sitting allows full motion. However, it is advisable to ask your health visitor or doctor to check your baby thoroughly.

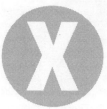

Xiphisternum, baby

The xiphisternum is a part of the sternum, or breastbone. It is seen, or felt, as a soft piece of cartilage that protrudes at the lower end of the ribcage, in the mid-line, just below the level of the nipples. This often causes anxiety as parents are worried about a lump on the chest which they think is abnormal. But it is quite normal and gradually becomes less obvious as the ribs and the cartilage around the ribs become firmer.

X-rays in pregnancy

Because X-rays involve the use of radiation – which may potentially harm a baby in the womb – it is safest to avoid an X-ray of your abdomen or pelvis in pregnancy. The harmful effects of X-rays are dependent on the dose you are exposed to. This includes the use of barium swallows/enemas (which may be used as part of tests for symptoms in the digestive system) and studies of your kidney or your lower spine. These use multiple exposures and relatively high doses of radiation and are not appropriate in pregnancy.

If your doctor or dentist recommends the use of X-ray investigations because establishing a clear diagnosis is a priority then it is safer if the X-rays are not pointing towards your uterus. It is also preferable to have a lead apron to lie across your abdomen to stop the rays from beaming towards your uterus.

If you have been exposed to X-rays during pregnancy consult your doctor about the doses and the risks to your baby.

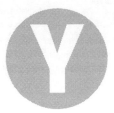

Yoga

See also Exercise, mother; Posture.

Yoga is an ideal form of exercise and relaxation during and after pregnancy. It is safe providing you work within your own personal limits and do not stretch excessively. Yoga illuminates a path from a hectic, outwardly focused life to a calmer, more peaceful and centred existence: a great preparation for each day in pregnancy and when you are with your baby and family after birth.

A practice begun in India thousands of years ago, yoga means 'yoking' or 'union', and refers to the link between mind and body. The aim of yoga practice is to restore the balance between the two in order to bring a feeling of peace and to develop physical ease and mental calm that is an ideal foundation for meditation and physical health. The postures both stretch and tone muscles and organs, and the breathing practices are calming and energising. Together they improve energy and relieve stress.

A vast collection of postures, movements and breathing exercises has been devised over thousands of years. With the guidance of a teacher you can use general postures and vary them according to the way you feel on any day. Many can be used to ease aches and pains and improve digestion. And if you practise regularly, your strength and flexibility may help you to have an active birth. After the birth, yoga is an ideal exercise when your body is recovering and you are caring for your new baby.

Breathing (Pranayama)

Yoga practitioners have used 'Pranayama' meditation for centuries. Breathing awareness is an integral part of yoga postures but a separate time devoted to breathing is a powerful way to connect with 'prana', your life force. Your breath is always there, a tool to centre and calm you. When you breathe deeply you oxygenate your body – and pass oxygen-rich blood to your baby in pregnancy – and your lungs massage your abdominal organs. Insufficient breathing can contribute to a range of ailments from lethargy to digestive disorders. Simple breathing exercises, including regular deep breathing, are very effective. You may want to spend time focusing on your breath each day (page 105) and in labour, breathing is a powerful tool (page 362).

■ SAFETY

In addition to the guidelines for exercising safely on page 227:

* Seek advice from a qualified teacher who is experienced in guiding women during pregnancy.
* Gentle yoga done with awareness will cause no harm to your baby or your pregnancy and will not bring on PREMATURE BIRTH. High energy yoga classes are not appropriate.
* If you experience HEARTBURN, avoid forward-leaning positions.
* Circulatory problems such as varicose veins or PILES can be alleviated with daily pelvic floor exercises (page 438) done in the all-fours or knee-chest position. Avoid positions such as squatting that put pressure on the pelvic region.

- If you experience pelvic pain (page 43) avoid open-legged positions with tension on your pubic joint. Instead, kneel on or between your feet, sit with legs crossed or straight out.
- Use cushions to make yourself comfortable and ease pressure on your joints (for example, under your bottom while kneeling).
- If your back gets tired or aches, sit with your lower back flush against a wall.
- If you have been advised to rest in bed, you can still do a number of the upper body and leg yoga stretches, which can help maintain your energy and sense of wellbeing.

✚ Red flag

- Stop any exercise and seek immediate medical care if you have vaginal BLEEDING.
- If you feel dizzy or light-headed in any position, and particularly while standing or lying on your back, lie down on your left side and rest until it passes.

▓ WITH YOUR BABY

It becomes harder to make time for quiet yoga practice once your baby is born, or during a subsequent pregnancy when you already have children. You will be distracted but you can still benefit from a few minutes of stretching and relaxing. Your baby may be happy to lie down and watch and you can hold him for some postures. If you have a toddler, he may enjoy imitating your movements and playing around you. For more focused practice, use the time when your baby (or children) are asleep or enrol someone to care for them or take them out for a walk while you have 30 minutes to yourself or attend a local class. There may be a mum and baby class near you.

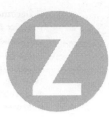

Zinc deficiency

See also Food and eating, mother, vitamins, minerals, EFAs and supplements.

Zinc is an essential nutrient for you and your baby. There are various sources, explored on page 264, and you may wish to take supplements. It is important to ensure you get sufficient as normal zinc levels aid conception and the early development of your baby. In the later stages of pregnancy your baby draws heavily on your stores. A deficiency may interfere with optimal growth for your baby and contribute to depression. Severe deficiency can also result in difficulty to treat sore skin rashes around the bottom and mouth.

Acknowledgements

The journey that has led to *Mother and Baby Health* has spanned a decade, beginning with the creation of a booklet 'Journey into Parenthood' for the Birth Unit at the Hospital of St John and St Elizabeth in London. This booklet was like a seed that grew with our own experience and with further input from midwives, doctors and complementary professionals. This enabled us to write *Birth and Beyond* in 2002.

Birth and Beyond was holistic and was based on the principle of integrating various methods of healthcare and lifestyle choices. It acknowledges the importance of physical, emotional and spiritual wellbeing, for mums, babies and dads, through pregnancy, birth, and beyond. The information in *Mother and Baby Health* rests on this same principle, and we are indebted to the many people who were involved in the creation of *Birth and Beyond* – your input is reflected in this new book.

Mother and Baby Health has been created by: Yehudi Gordon, father, grandfather and obstetrician; Harriet Sharkey, mother, writer and doula; Andrew Raffles, father and paediatrician; and Felicity Fine, mother and homeopath. The incredible range of the book's contents is also due to the input of many professionals who worked with us. This book got off the ground because of the encouragement from Random House, particularly Fiona MacIntyre, Clare Hulton and Julia Kellaway, and our devoted agent, Michael Alcock. Thank you.

The beginnings of *Mother and Baby Health* go much further back. Yehudi's vision for integrating numerous modes of healthcare has been a core aspect of his practice in gynaecology and obstetrics for over 30 years. The philosophy outlined in these pages is practised on the Birth Unit, which was established by Yehudi in 1981, and is now at the Hospital of St John and St Elizabeth. The Birth Unit is well known for active and water birth and the midwives and consultants all believe in integrated family support combining conventional and complementary care. Many of the midwives have additional complementary training and have made a valuable contribution to this book. Yehudi also founded Viveka, an integrated healthcare practice in London and many of the specialists working with him at Viveka have been involved in this book.

Mother and Baby Health also owes much to our own experiences with parents and babies whom we have had the pleasure of meeting over the decades, sometimes on several occasions as more children arrived and families have grown. Our personal lives have of course been crucial, and our own experiences as babies and as parents and grandparents have profoundly informed our writing and influenced our research. One of the key elements of this book is a respect for babies as sensitive, feeling and aware people. We are immensely grateful to Kitty Hagenbach for her insights, love and encouragement that have helped us celebrate these qualities in ourselves and in every baby. Kitty's friendship and generosity in sharing her views have been instrumental in the way this book has evolved. Glenn and Caron Barruw and Fran Riley have inspired us to value and have the courage to write about parents' and baby's emotions and feelings. Our insights have also been encouraged by Ann Herreboudt who provides family support at Viveka and by Peter Walker who passionately advocates touch and massage.

The Birth Unit team

The Birth Unit team has always been there for us. We would like to thank all the midwives, obstetric and paediatric consultants on the Birth Unit for their encouragement and care. Particular thanks to: Anne Herreboudt, for her advice on parenthood, and for first aid and accident prevention; Julie Whitehead, for her attention to detail regarding breast- and bottle-feeding; and Patricia Scott and Sandra Dick, Pratibha Patel and Kirstie Fletcher for their exemplary midwifery care. Bill Smith and Peter Twining have provided state-of-the-art ultrasound scanning. Christopher Board heads the hospital of St John and St Elizabeth and his support and that of his team, including Christine Malcolmson and Judith Pickersgill, has always been unwavering.

For complementary care and lifestyle advice

We would like to thank: Alison Belcourt and Marilyn Glenville for their nutritional advice; Anita O'Neill, for practical aromatherapy tips; Barbara Moss, for insight into acupuncture; Delphine Sayre, who gave advice on using herbs; Gowri Motha, for her inspiration on visualisations and preparing for birth; Jill Benjoya-Miller, for guidance on yoga; Jonty Hurwitz, whose honesty about fathering is refreshing; Kitty Hagenbach for insight into the emotional life of babies, adults and families; Lynda Leach, Karen Eichorn and Tanya Savage, for baby massage; Lynn Haller and Barbara Gough, whose osteopathic skill with newborn babies and with mums is always an inspiration; Malcolm Levinkind, for insight into baby and child dental health; and Shirel Stemmons, for advice on exercise.

Other advice

For insight into babies' perception and development we thank Professor Hugh Johnson and Eileen Mansfield at the Babylab at Birkbeck College, London; Professor Annette Karmiloff-Smith; and Giep Franzen, Margot Bouwman and Dr Gill Harris. We also thank Margot Sunderland, whose exploration of babies' emotions has greatly enriched our own understanding.

The photography

Genna Naccache provided the photographs for *Birth and Beyond* and the wonderful pictures for this cover. It is a real pleasure to have someone like Genna who can capture a moment so well – so thank you! Thank you also, Tanya and Toni-Rae, for the time you spent with Genna and for being so beautiful.

Book production

We would like to thank all those who have been involved in producing this book at Vermilion. From the original conception until the very last full stop, Julia Kellaway has been amazing – supportive, considerate and firm when it counts. Clare Hulton has been with us along the way too, giving us encouragement and support at all stages. We are also very grateful to the other members of the team.

The essential foundation

Behind the scenes we have had tremendous support from our partners and families, who have loved and nurtured us; their concepts and approaches to life and to parenting and health have informed our thoughts. Particularly, we thank Wendy Gordon, Dee Sharkey, Jo Raffles and Barry Fine. Of course, none of this would have been possible without our children and grandchildren, who have helped us to come from the heart: Gabi, Tanya and Nick, Patrick and Rosa, Michael, Ben and Suzanne, Adam and Nina, Max, Jura and Noah, and Toni-Rae. You bring so much joy, and teach us so much.

Amazing families

We thank all the parents who have honoured us by asking us to be present for the births of their babies, and the families whose experiences, feedback and stories have helped us create this book. You and your wonderful babies have inspired us.

Index

100-day cough 568

abdominal pain during
    pregnancy 1–2
ABO incompatibility 67
abscesses and mastitis 95–7
abuse *see* child protection and
    abuse; violence and abuse,
    mother
accident prevention and safety
    11–13
accidents and first aid, baby
    3–13
    ABC of resuscitation 3
    emergency situations 4
aching hips (sciatica) 44, 45
acidophilus 34–5, 118
acidosis 179, 250, 252
acne, baby 459
acquired immune deficiency
    syndrome (AIDS) 311–14
acrocyanosis 482
active birth 349–51
    in water 351–3
acupuncture 14, 382
acyclovir 129, 130
adenosyl methionine 139
adipocytes 563
adrenal glands 268, 310–11
adrenalin syringe 17
adrenaline 292, 310–11
afterpains 368, 393–4
albinism 478
albus oil 157
alcohol 188–92
allergy and intolerance 14–21
ALTE (apparent life-
    threatening event) 102–3
ambiguous genitalia 267–8
ammoniacal dermatitis 419
amniocentesis and CVS
    (chorionic villus sampling)
    21–3

amniotic fluid 23–5
amphetamines 188, 192, 193
ampicillin 270
anaemia
    baby 25–6
    mother 26–8
    sickle cell 476–8
    thalassaemia 476–8
anal fissure 441–2
anal pain 2
analgesic medications 408–9
anaphylactic shock 16–17
anencephaly 149
anger and rage 218
ankyloglossia (tongue tie)
    516–17
anorexia 200–2
anorexia athletica 230
antacids 293, 299
antenatal tests 28–34
antepartum haemorrhage 64
anti-anxiety drugs and
    antidepressants 176–7,
    407
anti-clotting drugs 407
antibiotic allergy, and
    vaccination 540
antibiotics 34–5, 407, 537
anticancer drugs 407
anticonvulsant drugs 407
antidepressants and anti-
    anxiety drugs 176–7, 407
antihistamines 205
antioxidants, in mother's diet
    263
antiphospholipid syndrome 59
anxiety and fear 212–13
aortic stenosis 290
APGAR test 337
apnoea 102
apparent life-threatening event
    (ALTE) 102–3
apthous ulcer 416

arched neck (meningitis
    symptom) 410
arhythmia 291
aromatherapy 35–6
    during labour 364
Artemesia vulgaris 14
aspartame 440
Asperger's syndrome *see*
    autism spectrum disorders
    (ASD) and developmental
    concerns
asphyxia and foetal distress
    249–53
aspiration pneumonia 383
aspirin 408–9
asthma, mother 38–9
asthma and wheezing, baby
    36–8
ataxic cerebral palsy 126, 127
athetoid cerebral palsy 126–7
atopic dermatitis, mother 484
atrial septal defect 290
atrioventricular canal defect
    290
attention deficit disorder
    (ADD) 39–40
attention deficit hyperactivity
    disorder (ADHD) 39–40
au pairs 135
augmentation of labour 374–8
autism, and vaccinations 537,
    540
autistic spectrum disorders
    (ASD) and developmental
    concerns 39–42
autoimmune thyroiditis
    (Hashimoto's disease) 515
azithromycin 137
AZT (zidovudine) 313

Babinski reflex 339
back pain 2, 43–5
bacteria

in the mouth 507
in the vagina 375, 377
bacterial food poisoning 399
bacterial meningitis 409
bacterial vaginosis 392, 393
bad news 45–6
Balaskas, Janet 349
barberry 296
barium enema, baby 62, 152
barium swallow, baby 103
Barlow and Ortolini's test 304
bat ear 199
BCG 523–4
bee sting 10
behaviour, baby
  advice 46–8
  difficult 48–51
benzodiazepines 408
beta-blockers 514
bicornuate uterus 534–5
bifidobacteria 34–5
big feelings 208–10
biliary atresia 327, 328
bilirubin 26, 54, 138
binge eating 201–2
bipolar disorder 176
birth see labour and birth
birthmarks 52
birth partner 358–9
birth plan 359–60
birth, reactions to 395–6
birth trauma/injuries to baby
  53–6
birthing ball 351
birthing stool 351
Bishop score 376
biting, hitting or pinching by
  baby 51–2
bladder pain 2
bleeding, baby 61–3
  and blood-clotting disorders
  56–8
bleeding, mother 63–4, 360,
  361–2
bleeding, mother
  and blood-clotting disorders
  58–61
  during labour 360
  during pregnancy 63–4
  following birth 361–2
bloating and flatulence 64–6
blocked milk ducts 91–2

blocked nose, baby 66–7
blocked tear ducts 232
blood-clotting disorders 56–61
blood group and rhesus factor,
  mother 67–8
blood pressure
  high and pre-eclampsia
  68–71
  low and fainting 71–2
blood screening, baby 72
blood tests, antenatal 30
blood tests, baby after birth
  338
blood transfusion, mother 72
blue baby (cyanotic heart
  defects) 289–90
blue cohosh 296
blues 218–20
body and mind, interrelation
  73–4
body development 271–5
body image and self-esteem
  72–3
body mass index (BMI) 34
'bodymind' 73–4, 393–4
bonding and attachment
  210–11
bonding and love, hormones
  307–9
bonding with your baby, father
  235–6
bones, broken, baby 4
  caused by birth trauma 53–4,
  346
Bordetella pertussis 568–9
bottle-feeding 74–80
boundaries see parenting
bow legs 80
bowel pain 2
brain, developmental stages
  273–4
brain injury at birth 55, 56
Braxton-Hicks contractions
  367
breast lumps 80
breast pain
  during breastfeeding 98–9
  in pregnancy 80–1
breastfeeding
  advice 81–91
  difficulties 91–100
breasts, caring for 83

breath holding, baby 101–2
breathing
  baby, difficulties 102–5
  mother 105–6, 362–3
breathlessness, mother 106–7
breech baby 342–4
brittle bone disease 54
broken bones and fractures,
  baby 4
  caused by birth trauma 53–4,
  346
bromocriptine 93
bronchioles 38
bronchiolitis (RSV) 107
bronchitis 160, 194
bronchodilator 38
bronchospasm 38
bulimia nervosa 201–2
bumps and bruises, baby 5
burns and scalds, baby 5–6

caesarean section ('C' section)
  108–16
caffeine 193
calcium, in mother's diet 263
calculi (stones) 534
Calpol 429
camomile 145, 153, 258, 161
candida (thrush) 117–20
canker ulcer 416
cannabis/marijuana 193
caput succedaneum 54
car seats 12–13, 522
cardiotocograph (CTG) 250–1
caring and nurturing 211
caring for baby 120–1
caring for you 121–4
carpal tunnel syndrome
  279–80
cascara sagrada 296
castor oil 296
cat scratches, baby 6
cataracts, congenital 478–9
catarrh 155, 199
caul, born in 24
celery seed 296
cephalohaematoma 54
cephalosporins 537
cerebral palsy (CP) 56, 124–7
cerebrospinal fluid (CSF) 385,
  386, 409, 410–11
cervical cancer 127

cervical erosion 127
cervical incompetence 127–8
chickenpox 128–31
chickenpox vaccine 539
child protection and abuse 131–4
childcare 134–7
childhood vaccination programme 537–9
childminders 135–6
Chinese herbal medicine 297
chlamydia 137–8
chloramphenicol 407
chloroform 381
chlorpheniramine 205
choking, baby 6
cholestasis 138
cholestyramine 139
chordee, baby 439
chorionic villus sampling (CVS) and amniocentesis 21–3
Christmas disease 57
chromium supplement 265
chronic secretory otitis media 198–9
circumcision 140–2
cleft lip and palate 142–3
clindamycin 270
cloasma 482
club foot (talipes equinus) 143
cocaine and crack 193
cochlear implant 287
codeine 160, 185, 408
coeliac disease (gluten intolerance) 20
coffee 258
coil 154, 155
colas, diet and fizzy drinks 258
cold injury, baby 6 see also hypothermia
cold sores see herpes
colds and coughs 155–62
colic 144–6
Colief (lactase) drops 21
colitis 61
colonoscopy 320
complementary therapies 147–8, 222–5, 363–6
complex carbohydrates 180, 261
compliant baby 121
computerized tomography (CT) 125

condoms 154
congenital abnormalities 148–9
congenital dislocation of the hip (CDH) 304–5
conjunctivitis (sticky eye) 232–3
constipation 149–54
contented baby 120–1
Continuous Positive Airway Pressure (CPAP) 105
contraception 154–5
contraceptive pill in pregnancy 407
contractions 367–8
cord compression and prolapse 339–40
cordocentesis see amniocentesis and CVS
corticosteroid medications 408
cortisol and stress 310
cortisone 38 see also hydrocortisone
coughs and colds 155–62
counselling and psychotherapy 162–3
couples see relationships
cow's milk allergy/intolerance 19–20
CPAP (Continuous Positive Airway Pressure) 105
cracked nipples 97–8
cradle cap 163–4, 459
cramp hips (sciatica) 44, 45
cranial osteopathy 424–5
cravings and pica 255–6
crèche 136
Crohn's disease 185, 540
crossed extensor response 339
croup 164–5
crying 165–170 see also colic
cryotherapy 231
cryptorchidism 511
cryptotia 199
curry to induce labour 378
cutis marmorata 482
cuts and abrasions, baby 6–7
cyanosis 246
cyanotic heart defects (blue baby) 289–90
cycling exercise 227, 229, 255
cypress oil 94

cystic fibrosis 152, 170
cystitis, mother 170–2
cystocoele 318
cytokines 16
cytomegalovirus (CMV) 172–3
cytotoxic drug 204

dad see father
dairy in weaning 20, 182, 183–4
deafness see hearing difficulties, baby
death of a baby 399–403, 501–4
deep vein thrombosis and pulmonary embolism 545–6
DEET (diethyltoluamide) 520–1
dehydration, baby 181, 182
dental care 508
depression and anxiety 174–7
development, baby see growth and development
developmental concerns and autistic spectrum disorders (ASD) 39–42
developmental dysplasia of the hip (DDH) 305
dexamethazone 139
diabetes 177–81
diaphragmatic hernia 297–8
diarrhoea 181–5
diet see eating difficulties, mother; food and eating, mother
dieting, mother 256–7
dihydrocodeine 192
dilatation and curettage (D&C) 185
diphenoxylate 185
diphtheria vaccination 537
Diprobase lotion/cream 139
discipline see parenting
disproportion (tight fit) in labour 368–9
divarication of the rectus muscles 299
dive reflex 339
dog bites, baby 7
dopamine antagonist drugs 552

Doppler ultrasound scans 34
double uterus 534
double vagina 534
doulas (paramana doulas) 186
Down's syndrome (trisomy 21) 30–1, 186–7
doxycycline 137
drinking see alcohol; food and eating, mother
drowning and near drowning, baby 7
drugs 188–94 see also medications in pregnancy
dummies 194–5
dyad, mother–baby 210
dysfunction of symphysis pubis (DSP) 43

ears, baby
  bleeding from 62
  infection and pain 196–9
  injury to 8
  piercing 199
  shapes 199–200
eating, mother 257–65
  difficulties 200–2
echinacea 119, 158, 258
echocardiogram, baby 103–4
echocardiography, foetal 291
ectopic pregnancy 202–4
eczema 204–6, 484
EFAs (essential fatty acids), in mother's diet 263–4, 265
egg allergy, and vaccination 540
Eisenmenger's complex 290
elbows that click 330
electrocardiogram (ECG) 104, 289, 292
electroencephalogram (EEG) 125, 249
EMDR (eye movement desensitisation and reprocessing) 450–1
emotions 206–10
  support and treatment 162–3, 222–5
energy, accessing in labour 346–9
encephalitis 130, 247
encephalocoele 500
endorphins 309, 331–2, 428
Enfamil 554

engaged and non-engaged head 340–1
engorgement of breasts 92–4
entonox (gas and air) 386
epi-pen 17
epidural 383–6
epigastric hernia 298
epilepsy 243–6
epinephrine injection 17
episiotomy and tears 369–73
Epstein-Barr virus (EBV) 225–6
Erb's palsy 56
ergometrine 391
erythema toxicum 459
erythromycin 137, 138
ethyl mercury 536
eucalyptus 157, 158, 160, 161
exercise, mother 226–30
exomphalos 298
explorative urge 211–12
expressing milk 89–90
extra digits 230
eye movement desensitisation and reprocessing (EMDR) 450–1
eyes, baby
  blocked tear ducts 232
  conjunctivitis (sticky eye) 232–3
  crossing and squinting 230–1
  development of visual sense 277–8
  infection and swelling 231–3
  injury to 8–9
  pupils of different sizes 231
  retinoblastoma 231
  sight problems and blindness 478–80
  styes 233
  see also vision, baby

facial nerve palsy 56
factor V (Leiden) 59
factor VIII deficiency 57
factor IX deficiency 57
factor XI deficiency 57
failure to thrive (low weight gain) 559–62
fainting, and low blood pressure 71–2
falling down stairs 8

false and pre-labour 357–8
family see parenting
family of origin influence 207
father 87, 234–8, 472–3
fear and anxiety 212–13
fear and stress, hormones 310–11
febrile seizures 241–2, 246–7
feeding see breastfeeding, advice; bottle-feeding; weaning
feel good hormones/ endorphins 309
feelings see emotions
feet, baby 9, 143, 249
femoral hernia 298
fencing reflex 339
fennel 258
ferritin 28
fever, baby 239–42
fibroids 242–3
finances 415–16
fingers, baby 9, 230
first aid and accidents, baby 3–13
  ABC of resuscitation 3
  emergency situations 4
first aid kit 11
  homeopathy 306
fits and epilepsy
  baby 241–2, 245–9
  mother 243–5
flat feet 249
flattened head (plagiocephaly) 281
flatulence and bloating 64–6
flying
  in pregnancy 520, 521
  with baby 523
flu (influenza) 320–2
foetal alcohol effect 191–2
foetal alcohol syndrome (FAS) 191–2
foetal distress and asphyxia 249–53
foetal echocardiography 291
foetal heart monitoring 335–7
foetoscopy 22, 23
folic acid, in mother's diet 264
fontanelle 181, 410, 281
food allergy see allergy and intolerance

food and eating, mother 253–61
foot problems see feet, baby
forceps 373–4
foreign body in the nose 8
formula milk types 79–80
fruit juices 258

ganciclovir 173
gardnerella vaginitis 543
gas and air (entonox) 386
gastro-oesophageal reflux 554
gastroenteritis see diarrhoea, baby
gastroschisis 298
Gaviscon 79
Gavison Infant 554
genes and genetics 266–7
genetic counselling 267
genetic testing 266–7
genital touching, baby 49
genitalia, ambiguous 267–8
gentian violet 119
German measles (rubella) 466–7 see also MMR vaccine
ginger tea 258, 552
gingivitis 507–8
glaucoma 479, 480
glue ear 198–9, 286–7
gluten intolerance (coeliac disease) 20
goitre 513
golden seal 296
gonorrhoea 268–9
Gordon, Yehudi 351
grasp reflex 338
Graves disease 513
gripe water 145
Group B streptococcus (Group B strep, GBS) 269–70
growth and development, baby 270–8
growth charts 274–5
growth spurts 86
guilt 213–15
Guthrie test 338

H2 blockers 293, 553
HAART (highly active antiretroviral therapy) 311
haemangioma (strawberry mark) 52

haemarthroses 57
haematuria 534
haemoglobinopathy screening, baby 72
haemophilia 56–7
Haemophilus influenzae Type b (Hib) vaccination 537
haemorrhagic disease of the newborn (vitamin K dependent bleeding) 62–3
haemorrhoids (piles) 440–2
hair, during and after pregnancy 279
hair pulling, baby 49–50
hand pain and carpal tunnel syndrome 279–80
hand, foot and mouth disease (HFMD) 280
hands, injury 9
happiness and sadness 218–20
Hashimoto's disease 515
hay fever see allergy and intolerance
head and head shapes 280–1
head banging 50–1
head injury, baby 9–10
during birth 54–6
head pain, mother 282–4
healing (healers) 284
health checks, baby
after birth 284–6
during labour 335–7
health checks, mother
after birth 284–6
antenatal 28–34
hearing development 275–6
hearing difficulties, baby 286–8
hearing screening/tests, baby 288
heart defects, baby 288–90
heart disease, mother 290–1
heart-shaped uterus 534–5
heart rhythms and murmurs
baby 291
mother 291–2
heartburn and indigestion 292–4
heat rash 459–60
heel prick test 338
heparin 407
hepatitis 294–6

herbal medicine 296–7
herbal teas and drinks 258
hermaphroditism 268
hernia 297–9
heroin and methodone 193
herpes 300–1
herpes gestationis 483
HIE (hypoxic ischemic encephalopathy) 301–2
high blood pressure (pre-eclampsia) 68–71
high-risk pregnancy 302–4
highly active antiretroviral therapy (HAART) 311
hips, baby
clicky 304–5
congenital dislocation 304–5
hips, mother, painful (sciatica) 44, 45
Hirschsprung disease 152
histamine 10
hitting, biting or pinching by baby 51–2
'hole in the heart' (ventricular septal defect) 289, 290
home birth 353–5
homeopathy 305–7, 364–6, 536
in labour 364–6
hormones 307–11
human immunodeficiency virus (HIV) 311–14
hydrocephalus 281–2
hydrocortisone cream 6, 10, 117, 164
hydrops foetalis 314–15
hypoglycaemia
in the newborn 315
mother 261–2
hypoplastic left heart syndrome 290
hypospadias, baby 439
hypothermia, baby 315–16
hypoxic ischemic encephalopathy (HIE) 301–2

IBD (inflammatory bowel disease), mother 320
IBS (irritable bowel syndrome), mother 326
ibuprofen 408, 409

ichthyosis 460
idiopathic thrombocytopaenic
    purpura (ITP) 58, 60
immunisation *see* vaccinations,
    baby
in-toeing and tibial torsion 322
incontinence 317–20
indigestion and heartburn
    292–4
induction of labour 374–8
Infacol 145
Infant-led parenting 432
infectious mononucleosis
    225–6
inflammatory bowel disease
    (IBD), mother 320
influenza (flu) 320–2
inguinal hernia 298–9
inhaled and swallowed objects
    or liquids 8
injury
    at birth, mother 395
    birth trauma/injuries to baby
    53–6
    see also accidents and first
    aid, baby
insect bites and stings 10
insomnia, mother 497
interferon 295
internal examination in
    pregnancy 32
intestinal atresia 554
intestinal malrotation 554
intimacy *see* sex
intolerance and allergy 14–21
intrauterine growth restriction
    (IUGR) 322–6
intussception 61–2
iron, in mother's diet 264, 265
irritable bowel syndrome (IBS),
    mother 326
isoniazid 524

jaundice, baby 327–9
jogging, in pregnancy 227
Junifen 429
juniper 296

kangaroo care 518
keloids 115, 119
kernicterus 329
kidney pain 2

Klumpke's palsy 56
knees or elbows that click 330
knock knees 330
Koplik's spots 406

labour and birth
    baby 331–46
    father's presence 234–5
    mother 346–96
Lactobacilli 34–5, 118
lactose intolerance 20–1
lady's mantle 258
Lammers, Lilliana 186
large babies 396–8
large head (megancephaly) 282
laryngomalacia (floppy larynx)
    104
laxatives 153
leg pain and cramps, mother
    398–9
lemon balm 65, 153, 258
lemongrass 95, 223
listening, tips for 462–3
listeria 399
lithium 177
loperamide 185
loss of a baby 399–403, 501–4
love 215–17
low blood pressure and
    fainting 71–2
low milk flow 94–5
lumbar pain 43
lupus (autoimmune disorder)
    59

macrosomic baby 396
magnesium 39, 118, 178, 244,
    255
magnesium sulphate 70
magnetic resonance imaging
    (MRI) 125
malpresentation 342–5
mammalian brain and
    emotions 207
MAOIs (monoamine oxidase
    inhibitors) 176
marbled skin 482
marigold tonic 258
massage 404–5
    breasts 83
mastitis and abscesses 95–7
maternity nurse 135

measles 406–7
measles, mumps, rubella
    (MMR) vaccine 539–40
meconium 251, 253, 447
medications in pregnancy
    407–9
megancephaly (large head) 282
melasma 482
meningitis, baby 409–11
meningococcal rash 460
meningococcus Type C
    vaccination 537
meningocoele 500
mercury in the diet 260
Metanium cream 419
metatarsus adductus 143
methotrexate 204
metoclopramide 552
metronizadole 523, 543
microcephaly (small head)
    282
milia rash, baby 459
milk types (formula milk)
    79–80
minerals, in mother's diet 263,
    264–5
miscarriage 411–15
MMR (measles, mumps,
    rubella) vaccine 539–40
money 415–16
Mongolian blue spots 460
monoamine oxidase inhibitors
    (MAOIs) 176
morhulin 419
morning sickness *see* vomiting
    and nausea, mother
moro reflex 338
mother baby dyad 210
mouth injury, baby 10
mouth ulcers, mother 416
movement of baby in
    pregnancy 416–17
moxibustion 14
multiple births 525–8
mumps 417

naevus (birthmark) 53
nannies 135
nappies 418
nappy rash 418–20
naproxen 408, 409
nasal congestion, baby 66–7

natural birth 349–50
nausea *see* vomiting and nausea, mother; vomiting, baby
neck arching (meningitis symptom) 410
Neocate formula milk 20
neonatal abstinence syndrome 192
neonatal asphyxia 250
neonatal death 420
neonatal herpes 301
neonatal intensive care unit (NICU) 497–500
neural tube defects and spina bifida 500–1
Neurolinguistic Programming (NLP) 163
nicotine 188–90, 193–4
NICU (neonatal intensive care unit) 497–500
night feeds 86
nipples
  cracked 97–8
  flat or inverted 98
nitrazine 392
noisy breathing (stridor) 103–4
non-engaged head 340–1
non-steroidal anti-inflammatory drugs (NSAIDS) 408–9
noradrenaline 175, 310, 323
nose, baby 8, 10, 62, 66–7
nuchal scan 31, 34, 187
nursery care 136
nut allergy 21
nutrition, baby 420–1 *see also* food and eating, mother
nutritional therapy 421
nystatin 117, 119

obesity 562–4, 566–7
obsessive behaviour 176
occipito anterior position 344
occipito posterior position 344
Odent, Michel 186, 351
oedema (swelling), mother 504–6
oesophageal atresia and tracheo-oesophageal fistula 422–3

older parents 423–4
omega oils (EFAs), in mother's diet 263–4, 265
opiates 193
osteopathy 424–5
osteoporosis 425–6
otitis externa 196
otitis media 196
overactive thyroid *see* thyroid, baby; thyroid, mother
overdue (post-maturity) 378–80
overeating, compulsive 201–2
overweight 562–4, 566–7
oxalate stones 538
oxytocin 391

pain
  baby 427–8
  in labour 380–1
  mother 430–1
pain relief
  baby 428–30
  in labour 381–6
  mother 381–6, 408–9
pale skin and cool limbs, baby 410
palmar grasp reflex 338–9
palpitations, mother 291–2
papular dermatitis of pregnancy 483
paracetamol 408, 429–30
paramyxovirus 406
parenting 432–7
parvovirus 25, 437–8
patent ductus arteriosus (PDA) 290
pelvic floor exercises (Kegel) 438–9
pelvic pain 43–5
penicillin 269, 170, 399, 407
penicillin allergy 15
penis, baby, hypospadias and chordee 439
pennyroyal 296
peppermint 153, 258
Pepti 20
perineum 370–1, 438
  episiotomy 370–1
  preparing for birth 438
  stitching 371
  tears 370–1

pertussis (whooping cough) vaccination 537
pethidine 352, 454
pets 6, 7, 13
Phenergan 205
phenobarbital 244
phenylalanine 440
phenylketonuria (PKU) 338, 439–40
phenytoin 244
phimosis 140
phlebitis 544, 545–6
pica 255–6
pilates 440
piles (haemorrhoids) and anal fissure 440–2
Piriton 205
PKU (phenylketonuria) 338, 439–40
placenta, retained 361, 391, 412, 442
placenta accreta 442
placenta praevia (low-lying placenta) 442–4
placental abruption 444–6
plagiocephaly (flattened head) 281
plantar grasp reflex 339
plaque (dental) 507–8
play 446
playfulness 217
pneumococcal vaccination 538
pneumococcus 410
pneumonia, baby 446–7
pokeroot 296
polio 538
polydactyly 230
polyene antifungal remedy 119
polyhydraminios 24–5
Ponseti method 143
poo, baby 61–2, 182, 447–8
  blood in 61–2
  colourless 328
  frothy 14, 20, 183, 448
  green frothy 448
  hard 448
  putty-coloured 20
  red-currant jelly apprearance 182
  white 328
port wine stain (birthmark) 52
positions

baby 341–5
for birth 350–3
positron emission tomography (PET) 125
posseting 421
post maturity (overdue) 378–80
post traumatic stress disorder (PTSD) 448–51
posture 451–2
potty, early encouragement to use 150
pre-eclampsia, and high blood pressure 68–71
Pregestamil 20
pregnancy testing 452–3
premature birth 453–7
premature labour *see* premature birth
Prevnar 538
prickly heat 459–60
primodone 244
probiotics 34–5
prochlorperazine 552
progesterone
low and miscarriage 411, 414, 423
supplementation 413
vaginal pessaries 177
prolactin 76, 93
prolapse
umbilical cord 339–40
vaginal 318–19
propylthiouracil 514
Prozac 176
prune juice for baby 150
prurigo of pregnancy 483
pruritic urticarial papules of pregnancy (PUPP) 483
pruritis 138
pseudoephedrine 199
psoriasis, mother 484
psychotherapy and counselling 162–3
puerperal psychosis 176
pulmonary atresia 289
pulmonary embolism 545–6
pulmonary stenosis 290
PUPP (pruritic urticarial papules of pregnancy) 483
purpura 62
pyelonephritis 171

pyloric stenosis 554
pyogenic granuloma 530

rage and anger 218
rashes and spots, baby 458–61
rashes in pregnancy 483–4
raspberry tea 258
RAST blood test for allergy 18
Raynaud's disease 482
recreational drugs 188–90, 193
rectocoele 218
red clover 258
reflexes at birth 338–9
reflexology 461
reflux, baby
and colic 144
food, baby 554
urinary 532
rejection of breast by baby 99–100
relationships 461–4
reptilian brain 206
resentment 123, 214, 382, 396, 415–16, 433, 470, 472
respiratory distress syndrome (RDS) 105
restless leg syndrome 464–5
resuscitation, baby 3
retained placenta, 361, 391, 412, 442
retinoblastoma 231
retinopathy of prematurity 479
retrolental fibroplasias 479
Reye's syndrome 240
rhesus factor 67–8
ribavirin 295
rickets 465
rooibos tea 258
rooting reflex 338
roseola infantum (sixth disease) 465–6
routine and structure 435–7
RSV (respiratory syncitial virus) 107
rubella (German measles) 466–7 *see also* MMR vaccine
rubeola 406
rue 296
running exercise 227
rupture of membranes,

spontaneous and premature 391–3

sacral dimples, baby 468
sacroiliac joint pain 43
sadness and happiness 218–20
safety and accident prevention 11–13
safety in pregnancy 468–70
sage 296
salbutamol 17, 18, 107
scar tissue, mother 371
SCBU (special care baby unit) 497–500
sciatica 44
security objects 52
self-esteem and body image 72–3
senna 296
Senokot syrup 151
separation anxiety 220–1
septate uterus 534
serotonin re-uptake inhibitors (SSRIs) 176
sex 470–5
sex hormones, treatments 407
sexually transmitted diseases 476
shingles in pregnancy 476
shoulder dystocia 53, 345–6
sickle cell disease 476–8
SIDS (sudden infant death syndrome) 503–4
sight problems and blindness, baby 478–80
sign language
baby 76, 169
single parenting 480–1
sinusitis, mother *see* coughs and colds, mother
sixth disease 465–6
skin, baby 62, 481–2
skin in pregnancy 482–5
skin-to-skin contact 517–18
skin treatments in pregnancy 407–8
slapped cheek disease (parvovirus) 437–8
sleep
baby 485–95
mother 495–7
sleeping pills 408

small head (microcephaly) 282
smell, development of sense 276
smiling, baby 277
smoking 188–90, 193–4
southernwood 296
soya milk, baby 20, 79, 145, 184, 197
spastic cerebral palsy 126
special care baby unit (SCBU) 497–500
spider veins 545
spina bifida and neural tube defects 500–1
spiritual life 501
spontaneous abortion 411–15
spontaneous and premature rupture of membranes 391–3
spots and rashes, baby 458–61
squinting 230–1
SSRIs (serotonin re-uptake inhibitors) 176
startle reflex 338
stem cells 530–1
stepping reflex 339
steroid medications 408
sticky eye 231–3
stillbirth 501–3
stomach pain 2
stools, baby 61–2, 182, 447–8
  blood in 61–2
  colourless 328
  frothy 14, 20, 183, 448
  green frothy 448
  hard 448
  putty-coloured 20
  red-currant jelly appearance 182
  white 328
stopping breast feeding 90–1
strabismus 230–1
strawberry mark (haemangioma) 52
streptomycin 34, 407
stress 221–2
stress and fear, hormones 310–11
stress incontinence 317
stretch and sweep (membranes) 378
stye 233

sub-aponeurotic haematoma 55
sucking reflex 338
sudden infant death syndrome (SIDS) 503–4
sudden unexpected death in infancy (SUDI) 503–4
Sudocreme 419
sugar, in mother's diet 261–2
supplements, dietary 263–5
support tights, varicose veins 544
supra ventricular tachycardia (SVT) 291
surfactant produced by lungs 105, 178
surgery, homeopathic support 504
swallowed and inhaled objects or liquids 8
sweeping the membranes 378
swelling (oedema), mother 504–6
swollen testicles (hydrocoeles) 510
symphysis pubis dysfunction 43
syntocinon 391
syntometrine 391
syphilis 506

tamazepam 192
tansy 296
taste, development of 277
Tay-Sachs disease 507
Tcharkovsky, Igor 351
tea 258
tears and episiotomy 369–73
teeth, baby 508–10
teeth and gums, mother 507–8
teething 509–10
temperature, taking baby's 239–40
TENS pain relief 386
tentorial tears 55
testicles 510–12
testicular torsion 510–11
tetanus ('lockjaw') 537
tetrachloroethylene 470
tetracycline 34, 138, 407
tetralogy of Fallot 289
thalassaemia 476–8

thermometers/taking temperatures 239–40
thiomersal in vaccines 536–7
thrombocytopaenia 57–8, 60–1
thrombophilia, mother 59
thrombosis and pulmonary embolism 545–6
thrush (candida) 117–20
thuja 296
thumb sucking 512
thyroid 513–15
thyroid function 512
tibial torsion and in-toeing 322
tiger in the tree pose 145
time and space for parenting 436–7
tingling in thighs or feet 44
tiredness 238, 515–16
tocolytic medication 454
toes, baby 9, 230
tongue tie (ankyloglossia) 516–17
tonic neck reflex 339
torticollis (wry neck) 569
total serum bilirubin (TSB) 328
touch, skin-to-skin contact 517–18
toxaemia 29, 68–71
toxoplasmosis 518–19
tracheo-oesophageal fistula 422–3
tranquillisers 408
transcutaneous bilirubin (TCB) test 328
transfusion, blood
  baby 329
  mother 72
transient tachypnoea of the newborn (TTN) 104–5
transverse lie 345
trauma after birth
  baby 53–6
  mother 395
travel 519–22
Treponema pallidum 506
trichomoniasis 523
tricyclics 176
trimethoprim 407
tuberculosis (TB) 523–4
tuina 14
twins and higher multiples 525–8

twin-to-twin transfusion syndrome 528

ulcerative colitis 61, 185
ultrasound scanning 33–4
umbilical cord 529–30
  blood banking and stem cells 530–1
  compression and prolapse 339–40
  cutting 334–5
umbilical hernia 299
underactive thyroid see thyroid, baby; thyroid, mother
underweight 559–62, 567–8
undescended and retractile testicles 511–12
upright positions for birth 350–1
urinary tract infection 170–2, 531–3
urine
  baby 533
  mother, blood and stones 533–4
urine tests, antenatal 32
ursodeoxycholic acid 139
urticarial rash 460
uterus, abnormal shape 534–5
uterus and ovaries, pain during pregnancy 1–2

vaccinations, baby 536–41
vaccinations in pregnancy 408
  see also influenza (flu), mother; travel in pregnancy
vagina, baby, bleeding from 62
vagina, mum

preparing for birth 438
  tears and cuts 370–1
vaginal birth after caesarean (VBAC) 115
vaginal discharge and infection 541–2
vaginal laxity 317–20
vaginal pain 542–3
vaginal prolapse 318–19
vaginosis 543
Valium 70, 188
varicella immune globulin (VZIG) 129, 130
varicella zoster see chickenpox
varicose veins 544
Vaseline 419
VBAC (vaginal birth after caesarean) 115
veins, mother 543–6
venous thrombosis 545
Ventolin 17, 18
ventouse 373–4
ventricular septal defect ('hole in the heart') 289, 290
violence and abuse 546–9 see also child protection and abuse
viral meningitis 409
vision, baby 277–8, 478–80 see also eyes, baby
visualisation and self-hypnosis 549–50
vitamin A, in mother's diet 263
vitamin C, in mother's diet 263
vitamin E, in mother's diet 263
vitamin K, in mother's diet 264
vitamin K dependent bleeding (haemorrhagic disease of the newborn) 62–3
vitamin supplements, baby 559
vitamins, minerals, EFAs and

supplements, mother 263–5
vomiting, baby 553–6
vomiting and nausea, mother 551–3
vomiting blood, baby 63
von Willebrand's disease 58

warfarin 407
wasp sting 10
water, types of drinking water 257–8
water birth 351–3
weaning, baby 557–9
webbed toes 559
weight
  baby 559–64
  mother 564–8
West Nile virus 522
Wharton's jelly 339
wheezing, baby 36–8
whooping cough (pertussis) 537, 568–9
World Health Organization (WHO) Child Growth Standards 274
wormwood 296
wry neck (torticollis) 569

X chromosomes 266
X-rays in pregnancy 570
xiphisternum, baby 570

Y chromosome 266
yoga 571–2

zidovudine (AZT) 313
zinc
  deficiency 573
  in diet 27, 79, 118, 244, 258, 263, 264, 265
zinc cream 419